Minimally Invasive Spinal Deformity Surgery

Michael Y. Wang • Yi Lu
D. Greg Anderson
Praveen V. Mummaneni
Editors

Minimally Invasive Spinal Deformity Surgery

An Evolution of Modern Techniques

Springer

Editors
Michael Y. Wang, M.D., M.S.
Department of Neurological Surgery
University of Miami Miller
School of Medicine
Miami, FL
USA

Yi Lu, M.D., Ph.D.
Department of Neurosurgery
Brigham and Women's Hospital
Harvard Medical School
Boston, MA
USA

D. Greg Anderson
Department of Orthopaedics
Thomas Jefferson University
Philadelphia, PA
USA

Praveen V. Mummaneni, MD
Department of Neurological Surgery
University of California
San Francisco, CA
USA

ISBN 978-3-7091-1406-3 ISBN 978-3-7091-1407-0 (eBook)
DOI 10.1007/978-3-7091-1407-0
Springer Wien Heidelberg Dordrecht London New York

Library of Congress Control Number: 2013957182

Printed on acid-free paper

Springer is part of Springer Science+Business Media (www.springer.com)

Foreword

Minimally Invasive Spinal Deformity Surgery: An Evolution of Modern Techniques is intended to provide an educational resource for surgeons in an area where there has until now been a paucity of literature. Many advances in the area of minimally invasive spine surgery (MISS) are occurring through small series of patients operated on by innovative thought leaders. This book provides the opportunity to put this collection of surgical techniques and early outcomes into one place so that the student of this advancing field may gain a broader exposure to the current knowledge base.

With the increasingly aging patient population, it is now common to see in one's practice older patients with advanced degenerative spine disease and deformity. These issues can be incapacitating, causing pain and immobility, and reducing the patient's quality of life. Multiple medical comorbidities often exist in these patients, along with osteoporosis, causing challenges and often complicating treatment. As a consequence, surgical treatment of adult spinal deformities is fraught with hazards and complications, which has led thought leaders to seek better solutions. Contemporary spine surgeons, both orthopedic surgeons and neurosurgeons, are recognizing that MISS is an increasingly desirable option for managing this difficult patient population. MISS techniques are reported to minimize blood loss and surgical site pain and to speed up recovery. Recent work by McGirt et al. [1] showed that the number of surgical site infections with two-level fusions performed via MISS was significantly reduced as compared to that seen with open lumbar two-level fusions.

This book is divided into sections that will help provide good background information to readers wishing to become knowledgeable in all areas of MISS. The "Deformity Surgery Principles" section includes not only epidemiology and classification but important issues for adult deformity surgery, such as sagittal balance and lumbopelvic parameters. The next section, "Percutaneous Segmental Fixation," reviews techniques of screw insertion with a subsection on osteoporotic bone. The use of interbody fusion devices is separately discussed in the more popular "Posterior Approaches" and a section covering "Lateral Approaches." The lateral approach section includes a chapter on the role of neuromonitoring, the use of which is vitally important in making this procedure safe. "Dealing with the Lumbo-Pelvic Junction" discusses the importance of good distal fixation, not only to S1 but also to the ilium, and the minimally invasive techniques to accomplish this fixation are also well discussed. "Achieving Intersegmental Arthrodesis" discusses the very important issue of bone grafting techniques. Much of what has been learned in adult deformity surgery is being incorporated into MISS approaches for posterior adolescent idiopathic scoliosis surgery and is covered in the "Future Directions" section.

I applaud the editors of this book for soliciting highly relevant information on this subject; they have done an outstanding job to make sure that significant, new information is available to surgeons wishing to learn some of these techniques in order to take care of this increasing patient population.

Reference

1. McGirt MJ, Parker SL, Lerner J, Engelhart L, Knight T, Wang MY. Comparative analysis of perioperative surgical site infection after minimally invasive versus open posterior/transforaminal lumbar interbody fusion: analysis of hospital billing and discharge data from 5170 patients. J Neurosurg Spine 2011;14(6):771–8.

Philadelphia, PA Randal R. Betz, M.D.

Contents

Part I

Deformity Surgery Principles

The Epidemiology of Adult Spinal Deformity and the Aging Population

1

Joseph S. Cheng, Jonathan Forbes, Cyrus Wong, and Edward Perry

1.1 The Aging Population

The American population is aging, and aging is associated with a rise in the prevalence of degenerative spinal disorders. According to the 2010 Census, while the percentage of younger people in the USA between the working ages of 25–44 years old declined by 3.4 %, the older population within the working age, that is, ages 45–64 years old, increased by 31.5 % and now make up 81.5 million people in the US population [1]. The growth of people within the retirement age bracket, age 62 years and older, in the US population grew by 21.2 % from 2000 to 2010. Overall, people over the age of 65 years and considered typically retired from the work force make up 40.3 million people and represent 39 % of the total US population. Between 2000 and 2010, this older age group represented the fastest growth sector in the USA and has been associated with the increase in spinal care needed, including adult degenerative spinal deformities (Table 1.1).

In addition to these statistics of the growing number of "baby boomers" nearing retirement age, the increase in our older US population is also related to a trend for longer life expectancy as noted with the fastest growing segment of the US population being those 90 years and older [1]. The number of people in the US who are 90 years and older has tripled over the past three decades reaching 1.9 million in 2010 and is expected to quadruple over the next four decades, thanks to advances in medicine and healthcare [2]. Due to increasing life expectancy in the USA, those over the age of 90 years now represent 4.7 % of the population over the age of 65 as compared to only 2.8 % in 1980 with a projected increase to 10 % of the older population in the USA by the year 2050 [1, 2].

As the number of our senior citizens increases, so too will the need for age-appropriate medical care. The majority of the older population in the USA has one or more disabilities, with lumbar spondylosis and low back pain being the most frequently reported musculoskeletal problems [2–4]. Compared to other medical problems, the disability associated with degenerative spine disease is significant with a lower quality of life based on EQ-5D, which is a standardized measure of health status developed by the EuroQol Group (Table 1.2). Based on a review of the literature, it would appear that the disability associated with lumbar spondylosis is more than twice that of prostate cancer and is more disabling than diseases such as congestive heart failure, chronic obstructive pulmonary disease, and diabetes.

The disability associated with degenerative spine disease and adult deformity becomes more significant as a patient becomes older. For example, those over 90 years old typically do not live with their families and live either alone or in a nursing facility. Their ability to live independently versus being institutionalized in a skilled nursing facility is

J.S. Cheng, M.D., M.S. (✉) • J. Forbes, M.D.
C. Wong, M.D. • E. Perry, M.D.
Vanderbilt University Medical Center,
Nashville, TN, USA
e-mail: joseph.cheng@vanderbilt.edu

M.Y. Wang et al. (eds.), *Minimally Invasive Spinal Deformity Surgery*,
DOI 10.1007/978-3-7091-1407-0_1, © Springer-Verlag Wien 2014

Table 1.1 Population table of age and sex composition comparing 2000–2010 data

Population by Sex and Selected Age Groups: 2000 and 2010
(For information on confidentiality protection, nonsampling error, and definitions, see *www.census.gov/prod/cen2010/doc/sfl.pdf*)

Sex and selected age groups	2000		2010		Change, 2000 to 2010	
	Number	Percent	Number	Percent	Number	Percent
Total population................	281,421,906	100.0	308,745,538	100.0	27,323,632	9.7
SEX						
Male..........	138,053,563	49.1	151,781,326	49.2	13,727,763	9.9
Female..........	143,368,343	50.9	156,964,212	50.8	13,595,869	9.5
SELECTED AGE GROUPS						
Under 18 years..........	72,293,812	25.7	74,181,467	24.0	1,887,655	2.6
Under 5 years..........	19,175,798	6.8	20,201,362	6.5	1,025,564	5.3
5 to 17 years..........	53,118,014	18.9	53,980,105	17.5	862,091	1.6
18 to 44 years..........	112,183,705	39.9	112,806,642	36.5	622,937	0.6
18 to 24 years..........	27,143,454	9.6	30,672,088	9.9	3,528,634	13.0
25 to 44 years..........	85,040,251	30.2	82,134,554	26.6	−2,905,697	−3.4
45 to 64 years..........	61,952,636	22.0	81,489,445	26.4	19,536,809	31.5
65 years and over..........	34,991,753	12.4	40,267,984	13.0	5,276,231	15.1
16 years and over..........	217,149,127	77.2	243,275,505	78.8	26,126,378	12.0
18 years and over..........	209,128,094	74.3	234,564,071	76.0	25,435,977	12.2
21 years and over..........	196,899,193	70.0	220,958,853	71.6	24,059,660	12.2
62 years and over..........	41,256,029	14.7	49,972,181	16.2	8,716,152	21.1

Sources: U.S. Census Bureau, *Census 2000 Summary File 1* and *2010 Census Summary File 1*.
From: Howden and Meyer [1]

Table 1.2 Overview of baseline EQ-5D indices, number of studies, and number of patients for selected disease states

Disease state	Number of studies	Number of patients	Mean EQ-5D index (SD)
Prostate cancer	6	2,317	0.79 (0.23)
Diabetes type II	32	35,348	0.76 (0.22)
IBD	5	1,229	0.75 (0.23)
COPD	11	7,495	0.70 (0.24)
ERSD/RF	8	2,126	0.66 (0.26)
Rheumatoid arthritis	24	28,569	0.66 (0.22)
CHF	12	5,067	0.63 (0.25)
Knee OA	10	3,029	0.52 (0.26)
PVD	9	1,824	0.50 (0.28)
OA of the hip	9	36,301	0.41 (0.31)
Lumbar spondylosis	**24**	**11,801**	**0.39 (0.26)**
Total	**137**	**135,106**	

related to the management of their disabilities affecting their independent function [2]. Given the prevalence of spinal disorders in the elderly population and their associated disability, it can be expected that the need for medical care, including surgery, to promote a higher quality of life or increase their quality-added life years (QALYs), is expected to exponentially increase in an attempt to maintain the function and overall quality of life in our older patients.

1.2 Incidence of Spinal Disorders and Deformity in Our Aging Population

Low back pain (LBP) is a highly prevalent and disabling condition that is associated with significant healthcare resource utilization in the USA [5, 6]. The incidence of LBP is high in older people with 42 % of this population reporting at least one episode of low back pain within the past year; as a result, those over the age of 64 years represent 20 % of all visits to physicians for LBP [7–9]. While Medicare data (1991–2002) showed that there was a 32 % increase in LBP patients and a 387 % increase in related charges for LBP, there is a paucity of research data focused on LBP in older people over the age of 65 [10, 11]. However, there is data noting that the majority of low back pain associated with underlying structural pathology from degenerative spine disease such as spinal stenosis, with associated etiologies such as spondylosis or scoliosis, is what necessitates medical management [12, 13].

Adult degenerative scoliosis is typically defined as a curvature greater than 10° in an adult patient associated with spondylosis and degenerative changes of the spine. While this may occur as a process of aging in a patient with a preexisting adolescent idiopathic scoliosis, this is typically associated with a de novo spinal deformity from age-related degenerative spine disease but can also be associated with iatrogenic etiologies such as post-laminectomy syndrome or asymmetric insufficiency fractures from osteoporosis. In 2006, Kobayashi reported an incidence of 37 % de novo development of degenerative scoliosis in a study of 60 subjects 50–84 years old followed over 12 years [14]. This work supported the data reported by Schwab in 2005, looking at the incidence of scoliosis in those age 60 years or older. Schwab studied 75 people with an average age of 70.5 years old who had no known history of scoliosis or prior spine surgery. He determined that 68 % of people in the study had a Cobb angle of greater than 10° and thus met the definition of scoliosis [15]. Given the inherent relationship between age and the progression of degenerative spine disease, it is not surprising that this is one of the most frequent indications for surgery among patients older than age 65 [12, 13, 16–19].

1.3 Incidence of Spinal Surgery for Adult Spinal Deformity in Our Aging Population

Surgery to correct spinal deformity secondary to age-related degeneration is one particular discipline that has experienced considerable growth in recent years. As noted previously, much of this growth can be attributed to the aging American population. While conservative management of adult deformity is the primary method of management in elderly patients, surgery is increasingly being chosen due to the severity of the disability [20]. There are a number of factors associated with the increased prevalence of spinal deformity in an aging population, and previous studies have sought to elucidate the relationship between advancing age and progression of thoracic kyphosis and associated increases in positive sagittal imbalance [19, 21]. The degenerative spinal deformity seen in older patients affects the spinal balance in inherent load-bearing capacity of the spine, associated with a shift of their center of gravity as estimated by their plumb line anteriorly outside Dubousset's cone of economy with associated progressive disability [21–23].

The incidence of spinal surgery for adult degenerative spinal deformities appears to be increasing due to reported outcomes of older patients being equivalent with their younger counterparts given adjustments for associated medical conditions [24]. A large retrospective series with at least a 5-year average follow-up showed significant improvement of visual analogue scale (VAS) scores, and 70 % of patients reported excellent to good clinical outcome [25]. Rageb also reported a large series of 118 patients and found excellent to good patient reported outcomes in over 90 % of patients, although they did not formally collect VAS or Oswestry Disability Index (ODI) data [26]. Total complication rates varied among studies but collectively appear to occur in about 38 % of patients. Even accounting for perioperative complications, outcomes have been shown to be good with regard to reduced pain and disability scores with proper patient selection and preoperative screening considerations [27], especially in patients who had more significant preoperative disability [28]. As pre- and postoperative outcome assessment improves among practitioners, the validity of the data and thereby the efficacy of spinal surgery in the elderly population may further solidify. The role of MIS techniques in deformity surgery for the elderly population has been reported [29] but not been fully elucidated. While more technically challenging, the reduced blood loss may prove beneficial for older patients in further reducing perioperative morbidity.

While the incidence of spinal degenerative disease and treatments from individual centers or small cohort analyses have been noted in the past, there remains a paucity of data in looking at the incidence of spinal surgery for adult spinal deformity from a population standpoint in the USA. Part of the difficulty in tracking the overall surgical incidence is the variations in nomenclature for diagnosis using the Ninth Revision of the International Classification of Diseases (ICD-9). While some surgeons will document ICD-9 code 737, Curvature of the Spine, as a preoperative

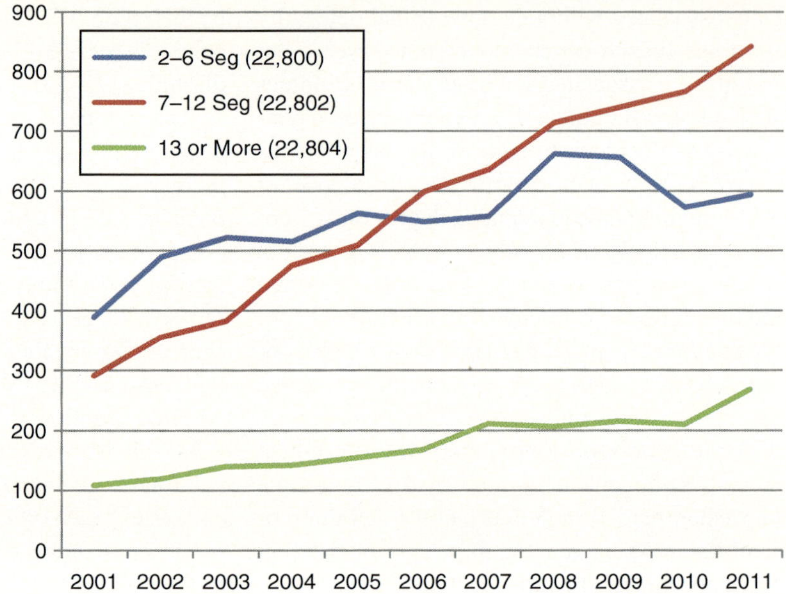

Fig. 1.1 Increase in posterior spinal arthrodesis (fusion) for spinal deformity by CPT code based on Medicare data for 2001–2011

indication for spinal surgery for adult degenerative scoliosis, the majority will use ICD-9 code 722, Intervertebral Disc Disorders. While this is technically the correct documentation of the degenerative disease being treated, it becomes difficult to distinguish those who have associated deformities that meet the criteria of scoliosis from those without a curve greater than 10°.

In addition, documentation of the surgical technique for treatment of adult scoliosis may also vary based on the Current Procedural Terminology (CPT) code used. For posterior approaches, a surgeon may use CPT codes 22800, 22802, or 22804, depending on the number of spinal segments:

- **CPT 22800** Arthrodesis, posterior, for spinal deformity, with or without cast; up to six vertebral segments
- **CPT 22802** Arthrodesis, posterior, for spinal deformity, with or without cast; 7–12 vertebral segments
- **CPT 22804** Arthrodesis, posterior, for spinal deformity, with or without cast; 13 or more vertebral segments

The growth rate of these surgical codes have been significant, especially for CPT 22802 which had increased 289 % in the 10-year period from 2001 to 2011 based on the Medicare data of typically older adults and those with disabilities (Fig. 1.1). The growth rate of spinal surgery for deformity of six vertebral segments or less was noted to be 153 % while the rate for deformities requiring arthrodesis or fusion of 13 or more vertebral segments was 248 % in this adult population (Fig. 1.1).

However, instead of using the deformity CPT codes above which typically have been used for flexible adolescent curves, surgeons may also code their surgeries for adult deformities using the CPT primary codes of CPT 22610 or CPT 22612 for posterior spinal fusions. With these primary codes, the surgeon would then be able to add on CPT 22614 for each additional vertebral segment after the first two in which arthrodesis had been performed:

- **CPT 22600** Arthrodesis, posterior or posterolateral technique, single level; thoracic (with or without lateral transverse technique)
- **CPT 22612** Arthrodesis, posterior or posterolateral technique, single level; lumbar (with or without lateral transverse technique)
- **CPT 22614** Arthrodesis, posterior or posterolateral technique, single level; each additional vertebral segment (list separately in addition to code for primary procedure)

While these surgical procedure codes may be used for de novo age-related deformity, these

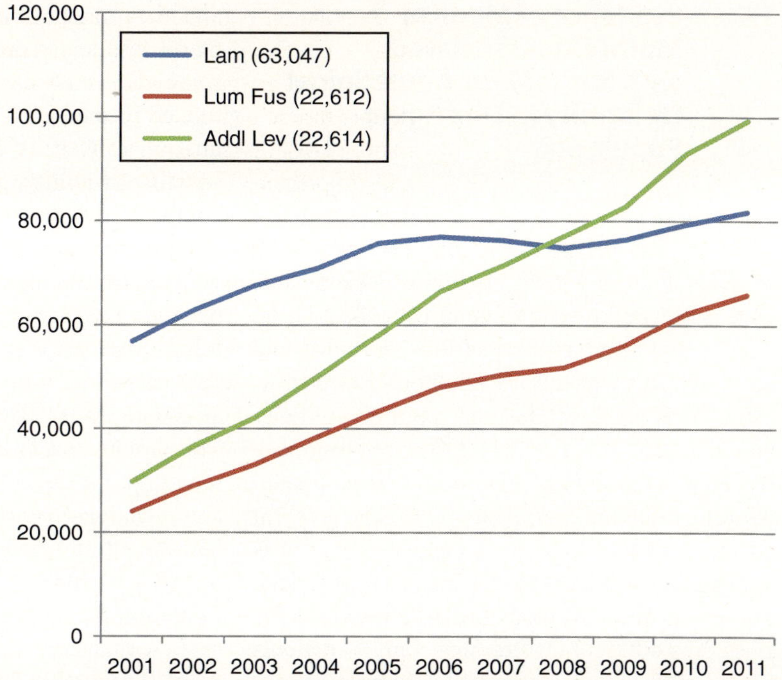

Fig. 1.2 Increase in lumbar laminectomies and lumbar fusion by CPT code based on Medicare data for 2001–2011

procedure codes may also be used for arthrodesis and stabilization of adult iatrogenic deformities such as associated with wide decompression of pathologies such as spinal stenosis (Fig. 1.2). The incidence of lumbar laminectomies based on Current Procedural Terminology (CPT) code 64037 has increased from 56,840 procedures reported to CMS in the year 2000 to 81,700 procedures reported in 2010 in the Medicare population, indicating a 144 % growth in procedures. As one would expect, the increase in post-laminectomy syndrome as documented by the Ninth Revision of the International Classification of Diseases (ICD-9) code 722 has led this to be one of the top five preoperative diagnoses for the use of lumbar fusion based on CPT code 22612, with a growth curve of utilization that follows that of the spinal decompression (Fig. 1.2). While the rate of growth of CPT 22612 is much higher at 274 %, rising from 24,032 procedures in 2001 to 65,834 procedures in 2011, this procedure code also includes treatment of other spinal disorders ranging from degenerative diseases such as spondylolisthesis to traumatic injuries such as lumbar burst fractures.

Although recognition of methods to prevent iatrogenic destabilization and flat back syndrome has improved, the increase in the number of patients with lumbar stenosis who had prior spinal surgeries is likely to increase the number of patients in need of deformity correction. Over the past two decades, there has been a significant increase in the number of spinal procedures for disorders such as stenosis in older patients as well as in the overall Medicare expenditure for spine-related pathologies [12, 13, 19]. Our current analysis of the Medicare data correlates with the study of Medicare beneficiaries over or equal to 65 years old by Deyo and colleagues, who demonstrated a 230 % increase in the rates of index spinal surgery over a 10-year period [12, 13]. The concerns about the problem of growing healthcare costs in the care of this aging group of patients are noted by a recent 2008 report by Martin in which spine-related healthcare expenditures totaled $86 billion in 2005 alone, which was a 65 % increase from 1997 [30]. This has renewed focus on the value of medical and surgical intervention for our patients with adult spinal deformity with assessment of the relative risks and morbidity associated with the treatments compared to the natural history of the disease.

1.4 Incidence of Medical Morbidity Associated with Surgery for Adult Spinal Deformity in Our Aging Population

While statistics indicate an anticipated increase in the number of surgeries required for correction of spinal deformity in the upcoming decades, surgical correction of adult spinal deformity is not without significant risks of serious morbidity and mortality. A review of 361 adult deformity cases from Johns Hopkins Hospital reported a 30-day mortality rate of 2.4 % [31]. Causes of mortality included myocardial infarction, sepsis-related multiorgan failure, pulmonary embolus, cerebral edema, and hypovolemic shock, and risk was strongly associated with preoperative American Society of Anesthesiology (ASA) physical status class. In a different institutional study of patients 75 and older undergoing spinal deformity correction involving fusion across a minimum of five levels, an overall complication rate of 62 % and a major complication rate of 38 % were reported, with major complications being life-threatening or with significant impact on outcome (i.e., deep wound infections, renal failure, myocardial infarction) [32]. The authors found that morbidity, but not mortality, was significantly associated with increased age. In addition, hypertension was associated with a ten times greater risk for major perioperative complication. Likewise, a multicenter study out of the Spinal Deformity Study Group reported an overall complication rate of 71 % among elderly patients 65–85 years old, with 42 % minor and 29 % major complications, indicating that relatively high rates of morbidity following adult spinal deformity correction occur even in the best hands at expert centers [33]. This multicenter review also found a similar correlation between age and morbidity with elderly patients having roughly four to five times higher complication rates than younger patients.

The high risk of complications is in part due to the nature of the surgery itself as well as the characteristics of the patient population. Deformity correction requires extensive surgery typically involving multiple level osteotomies and instrumentation with greater associated blood loss and risk of neurologic injury. Adult spinal deformity patients also present challenges related to their rigid deformities and poor bone quality as well as risk factors related to their baseline disability, deconditioning, and medical comorbidities given their advanced age and limited mobility [34, 35].

Risk stratification, especially among elderly patients, is exceedingly important when considering surgery for spinal deformity. The various medical comorbidities can and should be evaluated preoperatively to assist in risk stratification. The Goldman Cardiac Risk Index is one such measure and has documented increased cardiac complications in patients with a history of diabetes mellitus, non-sinus rhythm greater than 5 PVCs a minute, aortic stenosis, myocardial infarction during the past 6 months, uncompensated congestive heart failure, or age greater than 70 years [36, 37]. Pulmonary complications are also not uncommon in this population. The preoperative baseline Pco2 provides a useful metric—as patients with chronic obstructive pulmonary disease and a Pco2 greater than 50 are more likely to require postoperative mechanical ventilator support [38]. Early mobilization with incentive spirometry in the deformity population is important to minimize postoperative pulmonary complications. The large amount of fluid shifting encountered during large open procedures in deformity reduction is relevant when considering complications related to the renal system. Advanced age is associated with a decrease in creatinine clearance and glomerular filtration rate [39]. This can lead to fluid and electrolyte imbalance following volume repletion with hypotonic fluids. Postoperative hyponatremia in this population is not uncommon. Morbidity involving the gastrointestinal system is also common following open surgical reduction—many authors quote that a postoperative ileus of at least 2–3 days is to be expected [40]. Wound infection is one final category of postoperative morbidity that deserves mention. Advanced age is associated with a risk of wound infection that is approximately three to six times that of younger patients [41].

Many of the morbidities described above are exacerbated by extended length of the surgery, increased operative blood loss, and prolonged immobilization relating to postoperative pain associated with open reduction of spinal deformity. Contemporary technological advances have recently made possible the use of minimally invasive techniques for internal segmental fixation and reduction of deformity [34, 42]. Previous applications of minimally invasive surgery have been associated with reductions in postoperative pain, blood loss, and operative time when compared to similar open procedures [43–45]. As the population ages and the need for spinal deformity correction increases, the role of minimally invasive deformity correction in years ahead is expected to exponentially increase.

Conclusion

Many authors have identified a trend of rising medical care for the treatment of degenerative spinal disorders in our Medicare population, and assuming a stable incidence of spinal disease, concluding that there is too much inappropriate medical and surgical care being delivered. However, the population data would indicate that we have a rapidly growing older US population and that this is associated with age-appropriate degenerative spinal disorders including spinal deformities needing medical and surgical care.

Concern about our growing healthcare costs had led to discussions on the cost-effectiveness of treatment options including the use of minimally invasive surgical techniques. As spinal disorders are associated with some of the highest rates of disability and loss of independence for our patients, understanding the epidemiology of adult spinal deformity and our aging population is needed to avoid inappropriate rationing of care. The only way to assess the appropriateness of these spinal treatments is to analyze the clinical variables and outcome measurements for the effectiveness, rather than looking at absolute costs or rate of growth data alone, as overinterpretation of any subset of data is potentially misleading and dangerous.

References

1. Howden LM, Meyer JA. Age and sex composition: 2010–2010 census briefs. 2011. http://www.census.gov/prod/cen2010/briefs/c2010br-03.pdf
2. He W, Muenchrath MN. 90+ in the United States: 2006–2008-American Community Survey Reports. 2011. http://www.census.gov/prod/2011pubs/acs-17.pdf
3. Bressler HB, Keyes WJ, Rochon PA, et al. The prevalence of low back pain in the elderly: a systematic review of the literature. Spine. 1999;24:1813–9.
4. Koch H, Smith MC, DHHS publication (PHS). Office-based ambulatory care for patients 75 years old and over, National Ambulatory Medical Care Survey, 1980 and 1981. Hyattsville: Advance Data from Vital and Health Statistics, National Center for Health Statistics (NCHS); 1985. p. 85–1250.
5. Dagenais S, Caro J, Haldeman S. A systematic review of low back pain cost of illness studies in the United States and internationally. Spine J. 2008;8:8–20.
6. Deyo RA, Mirza SK, Martin BI. Back pain prevalence and visit rates: estimates from U.S. national surveys, 2002. Spine (Phila Pa 1976). 2006;31:2724–7.
7. Weiner DK, Haggerty CL, Kritchevsky SB, et al. How does low back pain impact physical function in independent, well-functioning older adults? Evidence from the Health ABC cohort and implications for the future. Pain Med. 2003;4:311–20.
8. Cypress BK. Characteristics of physician visits for back symptoms: a national perspective. Am J Public Health. 1983;73:389–95.
9. Hart LG, Deyo RA, Cherkin DC. Physician office visits for low back pain. Frequency, clinical evaluation, and treatment patterns from a US national survey. Spine. 1995;20:11–9.
10. Weiner DK, Kim Y, Bonino P, et al. Low back pain in older adults: are we utilizing healthcare resources wisely? Pain Med. 2006;7:143.
11. Bigos SBO, Braen G, et al. Acute low back problems in adults. Rockville: Agency for Health Care Policy and Research, Public Health Service, US Department of Health and Human Services; 1994.
12. Deyo RA, Mirza SK, Martin BI. Error in trends, major medical complications, and charges associated with surgery for lumbar spinal stenosis in older adults. JAMA. 2011;306:1088.
13. Deyo RA, Mirza SK, Martin BI, Kreuter W, Goodman DC, Jarvik JG. Trends, major medical complications, and charges associated with surgery for lumbar spinal stenosis in older adults. JAMA. 2010;303:1259–65.
14. Kobayashi T, Atsuta Y, Takemitsu M, Matsuno T, Takeda N. A prospective study of de novo scoliosis in a community based cohort. Spine (Phila Pa 1976). 2006;31(2):178–82.
15. Schwab F, Dubey A, Gamez L, El Fegoun AB, Hwang K, Pagala M, Farcy JP. Adult scoliosis: prevalence, SF-36, and nutritional parameters in an elderly volunteer population. Spine (Phila Pa 1976). 2005;30(9):1082–5.

16. Carreon LY, Puno RM, Dimar 2nd JR, Glassman SD, Johnson JR. Perioperative complications of posterior lumbar decompression and arthrodesis in older adults. J Bone Joint Surg Am. 2003;85-A:2089–92.
17. Cassinelli EH, Eubanks J, Vogt M, Furey C, Yoo J, Bohlman HH. Risk factors for the development of perioperative complications in elderly patients undergoing lumbar decompression and arthrodesis for spinal stenosis: an analysis of 166 patients. Spine (Phila Pa 1976). 2007;32:230–5.
18. Zheng F, Sandhu HS, Cammisa Jr FP, Girardi FP, Khan SN. Predictors of functional outcome in elderly patients undergoing posterior lumbar spine surgery. J Spinal Disord. 2001;14:518–21.
19. Amundsen T, Weber H, Nordal HJ, Magnaes B, Abdelnoor M, Lilleas F. Lumbar spinal stenosis: conservative or surgical management? A prospective 10-year study. Spine (Phila Pa 1976). 2000;25:1424–35. discussion 1435–1426.
20. Glassman SD, Berven S, Kostuik J, Dimar JR, Horton WC, Bridwell K. Nonsurgical resource utilization in adult spinal deformity. Spine (Phila Pa 1976). 2006;31:941–7.
21. Schwab F, Lafage V, Boyce R, Skalli W, Farcy JP. Gravity line analysis in adult volunteers: age-related correlation with spinal parameters, pelvic parameters, and foot position. Spine (Phila Pa 1976). 2006;31(25):E959–67.
22. Dubousset J. Three-dimensional analysis of the scoliotic deformity. In: Weinsteid SL, editor. The pediatric spine: principles and practice. New York: Raven Press; 1994.
23. Glassman SD, Bridwell K, Dimar JR, Horton W, Berven S, Schwab F. The impact of positive sagittal balance in adult spinal deformity. Spine (Phila Pa 1976). 2005;30(18):2024–9.
24. Drazin D, Shirzadi A, Rosner J, Eboli P, Safee M, Baron EM, Liu JC, Acosta FL. Complications and outcomes after spinal deformity surgery in the elderly: review of the existing literature and future directions. Neurosurg Focus. 2011;31(4):E3.
25. Best NM, Sasso RC. Outpatient lumbar spine decompression in 233 patients 65 years or older. Spine (Phila Pa 1976). 2007;32:1135–40.
26. Rageb AA, Fye MA, Bohlman HH. Surgery of the lumbar spine for spinal stenosis in 118 patients 70 years of age or older. Spine (Phila Pa 1976). 2003;28:348–53.
27. Glassman SD, Hamill CL, Bridwell KH, Schwab FJ, Dimar JR, Lowe TG. The impact of perioperative complications on clinical outcome in adult deformity surgery. Spine (Phila Pa 1976). 2007;32:2764–70.
28. Li G, Passias P, Kozanek M, Fu E, Wang S, Xia Q, Li G, Rand FE, Wood KB. Adult scoliosis in patients over sixty-five years of age: outcomes of operative versus non-operative treatment at a minimum of two-year follow-up. Spine (Phila Pa 1976). 2009;34(20):2165–70.
29. Scheufler KM, Cyron D, Dohmen H, Eckardt A. Less invasive surgical correction of adult scoliosis. Part II: complications and clinical outcome. Neurosurgery. 2010;67(6):1609–21.
30. Martin BI, Deyo RA, Mirza SK, et al. Expenditures and health status among adults with back and neck problems. JAMA. 2008;299:656–64.
31. Pateder DB, et al. Short-term mortality and its association with independent risk factors in adult spinal deformity surgery. Spine (Phila Pa 1976). 2008;33(11):1224–8.
32. Acosta Jr FL, et al. Morbidity and mortality after spinal deformity surgery in patients 75 years and older: complications and predictive factors. J Neurosurg Spine. 2011;15(6):667–74.
33. Smith JS, et al. Risk-benefit assessment of surgery for adult scoliosis: an analysis based on patient age. Spine (Phila Pa 1976). 2011;36(10):817–24.
34. Wang MY. Percutaneous iliac screws for minimally invasive spinal deformity surgery. Minim Invasive Surg. 2012;2012:173685.
35. Fehlings MG, Ibrahim GM. Spinal deformity. J Neurosurg Spine. 2010;13(6):663–4. discussion 664–5.
36. Goldman L. Multifactorial index of cardiac risk in noncardiac surgery: ten-year status report. J Cardiothorac Anesth. 1987;1(3):237–44.
37. Ford MK, Beattie WS, Wijeysundera DN. Systematic review: prediction of perioperative cardiac complications and mortality by the revised cardiac risk index. Ann Intern Med. 2010;152(1):26–35.
38. Milledge JS, Nunn JF. Criteria of fitness for anaesthesia in patients with chronic obstructive lung disease. Br Med J. 1975;3(5985):670–3.
39. Rowe JW, et al. The effect of age on creatinine clearance in men: a cross-sectional and longitudinal study. J Gerontol. 1976;31(2):155–63.
40. DeWald RL. Spinal deformities: the comprehensive text. 1st ed. New York: Thieme; 2003.
41. Nicolle LE, Huchcroft SA, Cruse PJ. Risk factors for surgical wound infection among the elderly. J Clin Epidemiol. 1992;45(4):357–64.
42. Wang MY, Mummaneni PV. Minimally invasive surgery for thoracolumbar spinal deformity: initial clinical experience with clinical and radiographic outcomes. Neurosurg Focus. 2010;28(3):E9.
43. Deutsch H, Boco T, Lobel J. Minimally invasive transpedicular vertebrectomy for metastatic disease to the thoracic spine. J Spinal Disord Tech. 2008;21(2):101–5.
44. Foley KT, Holly LT, Schwender JD. Minimally invasive lumbar fusion. Spine (Phila Pa 1976). 2003;28(15):S26–35.
45. Schwender JD, et al. Minimally invasive transforaminal lumbar interbody fusion (TLIF): technical feasibility and initial results. J Spinal Disord Tech. 2005;18(Suppl):S1–6.

Classification Schema for Scoliosis

2

Olaolu C. Akinbo, Tsung-Hsi Tu, John E. Ziewacz, and Praveen V. Mummaneni

2.1 Introduction

Scoliosis classifications serve as a guide for treatment decisions [1, 2]. An ideal classification system should be comprehensive and easy to utilize [3].

2.1.1 Definitions

Definitions of the Scoliosis Research Society (SRS) are presented here for clarity. The central sacral vertical line (CSVL or CSL) is the vertical line in an anteroposterior radiograph that passes through the center of the sacrum (Fig. 2.1). The vertebra or disc of a scoliotic curve which is most deviated laterally from the central sacral line is the apical vertebra. A thoracic curve must have its apex between the T2 and T11 vertebra, a thoracolumbar curve must have its apex at the T12–L1 vertebra, and a lumbar curve must have its apex between the L1 and L5 vertebra. The cephalad end vertebra is the vertebra in the cephalad direction from a curve apex whose superior surface is maximally tilted toward the concavity of the curve. Similarly, the caudad end vertebra is the vertebra in the caudad direction from a curve apex whose inferior surface is maximally tilted toward the concavity of the curve. The magnitude of the curve is assessed by the Cobb method, and this is the angle between lines drawn on end plates of the end vertebrae (superior end plate of the cephalad end vertebra; inferior end plate of the caudad end vertebra). In a patient with multiple curves, the major curve is that which has the largest Cobb measurement on an upright long cassette coronal x-ray of the spine; any smaller curve is termed a minor curve. The neutral vertebra is that which has no axial rotation. A stable vertebra is the thoracic or lumbar vertebra which is adjacent to a scoliotic curve and it is most closely bisected by the CSVL (assuming the pelvis is level). See Fig. 2.1. A curve is described as structural if its coronal plane Cobb measurement does not correct past zero on supine maximal voluntary lateral side-bending x-ray film. This measures the flexibility of the curve. Kyphosis is a posterior convex angulation of the spine [4].

2.2 Adolescent Idiopathic Scoliosis Classification Systems

Based on etiology, scoliosis has been broadly subdivided into idiopathic, neuromuscular, syndromic, congenital, and degenerative types. The idiopathic type (which is most common) can be

O.C. Akinbo, MBBS • T.-H. Tu, M.D.
J.E. Ziewacz, M.D., MPH • P.V. Mummaneni, MD (✉)
Department of Neurological Surgery,
University of California, San Francisco,
San Francisco, CA, USA
e-mail: mummanenip@neurosurg.ucsf.edu

M.Y. Wang et al. (eds.), *Minimally Invasive Spinal Deformity Surgery*,
DOI 10.1007/978-3-7091-1407-0_2, © Springer-Verlag Wien 2014

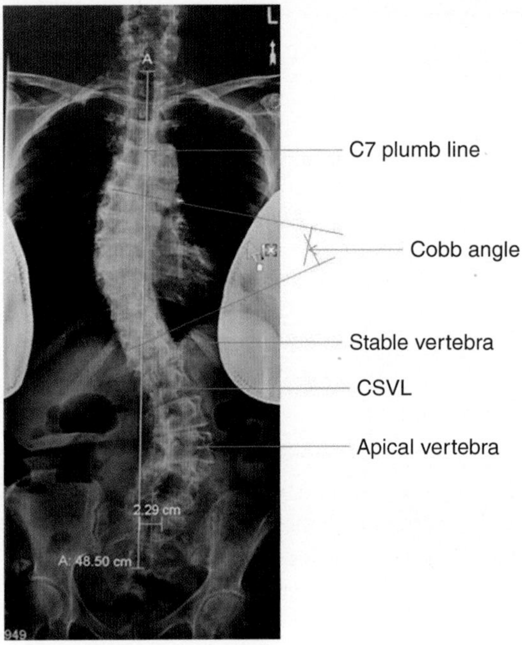

Fig. 2.1 36-in. antero-posterior X-ray illustrating scoliosis terms. *CSVL* Central Sacral vertical line

subclassified further according to the patient's age at diagnosis into infantile, juvenile, adolescent, and adult groups [5]. The early efforts at classification of scoliosis were essentially focused on the adolescent idiopathic scoliosis (AIS) subtype.

Schulthess in 1905 classified scoliosis into cervicothoracic, thoracic, thoracolumbar, lumbar, and combined double primary [6]. This classification was based on curve type and its location. Subsequent publications by James in 1954 [7] and Moe in 1970 [8] excluded the cervicothoracic type due to its rarity. However, they retained the fundamental principles of curve location and type in classifying the disorder. These features were noted to be constant for a curve even during its growth [9]. The early classifications were inadequate for making treatment decisions. Advancements in the understanding of the clinical features of scoliosis, investigative modalities, and surgical techniques led to more refined classification schemes. These include the classification systems of King [10], Coonrad [11], Lenke [12], and the Peking Union Medical College [3].

2.2.1 The King System

The King classification was aimed at choosing the patients who are suitable for selective thoracic fusion in the presence of combined thoracic and lumbar scoliosis and to identify the segments to be fused. A retrospective review of 405 patients who had undergone posterior spine fusion with Harrington rod instrumentation for thoracic AIS was done. They excluded the patients who had single lumbar or thoracolumbar curves, developmental delay, neuromuscular disease, and spondylolisthesis and those who were older than 25 years at the time of surgery. The following set of x-ray films were analyzed for each patient: preoperative standing anteroposterior (AP) or posteroanterior (PA) and a set of preoperative supine side-bending AP films. The curve types were assessed based on the CSL and the stable vertebra was noted. The term "flexibility index" was introduced. This is determined by measuring the percentage of flexibility of the thoracic and lumbar curves on maximum lateral bending x-ray films. The percentage correction of the thoracic curve is deducted from that of the lumbar curve; this difference is the flexibility index [10].

Type I is an S-shaped curve in which both the thoracic curve and the lumbar curves cross the midline. The lumbar curve is larger than the thoracic curve on the standing radiograph. The flexibility index is a negative value (i.e., the thoracic curve was more flexible on side bending). Type II is an S-shaped curve in which both the thoracic and lumbar curves cross the midline. The thoracic curve is equal to, or greater than, the lumbar curve and the flexibility index is ≥ 0. Type III is a thoracic curve in which the lumbar curve does not cross the midline (so-called overhang). A type IV long thoracic curve is one in which L5 is centered over the sacrum but L4 tilts into the long thoracic curve. In type V, there is double thoracic curve in which the T1 is tilted into the convexity of the upper curve and the first rib is elevated on this convexity.

The classification by King et al. did not include any consideration for the sagittal deformity; the curve types were determined only with coronal imaging. This classification was subsequently found to have poor interobserver and intraobserver reliability and it had limited reproducibility [12–14].

2.2.2 The Coonrad System

In 1998, Coonrad et al. noted the lack of a comprehensive, data-based, and user-friendly coronal pattern classification of idiopathic scoliosis [11]. They reviewed the records and radiographs of 2,000 consecutive patients with idiopathic scoliosis. These patients spanned a period of 30 years. Their aims were (1) to identify and categorize the spectrum of coronal curve patterns in a large sample of patients with idiopathic scoliosis according to the SRS definition of the apical vertebra and (2) to apply simple numerical nomenclature for classification. The classification was seen as a vital prelude to the consideration of the sagittal and three-dimensional variables of idiopathic scoliosis. The flexibility of the curves was determined by a supervised recumbent lateral bending coronal x-ray. Eleven types were described and these are summarized below.

Type 1A consists of thoracic and lumbar curves and both are structural. The lumbar curve is larger and/or less flexible, and its apex is at/or below the L1–L2 disc space. Type 1B consists of thoracic and thoracolumbar curves, both are structural. The thoracolumbar curve is larger and/or less flexible, and its apex is at T12, L1, or the disc space in between. Type 2A consists of thoracic and lumbar curves, both are structural. The thoracic curve is larger and/or less flexible and the apex of the lumbar curve is at or below the L1–L2 disc space. Type 2B consists of thoracic and thoracolumbar curves, both are structural. The thoracic curve is larger and/or less flexible. The apex of the lumbar curve is at T12, L1, or the disc space in between. Type 3 consists of a thoracic curve that is structural, and its apex is at T7–T9. Type 4 consists of a thoracic structural curve with the apex at either T10 or T11. The lower end vertebra is usually at L2 or L3 and the L4 is tilted into the curve. Type 5 consists of double thoracic curves and both are structural. The T1 or T2 vertebra is usually tilted into the upper curve. Both apices are located at the thoracic spine segment. Type 6 consists of a thoracolumbar curve, the apex of which is at T12, L1, or the disc space in between. Type 7 consists of a lumbar curve, and the apex is at the L1–L2 or L4–L5 disc spaces or between these. Type 8 consists of triple curves; the size of the largest of the three curves determines the laterality. Type 9 consists of multiple curves. The largest number in the Coonrad study was the quadruple.

This classification was based on the following characteristics of the curves: the location, number, relative Cobb angles, and flexibility of each curve when they are multiple. The sagittal and three-dimensional features of the deformity were not considered. It was however noted that these were necessary for the choice of treatment, fusion levels, and surgical approach. The identification and categorization of the spectrum of existing coronal pattern types is considered a mandatory prerequisite for any classification. This classification complemented the King's system. Its interobserver and intraobserver reliability was initially reported to be 98.7 % and 100 %, respectively. However, the former was subsequently found to be only 46 % ($\kappa = 0.38$) [15]. The Lenke classification system was introduced 3 years later.

2.2.3 The Lenke System

Lenke et al. in conjunction with the Scoliosis Research Society (SRS) introduced another classification system in 2001 which is based on both coronal and sagittal aspects of the scoliotic deformity. This method was designed to determine the appropriate vertebral levels that should be included in a fusion. They studied four x-ray films for each of their 27 patients, including the coronal and lateral views of the standing long cassette x-rays and the coronal views of the right and left supine side bending. The curve locations were defined as proximal thoracic (PT), main thoracic (MT), or thoracolumbar/lumbar (TL/L). The apex of the PT curve lies at T3, T4 or T5. That of the MT curve lies between T6 and the T11/T12 disc. The SRS definitions were applied

Curve type	I	II	III	IV	V	VI
Curve configuration	Main thoracic	Double thoracic	Double major	Triple major	Thoracolumbar/ lumbar	Thoracolumbar/ lumbar- main thoracic
Major structural curve	MT	MT	MT	MT or TL/L	TL/L	TL/L
Minor structural curve	Nil	PT	TL/L	MT or TL/L PT	Nil	MT
Minor non-structural curve	PT, TL/L	TL/L	PT	Nil	PT, MT	PT

Lumbar curve modifier
A: CSVL lies between the lumbar pedicles up to the stable vertebra
B: CSVL touches the concave border of the apex or lies between this and its concave pedicle
C: CSVL lies completely medial to the entire concave boarder of the apical vertebra

Thoracic sagittal modifier	
–	< 10° (Hypokyphotic)
N	+10° to +40° (Normal)
+	> +40° (Hyperkyphotic)

Fig. 2.2 The Lenke system. A structural curve has a Cobb angle of ≥25° on side-bending radiographs and/or kyphosis of at least +20°. The minor non-structural curves maybe present or not. *PT* Proximal Thoracic curve. *MT* Main Thoracic curve. *TL/L* Thoracolumbar/Lumbar curve. *CSVL* Central sacral vertical line (Adapted from, Lenke LG, Betz RR, Harms J, Bridwell KH, Clements DH, Lowe TG, Blanke K. Adolescent idiopathic scoliosis: a new classification to determine extent of spinal arthrodesis. J Bone Joint Surg Am 2001;83:1169–81, [12])

to distinguish between major and minor curves and also to define the apices of the thoracolumbar and lumbar curves. The flexibility of the minor curves was considered. They lacked normal flexibility if the Cobb angle is ≥25° on side-bending radiographs and/or kyphosis is at least +20°, and these were described as structural. The curve types were based on the identification of the major curve and the structural characteristics of the minor curves [12] as follows.

In type 1, the MT curve is the major curve; the PT and TL/L curves are minor and nonstructural. Type 2 consists of double thoracic curves; the MT curve is major, while the PT curve is minor and structural. The TL/L curve is minor and nonstructural. Type 3 consists of double major curves. The Cobb angle of the MT is ≥TL/L or it may be lesser, in which case the difference is not greater than 5°. Both curves are structural and the MT is regarded as the major curve, while the PT curve is nonstructural. Type 4 consists of triple major curves, the PT, MT, and TL/L. All are structural and either of the two latter curves may be the major curve. In type 5, the TL/L curve is structural and it is the major curve. The PT and MT curves are nonstructural. In type 6, the TL/L curve is the major curve, and it is at least 5° greater than the MT which is also structural. The PT curve is nonstructural. See Fig. 2.2.

Lumbar spine modifiers A, B, or C were introduced because the lumbar deformity alters spinal balance and affects proximal curves. Modifier "A" is applied when the CSVL runs between the lumbar pedicles to the level of the stable vertebra. The curve apex must be in the thoracic spine, at or cephalad to the T11/T12 disc. Thus, modifier

A can only be applied for a main thoracic curve (types 1–4). It is not applied for thoracolumbar/lumbar curves (types 5 and 6) or when the CSVL lies on the medial aspect of the lumbar apical pedicle. Modifier "B" is applied when the CSVL touches the concave margin of the lumbar curve apical vertebra body (or bodies if the apex is a disc) or when it lies between this border and the concave pedicle. The TL/L curves are excluded because the curves all have a thoracic apex. Modifier C is applied if the CSVL lies completely medial to the entire concave lateral aspect of the thoracolumbar or lumbar apical vertebral body or bodies (if the apex is a disc).

The kyphotic component of the thoracic spine deformity was described in this method of classification with another set of modifiers: –, N, or +. The mean normal sagittal thoracic alignment from the fifth to the twelfth thoracic vertebra is +30° with a range of +10° to +40° [16]. Patients who have adolescent idiopathic scoliosis tend to have decreased thoracic kyphosis or even thoracic lordosis in comparison with normal controls [16, 17]. The sagittal thoracic modifiers were determined by measurements from the superior end plate of the fifth thoracic vertebra to the inferior end plate of the twelfth thoracic vertebra on a standing lateral radiograph. Modifier "–" is applied if there is thoracic hypokyphosis, which is a curve <+10°. Modifier "N" is applied for normal thoracic kyphosis (+10° to +40°), while the "+" sign is applied for hyperkyphotic thoracic curves (>+40°). The recommendation for spinal arthrodesis is that it should include only the major curve and structural minor ones.

Lenke et al. noted inaccuracies in assessing axial plane deformity on biplanar radiographs; thus the axial components of the deformities were excluded from this system of classification. The authors stated that the mean interobserver reliability for determining curve type with this system was 93 % (range, 85–100 %), with a mean κ value of 0.92 (range, 0.83–1.00), while that of the King system was found to be 64 %, and the κ value was 0.49 [14]. Subsequently, other investigators reported moderate range interobserver reliability for the Lenke system [18, 19].

The Lenke system is more comprehensive than the earlier classifications; it also provides for objective curve assessments to aid surgical planning. The sagittal component of the deformity was included in the classification. However, the complexity must be noted. Forty-two curve patterns are derivable by the application of the modifiers to the six basic curve types. The rotational component of the deformity was also not addressed. The Lenke system is currently the most widely utilized classification scheme for AIS and it thus provides a basis for comparison of treatments and outcomes [20].

2.2.4 Peking Union Medical College System

Qiu et al. at the Peking Union Medical College (PUMC) proposed this system of classification in 2005. They reviewed the records of 427 idiopathic scoliosis patients who were managed operatively over 18 years. The curves were assessed with the preoperative supine side-bending radiograph and anteroposterior and lateral standing radiographs taken before and after surgery. The SRS definitions of scoliosis and curve apex locations were strictly applied. The flexibility of the curvature was calculated thus: (Cobb angle on standing – Cobb angle on convex bending)/Cobb angle on standing} × 100 % [3]. The rotation of the apical vertebra was recorded from 1° to 4° using the Nash-Moe method [21].

This method was designed to enable the selection of a surgical approach and of fusion levels. All the curves were classified into single, double, and triple curves according to the apex vertebra, and these were termed types I, II, and III, respectively. There were a total of 13 subtypes.

Type Ia is a thoracic curve, Ib is thoracolumbar, and Ic, a lumbar curve. Type II consists of thoracic (T) and thoracolumbar/lumbar (TL/L) curves. Subtype IIa consists of double thoracic curves. In subtype IIb, the T curve is at least 10° > TL/L curve. For IIc, the difference between the Cobb angles of T and TL/L curves is <10°, while in IId, the TL/L is 10° > T curve. Further subdivisions of these subtypes are based on the differences in flexibility of the curves, presence of TL/L kyphosis, and its degree of axial rotation. Subtype IIIa consists of triple curves; its thoracolumbar/lumbar component has a Cobb angle of ≤45°, rotation <2°, flexibility ≥70°, and no kyphosis. In subtype IIIb, distal lumbar curve is larger and more rigid.

The interobserver and intraobserver reliability that was stated by the authors for the PUMC system was 85 % (κ=0.83) and 91 % (κ=0.90), respectively [3]. This method has attempted to further simplify the classification of AIS into three major types, although there are 13 subtypes. It has also included the rotational component of the deformity. The reliability of this scheme requires further validation through independent prospective multicenter studies.

2.3 Adult Scoliosis Classifications

Adult scoliosis is an entirely distinct entity from AIS with respect to clinical features, radiological findings, treatment, and prognosis [22]. Degenerative changes are frequently associated with adult deformity. These include spinal stenosis, spondylolisthesis, rotational subluxation, lumbar hypolordosis, and rigidity [2]. There are also differences with respect to the patterns of the deformity, its progression, the clinical features, the goals, and strategies of treatment.

Until recently, the management of adult scoliosis was mostly nonoperative. This was due to the significant risks which were related to the patient's age, poor bone quality, and the lack of adequate instrumentation to enable and maintain correction. However, the increase in age and longevity of the population, coupled with advances in surgical techniques and anesthetic care, has stimulated substantial progress in the surgical care of adult scoliosis patients [23]. Adult scoliosis is generally considered as greater than 10° of coronal curvature in a skeletally matured spine. The health status and treatment options in adult scoliosis are significantly influenced by symptomatic degenerative changes and the global imbalance of the spine in the sagittal and coronal plane [2, 27]. These should be incorporated into a comprehensive adult scoliosis classification system. Also the principles that guide the choice of management such as operative, nonoperative, limited, or extensive instrumentation require detailed definition through an effective classification method. Four classification systems have been developed for adult scoliosis by Aebi [24], Schwab et al. [25], the Scoliosis Research Society (SRS) [2], and the hybrid SRS-Schwab system [26].

2.3.1 Aebi Classification System

The classification system of adult scoliosis developed by Max Aebi in 2005 is focused on etiology much more than specific details of the deformity. There are four types (I, II, IIIa, and IIIb). Type I consists of primary degenerative scoliosis and this is typically in the thoracolumbar or lumbar spine, with an apex between L2 and L4. The deformity was said to have resulted from asymmetric degenerative disc changes with asymmetric vertebral loading. There is attendant frontal deviation and rotation with the facet joints on one side acting as a pivot. Type II describes a progressive idiopathic thoracolumbar and/or lumbar scoliosis which has been present since adolescence or childhood but becomes progressive due to mechanical, bony, or degenerative changes. In type III there are two subgroups. Type IIIa consists of secondary adult scoliosis mostly at the thoracolumbar, lumbar, or lumbosacral segments. This type occurs secondary to an adjacent curve within the spine, lumbosacral anomaly such as hemisacralization, or pelvic obliquity which is secondary to a hip pathology or a leg length discrepancy. Type IIIb includes adult scoliosis that is caused by bony weakness, due to metabolic bone disease and osteoporosis [24].

The Aebi system offers a relatively simple means of classifying adult deformity based on the etiology. It may be useful in predicting the natural history of the disease. However, it does not reflect the complexity of specific deformities to a degree that is adequate for detailed surgical planning.

2.3.2 The Schwab System

Schwab et al. noted that the impact of the adult scoliotic deformity and treatment approaches is related to pain and disability and not to the skeletal age or the projected progression of the deformity [25]. Thus the pediatric and adolescent methods cannot be transposed on adult patients. Their hypothesis was that a reliable radiographic classification that consists of clinical groups could be developed. These clinical groups are to be segregated by the initial treatment modality (operative versus nonoperative) and quality of life.

The study recruited 947 adults from 11 centers. Modifiers were applied to grade the lumbar lordosis and subluxations (either in coronal or sagittal plane). This system has five major types of adult scoliosis, and these were distinguished according to the location of the apex vertebra. In type I there is single thoracic curve. Type II consists of a major upper thoracic curve with the apex at T4–T8 and also a thoracolumbar or lumbar curve. In type III, there is a lower thoracic major curve, whose apex is at T9–T10, and a thoracolumbar or lumbar curve. Type IV adult scoliosis consists of a thoracolumbar major curve, the apex is at T11–L1, and any other minor curve may be present. Type V has a major lumbar scoliotic curve with its apex at L2–L4 and any other minor curve. Major and minor curves were distinguished as defined by the SRS. If there are more than two curves with identical Cobb angle measurements, then the lower curve is selected as the major.

Lumbar lordosis modifiers (A, B, and C) were measured based on the T12–S1 sagittal Cobb angle. Modifier "A" implies marked lordosis which is >40°, modifier "B" implies moderate lordosis which ranged between 0° and 40°, while modifier "C" indicates no lordosis. A subluxation modifier was also added. The maximal intervertebral subluxation in the coronal or sagittal plane was measured to determine the subluxation modifier score. The "0"modifier was applied if there is no subluxation, "+" for moderate subluxation (1–6 mm), and modifier "++" for marked subluxation (>7 mm). Disability and pain were assessed with Oswestry Disability Index (ODI) and SRS function/pain scores and compared across the subtypes. Analysis of the treatment pattern across the subtypes was also performed.

Loss of lordosis was associated with significantly lower SRS pain/function and higher ODI scores (lordosis modifier A vs. C, $P<0.007$) in patients with thoracolumbar and lumbar curve patterns (types IV and V). However, this was contrary to its effect on the major thoracic types (I, II, and III), for which it had no statistically significant impact. The subluxation modifier was also associated with a marked impact for adult scoliosis types IV and V when measured with the SRS function score and ODI. The impact was not significant for the thoracic curves. The curve type was not predictive of surgical management, but there was a significant increase in the surgical rate with an increasing lordosis modifier (A vs. C; 36 % vs. 54 %, respectively; $P<0.04$) and with higher intervertebral subluxation (modifier "0" vs. "++"; 36 % and 52 %, respectively; $P<0.001$).

This classification method was focused on clinical impact parameters and it was not fully descriptive of the structural variations of the curves. This is quite contrary to the detailed radiographic parameters that were employed in the adolescent classification methods. However, it is known that in the management of adult scoliosis, pain and disability are major issues.

2.3.3 The SRS System

This adult scoliosis classification system was developed by the adult spinal deformity committee of the Scoliosis Research Society. It aims to provide a basis for an evidence-based approach to the management of adult spinal deformity as well as comparison of treatment modalities and outcomes between various centers. The classification is based on standing full-length radiographs in the coronal and sagittal planes. Global balance, regional deformity patterns, and focal degenerative changes within the deformity were assessed [2].

Six primary coronal curves were identified based on the apical levels and there is also a designation for primary sagittal-plane deformity in the absence of a significant coronal curve. The six primary curves were single thoracic (ST), double thoracic (DT), double major (DM), triple major (TM), thoracolumbar (TL), and lumbar (L) and a primary sagittal-plane deformity (SP). These curves were defined according to the criteria of the SRS. Significant primary thoracic curves must be ≥40° and the C7 sagittal plumb line must lie lateral to the apical vertebral body of the curve. The upper thoracic curves are structural if the first thoracic rib or clavicular tilt is ≥5° with the elevated side located ipsilateral to the apex of the deformity. The criteria for the thoracolumbar and lumbar curves are a Cobb angle which is ≥30° and the CSVL which is lateral to the apical vertebral body of the curve.

A sagittal modifier was applied because the kyphotic deformity in the sagittal plane is known to have significant impact on the health status and surgical strategies when correcting adult scoliosis. The sagittal modifier for the PT region is positive when the sagittal Cobb angle is ≥ 20°. The corresponding values for the MT region is Cobb angle ≥50°, TL region ≥20°, and L region ≥−40°. The lumbar degenerative modifier is only applied if radiographic evidence of disc narrowing, facet arthropathy, and degenerative spondylolisthesis or rotatory subluxation ≥3 mm in any plane is present. The global balance modifier describes the spinal column imbalance in either the coronal or sagittal plane. Loss of sagittal balance was significant if the C7 plumb line is ≥5 cm either anterior or posterior to the sacral promontory, while the loss of coronal balance is significant if the C7 plumb line is ≥3 cm to either side of the CSVL.

The authors reported a good interobserver reliability for curve type (κ=0.64), sagittal modifier (κ=0.73), degenerative lumbar modifier (κ=0.65), and global balance modifier (κ=0.92). This classification system does not account for the presenting symptoms, patient's age, and comorbidities such as osteoporosis and systemic diseases. These clinical parameters are important in treatment decisions for adult scoliosis. Further validation of this system will be required.

2.3.4 The SRS-System

A hybrid SRS-Schwab classification of adult scoliosis was recently published [26] (Fig. 2.3). The authors noted the substantial correlation of pelvic

Coronal curve type	Curve location	Curve apex	Cobb angle
T	Major thoracic	T9 and above	> 30°
L	Major lumbar or major thoraco-lumbar	T10 and below	> 30°
D	Double major curves	Double	Both curves > 30°
N	No coronal curve > 30°		

Sagittal modifier	PI-LL	SVA	PT
0	< 10°	< 4 cm	< 20°
+	< 10° to 20°	4 to 9.5 cm	20° to 30°
++	> 20°	> 9.5 cm	> 30°

Fig. 2.3 The SRS-Schwab system

parameters with pain and disability [27]. Thus they aimed to incorporate these clinically relevant spinopelvic parameters into the Schwab classification system and subsequently assess the reliability of the hybrid system. The relevant parameters include the sagittal vertical axis (SVA), the pelvic tilt (PT), and the difference between the pelvic incidence (PI) and the lumbar lordosis (LL), PI-LL. The PI is the angle between the line drawn perpendicular to the sacral end plate at its midpoint and the line drawn from the midpoint of the sacral end plate to the midpoint of the bicoxo-femoral axis. The LL is the sagittal Cobb angle measured between the superior end plate of L1 and the superior end plate of S1. The PT is the angle between the line connecting the midpoint of the sacral end plate to the midpoint of the bicoxo-femoral axis and the vertical. The SVA is the offset between the sagittal C7 plumb line and the posterosuperior corner of the sacrum. The measurements were done on full-length coronal and sagittal spine radiographs. The cutoff values for grades of the modifiers were determined using outcome scores that were previously reported to have a strong clinical impact [28, 29].

There are four basic curve types in this system. Type T is a major thoracic scoliotic curve with apex at T9 or higher and Cobb angle is >30°. Type L is a major lumbar or thoracolumbar major curve, its apex is at T10 or lower, and Cobb angle is >30°. Type D is a double major curve and each curve is >30°. While in type N, there is no coronal curve that is greater than 30° (i.e., no major coronal deformity).

The first sagittal modifier is the PI-LL measure; this parameter is important for the surgical planning of osteotomies in order to preserve an adequate LL. The "0" modifier is applied for patients with PI-LL values <10°. The "+" modifier is applied for values between 10° and 20°, while the "++" modifier is applied for values >20°. The PT is crucial in assessing spinal deformity; a high PT (increased pelvic retroversion) is a compensatory mechanism that can affect and also reduce the apparent extent of global sagittal malalignment. Modifier "0" is applied for a PT<20°, "+" is for PT values between 20° and 30°, while the "++" modifier is applied for PT values >30°. Patients with an SVA of less than 40 mm are classified with modifier "0," SVA between 40 and 95 mm had "+," and SVA of greater than 95 mm, "++."

The inter-rater reliability that was reported by the authors for the entire classification was 0.79. They concluded that its application is easy and consistent. A recent study has demonstrated that this system is descriptive, correlates with health-related quality of life (HRQOL) scores, and corresponds to treatment preference for adult spinal deformity [30].

Conclusion

The importance of scoliosis classification systems lies in its ability to standardize communication among health-care providers and to facilitate comparison of management approaches and outcomes. The classification of AIS which is essentially structural has gone through various stages. The initial efforts were descriptive of coronal curve types, their location along the spinal column, and the relative flexibility of the curves. Lenke et al. introduced modifiers that described the kyphotic component and the associated lumbar deformity. The axial rotation of the deformity was part of the modifiers used in the PUMC method in an attempt to address the three-dimensional configuration of the deformity. Adult scoliosis classification methods differ from that of the AIS because of the preponderant degenerative features and systemic diseases in this age group. Pain and disability are major factors in the management of adult scoliotic patients. These must all be factored into the classification methods to ensure a complete description of the adult scoliosis patient and the deformity. Such classification must also be useful for effective treatment decision-making.

References

1. Garbuz DS, Masri BA, Esdaile J, Duncan CP. Classification systems in orthopaedics. J Am Acad Orthop Surg. 2002;10:290–7.
2. Lowe T, Berven SH, Schwab FJ, Bridwell KH. The SRS classification for adult spinal deformity: building

on the King/Moe and Lenke classification systems. Spine. 2006;31:S119–25.
3. Qiu G, Zhang J, Wang Y, Xu H, Zhang J, Weng X, Lin J, Zhao Y, Shen J, Yang X, Luk KD, Lu D, Lu WW. A new operative classification of idiopathic scoliosis: a peking union medical college method. Spine. 2005;30:1419–26.
4. SRS Terminology Committee and Working Group on Spinal Classification. Revised Glossary of Terms, March 2000.
5. Breakwell LM, Lenke LG. The Lenke classification system of adolescent idiopathic scoliosis. In: Mummaneni PV, Lenke LG, Haid Jr RW, editors. Spinal deformity: a guide to surgical planning and management. St Louis: Quality Medical Publishing Inc; 2008. p. 47–68.
6. Schulthess W. The pathology and treatment of the spine. Joachimsthal handbook of orthopedic surgery [in German]. Berlin: Gustav Fischer; 1905–1907.
7. James JIP. Idiopathic scoliosis. The prognosis, diagnosis and operative indications related to curve patterns and age of onset. J Bone Joint Surg. 1954;36-B:36–49.
8. Moe JH, Kettleson DN. Idiopathic scoliosis. Analysis of curve patterns and the preliminary results of Milwaukee-brace treatment in 169 patients. J Bone Joint Surg. 1970;52-A:1509–33.
9. Ponseti IV, Friedman B. Prognosis in idiopathic scoliosis. J Bone Joint Surg Am. 1950;32-A:381–95.
10. King HA, Moe JH, Bradford DS, Winter RB. The selection of fusion levels in thoracic idiopathic scoliosis. J Bone Joint Surg Am. 1983;65:1302–13.
11. Coonrad RW, Murrell GA, Motley G, Lytle E, Hey LA. A logical coronal pattern classification of 2,000 consecutive idiopathic scoliosis cases based on the scoliosis research society-defined apical vertebra. Spine. 1998;23:1380–91.
12. Lenke LG, Betz RR, Harms J, Bridwell KH, Clements DH, Lowe TG, Blanke K. Adolescent idiopathic scoliosis: a new classification to determine extent of spinal arthrodesis. J Bone Joint Surg Am. 2001;83:1169–81.
13. Cummings RJ, Loveless EA, Campbell J, Samelson S, Mazur JM. Interobserver reliability and intraobserver reproducibility of the system of King et al. For the classification of adolescent idiopathic scoliosis. J Bone Joint Surg Am. 1998;80:1107–11.
14. Lenke LG, Betz RR, Bridwell KH, Clements DH, Harms J, Lowe TG, Shufflebarger HL. Intraobserver and interobserver reliability of the classification of thoracic adolescent idiopathic scoliosis. J Bone Joint Surg Am. 1998;80:1097–106.
15. Behensky H, Giesinger K, Ogon M, Krismer M, Hannes B, Karlmeinrad G, Michael O, Martin K. Multisurgeon assessment of coronal pattern classification systems for adolescent idiopathic scoliosis: reliability and error analysis. Spine. 2002;27:762–7.
16. Bernhardt M, Bridwell KH. Segmental analysis of the sagittal plane alignment of the normal thoracic and lumbar spine and thoracolumbar junction. Spine. 1989;14:717–21.
17. Bridwell KH, Betz R, Capelli AM, Huss G, Harvey C. Sagittal plane analysis in idiopathic scoliosis patients treated with Cotrel-Dubousset instrumentation. Spine. 1990;15:921–6.
18. Ogon M, Giesinger K, Behensky H, Wimmer C, Nogler M, Bach CM, Krismer M. Interobserver and intraobserver reliability of Lenke's new scoliosis classification system. Spine. 2002;27:858–62.
19. Richards BS, Sucato DJ, Konigsberg DE, Ouellet JA. Comparison of reliability between the Lenke and King classification systems for adolescent idiopathic scoliosis using radiographs that were not premeasured. Spine. 2003;28:1148–57.
20. Lam FC, Kanter AS, Okonkwo DO, Ogilvie JW, Mummaneni PV. Thoracolumbar spinal deformity: part II. Developments from 1990 to today: historical vignette. J Neurosurg Spine. 2009;11:640–50.
21. Nash Jr CL, Moe JH. A study of vertebral rotation. J Bone Joint Surg Am. 1969;51:223–9.
22. Smith JS, Shaffrey CI, Kuntz IV C, Mummaneni PV. Classification systems for adolescent and adult scoliosis. Neurosurgery. 2008;63:A16–24.
23. Mummaneni PV, Ondra SL, Haid RW. Principles of spinal deformity: part II. Advances in the operative treatment of thoracolumbar deformity. Contemp Neurosurg. 2002;24:1–10.
24. Aebi M. The adult scoliosis. Eur Spine J. 2005;14:925–48.
25. Schwab F, Farcy JP, Bridwell K, Berven S, Glassman S, Harrast J, Horton W. A clinical impact classification of scoliosis in the adult. Spine. 2006;31:2109–14.
26. Schwab F, Ungar B, Blondel B, Buchowski J, Coe J, Deinlein D, DeWald C, Mehdian H, Shaffrey C, Tribus C, Lafage V. Scoliosis Research Society—Schwab adult spinal deformity classification: a validation study. Spine. 2012;37(12):1077–82.
27. Glassman SD, Berven S, Bridwell KH, et al. Correlation of radiographic parameters and clinical symptoms in adult scoliosis. Spine. 2005;30:682–8.
28. Lafage V, Schwab F, Patel A, et al. Pelvic tilt and truncal inclination: two key radiographic parameters in the setting of adults with spinal deformity. Spine (Phila Pa 1976). 2009;34:E599–606.
29. Glassman SD, Bridwell K, Dimar JR, et al. The impact of positive sagittal balance in adult spinal deformity. Spine (Phila Pa 1976). 2005;30:2024–9.
30. Schwab F, Lafage V, Shaffrey CI, Smith JS, Moal B, Ames CP, Fu KG, Mummaneni PV, Burton DC, Gupta M, Deviren V, Mundis G, Hart R, Bess S, International Spine Study Group. The Schwab-SRS adult spinal deformity classification: assessment and clinical correlations based on a prospective operative and non-operative cohort. Neurosurgery. 2012;71(2):E556.

Indications for Adult Spinal Deformity Surgery

3

Jeffrey H. Weinreb, Kristina L. Bianco, Virginie Lafage, and Frank Schwab

3.1 Introduction

Shifting demographics and aging populations have resulted in a rise in adult spinal deformity (ASD). ASD refers to abnormal spinal curvature in the coronal, axial, or sagittal planes in patients over the age of 18. A recent publication found that the prevalence of ASD ranges from 2 % to 32 % in the general population but exceeds 60 % for adults greater than 60 years of age [1]. With a simultaneous shift in expectations for quality of life (QOL), the demand for treatment of ASD has dramatically increased. ASD is most commonly caused by untreated adolescent idiopathic scoliosis, adult-onset degenerative scoliosis, or primary sagittal imbalance [2]. While some cases of ASD can be managed with conservative care and nonoperative procedures, many ASD cases require surgical intervention. Unlike adolescent idiopathic scoliosis (AIS), there is no widely accepted classification system that provides guidelines for the surgical treatment of ASD [3]. Therefore, the decision to undergo surgical treatment of ASD must carefully consider clinical symptoms, radiographic parameters, coexisting medical comorbidities, and the patient's physiologic status. The potential benefits and risks associated with the surgical treatment of ASD must also factor into the treatment decision. This chapter provides an overview of current indications for the surgical treatment of ASD and highlights the significance of using a combination of both clinical symptomatology and radiographic imaging to propose the optimal treatment plan for patients with ASD.

J.H. Weinreb • K.L. Bianco • V. Lafage, Ph.D.
Department of Orthopaedic Surgery,
NYU Hospital for Joint Diseases,
New York, NY, USA

F. Schwab, M.D. (✉)
Division of Spine Surgery,
NYU Hospital for Joint Diseases,
301 East 17th Street, New York, NY 10003, USA
e-mail: fschwab@att.net

3.2 Symptom-Driven Treatment

Clinical symptomatology is one of the key factors in the treatment decision process for patients affected by ASD. While the evaluation for pediatric and adolescent spinal deformity is based on radiographic data, the evaluation of ASD is based both on radiographic data and clinical symptoms [4]. When presenting with spinal deformity, younger adult patients tend to seek coronal plane deformity treatment, while older patients are more likely to desire treatment for relief of pain and disability [4]. Through operative treatment, surgeons are tasked with alleviating pain, restoring spinal alignment, and improving functionality. This undertaking is complicated by the fact that the adult patient population has greater risks related to surgical care and a diminished healing potential compared to children or adolescents with spinal deformity [4]. It is important to note that a distinction exists between pain and disability, the primary treatment drivers in the adult population. Pain and disability are two separate clinical phenomena, with differing symptomatology and treatments.

M.Y. Wang et al. (eds.), *Minimally Invasive Spinal Deformity Surgery*,
DOI 10.1007/978-3-7091-1407-0_3, © Springer-Verlag Wien 2014

3.2.1 Pain

Both axial and radicular pain receive substantial attention as indicators for ASD surgery. Although both types of pain are mediated by the spinal cord and nerves, their etiologies, symptom patterns, and surgical indications differ considerably. Both types of pain may be managed with analgesics such as nonsteroidal anti-inflammatory drugs (NSAIDs) or narcotics, although continuous narcotic usage may lead to dependency or desensitization. Noninvasive conservative pain management methods, such as physical therapy or spinal injections, should be considered before operative treatment.

3.2.2 Axial Pain

Axial pain in the setting of ASD is most commonly a pain disorder of the lumbosacral region that is hypothesized to result from advanced intervertebral disc (IVD) degeneration and facet arthrosis. IVD degeneration results in physiologic disc changes, which in turn produce pain through instability, abnormal motion, or loss of stiffness. Pain may result from biochemical environment changes, such as inflammatory cytokines or nociceptive neurotransmitter release [5]. Although IVD is often implicated in axial pain, pain may also arise from the associated anatomy. The facet joints, ligaments, fascia, nerve roots, and dura are capable of transmitting pain. Progressive disc disease results in load cycling to surrounding structures, which may lead to increased arthropathy, ligamentous hypertrophy, and muscle fatigue. Studies performed on patients with similar symptoms demonstrate a wide range of pain sources, including the disc, facet joints, and sacroiliac joints, and it remains unclear whether the disc itself or other surrounding structures are the actual source of pain [5].

Spinal fusion may be indicated when axial lower back pain is present and is predicated on the theory that pain is related to abnormal movement and loading across a motion segment due to disc and facet degeneration. Spine surgeons have adopted fusion across a degenerated disc as a method for relieving pain, although the literature has failed to demonstrate consistent successful clinical outcomes after fusion surgery in this patient population [5].

3.2.3 Radicular Pain

Pain radiating into one or more extremities via a nerve dermatome is defined as radicular pain and implies inflammation, pressure, dysfunction, or stretch of a nerve root [6]. Discectomy is a common treatment method for radicular pain related to focal disc herniation; and success ranges from 48 % to 89 % in the literature [7]. Long-term follow-up reveals that 50–60 % will experience significant back pain after 10 years and 20–30 % will develop recurrent radicular pain [7]. Nerve decompression via foraminotomy or laminectomy is also used to treat intractable radicular pain that is unresponsive to nonsurgical symptom management [8, 9]. Additionally, when radicular pain occurs as a result of isthmic spondylolisthesis, instrumented fusion has shown to be effective in treating symptoms [9]. However, unsatisfactory outcomes following surgical intervention indicate ongoing degeneration, segmental instability, spinal stenosis, and recurrent disc herniation [10].

3.2.4 Disability

Disability, whether in conjunction with pain or not, is another important driver for ASD treatment and should be considered separately from pain syndromes described above. Disability implies functional limitation and may be caused by deformity, biomechanical insufficiency, and mechanical impediment. For example, a patient with marked pelvic retroversion may not have significant pain, but may be very limited in common tasks due to sagittal plane deformity and an inability to extend the hips (gait and standing disruption). Disability caused by pain may be managed through medication (as previously discussed), and mechanical disability may be managed with external walking aids, braces, or wheelchairs. The Oswestry Disability Index (ODI) is a widely used questionnaire to assess disability and can be used to track disability changes in a single patient or in a population [11].

3.3 Correlating Imaging with Symptomatology

Radiographic imaging, in addition to the evaluation of pain and disability, is critical in the diagnosis and treatment planning related to ASD. Studies have demonstrated that patients with more severe disability stand to gain the most from surgical intervention. Furthermore, patients with more severe radiographic deformity tend to exhibit more pain and score lower on disability surveys [12, 13]. However, ASD patients do not become uniformly disabled with age, and disability cannot be solely predicted by radiographic findings [4]. A recent classification system acknowledges the relationship between imaging and disability and defines radiographic goals for surgery.

3.4 SRS-Schwab Classification

While ASD has previously been described using pediatric classification systems, the SRS-Schwab classification has been established as an improved method to categorize patients according to drivers of pain and disability for adults with spinal deformities. The SRS-Schwab classification system uses radiographic imaging to assess the extent of spine deformity, evaluate whether spine deformity surgery is necessary, and establish a plan if surgical correction is needed. This classification system has shown excellent inter- and intra-observer reliability on pre-marked and unmarked x-rays and has proven to be essential for the assessment of spinal deformity and surgical planning [14]. The SRS-Schwab classification has recently been updated to incorporate pelvic parameters, which have been found to play a fundamental role in the radiographic evaluation of patients with spinal deformities [15–22].

Restoration of sagittal alignment is a fundamental goal of spinal surgery. Several key parameters, including sagittal vertical axis (SVA), pelvic tilt (PT), and pelvic incidence minus lumbar lordosis (PI-LL), have been identified as important

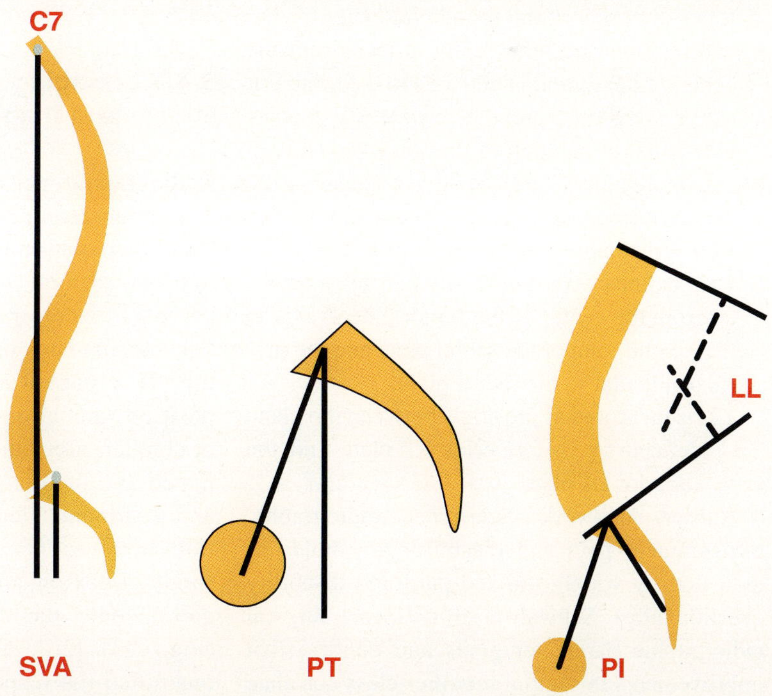

Fig. 3.1 Sagittal parameters that are important in the evaluation of ASD and can be used for surgical planning. Sagittal vertical axis (*SVA*), pelvic tilt (*PT*), and pelvic incidence minus lumbar lordosis (*PI-LL*) are correlated with the disability of patients

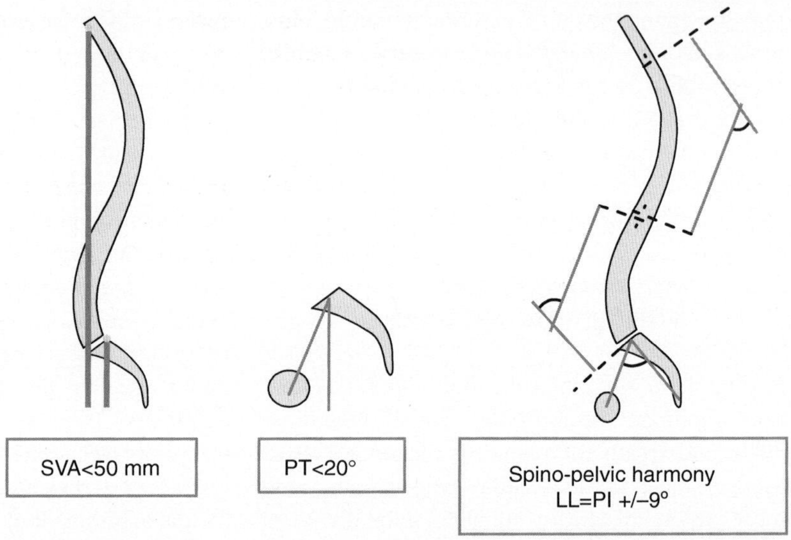

Fig. 3.2 Surgical parameter measurement goals based on correlations between these parameters and HRQOL survey scores

radiographic parameters used in the evaluation of ASD (Fig. 3.1.). These parameters have been found to be highly correlating with the disability of patients and provide a guide for patient assessment and surgical planning [21, 23].

SVA is used to determine global sagittal alignment and is the distance between a vertically drawn plumb line from the midpoint of the C7 vertebra and its offset from the posterior-superior corner of the sacral end plate.

PT is the angle between a line drawn from the center of the femoral head axis to the midpoint of the sacral plate and the vertical. PT denotes the spatial orientation of the spine.

PI-LL is a sagittal modifier that represents the difference between the angle measurement of PI and the angle measurement of LL.

- **PI** is defined as the angle between a line drawn from the center of the femoral head axis to the midpoint of the sacral plate and the perpendicular to the sacral plate.
- **LL** is measured as the angle between the plane defined by the superior S1 plate and the superior L1 plate.

Subsequent work determined radiographic measurement pain and disability thresholds as indicated by widely utilized pain and disability questionnaires. Schwab et al. delineate surgical radiographic parameter goals and confirm that improvements in sagittal modifier class correlate with pain and disability improvement. The threshold for disability is defined as an ODI score greater than 40, an SVA greater than 47 mm, a PT greater than 22°, and absolute value of PI minus LL greater than 11° [24]. Considering the radiographic parameter correlation with pain and disability, Schwab et al. define realignment objectives in the sagittal plane as an SVA less than 50 mm, a PT less than 20°, and LL equal to PI ± 9° (Fig. 3.2) [25].

3.4.1 Imaging Analysis and Diagnosis

Radiographic measures in the context of ASD evaluation require images obtained in a free-standing patient position. This patient positioning is essential to effectively evaluate key aspects of a deformity and potential compensatory mechanisms that a patient may be recruiting. If a patient is not in a weight-bearing position, global deformity, truncal inclination, or compensatory mechanisms can be underestimated and lead to improper patient evaluation and treatment. Ideal standing radiograph position involves natural foot position, forward shoulder flexion, and elbow flexion to bring fingertips onto the cheekbones or midclavicles (Fig. 3.3) [26]. CT and MRI studies have quantified the response of the lumbar spine to rotatory torque and have correlated increased

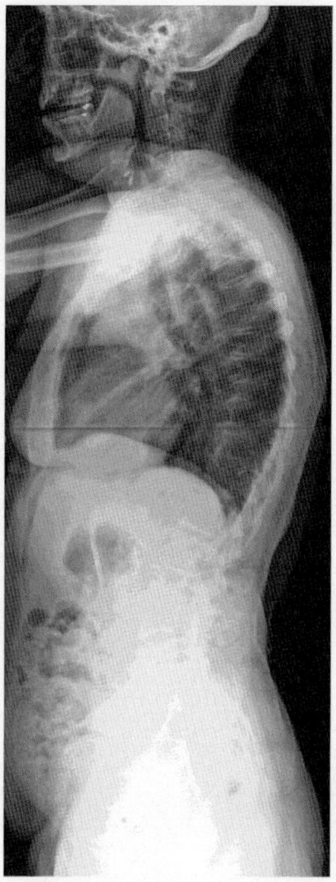

Fig. 3.3 Proper standing position for ASD evaluation radiography

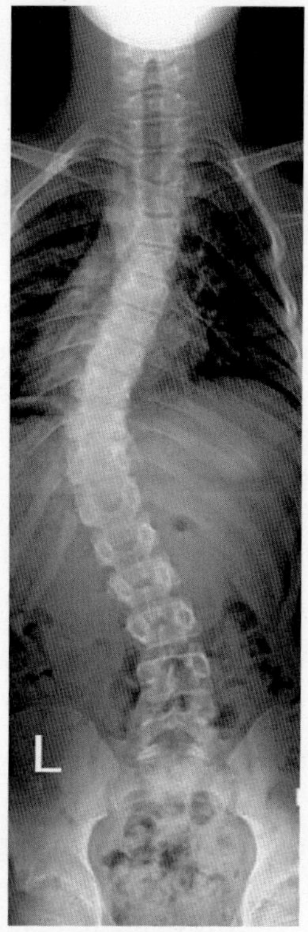

Fig. 3.4 Example of an AP X-ray image

axial rotation in degenerated discs with pain provocation on discography [27, 28]. Additionally plain radiographic findings in patients with axial low back pain may demonstrate characteristics consistent with degenerative disc disease. While radiography does not demarcate soft tissue disc, film may reveal decreased disc height consistent with a collapsed or dehydrated disc. Sclerotic end plates or bone-on-bone appearance are commonly seen with severely degenerated discs and may indicate pain origin [5]. A review of common imaging techniques applied in the evaluation of symptomatic ASD follows.

3.4.2 X-Ray

Conventional radiography with plain-film radiography is any easy procedure to perform. Whole spine images of the standing frontal (anteroposterior) and sagittal (lateral) view are required for adequate evaluation of the patient's deformity. Radiographs should include the occiput superiorly and the femoral heads inferiorly. This process allows spinal assessment in a freestanding position (Figs. 3.3 and 3.4). However, this method utilizes ionizing radiations and can be harmful with prolonged exposure. Newer technologies, such as those employed by EOS imaging, may offer low-dose alternatives to traditional single-beam radiographs.

3.4.3 MRI

MRI uses a strong magnetic field in the radio frequency range. This method is particularly useful for the visualization of soft tissue structures, especially the disc space and adjacent soft tissues. Nonetheless, major limitations of this process include the inability to obtain standing images and long acquisition times. The use of a strong magnetic field may also be problematic for patients with electronic devices such as a pacemaker or spinal cord stimulators.

3.4.4 CT

CT imaging produces tomographic slices of specific area of the body through the axial plane. Computer algorithms allow image reconstruction in the sagittal and coronal planes. This process is particularly useful for bone tissue visualization. Combination with myelography, which consists of an intrathecal contrast agent injection, allows a clear and accurate representation of the spinal anatomy. Results of this combination provide better osseous and joint anatomy than MRI. However, as with conventional radiographs, this method utilizes ionizing radiations that may be dangerous for patients (Fig. 3.5).

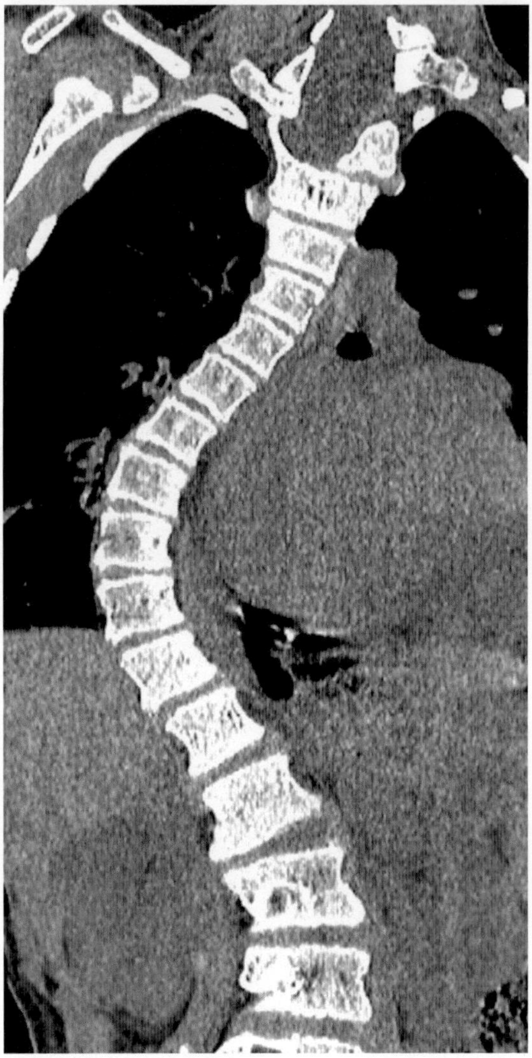

Fig. 3.5 Example of an AP CT scan in a scoliosis patient (Reprinted with permission from Ha et al. [53])

3.4.5 EMG

EMG may be helpful in identifying sources for radicular pain patterns and guide indications for surgery. EMG is defined as muscular electrical activity recording and forms a valuable aid in the neuromuscular function assessment. EMG and nerve conduction studies are routinely used to differentiate radiculopathy from peripheral symptoms and confirm the localization of radicular compression. Patients who present with abnormal EMG and signs of radiculopathy may be eligible for surgical decompression if focal pathology is confirmed on imaging.

Biomechanical studies have demonstrated that the spine itself cannot bear large loads and therefore recruits the paraspinal musculature to maintain shape [29]. In ASD evaluation, abnormal EMG recordings in one study were shown to be predictive relative to progression of deformity, as asymmetry in paraspinal EMG activity at the lower end vertebra of the curve was associated with deformity progression [30].

3.5 Operative Indications

The foremost indication for surgical ASD treatment is the lack of response to nonsurgical pain and disability management. Nonsurgical treatments include bracing, pain medication, exercise, and physical therapy. If these conservative treatments fail to provide satisfactory outcomes, ASD surgery may be indicated.

To determine whether or not a patient will likely benefit from surgical treatment for ASD, Schwab et al. describe a binary logistic regression method to build predictive models of certain independent variables including gender, age group, BMI, subluxation degree, osteotomy, and sagittal balance, among others [13]. The minimal clinically important difference (MCID) was determined by several widespread pain and appearance surveys. Patients most likely to benefit significantly from surgery had higher grades of deformity by the classification modifiers, more severe subluxation, and worse pain and disability scores. From a clinical perspective, patients with less morbidity before surgery have lower improvement potential in terms of disability and may be more affected by the difficulties associated with recovery than the clinical improvement realized by surgical correction of ASD.

A comparison study of matched pairs of operative and nonoperative ASD treatment by Glassman et al. demonstrated that nonsurgical patients have greater preoperative risk factors, while surgical patients have larger coronal curves and more frequent leg pain and more severe back pain [31]. Surgery is indicated in younger adult patients with large curvature of the spine accompanied by chronic pain or disability that is unrelieved by conservative management. Surgical correction may also be indicated when deformity is aesthetically unacceptable to the patient. Surgery is indicated in the elderly for the same reasons but is also indicated for significant loss of pulmonary function not attributable to underlying pulmonary disease [32].

The risks and potential benefits of any planned surgery must be carefully weighed and reviewed in open discussion with patients. The goal of ASD surgery is often not to completely restore function or remove all deformity and pain, but to offer improved alignment, halt progression, and provide stability to address the main components of deformity – disability and pain. The patient's expectations regarding the surgery must be clearly established and managed, as unrealistic patient expectations lead to dissatisfaction with the end result.

It is important to underline the capabilities of any given surgeon and medical team in performing corrective surgery. For example, in a given case, a transforaminal lumbar interbody fusion (TLIF) may be the preferred technique compared to a combined anterior/posterior interbody fusion because it is associated with shorter operating time, less blood loss, shorter hospital stay, and lower incidence of complications including infection and pseudoarthrosis [33]. However, a TLIF should not be attempted by a surgeon without experience in this technique if he/she is more experienced with anterior/posterior interbody fusion.

3.6 Benefits of Surgical Treatment

The surgical treatment of ASD has become an extensively studied topic and the potential benefits of surgery have been widely established. Surgical treatment of ASD has been found to significantly improve spinal alignment and improve factors associated with QOL. ASD patients treated surgically report a greater reduction of total pain, leg pain, and fatigue and significant improvements in self-image and daily function in comparison to ASD patients treated nonoperatively [34–39]. The benefits associated with surgery should be considered by patients and physicians in the decision to choose surgical treatment.

Reduction of pain and disability: The surgical treatment of ASD can significantly reduce pain associated with spinal deformities. In a study of surgical versus nonsurgical treatment of adults with idiopathic scoliosis, surgically treated patients reported a significantly greater decrease in back pain, leg pain, fatigue, and disability than patients who were treated nonsurgically [34, 36, 39]. The management of pain and disability is a critical factor to consider in treatment decisions.

Improvement of QOL measures: Patients with ASD demonstrate greater functional limitations and greater daily analgesic use and report worse QOL measures than matched patients without ASD [2, 34, 40]. Patients should also be counseled that a major complication is more likely with revision, staged, and anterior/posterior surgery to improve understanding of risk profiles [2]. Studies have found that surgical treatment results in many benefits associated with improving the QOL of patients. Surgically treated patients experience a greater improvement in self-image and the ability to perform physical, functional, and positional tasks than nonsurgically treated patients [34, 37]. In a cohort study of patients with adult symptomatic lumbar scoliosis, operative treatment significantly improved QOL, whereas nonoperative treatment, whether observation, treatment with medications, or combining medication with injections and physical therapy techniques, did not significantly improve QOL for patients [35]. Furthermore, a retrospective review of conservative and surgical treatment of degenerative lumbar scoliosis found that patients who were treated surgically had significantly improved walking ability and QOL and experienced very few complications [38]. Though surgical treatment is often considered for the reduction of pain and disability for ASD patients, it is also imperative to consider QOL factors into the treatment decision. The changes in health-related quality of life (HRQOL) after surgical treatment of ASD can be predicted by the SRS-Schwab classification system.

In a study by Schwab et al., operatively treated patients had significantly greater disability and poorer HRQOL scores than the nonoperatively treated group. The operatively treated group also had significantly greater baseline deformity, reflected by worse scores for the SVA and PT modifiers by the SRS-Schwab classification parameters. However, at 1-year follow-up, the operatively treated patients showed significantly greater improvements than the nonoperatively treated group. These findings further support the potential for surgical treatment to improve the quality of life for adults with spinal deformity.

Improvements for elderly patients: The potential benefits of surgical treatment for ASD apply to all adults; however, a recent study has illuminated the possibility that surgical treatment provides disproportionately greater benefits to elderly patients [41]. A retrospective review of patients undergoing surgical treatment revealed that compared to younger patients, older patients were shown to have significantly greater baseline disability, greater severity of back and leg pain, and worse health status. Furthermore, elderly patients experienced significantly more complications with surgical treatment than younger patients. However, despite the greater disability and higher complication rate, elderly patients were found to have statistically indistinguishable postoperative outcomes measures of disability, health status, and back and leg pain as the younger age groups. This suggests that elderly patients may have a greater improvement in disability and pain with surgery, in comparison to younger patients. Another study demonstrated the substantial benefit of surgical treatment for patients over 65 years old with degenerative disc disease who are treated with decompression and arthrodesis [42]. Patients over 65 years old showed a greater improvement in back and leg pain scores than patients under 65 years old. Due to the increased risk of complications, surgical treatment might not always be advised for elderly patients. However, the findings that elderly individuals may have disproportionately greater benefits from surgical treatment can aid in the decision-making process for this patient population.

3.7 Risks of Surgical Treatment

Despite the proven potential benefits of surgical correction of ASD, there are many risks and complications associated with surgery. Patients who are deciding to undergo surgical treatment for ASD must balance the possible improvement from surgery with the inherent risks of the procedure.

Surgical complications: While the risk of complications would appear significantly higher for surgical treatment than it is for nonsurgical treatment, even nonoperative care can lead to functional deterioration and poor outcome. The incidence of major complications of ASD surgery has been found to be around 10 %, and the incidence of minor complications has been found to be 14–34 % [2, 3, 43]. In the elderly population, complication rates have been found to be as high as 80 % [43]. These high complication rates should be considered for patients deciding to undergo surgical treatment for ASD.

Common complications related to ASD surgery include pulmonary, cardiac, renal, hematological, and gastrointestinal issues, as well as infections. These complications vary in severity [43, 44]. Excessive blood loss, deep wound infection, and pulmonary embolism have also been reported as frequent complications of ASD surgery [2].

Bridwell et al. examined a cohort of patients treated operatively and nonoperatively for lumbar scoliosis. HRQOL scores from patients who experienced minor complications (excessive bleeding, superficial infection, minor neurologic deficit, postoperative CSF leak, and seroma) or major complications (including cardiac arrest, spinal cord deficit, nerve root deficit, vascular or visceral injury, instrumentation failure or junctional breakdown, deep wound infection, myocardial infarction, and major neurologic and/or motor deficit) [45] improved significantly from baseline to postoperative. However, there was a trend toward a smaller incremental improvement in those patients with major complications compared to those patients with minor or no complications [35].

3.8 Risk Factors for Surgical Complications

Past medical history: In general, patients who experience major complications related to surgery have complex medical histories and comorbidities [3]. Diseases, such as osteoporosis, have been found to lead to surgical complications during ASD surgery. Osteoporosis complicates surgical treatment options given the poor bone quality of osteoporosis patients [46]. Other common medical comorbidities include hypertension, depression/anxiety, coronary artery disease, and gastroesophageal reflux disease [3]. The number of comorbidities is an independent risk factor for complications following surgery [47]. Past medical history and comorbidities should be considered when contemplating the decision to undergo surgery for the treatment of ASD.

Previous surgeries and surgical procedures: In a retrospective review of patients who were surgically treated for ASD, the majority of patients who developed major complications were undergoing revision surgery or a staged procedure [2]. Revision surgery patients had the greatest incidence of excessive blood loss and deep wound infections. Nutritional and metabolic disorders from the first intervention can limit physiologic resilience in the second procedure. For this reason, postoperative spine-related infections have been found to be correlated with staging and multiple surgical approaches [48]. In addition, the SRS morbidity and mortality database found that patients who underwent osteotomies or combined anterior/posterior approaches had significantly higher rates of complications than other surgical approaches [49]. These findings should factor into operative planning, if surgery is considered.

3.9 Minimizing Surgical Risk

Risk scoring: Risk scoring is commonly used to identify patients at risk for adverse outcomes. Risk scoring systems help identify risk factors, improve patient counseling on the risk versus benefit of surgery, and reduce perioperative complications [2]. Risk scoring approaches include the American Society of Anesthesiologists (ASA) physical status class, the Acute Physiology and Chronic Health Evaluation (APACHE), the Injury Severity Score (ISS), and the Glasgow Coma Scale (GCS) [50, 51]. These classification systems predict the risk for morbidity and mortality associated with surgery. The majority of patients that experience complications from surgical treatment of ASD are ASA grade III [3]. An improved patient-specific risk scoring system is essential in the decision to choose surgical treatment. A risk scoring system that quantifies the impact pain generators and particular surgical procedures have upon the complication risk profile must be developed [2].

Cost of surgery: In addition to physiologic complications from surgery, the high cost of surgery is a societal and health economic issue. The high cost of surgery is in part due to complication rates and resource utilization following surgical correction of ASD [3]. In order to reduce the complications and costs of surgery, improved patient selection and procedure selection must be made [52].

Conclusion

Indications for surgical treatment rely on a complex interplay between patient and physician, and the decision to proceed with surgical treatment for ASD is based on a wide array of personal, clinical, radiographic, and outcomes modeling information. The capabilities of the surgeon, medical team, and hospital are of paramount importance when deciding on a treatment plan. While radiographic imaging and classification systems have been found to be effective tools to evaluate spinal deformity, clinical symptomatology, physical examinations, and expectations are imperative for good decision making. The evaluation of pain and disability, in addition to radiographic imaging, has made predictive modeling by pathology and surgical planning possible. The SRS-Schwab classification, combined with proper technical execution, can help determine benefits and likelihood of achieving success from surgery. An improved risk scoring system to quantify patient-specific parameters and to identify the complication risks of a surgical procedure will aid in the decision for surgical treatment of ASD.

References

1. Schwab F, Dubey A, Gamez L, et al. Adult scoliosis: prevalence, SF-36, and nutritional parameters in an elderly volunteer population. Spine. 2005;30:1082–5.
2. Schwab FJ, Hawkinson N, Lafage V, et al. Risk factors for major peri-operative complications in adult spinal deformity surgery: a multi-center review of 953 consecutive patients. Eur Spine J. 2012;21(12):2603–10.
3. Lafage V, Hawkinson N, Schwab F, et al. Major complications following adult spinal deformity surgery: is there a high risk patient profile? Chicago: SRS; 2012.
4. Bess S, Boachie-Adjei O, Burton D, et al. Pain and disability determine treatment modality for older patients with adult scoliosis, while deformity guides treatment for younger patients. Spine (Phila Pa 1976). 2009;34:2186–90.
5. Benzel EC, Hoh DJ, Ghogawala Z, Schlenk R. Indications for spine fusion for axial pain. In: Benzel EC editor. Spine surgery: techniques, complication avoidance, and management. 2nd ed. 2005. Philadelphia: Saunders Elsevier.
6. Benzel EC, Lavelle WF, Bianco AJ, Kitab SA. Anatomy of nerve root compression, nerve root tethering, and spinal instability spine surgery: techniques, complication avoidance, and management. In: Benzel EC editor. Spine surgery: techniques, complication avoidance, and management. 2nd ed. 2005. Philadelphia: Saunders Elsevier.
7. Traynelis VC. Spinal arthroplasty. Neurosurg Focus. 2002;13:1–7.
8. Williams RW. Microcervical foraminotomy. A surgical alternative for intractable radicular pain. Spine (Phila Pa 1976). 1983;8:708–16.
9. de Loubresse CG, Bon T, Deburge A, Lassale B, Benoit M. Posterolateral fusion for radicular pain in isthmic spondylolisthesis. Clin Orthop Relat Res. 1996;323:194–201.
10. Benzel EC, Mazanec DJ, DeMicco RC. Management of a 45-year-old with mechanical low back pain with or without L4-5 spondylolisthesis and no neurologic findings. In: Benzel EC editor. Spine surgery: techniques, complication avoidance, and management. 2nd ed. 2005. Philadelphia: Saunders Elsevier.
11. Fairbank JCT, Pynsent PB. The Oswestry disability index. Spine. 2000;25:2940.
12. Glassman SD, Berven S, Bridwell K, Horton W, Dimar JR. Correlation of radiographic parameters and clinical symptoms in adult scoliosis. Spine (Phila Pa 1976). 2005;30:682–8.
13. Schwab FJ, Lafage V, Farcy JP, Bridwell KH, Glassman S, Shainline MR. Predicting outcome and complications in the surgical treatment of adult scoliosis. Spine. 2008;33:2243.
14. Deyo RA, Cherkin DC, Ciol MA. Adapting a clinical comorbidity index for use with ICD-9-CM administrative databases. J Clin Epidemiol. 1992;45:613–9.
15. Schwab F, Dubey A, Gamez L, et al. Adult scoliosis: prevalence, SF-36, and nutritional parameters in an elderly volunteer population. Spine (Phila Pa 1976). 2005;30:1082–5.
16. Duval-Beaupere G, Marty C, Barthel F, et al. Sagittal profile of the spine prominent part of the pelvis. Stud Health Technol Inform. 2002;88:47–64.
17. Legaye J, Duval-Beaupere G, Hecquet J, Marty C. Pelvic incidence: a fundamental pelvic parameter for three-dimensional regulation of spinal sagittal curves. Eur Spine J. 1998;7:99–103.
18. Roussouly P, Gollogly S, Berthonnaud E, Dimnet J. Classification of the normal variation in the sagittal alignment of the human lumbar spine and pelvis in the standing position. Spine (Phila Pa 1976). 2005;30:346–53.
19. Schwab F, Lafage V, Boyce R, Skalli W, Farcy JP. Gravity line analysis in adult volunteers: age-related correlation with spinal parameters, pelvic parameters, and foot position. Spine (Phila Pa 1976). 2006;31:E959–67.
20. Vialle R, Levassor N, Rillardon L, Templier A, Skalli W, Guigui P. Radiographic analysis of the sagittal alignment and balance of the spine in asymptomatic subjects. J Bone Joint Surg Am. 2005;87:260–7.
21. Lafage V, Schwab F, Patel A, Hawkinson N, Farcy JP. Pelvic tilt and truncal inclination: two key radiographic parameters in the setting of adults with spinal deformity. Spine. 2009;34:E599.
22. Lafage V, Schwab F, Skalli W, et al. Standing balance and sagittal plane spinal deformity: analysis of spinopelvic and gravity line parameters. Spine. 2008;33:1572–8.

23. Schwab F, Ungar B, Blondel B, et al. Scoliosis research society – Schwab adult spinal deformity classification: a validation study. Spine. 2012;37:1077.
24. Schwab FJ, Bess S, Blondel B, et al. Combined assessment of pelvic tilt, pelvic incidence/lumbar lordosis mismatch and sagittal vertical axis predicts disability in adult spinal deformity: a prospective analysis: PAPER# 20*. 2011, p. 65.
25. Schwab F, Patel A, Ungar B, Farcy JP, Lafage V. Adult spinal deformity – postoperative standing Imbalance: how much can you tolerate? An overview of key parameters in assessing alignment and planning corrective surgery. Spine. 2010;35:2224.
26. Horton WC, Brown CW, Bridwell KH, Glassman SD, Suk SI, Cha CW. Is there an optimal patient stance for obtaining a lateral 36" radiograph? A critical comparison of three techniques. Spine. 2005;30:427–33.
27. Haughton VM, Rogers B, Meyerand ME, Resnick DK. Measuring the axial rotation of lumbar vertebrae in vivo with MR imaging. Am J Neuroradiol. 2002;23:1110–6.
28. Blankenbaker DG, Haughton VM, Rogers BP, Meyerand ME, Fine JP. Axial rotation of the lumbar spinal motion segments correlated with concordant pain on discography: a preliminary study. Am J Roentgenol. 2006;186:795–9.
29. Lu WW, Hu Y, Luk KDK, Cheung KMC, Leong JCY. Paraspinal muscle activities of patients with scoliosis after spine fusion: an electromyographic study. Spine. 2002;27:1180–5.
30. Cheung J, Halbertsma JPK, Veldhuizen AG, et al. A preliminary study on electromyographic analysis of the paraspinal musculature in idiopathic scoliosis. Eur Spine J. 2005;14:130–7.
31. Glassman SD, Schwab FJ, Bridwell KH, Ondra SL, Berven S, Lenke LG. The selection of operative versus nonoperative treatment in patients with adult scoliosis. Spine. 2007;32:93.
32. Bradford DS, Tay BKB, Hu SS. Adult scoliosis: surgical indications, operative management, complications, and outcomes. Spine. 1999;24:2617.
33. Figueiredo N, Martins JWG, Arruda AA, et al. TLIF: transforaminal lumbar interbody fusion. Arq Neuropsiquiatr. 2004;62:815–20.
34. Dickson JH, Mirkovic S, Noble PC, Nalty T, Erwin WD. Results of operative treatment of idiopathic scoliosis in adults. J Bone Joint Surg Am. 1995;77:513.
35. Bridwell KH, Glassman S, Horton W, et al. Does treatment (nonoperative and operative) improve the two-year quality of life in patients with adult symptomatic lumbar scoliosis: a prospective multicenter evidence-based medicine study. Spine. 2009;34:2171.
36. Smith JS, Shaffrey CI, Berven S, et al. Operative versus nonoperative treatment of leg pain in adults with scoliosis: a retrospective review of a prospective multicenter database with two-year follow-up. Spine. 2009;34:1693–8.
37. Li G, Passias P, Kozanek M, et al. Adult scoliosis in patients over sixty-five years of age: outcomes of operative versus nonoperative treatment at a minimum two-year follow-up. Spine. 2009;34:2165.
38. Kluba T, Dikmenli G, Dietz K, Giehl JP, Niemeyer T. Comparison of surgical and conservative treatment for degenerative lumbar scoliosis. Arch Orthop Trauma Surg. 2009;129:1–5.
39. Smith JS, Shaffrey CI, Berven S, et al. Improvement of back pain with operative and nonoperative treatment in adults with scoliosis. Neurosurgery. 2009;65:86–94.
40. Berven S, Deviren V, Demir-Deviren S, Hu SS, Bradford DS. Studies in the modified Scoliosis Research Society Outcomes Instrument in adults: validation, reliability, and discriminatory capacity. Spine (Phila Pa 1976). 2003;28:2164–9. discussion 2169.
41. Smith JS, Shaffrey CI, Glassman SD, et al. Risk-benefit assessment of surgery for adult scoliosis: an analysis based on patient age. Spine. 2011;36:817.
42. Glassman SD, Polly DW, Bono CM, Burkus K, Dimar JR. Outcome of lumbar arthrodesis in patients sixty-five years of age or older. J Bone Joint Surg. 2009;91:783–90.
43. Carreon LY, Puno RM, DimarII JR, Glassman SD, Johnson JR. Perioperative complications of posterior lumbar decompression and arthrodesis in older adults. J Bone Joint Surg. 2003;85:2089–92.
44. Baron EM, Albert TJ. Medical complications of surgical treatment of adult spinal deformity and how to avoid them. Spine. 2006;31:S106–18.
45. Glassman SD, Berven S, Kostuik J, Dimar JR, Horton WC, Bridwell K. Nonsurgical resource utilization in adult spinal deformity. Spine. 2006;31:941–7.
46. Glassman SD, Alegre GM. Adult spinal deformity in the osteoporotic spine: options and pitfalls. Instr Course Lect. 2003;52:579–88.
47. Kalanithi PS, Patil CG, Boakye M. National complication rates and disposition after posterior lumbar fusion for acquired spondylolisthesis. Spine. 2009;34:1963.
48. Fang A, Hu SS, Endres N, Bradford DS. Risk factors for infection after spinal surgery. Spine. 2005;30:1460–5.
49. Sansur CA, Smith JS, Coe JD, et al. Scoliosis research society morbidity and mortality of adult scoliosis surgery. Spine. 2011;36:E593.
50. Baker SP, O'Neill B, Haddon Jr W, Long WB. The injury severity score: a method for describing patients with multiple injuries and evaluating emergency care. J Trauma. 1974;14:187–96.
51. Knaus WA, Wagner D, Draper E, et al.: The APACHE III prognostic system. Risk prediction of hospital mortality for critically ill hospitalized adults. Chest 1991;100:1619–36.
52. Weidenbaum M. Considerations for focused surgical intervention in the presence of adult spinal deformity. Spine. 2006;31:S139–43.
53. Ha HI, Seo JB, Lee SH, et al. Imaging of marfan syndrome: Multisystemic Manifestations. Radiographics. 2007;27(4):989–1004.

4 Sagittal Balance

Jeffrey B. Knox and Baron S. Lonner

In recent years, the importance of sagittal plane alignment in the energy-efficient functioning of the individual has been underscored. Sagittal plane malalignment is a principal cause of disability in patients with spinal deformity and other spinal pathologies. It is associated with numerous conditions including degenerative disc disease, Scheuermann's kyphosis, spondylolisthesis, posttraumatic kyphosis, ankylosing spondylitis, and iatrogenic flatback deformity. Regardless of surgical technique, whether traditional or MIS, restoration or maintenance of sagittal alignment is paramount to achieving optimal functional outcomes.

While the majority of conditions affect alignment of a limited segment of the spine, local changes may be accompanied by compensatory changes at distant segments of the spine. With inadequate compensatory mechanisms or with large deformities, global sagittal imbalance may arise with many resulting negative consequences. The compensatory changes, themselves, may cause unwanted consequences, which should be taken into consideration in evaluating and treating patients with spinal disease. In order to properly understand sagittal malalignment, it is important to first understand the normal sagittal curvature of the spine.

J.B. Knox, MD • B.S. Lonner, MD (✉)
New York University Hospital for Joint Diseases, New York, NY 10002, USA
e-mail: blonner@nyc.rr.com

4.1 Local Spinal Alignment

Segmental sagittal alignment has been shown to be highly variable with a wide range of normal values [1, 2]. Normal cervical alignment averages 13.9° ± 12.3° of lordosis when measured from C2 to C7 in asymptomatic individuals [3]. The lordosis is centered between C4 and C6. Cervical lordosis is impacted by thoracic kyphosis as a number of authors have shown [4]. Alignment transitions to a relatively neutral to slightly kyphotic angulation about the cervicothoracic junction with normal values ranging from 1 to 20° of kyphosis, depending on age with significantly higher values in older individuals.

Normal thoracic kyphosis ranges from 20° to up to 66° [2, 5] with the apex of the kyphosis occurring around T6–T8. Higher kyphosis values have been correlated with both older age and female gender. The thoracolumbar junction represents an area of transition. Alignment at this level becomes neutral as the spine transitions from the kyphotic thoracic to the lordotic lumbar spine

Lumbar lordosis is similarly variable with normal values ranging anywhere from 20° to 80° with apex of curvature located at the L3/L4 disc space [5, 6]. The vast majority of lordosis occurs in the lower lumbar spine with approximately 2/3 arising from L4–L5 to L5–S1. In addition to individual variability, increased age is associated with decreased lumbar lordosis, which can be a result of disc degeneration. The individual's

M.Y. Wang et al. (eds.), *Minimally Invasive Spinal Deformity Surgery*,
DOI 10.1007/978-3-7091-1407-0_4, © Springer-Verlag Wien 2014

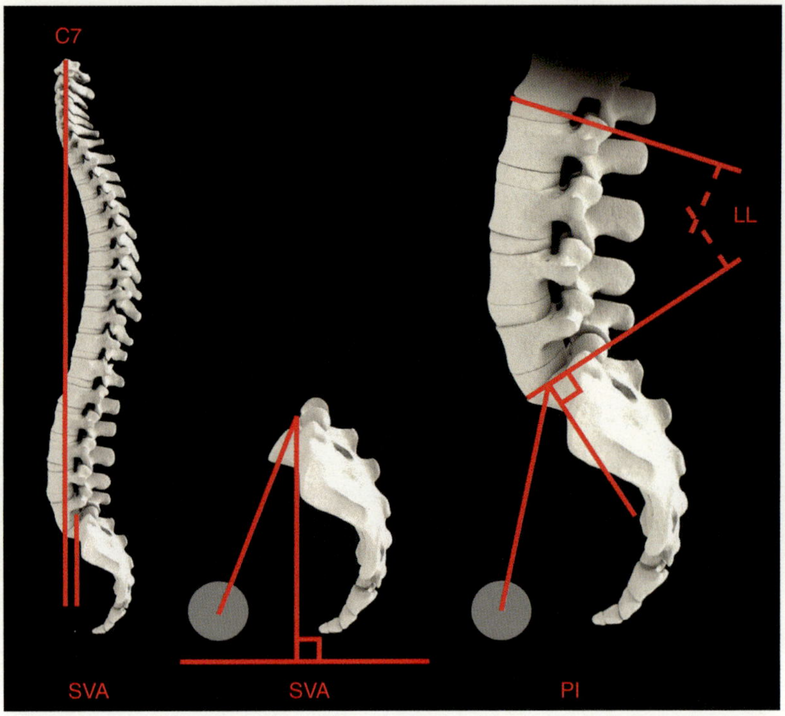

Fig. 4.1 Pelvic sagittal parameters

lordosis is determined by the innate pelvic morphology, namely, pelvic incidence [7].

Pelvic sagittal alignment represents an important component of the global sagittal alignment of the individual and is comprised of three primary parameters: pelvic incidence, pelvic tilt, and sacral slope (Fig. 4.1). Pelvic incidence represents a morphologic parameter, which reaches a fixed value by the time the patient reaches skeletal maturity. While this varies between individuals, this parameter does not change according to position or associated spinal deformity. Normal values range from 33° to 82° [2]. Pelvic incidence is the angle between a line from the center of the bicoxofemoral axis to the midpoint of the sacral endplate and a line perpendicular to the middle of the sacral endplate.

Contrary to pelvic incidence, pelvic tilt and sacral slope represent a positional parameter that varies with position and spinal deformity. Pelvic tilt is the angle between a line from the midpoint of the femoral heads to the midpoint of the sacral endplate and a vertical reference line. Sacral slope represents the angle between the sacral endplate and a horizontal reference line. These values are highly interrelated as pelvic incidence can be quantified as the summation of pelvic tilt and sacral slope (PI = PT + SS). Hence, alteration of PT or SS is associated with a proportional decrease in the other value to maintain a stable PI.

These values represent an important compensatory mechanism in spinal deformity in that patients with positive sagittal balance compensate increasing pelvic tilt in order to maintain upright posture. This mechanism relies on extension of the hip and intact and strong gluteal muscles and is an energy-inefficient process. As patients become older, their ability to compensate for spinal malalignment in the sagittal plane becomes compromised secondary to multiple factors including hip osteoarthritis, hip flexion contractures, and weak gluteal muscles (hip extensors). These factors all limit the pelvic compensatory mechanism.

As noted by Stagnara in 1982 and confirmed more recently, due to the wide variability of the so-called normal sagittal alignment, treatment is ideally tailored to the individual patient rather than creating a "one-size-fits-all" approach. The guiding principles are that the patient should be able to stand upright with minimum effort and the lumbar lordosis should closely match pelvic incidence within 10°. As such, proper attention to pelvic parameters is important to accurate understanding and planning of spinal deformity surgery and key to obtaining good results in these patients.

Sagittal pelvic alignment has also been shown to be important in spondylolisthesis. Patients with elevated pelvic incidence and its associated elevated lumbar lordosis place increased shear forces across the L5–S1 pars, thereby placing the patient at risk for development of spondylolysis. As such, a linear relationship has been shown between spondylolisthesis grade and PI. Sagittal pelvic alignment is important also in determining whether or not slip reduction is indicated. Despite the severity of slippage, normal posture is maintained if sacropelvic balance is maintained. When this becomes unbalanced with a retroverted pelvis, the patient develops forward sagittal balance and this may indicate a need for reduction [8].

4.2 Global Alignment

Numerous measurements exist to evaluate global sagittal plane alignment. The simplest and most commonly used reference point is the C7 sagittal vertical axis (C7SVA). This is drawn vertically down from the C7 vertebral body. The distance between this line and the posterosuperior corner of S1 is measured. Patients are considered to have positive sagittal balance when this line lies anterior to this point and negative when it lies posteriorly. This line normally lies 0.5 cm (±2.5 cm) from the posterosuperior corner of S1. The advantage of this measurement is that it is relatively simple and reliable and familiar to the majority of practitioners. An additional method of measuring overall balance is utilizing the T1 tilt angle. This is the angle between a line from the centroid of T1 to the center of the bicoxofemoral axis and the vertical plumb line. This measurement has the advantage of not requiring calibrated radiographs. T1 tilt angle has been shown to correlate with SVA with angles greater than 25° correlating with greater than 10 cm of positive sagittal imbalance and most importantly with patient-reported outcomes [9].

4.3 Imaging

Accurate measurement of these parameters depends on the ability to obtain high-quality radiographs. Full-length posteroanterior (PA) and lateral radiographs on 36-in. cassettes are crucial for complete radiographic evaluation of spinal alignment. Newer low-radiation biplanar radiography provides for excellent visualization with only 10 % of the radiation of conventional radiographs [10]. Visualization of the femoral heads is mandatory for calculation of pelvic parameters.

Patients should be instructed to stand with knees locked in extension to fully appreciate the sagittal plane while minimizing the effects of compensatory knee flexion. Additionally, position of the arms is key in obtaining quality radiographs. While arm flexion is required in order to properly visualize the spine, arm position also affects the apparent sagittal alignment of the spine. Such changes can be minimized using multiple techniques. One common method is to have the patient holding an IV pole or ski poles, which keeps the arms at a 45° angle with the weight of the arms supported by the poles [11]. This allows for passive elevation of the arms with minimal change in sagittal alignment. An alternative position is to have the patient hold the arms with their fists resting on the ipsilateral clavicles.

4.4 Outcomes

Sagittal plane imbalance is poorly tolerated and has dramatic implications for patients in terms of functional status and quality of life [12]. Patients with forward (indicated as +) sagittal balance must constantly exert energy to maintain a horizontal gaze and upright position. This results in markedly increased energy requirement during activities of daily living with increased oxygen consumption of up to 28 % and 60 % at 25° and 50°, respectively, of trunk flexion [13]. Part of this compensatory mechanism is knee flexion, which contributes to increased energy expenditure. Patients may complain of thigh and buttock fatigue as well as hip or knee pain in addition to their back complaints. In addition, pelvic retroversion and hyperextension of normal motion segments are utilized by the patient to maintain an erect posture and require muscular activity and energy expenditure.

What this means for the patient is a dramatic effect on quality of life and patient-reported health-related outcomes. Of the radiographic parameters, sagittal malalignment has been shown to be the most predictive factor correlated with adverse outcomes over coronal imbalance and coronal curve magnitude. This has been demonstrated via multiple indices including SF-12 physical health composite, SRS-29 pain, SRS-29 activity, SRS-29 total, and ODI questionnaires [9, 12, 14]. Such differences have been shown to be particularly pronounced past an SVA of 5 cm [9].

Another important factor is the location of sagittal deformity. While less important than overall sagittal balance, more distally based kyphosis is associated with worse prognosis. Patients with a regional kyphosis of the lumbar spine have been shown to experience significantly more pain and disability compared to those with neutral or lordotic lumbar alignment. Additionally, an elevated pelvic tilt (>25°) portends a poorer prognosis in terms of adverse health outcomes with increased pain and decreased function indicating that even well-compensated sagittal malalignment is poorly tolerated in many patients [9].

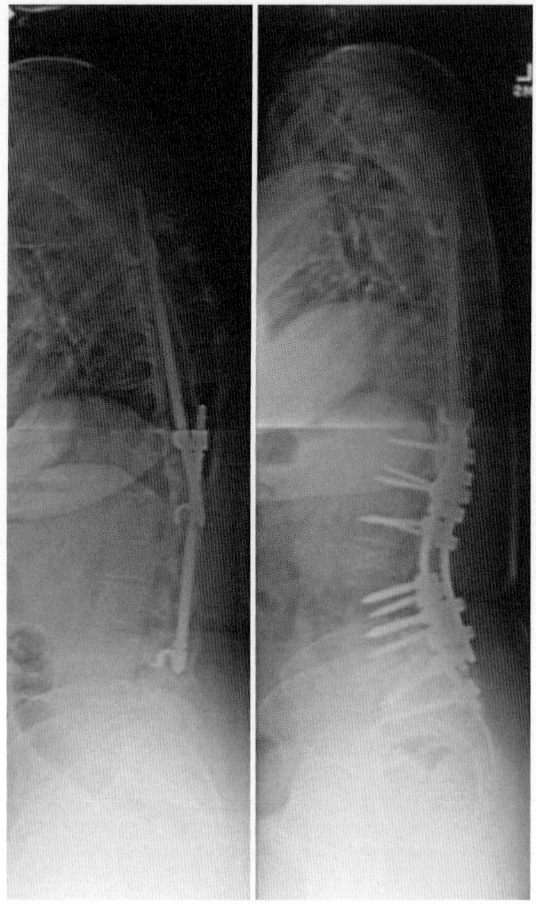

Fig. 4.2 Example of revision surgery for positive sagittal imbalance

Figure 4.2 demonstrates a representative case of a patient undergoing revision spinal fusion and instrumentation for positive sagittal imbalance. Preoperatively, the patient experienced severe disability with an ODI score of 24. However, at 4 months postop, the ODI had increased to 44 and the patient had improvement in all domains of the SRS (Table 4.1).

Table 4.1 Preoperative and postoperative SRS outcome score

	Activity	Pain	Image	Mental	Satisfaction	Mean
Preop	2.40	2	1.2	2.8	n/a	2.1
Postop	4.3	4.5	4.5	4.2	5	4.5

References

1. Stagnara P, De Mauroy JC, Dran G, et al. Reciprocal angulation of vertebral bodies in a sagittal plane: approach to references for the evaluation of kyphosis and lordosis. Spine. 1982;7(4):335–42.
2. Vialle R, Levassor N, Rillardon L, Templier A, Skalli W, Guigui P. Radiographic analysis of the sagittal alignment and balance of the spine in asymptomatic subjects. J Bone Joint Surg Am. 2005;87(2):260–7.
3. Yukawa Y, Kato F, Suda K, Yamagata M, Ueta T. Age-related changes in osseous anatomy, alignment, and range of motion of the cervical spine. Part I: Radiographic data from over 1,200 asymptomatic subjects. European Spine Journal: official publication of the European Spine Society, the European Spinal Deformity Society, and the European Section of the Cervical Spine Research Society 2012;21(8):1492–8.
4. Erkan S, Yercan HS, Okcu G, Ozalp RT. The influence of sagittal cervical profile, gender and age on the thoracic kyphosis. Acta Orthop Belg. 2010;76(5):675–80.
5. Bernhardt M, Bridwell KH. Segmental analysis of the sagittal plane alignment of the normal thoracic and lumbar spines and thoracolumbar junction. Spine. 1989;14(7):717–21.
6. Roussouly P, Pinheiro-Franco JL. Sagittal parameters of the spine: biomechanical approach. European Spine Journal: official publication of the European Spine Society, the European Spinal Deformity Society, and the European Section of the Cervical Spine Research Society. 2011;20(5):578–85.
7. Korovessis PG, Stamatakis MV, Baikousis AG. Reciprocal angulation of vertebral bodies in the sagittal plane in an asymptomatic Greek population. Spine. 1998;23(6):700–4. discussion 704–705.
8. Hresko MT, Labelle H, Roussouly P, Berthonnaud E. Classification of high-grade spondylolistheses based on pelvic version and spine balance: possible rationale for reduction. Spine. 2007;32(20):2208–13.
9. Lafage V, Schwab F, Patel A, Hawkinson N, Farcy JP. Pelvic tilt and truncal inclination: two key radiographic parameters in the setting of adults with spinal deformity. Spine. 2009;34(17):E599–606.
10. Deschenes S, Charron G, Beaudoin G, et al. Diagnostic imaging of spinal deformities: reducing patients radiation dose with a new slot-scanning X-ray imager. Spine. 2010;35(9):989–94.
11. Marks M, Stanford C, Newton P. Which lateral radiographic positioning technique provides the most reliable and functional representation of a patient's sagittal balance? Spine. 2009;34(9):949–54.
12. Glassman SD, Bridwell K, Dimar JR, Horton W, Berven S, Schwab F. The impact of positive sagittal balance in adult spinal deformity. Spine. 2005;30(18):2024–9.
13. Saha D, Gard S, Fatone S, Ondra S. The effect of trunk-flexed postures on balance and metabolic energy expenditure during standing. Spine. 2007;32(15):1605–11.
14. Glassman SD, Berven S, Bridwell K, Horton W, Dimar JR. Correlation of radiographic parameters and clinical symptoms in adult scoliosis. Spine. 2005;30(6):682–8.

Lumbopelvic Parameters

5

Manish K. Kasliwal, Justin S. Smith, Manish Singh, and Christopher I. Shaffrey

5.1 Introduction

The demographic shift toward an older population in the United States has led to an increased prevalence of adult scoliosis, with reported rates as high as 70 % among the elderly [1]. Although the disease may have a relatively benign course, some patients experience significant symptoms as a result of disc degeneration, facet arthropathy, and/or nerve root compression. Patients with symptomatic adult scoliosis typically present with pain and disability, and back pain and radiculopathy are the most common presentations [2]. Complete understanding of adult scoliosis requires assessment of lumbopelvic parameters, which have recently been shown to correlate with health-related quality of life (HRQOL) and have proven to be important in surgical planning for patients with adult spine deformity [3–6].

The spinal column performs a number of critical functions in the human body. As a structure, the spine is frequently defined by the vertebrae, discs, and surrounding soft tissues. It has been recently understood that when one considers the role of the spine in terms of balance and alignment, an isolated analysis of the spine is insufficient, and the spinal balance and alignment are intimately linked with the pelvis and lower extremities [7–14]. In fact, Dubousset considered the pelvis as a separate vertebra such that the marked importance of the pelvis is included in the analysis of the spine [15]. The pelvis, with its static morphology, serves as the base of the spine and articulates with it through the sacrum and sacroiliac joints; its morphology determines the position of the sacrum. The mobile spine adapts to the sacral position, adjusting the degree of curvature to achieve a mechanically efficient posture [16]. Since pelvic morphology is constant, or at least relatively static after adolescence for each individual, the morphology of the pelvis can be considered the foundation on which the rest of the spine derives its sagittal orientation [17]. In a normal, asymptomatic state, a balance occurs between the spine and the pelvis: spinopelvic balance. This term was first introduced by Vaz et al. [14] as a means of describing the relationship between pelvic morphology and the curvature of the spine.

Although the coronal component of adult deformity is often the most apparent and traditionally has been the target for surgical correction, it has been shown in multiple studies that sagittal balance plays a more important role in predicting the symptomatology and HRQOL in adults with scoliosis both before and after surgery [4, 6, 18, 19]. The ability to effectively maintain an upright standing posture is fundamental to normal human function, with spinal deformities often impairing the ability to maintain an upright posture. Recent studies of

M.K. Kasliwal, M.D. M.Ch. (✉)
J.S. Smith, M.D. Ph.D. • M. Singh, M.D.
C.I. Shaffrey, M.D.
University of Virginia Medical Center,
Charlottesville, VA, USA
e-mail: manish_kasliwal@rush.edu

M.Y. Wang et al. (eds.), *Minimally Invasive Spinal Deformity Surgery*,
DOI 10.1007/978-3-7091-1407-0_5, © Springer-Verlag Wien 2014

patients with spinal deformity have demonstrated that global spinal misalignment is a strong predictor of disability [4]. The concept of *cone of economy* was introduced by Dubousset to describe the fundamentals of optimal standing balance and posture, which is based on a cone, centered at the feet of a standing individual, projecting upward and outward, which defines the range of standing postures for which the body can remain balanced with minimal effort and free from external support [20]. As the body moves toward the periphery of this cone, often seen in patients with spinal deformities, additional effort and energy expenditure are necessary to maintain balance, and beyond the periphery, external support, such as a cane, crutch, or walker, may be necessary to prevent a person from falling. The substantially greater energy required to maintain an unsupported standing posture that approaches the periphery of the cone of economy or beyond can produce fatigue, pain, and disability, often seen in patients with spinal deformity [20]. Several radiographic measures have been defined for the assessment of spinal alignment, including coronal, sagittal, and pelvic measures, which if ideal should lead to maintenance of upright posture in the zone of economy, allowing for painless upright posture at rest and during motion [7]. There has been increasing recognition of the important role of the pelvis in influencing spinal alignment and parameters for evaluation of spinopelvic balance have been defined.

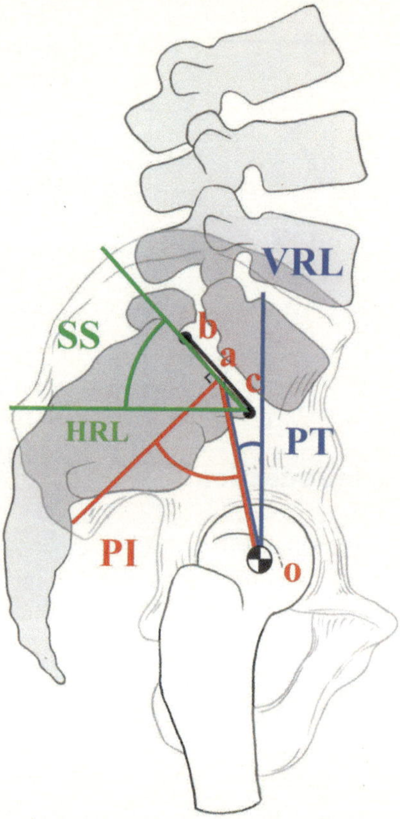

Fig. 5.1 Pelvic incidence (PI) is described as an angle subtended by a line which is drawn from the *center* of the femoral heads to the midpoint of the sacral endplate and a line perpendicular to the *center* of the sacral endplate. The sacral slope is the angle between the superior sacral endplate and a horizontal reference line, and the pelvic tilt is the angle between the line connecting the midpoint of the superior sacral plate to the center axis of the femoral heads and a vertical reference line. PI is the sum of the sacral slope (SS) and the pelvic tilt (PT). SS and PT vary based on pelvic position, while PI is a fixed parameter (Image reproduced with permission from Medtronic. Radiographic Measurement Manual. Memphis, TN: Medtronic Sofamor Danek; 2004)

5.2 Pelvic Incidence

Pelvic incidence (PI) is defined as the angle subtended by a line drawn between the center of the femoral head and the sacral endplate and a line drawn perpendicular to the center of the sacral endplate (Fig. 5.1) [21]. Pelvic incidence is a morphological parameter that remains consistent during a patient's lifetime, with slight changes occurring during prepubertal development [17]. Following puberty, PI is generally considered to be a fixed morphological parameter, reflecting the relationship of the sacrum to the pelvis [17]. Although the PI is fixed, it regulates and attempts to maintain sagittal balance primarily with changes of lumbar lordosis (LL). Recently, Schwab et al. reported on the role of PI in determining the degree of LL and supported a formula, based on the work of Duval-Beaupère and colleagues, in which lumbar lordosis (LL) = PI + 9° (± 9°) [13, 22].

5.3 Pelvic Tilt

Pelvic tilt (PT) is defined as the angle subtended by a line drawn from the midpoint of the sacral endplate to the center of the bicoxofemoral axis and a vertical plumb line extended from the bicoxofemoral axis (Fig. 5.1) [6]. When the spine tilts forward (age-related change, sagittal imbalance, loss of lordosis, increase of kyphosis), one way to maintain the spinopelvic alignment is to retrovert the pelvis with increase in PT to maintain an economic posture and to keep the spine as vertical as possible. In a review of 125 cases involving adults with spinal deformity by Schwab et al, there was a significant correlation between HRQOL measures and PT [13]. A high PT is indicative of pelvic retroversion in an attempt to compensate for sagittal-plane deformity, and it compensates for decreased LL (Fig. 5.2) [13]. While PT is an important parameter and does correlate with HRQOL, it should also be remembered that PT is a posture-dependent measurement [6, 13]. Correction of deformity by performing an osteotomy without accounting for an increased PT has the potential to result in incomplete correction of positive sagittal imbalance and persistent clinical symptoms of sagittal imbalance [7]. Pelvic realignment should attempt to obtain a postoperative PT<20° [19]. PT realignment restores appropriate femoral-pelvic-spinal alignment required during efficient ambulation. This parameter independently has been shown to correlate to impairment in walking tolerance; therefore, it should be considered in surgical planning [6, 13, 15].

5.4 Sacral Slope

Sacral slope (SS) is defined as the angle subtended by a line drawn along the endplate of the sacrum and a horizontal reference line extended from the posterior superior corner of S1 (Fig. 5.1) [23]. A mathematical relationship exists such that PI is the sum of PT and SS (PI = PT + SS) [5–7, 19, 23]. As PT increases, the SS decreases because the sacrum assumes a more vertical position about the femoral head axis (pelvic retroversion) [6].

5.5 Lumbar Lordosis

Lumbar lordosis (LL) is measured from the superior endplate of L1 to the superior endplate of S1 and plays an important role in maintenance of

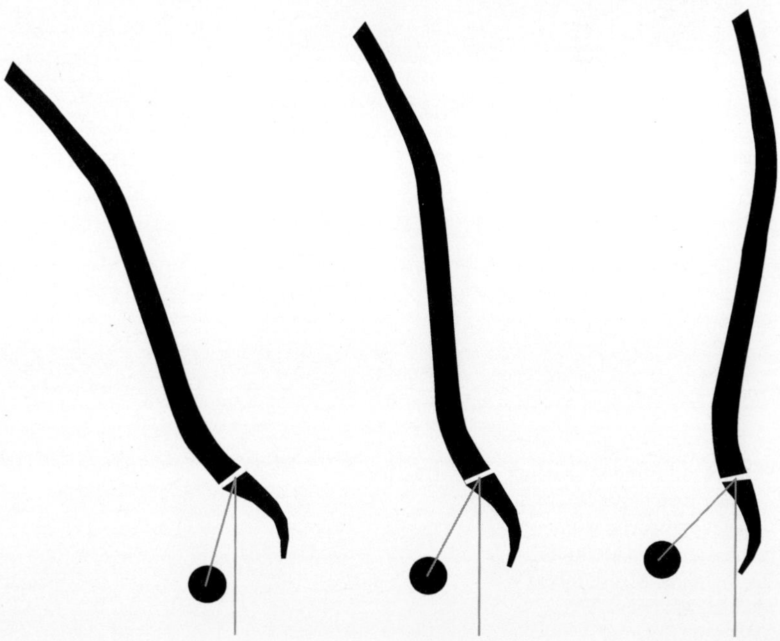

Fig. 5.2 Schematic diagram demonstrating for a given structural deformity, how pelvic retroversion compensates for spinal deformity. *Left*, no pelvic retroversion and high sagittal vertical axis (SVA). *Middle*, moderate pelvic retroversion and SVA. *Right*, high pelvic retroversion and no SVA

upright posture (Fig. 5.3) [13]. Loss of lumbar lordosis or flat back syndrome has been associated with clinical symptoms of back pain and inability to maintain upright posture [24]. Normal values of LL have been described for the adult population and typically range from 40° to 60°. However, the role of pelvis cannot be underestimated in influencing the LL, since every individual has an LL which is dependent on the PI [11, 17, 23, 25]. A study by Duval-Beaupère and colleagues demonstrated that there is a relationship between the LL and PI and that relationship must be maintained in order to optimize the spinopelvic balance [22]. A larger-than-normal PI needs to be balanced with a larger-than-normal SS and LL. Although the spine can be balanced even with a lower LL as compared to PI, the PT is often elevated in that case and signifies a sign of sagittal imbalance, highlighting the complex role the pelvis can play in determining the overall spinal balance [10].

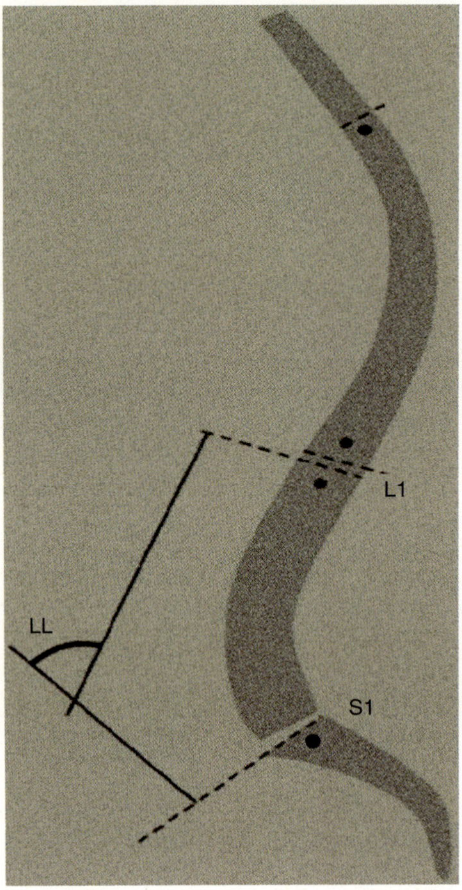

Fig. 5.3 Sagittal spinal parameters. Lumbar lordosis (LL) measured from the superior endplate of L1 to the superior endplate of S1

5.6 Pelvic Obliquity

Pelvic obliquity is a coronal plane parameter which often plays a crucial role in surgical planning. Pelvic obliquity is estimated by measuring the angle formed between a horizontal reference line and a line drawn between the 2 inferior points of the sacral ala on an anteroposterior radiograph (Fig. 5.4) [7]. Pelvic obliquity can be a result of leg length discrepancy from congenital or acquired conditions or from sacropelvic deformity, either of which may produce a compensatory lumbar curve to balance the spine. Correction of this lumbar curve without correction of the

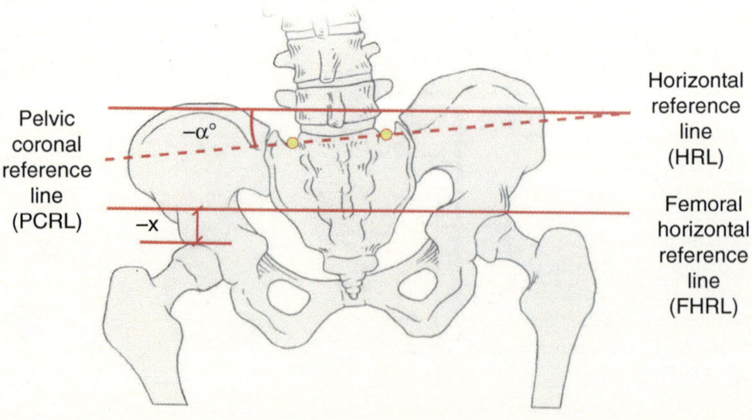

Fig. 5.4 Illustration showing measurement of pelvic obliquity (Image reproduced with permission from Medtronic. Radiographic Measurement Manual. Memphis, TN: Medtronic Sofamor Danek; 2004)

underlying pelvic obliquity may lead to coronal decompensation. Similarly, pelvic obliquity can be secondary (e.g., resulting from attempts to compensate for a spinal scoliotic curve), and in these cases, the curve correction strategies must be of sufficient magnitude to allow the pelvis to relax in the coronal plane following surgery. All patients should be evaluated clinically and radiographically for a leg length discrepancy, and if one is identified, the patient should be reevaluated both clinically and radiographically after fitting with a shoe lift to assess how the spine and pelvis respond to correction of the discrepancy. Patients with a flexible curve due to pelvic obliquity as a result of a leg length discrepancy may respond well to the addition of a shoe lift only or surgical treatment of the leg length discrepancy. If the spinal curve is rigid, it will not correct after the addition of a shoe lift, and surgical planning should take this into account.

5.7 The Spinopelvic Relationship and Pelvic Translation

Initially, treatment of scoliosis commonly remained restricted to correction of LL and thoracic kyphosis (TK). Recently, several studies have underscored the importance of pelvic morphology in the standing balance in normal adults and children, particularly through effect on LL [8, 9, 11, 12, 26]. It has been suggested that parameters across adjacent zones of the spinopelvic axis (pelvis/lumbar spine; lumbar spine/thoracic spine) are interdependent. These relationships result in the sagittal balance of an individual and the use of compensatory mechanisms. It has been shown that the center of mass of the standing person should be balanced within a narrow relationship to the feet for all subjects (adult patients with spinal deformity and asymptomatic adult subjects) as described by Dubousset's cone of economy concept [20]. In order to maintain the gravity line, it is evident that spinal deformity will lead to recruitment of balancing mechanisms [12]. One of the ways to measure this is to analyze the PT which indirectly measures the pelvic location regarding the heel line and increases when the sagittal vertical axis (SVA) increases to shift the pelvis posteriorly to maintain the overall balance [6]. These findings confirm the critical role of the pelvis in maintaining balance of the spinopelvic axis.

5.8 Clinical Relevance

It has been shown recently in a number of studies that proper sagittal alignment is the single most important factor affecting outcome for adults undergoing spinal deformity surgery [4, 19, 27]. Patients with spinal deformity with a positive sagittal alignment and inadequate LL have worse physical and social function, self-image, and pain scores [4]. While clinically effective, one of the shortcomings of the sagittal balance concept is that it does not address how balance should be achieved. This is where the concept of spinopelvic balance impacts adult spinal deformity surgery. Spinopelvic balance is based on the concept that there exists a normal, harmonious relationship between the pelvis and the spine [7–9, 11, 12, 26]. Restoring this relationship during adult spinal deformity correction may play an important role in determining the surgical outcomes of these patients, independent of sagittal balance. The results of a large study by Lafage et al. demonstrated that pelvic position, measured by PT, correlated with HRQOL measures in adult patients with spinal deformity [6]. Additionally, the abnormally high values for PT reflect pelvic retroversion, which is a compensatory mechanism for sagittal imbalance. This may affect the surgical decision on osteotomy type and location, as well as how and where correction is achieved along different segments of the spine [7]. Spinopelvic balance should be differentiated from sagittal balance; the latter describes the overall sagittal-plane relationship between spine and the pelvis, while the former describes how the components of the sagittal plane, the regional curves, affect and relate to each other. Vaz et al., [14] noted that the PI remains constant, while LL, TK, SS, PT, and knee position all vary. PI, which is constant in each individual, dictates the position of the sacrum, which is balanced by the degree of LL, which then impacts the amount of TK. Recently, a new classification system has been developed for adult deformity, the SRS-Schwab classification, which incorporates spinal and pelvic parameters with very high interobserver and intraobserver reliability and might be useful for classifying this group of patients [28].

Studies have demonstrated that patients who developed flat back or sagittal decompensation after spinal fusion tended to have a high PI and that decompensated patients had less LL in relation to PI. Gottfried et al. [29] reported a spinopelvic profile in patients who developed fixed sagittal imbalance after spine fusion, which consisted of a high PI and an extremely elevated PT and reduced LL and TK due to compensation for fixed sagittal imbalance with reduced TK and increased pelvic retroversion. This again highlights the importance of identifying abnormal sagittal spinopelvic parameters before surgery and appreciating that patients with elevated PI require more LL and that presence of high PT after surgery often indicates inadequate correction of sagittal spinal alignment. [6, 13, 18, 19, 21]

Conclusions

To conclude, the pelvis plays a critical role in balanced upright sitting and standing postures. Apart from the traditional measures such as SVA, LL, TK, and regional scoliotic curves, evaluation of pelvic parameters is paramount to develop a surgical strategy that maximizes the chances of optimal surgical outcome. When planning spinal reconstructive procedures, it is important to consider that preoperative planning formulas that do not evaluate pelvic parameters especially PI and PT may be inaccurate and increase the risk for postoperative misalignment. [30] Normalization of PT requires more angular correction than predicted by the formula of Ondra et al. [31] Pelvic obliquity and the associated etiology should also be taken into account as the etiology of pelvic obliquity and whether it is primary or is compensatory significantly affect the overall surgical planning. A number of studies have examined the relationship between position of the pelvis and alignment of the spine. It is important to understand this relationship in healthy subjects such that proper diagnostic evaluation and optimal treatment approaches for spinal deformity can be pursued. Poor integration of the spinopelvic relationship can lead to suboptimal outcome and iatrogenic pathology such as flat back and kyphotic decompensation syndromes, also termed "fixed sagittal imbalance."

References

1. Schwab F, Dubey A, Pagala M, Gamez L, Farcy JP. Adult scoliosis: a health assessment analysis by SF-36. Spine. 2003;28:602–6.
2. Smith JS, Fu KM, Urban P, Shaffrey CI. Neurological symptoms and deficits in adults with scoliosis who present to a surgical clinic: incidence and association with the choice of operative versus nonoperative management. J Neurosurg Spine. 2008;9:326–31.
3. Bridwell KH, Glassman S, Horton W, et al. Does treatment (nonoperative and operative) improve the two-year quality of life in patients with adult symptomatic lumbar scoliosis: a prospective multicenter evidence-based medicine study. Spine. 2009;34:2171–8.
4. Glassman SD, Bridwell K, Dimar JR, Horton W, Berven S, Schwab F. The impact of positive sagittal balance in adult spinal deformity. Spine. 2005;30:2024–9.
5. Lafage V, Bharucha NJ, Schwab F, et al. Multicenter validation of a formula predicting postoperative spinopelvic alignment. J Neurosurg Spine. 2012;16:15–21.
6. Lafage V, Schwab F, Patel A, Hawkinson N, Farcy JP. Pelvic tilt and truncal inclination: two key radiographic parameters in the setting of adults with spinal deformity. Spine. 2009;34:E599–606.
7. Ames CP, Smith JS, Scheer JK, et al. Impact of spinopelvic alignment on decision making in deformity surgery in adults: a review. J Neurosurg Spine. 2012; 16:547–64.
8. Labelle H, Roussouly P, Berthonnaud E, Dimnet J, O'Brien M. The importance of spino-pelvic balance in L5-s1 developmental spondylolisthesis: a review of pertinent radiologic measurements. Spine. 2005;30: S27–34.
9. Legaye J, Duval-Beaupère G. Sagittal plane alignment of the spine and gravity: a radiological and clinical evaluation. Acta Orthop Belg. 2005;71:213–20.
10. Neal CJ, McClendon J, Halpin R, Acosta FL, Koski T, Ondra SL. Predicting ideal spinopelvic balance in adult spinal deformity. J Neurosurg Spine. 2011;15:82–91.
11. Roussouly P, Gollogly S, Berthonnaud E, Dimnet J. Classification of the normal variation in the sagittal alignment of the human lumbar spine and pelvis in the standing position. Spine. 2005;30:346–53.
12. Schwab F, Lafage V, Boyce R, Skalli W, Farcy JP. Gravity line analysis in adult volunteers: age-related correlation with spinal parameters, pelvic parameters, and foot position. Spine. 2006;31:E959–67.

13. Schwab F, Lafage V, Patel A, Farcy JP. Sagittal plane considerations and the pelvis in the adult patient. Spine. 2009;34:1828–33.
14. Vaz G, Roussouly P, Berthonnaud E, Dimnet J. Sagittal morphology and equilibrium of pelvis and spine. Eur Spine J Off Publ Eur Spine Soc Eur Spinal Deform Soc Eur Sect Cerv Spine Res Soc. 2002;11:80–7.
15. Skalli W, Zeller RD, Miladi L, et al. Importance of pelvic compensation in posture and motion after posterior spinal fusion using CD instrumentation for idiopathic scoliosis. Spine. 2006;31:E359–66.
16. Labelle H, Roussouly P, Berthonnaud E, et al. Spondylolisthesis, pelvic incidence, and spinopelvic balance: a correlation study. Spine. 2004;29:2049–54.
17. Mac-Thiong JM, Berthonnaud E, Dimar 2nd JR, Betz RR, Labelle H. Sagittal alignment of the spine and pelvis during growth. Spine. 2004;29:1642–7.
18. Schwab FJ, Patel A, Shaffrey CI, et al. Sagittal realignment failures following pedicle subtraction osteotomy surgery: are we doing enough?: clinical article. J Neurosurg Spine. 2012;16:539–46.
19. Schwab F, Patel A, Ungar B, Farcy JP, Lafage V. Adult spinal deformity-postoperative standing imbalance: how much can you tolerate? An overview of key parameters in assessing alignment and planning corrective surgery. Spine. 2010;35:2224–31.
20. Dubousset J. Three-dimensional analysis of the scoliotic deformity. In: Weinstein SL, editor. The pediatric spine: principles and practice. New York: Raven; 1994. p. 479–96.
21. Legaye J, Duval-Beaupère G, Hecquet J, Marty C. Pelvic incidence: a fundamental pelvic parameter for three-dimensional regulation of spinal sagittal curves. Eur Spine J Off Publ Eur Spine Soc Eur Spinal Deform Soc Eur Sect Cerv Spine Res Soc. 1998;7:99–103.
22. Boulay C, Tardieu C, Hecquet J, et al. Sagittal alignment of spine and pelvis regulated by pelvic incidence: standard values and prediction of lordosis. Eur Spine J Off Publ Eur Spine Soc Eur Spinal Deform Soc Eur Sect Cerv Spine Res Soc. 2006;15:415–22.
23. Berthonnaud E, Dimnet J, Roussouly P, Labelle H. Analysis of the sagittal balance of the spine and pelvis using shape and orientation parameters. J Spinal Disord Tech. 2005;18:40–7.
24. Lu DC, Chou D. Flatback syndrome. Neurosurg Clin N Am. 2007;18:289–94.
25. Mac-Thiong JM, Labelle H, Berthonnaud E, Betz RR, Roussouly P. Sagittal spinopelvic balance in normal children and adolescents. Eur Spine J Off Publ Eur Spine Soc Eur Spinal Deform Soc Eur Sect Cerv Spine Res Soc. 2007;16:227–34.
26. Benner B, Ehni G. Degenerative lumbar scoliosis. Spine. 1979;4:548–52.
27. Glassman SD, Carreon L, Dimar JR. Outcome of lumbar arthrodesis in patients sixty-five years of age or older. Surgical technique. J Bone Jt Surg Am Vol 2010;92 Suppl 1 Pt 1:77–84.
28. Schwab F, Ungar B, Blondel B, et al. Scoliosis research society-Schwab adult spinal deformity classification: a validation study. Spine. 2012;37:1077–82.
29. Gottfried ON, Daubs MD, Patel AA, Dailey AT, Brodke DS. Spinopelvic parameters in postfusion flatback deformity patients. Spine J Off J North Am Spine Society. 2009;9:639–47.
30. Smith JS, Bess S, Shaffrey CI, Burton DC, Hart RA, Hostin R, Klineberg E, International Spine Study Group. Dynamic changes of the pelvis and spine are key to predicting postoperative sagittal alignment following pedicle subtraction osteotomy: a critical analysis of preoperative planning techniques. Spine. 2012;37:845–53.
31. Ondra SL, Marzouk S, Koski T, Silva F, Salehi S. Mathematical calculation of pedicle subtraction osteotomy size to allow precision correction of fixed sagittal deformity. Spine. 2006;31:E973–9.

The Importance of the Fractional Curve

6

Michael Y. Wang

6.1 Introduction

The last decade has witnessed the proliferation of techniques and technologies for minimally invasive spinal surgery (MIS). Many of these methods have now been effectively applied to treat spinal deformities, with the end result being that modern MIS surgeons have had to develop an understanding of traditional deformity principles. It cannot be overstated that deformity surgeons have spent the past 70 years developing an understanding of the principal tenets and goals of surgical intervention. This level of understanding, while continually in evolution, has been the result of tireless research, with the primary goal of improving patient outcomes. Needless to say, the application of MIS techniques should be applied with these principles foremost in mind. Examples of these tenets would include achieving a successful arthrodesis, respect for neural tissues, not stopping a fusion at the apex of a curve, and restoration/maintenance of coronal and sagittal balance.

One of the areas where MIS surgery has proven less than adequate has been the management of fractional curves in adult spinal deformity surgery. Because the development of scoliosis typically occurs gradually, the "major" curve is compensated for at least in part by one or two other "minor" curves as the body attempts to maintain coronal balance. As the typical major curve lies in the mid-lumbar spine, some compensation will also occur below this major curve. This scoliosis, which typically resides at the lumbosacral junction, is called the fractional curve (Fig. 6.1). In addition, a coronal imbalance at the L5/S1 level can actually produce a compensatory major curve above it.

6.2 Biomechanics of the Fractional Curve

Surgeons treating scoliosis should pay special attention to the lumbosacral junction. In traditional open surgery, fusions will often involve the lumbosacral junction, and successful operations need not pay special attention to this area as an open exposure will allow for neural decompression, fusion, instrumentation, and segmental manipulation to correct any local deformity. For example, due to difficulties in achieving an L5–S1 fusion, many surgeons will perform an adjunct anterior lumbar interbody fusion. While this approach adds the risks and morbidity of a second surgical approach, it offers several distinct advantages: (1) The ample exposure of the disc space unencumbered by neural elements allows the surgeon to place a graft with a large surface area for fusion. (2) The ability to place this large interbody spacer or graft improves

M.Y. Wang, MD, FACS
Departments of Neurological Surgery
and Rehab Medicine, University of Miami Miller
School of Medicine, 1095 NW 14th Terrace Lois
Pope Life Center, D4-6, Miami, FL 33136, USA
e-mail: mwang2@med.miami.edu

M.Y. Wang et al. (eds.), *Minimally Invasive Spinal Deformity Surgery*,
DOI 10.1007/978-3-7091-1407-0_6, © Springer-Verlag Wien 2014

anterior load sharing, off-loading stress from the posterior fixation hardware. (3) Distraction of the disc space also opens the neural foramen, indirectly decompressing the neural elements. (4) Removal of the anterior longitudinal ligament allows for application of significant forces to distract the disc space. This affords the opportunity to add up to 15° degrees of lordosis to the spine. (5) Improving sagittal and coronal alignment at the lumbosacral junction translates into greater effects up the spinal column than an equal correction in the mid-lumbar spine. In essence, then, the addition of a L5–S1 or L4–S1 ALIF will effectively deal with any fractional curve issues. Other methods for handling the fractional curve in open surgery include PLIF or TLIF, posterior decompression, and segmental manipulation of the screws and rods to achieve deformity correction.

In a review by McPhee and Swanson, correction of the fractional curve via a staged procedure resulted in a substantial correction of scoliosis, lordosis maintenance, and high arthrodesis rates. Furthermore, these radiographic findings were correlated with a greater more improvement in function than with posterior surgery alone [1]. Given these factors, both traditional and MIS surgeons should pay special attention to the fractional curve. Preoperatively, an assessment of the fractional curve's role in compensating for the major curve, its degree of flexibility, the amount of sagittal correction needed in this area, and any local neural element compression in this area is all critical in preoperative planning. Preoperative MRI, lateral bending X-rays, and 36 in. standing films can be helpful for preoperative patient evaluation.

6.3 Neural Entrapment at the Fractional Curve

In a study by Fu et al. of 36 patients with adult scoliosis, at least one level of severe foraminal stenosis was identified in 97 % of patients, and all but one of these patients had significant radicular pain. 19 % of patients presented with multiple levels of symptomatic nerve root entrapment, 76 % had pain corresponding to areas of the most severe foraminal stenosis, and 24 % had pain corresponding to areas of moderate stenosis [2]. During the preoperative evaluation, it is critical to identify the symptomatic level(s) of nerve entrapment, if there is concomitant leg pain. Fractional curve radiculopathies will typically involve L5 or S1, thus radiating down the posterior thigh and into the dorsum or sole of the foot (Fig. 6.1). Pain that is more localized to the anterior thigh or groin is typical of mid- and upper-lumbar radiculopathy and thus associated with the major curve.

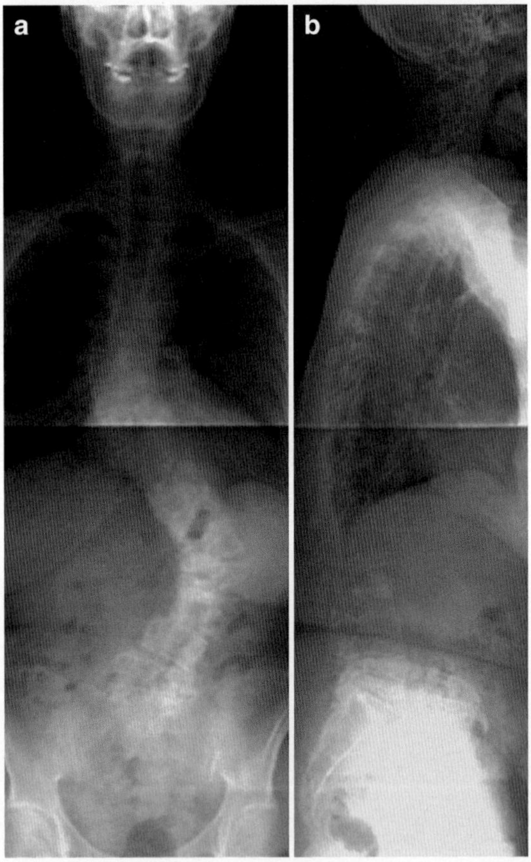

Fig. 6.1 (**a**) Typical adult degenerative scoliosis demonstrating the major curve in the mid-lumbar spine with a compensatory fractional curve at the lumbosacral junction. (**b**) Also note the loss of normal lordosis at the lumbosacral junction. (**c**) The patient's preoperative pain drawing showing symptoms of an L5 radiculopathy due to foraminal stenosis associated with the fractional curve

Fig. 6.1 (continued)

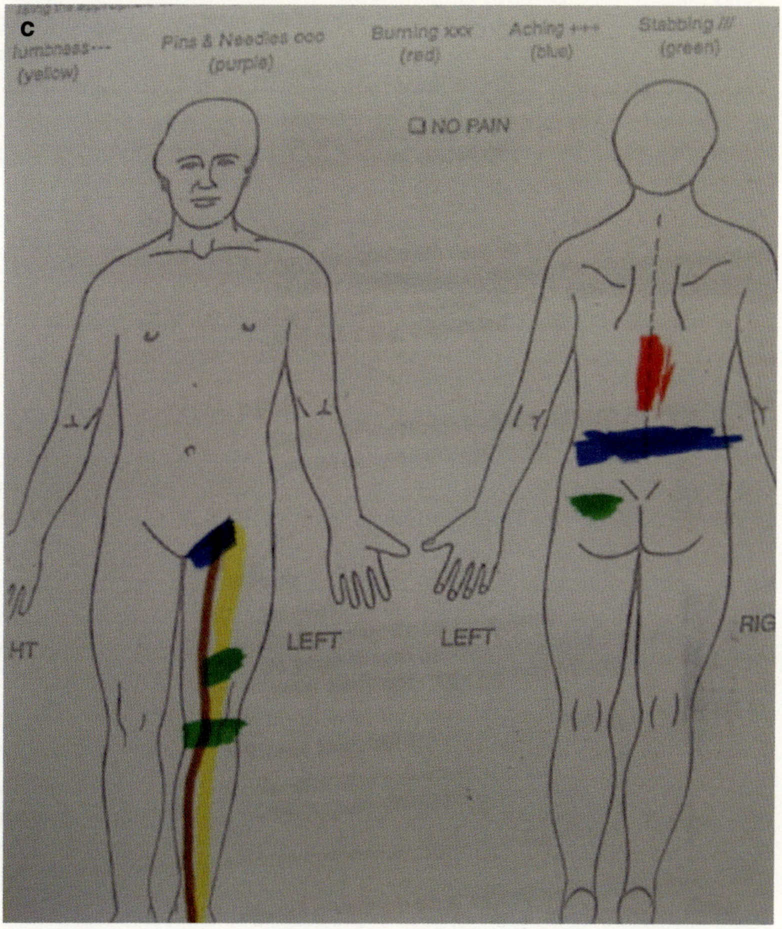

6.4 Delayed Adjacent Degeneration at the Lumbosacral Junction

Stopping a surgical construct before the lumbosacral junction is undertaken when the surgeon wishes to minimize the number of levels fused. Maintenance of motion at either L4/L5 and L5/S1 preserves a patient's ability to compensate for any over- or under-correction of deformity. This strategy requires a healthy disc at the interspace. In a study by Brown et al., six out of 16 adult scoliosis patients who had a long fusion stopping at L5 had significant adjacent segment degeneration on radiographic studies (38 %). Three of these (19 %) underwent revision surgery. Patients with good preoperative sagittal balance, preserved lumbar lordosis, good postoperative fractional curve correction, and L5–S1 disc height preservation were the most likely to benefit from stopping the fusion at L5 [3]. Patients with a preexisting fractional curve at the L5–S1 area who do not have the area fused surgically are thus at high risk for adjacent segment breakdown and the need for revision surgery.

6.5 Deficiencies with MIS Surgery

The use of MIS techniques to treat spinal deformity poses unique challenges. Some of the commonly used methods, such as trans-sacral screws or trans-psoas interbody fusion, are more easily applied at certain spinal levels. For example, the superior aspect of the iliac crest can render lateral access to the L5–S1 disc space highly problematic, without drilling through the iliac wings. Thus, surgeons employing this technique will have to either leave the lumbosacral curve untreated or employ a different route of access for deformity correction and fusion/fixation.

In addition, access to the low lumbosacral levels through the psoas muscles poses substantially more risk of a neurological complication, such as a femoral nerve injury or lumbosacral plexopathy [4]. The psoas muscle is also thicker and more prone to retraction-related injury in these areas. As such, some surgeons elect not to fuse L4–L5 through a lateral access route unless they go anterior to the psoas muscle.

Routes of access to accompany a trans-psoas approach include trans-sacral screws or MIS TLIF. Both of these approaches require prone positioning, thereby lengthening the surgical procedure and anesthetic time. In cases where prone positioning would be needed for supplemental MIS screw fixation, these may be acceptable options.

6.5.1 Curve Under-Correction

While the MIS surgeon may approach the patient with good intentions for deformity correction, under-correction of curves can be problematic. Open surgical procedures allow the surgeon to perform specific maneuvers to destabilize the spine, including facet osteotomies, placement of large interbody grafts, and removal of any posterior osteo-ligamentous structures. This allows for mobilization of the spine and later deformity correction and can be critical given the stiffness of adult deformities. Furthermore, the lumbosacral junction tends to be particularly rigid and may already be fused into an abnormal position. Open surgery also allows for application of forces more directly to the spine to manipulate it under direct visualization. For example, compression and distraction between pedicle screw heads in open surgery is more efficient as a force vector can be applied directly between the screw heads with the rod already in place. MIS techniques do not strip all the overlying soft tissues and make direct force application along the long axis of the rod problematic.

Thus, when performing MIS deformity surgery, the surgeon should realistically gauge his or her ability to destabilize and then fixate the lumbosacral junction into an acceptable alignment. Failure to do so can lead to clinical worsening, as a solid fusion/fixation can reduce the patient's ability to compensate for a fractional curve by stiffening the midlumbar spine (Figs. 6.2 and 6.3).

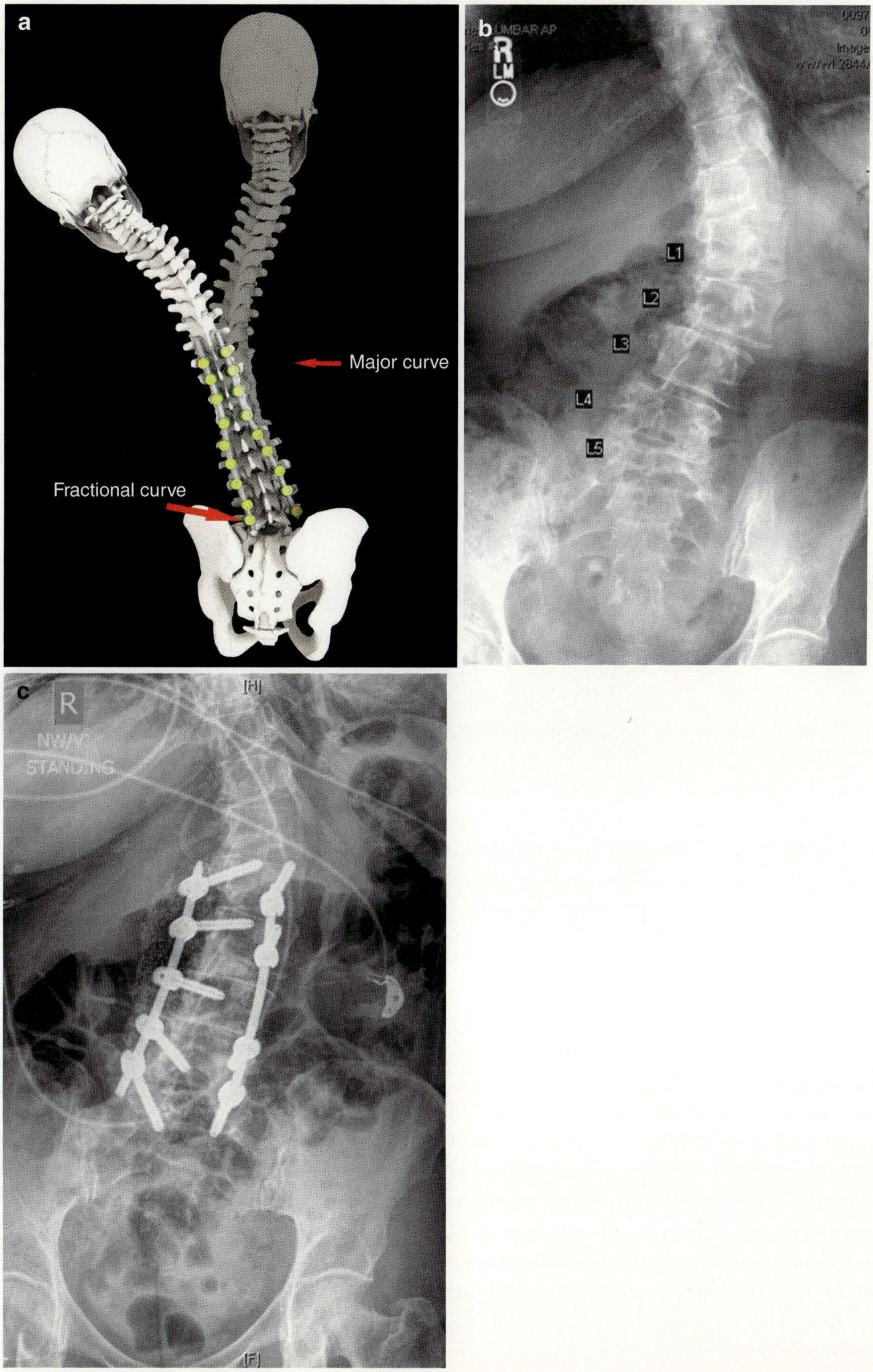

Fig. 6.2 (**a**) Consequences of correction of the *major curve* without proper attention to a fixed *fractional curve*, leading to a worsening of coronal balance after surgery. (**b** and **c**) Case example

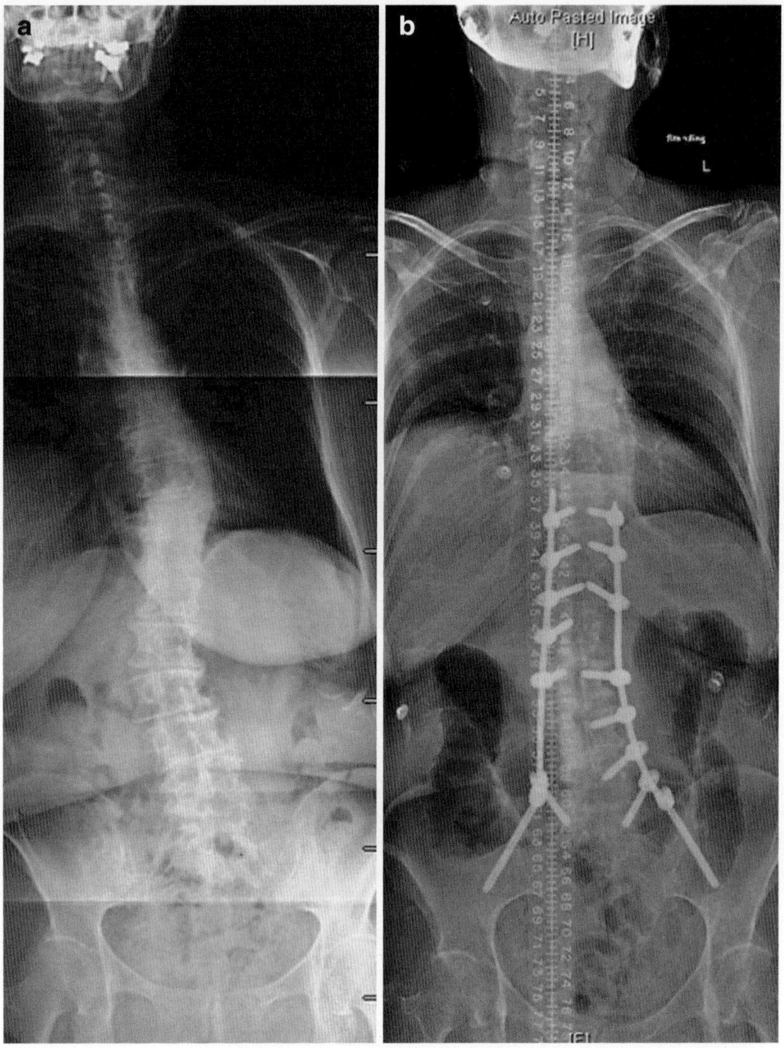

Fig. 6.3 (**a** and **b**) Proper attention paid to rigid major and fractional curves, resulting in neural decompression of the lower lumbar nerve roots, improvement of sagittal balance, and maintenance of coronal balance while correcting the scoliosis. This procedure was performed with a multilevel MIS TLIF at T11–iliac in concert with percutaneous screw-rod placement and facet fusion of the thoracolumbar area

Conclusions

The field of MIS spinal surgery is still in its infancy. In the past, minimal scientific communication between traditional open deformity surgeons and MIS surgeons has led to recognition that MIS techniques must still respect the established and validated goals of deformity surgery in general. Recognition and management of fractional curves is an example of one area where MIS deformity surgery can be deficient. Failure to recognize the limitations of MIS surgery can lead to suboptimal patient outcomes.

References

1. McPhee I, Swanson C. The surgical management of degenerative lumbar scoliosis. Posterior instrumentation alone versus two stage surgery. Bull Hosp Jt Dis. 1998;57:16–22.
2. Fu K, Rhagavan P, Shaffrey C, Chernavvsky D, Smith J. Prevalence, severity, and impact of foraminal and canal stenosis among adults with degenerative scoliosis. Neurosurg. 2011;69:1181–7.
3. Brown K, Ludwig S, Gelb D. Radiographic predictors of outcome after long fusion to L5 in adult scoliosis. J Spinal Disord. 2004;17:358–66.
4. Cahill K, Martinez J, Wang MY, Vanni S, Levi A. Motor nerve injuries following the minimally invasive lateral trans-psoas approach. J Neurosurg Spine. 2012;17:227–31.

Radiation Safety

7

D. Greg Anderson

7.1 Introduction

Radiation is a form of energy. There are **two basic types of radiation**: particulate radiation and electromagnetic radiation [1].

Particulate radiation is produced by the disintegration of an unstable atom and includes alpha and beta particles. These particles have both energy and mass [1]. Alpha particles are larger subatomic structures with two protons and two neutrons, which are capable of traveling only short distances with minimal tissue penetration. Alpha particles can, however, cause substantial biologic damage when inhaled or ingested. Beta particles are fast-moving electrons (or positrons) and are capable of traveling longer distances, penetrating deep into or through tissue [1]. Beta particles (positrons) are used in positron emission tomography (PET) scans.

The second basic type of radiation is **electromagnetic radiation (EMR),** which includes (in order of increasing energy) radio waves, microwaves, infrared waves, visible light, ultraviolet light, X-rays, and gamma rays. EMR is pure energy with no mass and has characteristics of both an electric and magnetic field. EMR is emitted by charged particles and travels in an oscillating wave with a wavelength that is inversely proportional to the energy of the wave. Electromagnetic waves contain photons, or small packets of energy, which travel (in a vacuum) at the speed of light [1].

Ionizing radiation includes forms of radiation that carry enough energy to liberate electrons from atoms, thus ionizing the atom. In the electromagnetic spectrum, wavelengths shorter than visible light are capable of ionizing atoms. Ionizing radiation can exert a major effect on human health by damaging DNA and causing genetic mutations. There are many sources of ionizing radiation in the environment including both natural and man-made sources. The average background radiation worldwide is about 3 mSv (0.3 rem) per year. Natural sources of ionizing radiation account for about 80 % of the background radiation to humans and include cosmic radiation, solar radiation, ingestion of radioactive elements, radon gas, and ground sources of radiation. Medical radiation accounts for the greatest component of man-made radiation exposure to humans and includes various diagnostic and therapeutic modalities [2].

In an occupational setting, exposure to ionizing radiation should be limited to the greatest extent possible to limit the potential health impacts of radiation exposure. Unfortunately, there is no threshold effect for ionizing radiation exposure, meaning that there is no exposure level with zero health risks below it. The sievert (Sv) is the primary unit utilized to discuss the effects of medical radiation exposure and is defined as 1 J of energy per kilogram of body tissue, averaged over the whole body. In occupational settings, radiation is generally measured in millisieverts

D.G. Anderson
Thomas Jefferson University, Philadelphia, USA
e-mail: greg.anderson@rothmaninstitute.com

M.Y. Wang et al. (eds.), *Minimally Invasive Spinal Deformity Surgery*,
DOI 10.1007/978-3-7091-1407-0_7, © Springer-Verlag Wien 2014

(mSv), or 1/1,000 Sv. The effects of ionizing radiation are reduced by the distance from the source according to the inverse square law: intensity = 1/distance [3].

Ionizing radiation has become an indispensable tool in modern medicine. Radiation is used in medicine in two primary ways: to diagnose disease or injury and to kill unwanted (generally cancerous) cells. The oldest and still most commonly used radiation modality is the plain radiograph. In this study, X-rays are passed through body tissues and collected on a photosensitive detector (film) producing an image of the tissues traversed by the X-ray beam. Less commonly performed diagnostic studies in the field of nuclear medicine involve the injection, swallowing, or inhalation of a radioisotope which emits particles which can be detected (by a gamma camera) for diagnostic purposes [2]. In general, the radioisotope chosen preferentially localizes to the specific tissues or organ where diagnostic information is required.

Due to the potential negative health impact of ionizing radiation, the Federal and State Governments impose strict controls on ionizing radiation exposure in an occupational setting [4]. The two primary bodies which oversee and provide recommendations on occupational exposure limits for radiation include the International Commission on Radiological Protection (ICRP) and The National Council on Radiation Protection (NCRP). In general, the guidelines established by these organizations have two principle objectives: (1) to prevent acute unhealthful radiation exposure and (2) to limit chronic radiation exposure to "acceptable" levels [5]. The general philosophy of occupational radiation exposure is to maintain exposure levels "**as low as reasonable achievable.**" This means that all radiation workers should make every reasonable effort to reduce radiation exposure to humans, far below the required limits whenever possible [5]. When considering diagnostic medical radiation exposure, the primary variables to consider are the following: exposure time, distance from the source, and the presence of shielding [6].

In the United States, the ICRP and NCRP recommendations include: [7–9]

1. **Occupational Exposures**
   - Annual effective dose limit: 50 mSv per year
   - Cumulative effective dose limit: 10 mSv X age (years)
2. **Equivalent Dose Limits for Specific Tissues**
   - Lens of eye: 150 mSv
   - Skin, hands, and feet: 500 mSv
   - Thyroid: 20 mSv

The primary risk from occupational radiation exposure is an increased risk of cancer, although other diseases such as cataracts and teratogenesis are also of concern. The risk depends on the amount of radiation received, the time over which the dose is received, and the body parts exposed. Although scientists assume low-level radiation exposure increases one's risk of cancer, medical studies have not demonstrated adverse health effects in individuals exposed to small chronic radiation doses (i.e., up to 10,000 mrem above background). Also, the increased risk of cancer from occupational radiation exposure is small when compared to the normal cancer rate in modern society [3].

As mentioned, there is no threshold effect, which means that there is no radiation dose with a zero risk of excess tumor formation. For instance, one study documented an increased rate of DNA translocation and certain cancers in pilots, which were exposed to radiation from flying at high altitudes [10]. Cancer risk was found to increase with more years of flight, showing the cumulative effects to radiation workers [10].

Among hospital workers, orthopedic surgeons have been shown to have as high as a fivefold increased chance of tumor formation, presumably caused by the prolonged occupational exposure to ionizing radiation [4, 11]. The most common modality to expose the spine surgeon to radiation is the C-arm used during spinal procedures. Unfortunately, spinal procedures using fluoroscopy may expose the surgeon to radiation doses 10–12 times higher than that of other nonspinal musculoskeletal procedures [12].

Patient exposure should also be considered. The relative radiation exposures of common diagnostic imaging modalities are: [9]

– Lumbar AP and lateral radiograph ⇒ 1.8 mSv
– Percutaneous insertion of 4 pedicle screws ⇒ 0.5 mSv
– Spiral CT scan of chest or abdomen ⇒ 10–20 mSv
– Cardiac ablation procedure ⇒ 10–300 mSv

As mentioned above, radiation exposure to the cornea can cause cataracts. Cataract formation is 4.6 times more frequent in radiation workers compared with nonradiation workers [13]. One study involving kyphoplasty found that radiation exposure to the eye was 0.271±0.200 mSv per vertebra when eye shields were not used [14].

Radiation scatter from the X-ray beam hitting the patient, metal retractors, and the OR table is the primary source of radiation exposure to the surgeon. The dose of radiation scatter is much higher on the side of the X-ray emitter as compared to the receiver (Fig. 7.1). To minimize the effects of radiation exposure, the following steps should be taken: [15]

1. Shielding: The surgical team should use personal protective equipment in the operating room (Fig. 7.2).
2. Distance: As dictated by the inverse square law, the exposure to radiation is inversely proportional to the square of the distance to the source. Therefore, the surgeon and other personnel should be located as far away as practical from the radiation source during fluoroscopic procedures [15]. When possible, the surgeon should work on the side of the X-ray source and not the X-ray emitter.
3. Fluoro Time: Minimize the beam-on time when using fluoroscopy. Use good coning techniques to narrow the beam and avoid magnification mode which has a higher radiation output. Use spot images, rather than continuous fluoroscopic images, whenever possible [15].

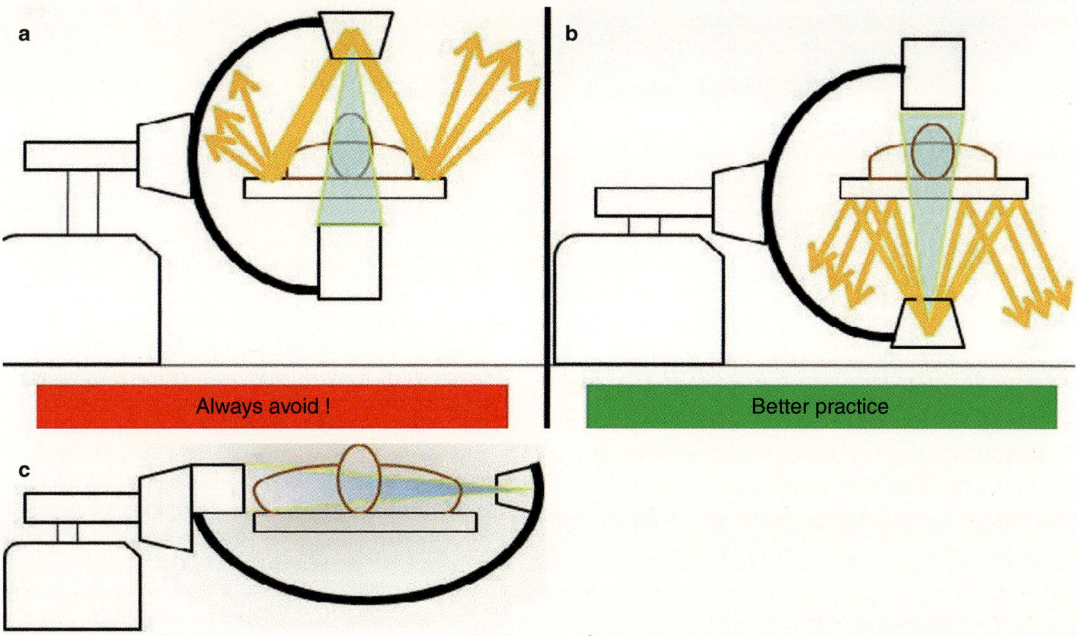

Fig. 7.1 Illustration of how the largest amount of radiation is produced by scatter near the X-ray source: (**a**) position of the X-ray tube above should be avoided; (**b**) by positioning the X-ray tube below the patient, the amount of scatter to the surgical team is reduced; (**c**) in the lateral position, the radiation scatter is less on the side of the X-ray receiver

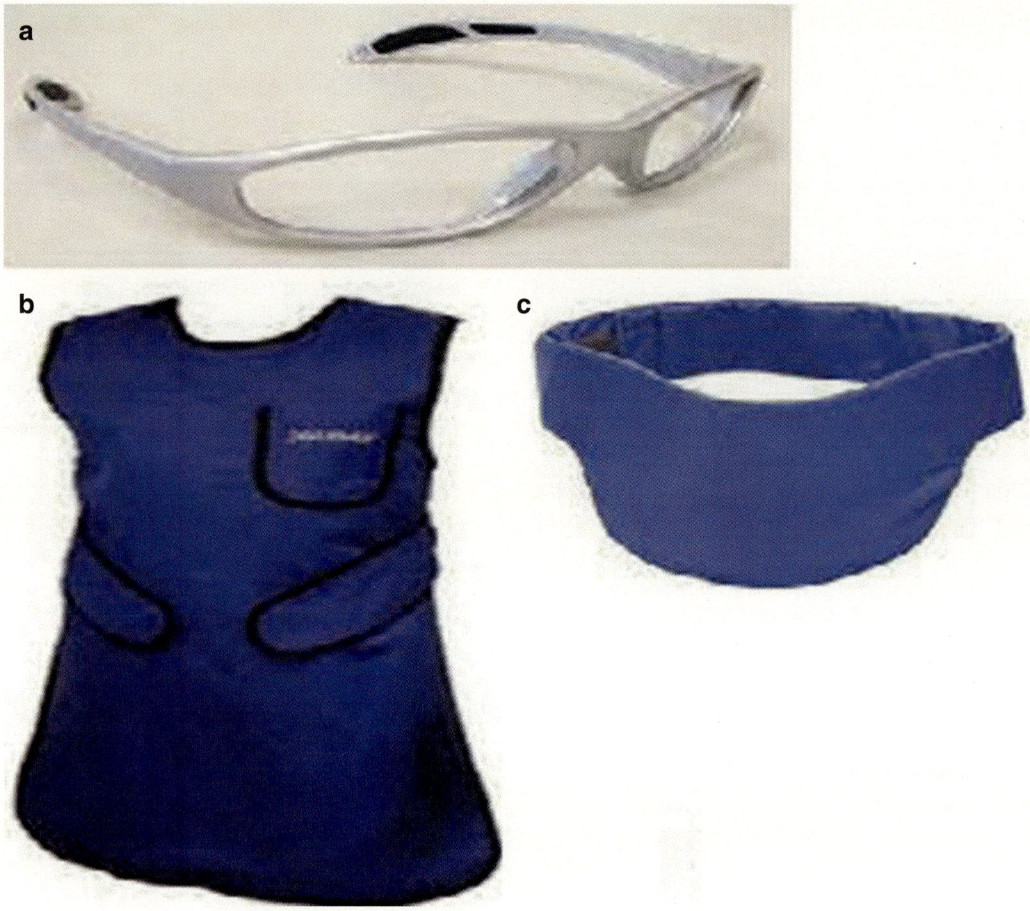

Fig. 7.2 Personal protective equipment used in operating room: (**a**) Leaded glasses (0.75 mm of lead equivalent), (**b**) leaded apron (0.5 mm of lead equivalent), (**c**) thyroid shield (0.5 mm of lead equivalent)

Conclusion

Understanding the physics of radiation and the biologic effects of radiation exposure, a surgeon can minimize the health risks to himself/herself and reduce the risks to the surgical team and patient. Proper personal protective equipment should always be utilized and specific steps should be taken to reduce fluoroscopic time and increase the distance from the radiation source when performing spinal procedures.

References

1. NDT Education Resource Center, 2001–2012, The Collaboration for NDT Education, Iowa State University. Available at www.ndt-ed.org/EducationResources/CommunityCollege/RadiationSafety/theory/nature.htm
2. Available at www.iaea.org/Publications/Booklets/Radiation/radsafe.html
3. NDT Education Resource Center, 2001–2012, The Collaboration for NDT Education, Iowa State University. Available at www.ndt-ed.org/EducationResources/CommunityCollege/RadiationSafety/introduction/backround.htm
4. ISIS Annual Meeting Radiation Safety for the Spine Interventionalist. Available at http://www3.gehealthcare.com/en/Products/Categories/Surgical_Imaging/~/media/Downloads/us/Product/Product-Categories/Surgical-Imaging/GEHealthcare-Radiation-Safety-Spine-Interventionalist-SafetyData.pdf
5. NDT Education Resource Center, 2001–2012, The Collaboration for NDT Education, Iowa State University. Available at www.ndt-ed.org/EducationResources/CommunityCollege/RadiationSafety/safe_use/exposure.htm
6. Grover SB, Kumar J. A review of the current concepts of radiation measurement and its biological effects. Indian j Radiol Imaging 12:21–32, 2002. Available at www.Ijri.org/text.asp?2002/12/1/21/28413

7. Balter S. An overview of radiation safety regulatory recommendations and requirements. Catheter Cardiovasc Interv. 1999;47:469–74.
8. Giordano BD, Baumhauer JF, Morgan TL, et al. Cervical spine imaging using standard C-arm fluoroscopy. Spine. 2008;33:1970–6.
9. Jone DP, Robertson PA, Lunt B, et al. Radiation exposure during fluoroscopically assisted pedicle screw insertion in the lumbar spine. Spine. 2000;25:1538–41.
10. Young LC, Sigurdson AJ, Ward EM, et al. Increased frequency of chromosome translocations in airline pilots with long-term flying experience. Occup Environ Med. 2009;66:56–62.
11. Mastrangelo G, Fedeli U, Fadda E. Increased cancer risk among surgeons in an orthopaedic hospital. Occup Med. 2005;55:498–500.
12. Kim CW, Lee YP, Taylor W, et al. Use of navigation-assisted fluoroscopy to decrease radiation exposure during minimally invasive spine surgery. Spine J. 2008;8:584–90.
13. Milacic S. Risk of occupational radiation-induced cataract in medical workers. Med Lav. 2009;100:178–86.
14. Mroz TE, Yamashita T, Davros WJ, et al. Radiation exposure to the surgeon and the patient during kyphoplasty. J Spinal Disord Tech. 2008;21: 96–100.
15. Radiologic science for technologists: physics, biology and protection: 4th Edition. Stewart Bushong. Available at www.gehealthcare.com/dose/media/4555/radiation_guide2__2_.pdf

8 Costs of Minimally Invasive Spine Surgery

Kevin S. Cahill

8.1 Introduction: Costs of Spinal Surgery

It is well known that the US healthcare system devotes significant resources to the evaluation and treatment of patients with spinal disorders. Back pain continues to be one of the leading causes of disability in the USA and has been reported to be the most common reason for seeking evaluation by a physician, second only to the common cold [1–4]. It is estimated that over 33 million US adults suffered from spine-related disorders in 2005 [4]. In addition, it has been shown that the average expenditure for medical care by US adults with spinal disorders is 73 % higher than adults without back and neck problems [4]. This corresponded to a national total expenditure of over 89 billion dollars in 2005 on spine-related care [4].

Given the high prevalence of spinal disorders in the US society and these associated costs, the costs and utilization of surgical procedures in the treatment of patients with spinal disorders have been under scrutiny. Although surgical costs are only one component in the complex array of healthcare resources that are consumed during the treatment and evaluation of patients with spinal disorders, they have received great interest in academia and the lay press [5]. A primary reason for this increased scrutiny has likely been the dramatic increase in utilization of surgical procedures for the treatment of spinal disorders.

There has been significant interest in the increased utilization of spinal decompression and fusion procedures in the treatment of cervical and lumbar spinal disorders over the past two decades [6–10]. It is well documented that the utilization of surgical procedures for the treatment of spinal disorders has been on the rise, although more recent evidence in Medicare patients suggests that overall surgical rates have slightly declined from 2002 to 2007 [7]. The majority of interest has been on the utilization of more costly spinal fusion procedures, with reports demonstrating a dramatic increase in spinal fusion rates over the past 15 years. For example, one report demonstrated that there has been an increase greater than 100 % in the number of fusion procedures performed for degenerative spine disease seen from 1996 to 2001 [6]. More recent data has indicated that the yearly total number of fusion procedures has stabilized since 2002, although the performance of complex surgical fusions has increased [7].

There is substantially less known about the utilization of minimally invasive techniques in spinal surgery. A variety of minimally invasive techniques have been developed for spinal procedures over the past decade. Many are now readily employed in routine spinal procedures. Details of these techniques can be found throughout the remainder of this comprehensive minimally invasive spinal surgery text. One of the first minimally invasive techniques developed for lumbar

K.S. Cahill, M.D. Ph.D. M.P.H.
Carolina Neurosurgery and Spine Associates,
Charlotte, NC, USA
e-mail: kevin.cahill@cnsa.com

M.Y. Wang et al. (eds.), *Minimally Invasive Spinal Deformity Surgery*,
DOI 10.1007/978-3-7091-1407-0_8, © Springer-Verlag Wien 2014

surgery was the muscle-splitting approach for lumbar micro-discectomy. This procedure is performed through a tubular retractor and has been described for initial as well as revision discectomy [11, 12]. More complex procedures involving minimally invasive fusion techniques have been more recently described for single-level as well as multilevel thoracolumbar pathologies [13–15].

Given the high prevalence of spinal disorders in the USA, the significant costs to the healthcare system associated with treatment of back pain, and the increasing utilization of certain surgical treatments for spinal disorders, determination of the economic value of surgical treatments for spinal disorders is of great significance to the population's health and healthcare finances. Minimally invasive surgical procedures are an example of a novel technology with a yet unknown cost profile and economic value. The evaluation of the cost profile of minimally invasive spinal procedures and the corresponding clinical outcomes has the potential to significantly improve outcomes in spinal fusion as well as help determine the most cost-effective treatments. The remainder of this chapter will provide an overview of the relevant components of a cost analysis of minimally invasive spinal surgery and summarize the available data.

8.2 Cost Analysis

There are several different categories of costs to consider when evaluating a novel surgical procedure. In general, most cost and cost-effectiveness analyses will be performed from the perspective of the society. Societal costs will consider everyone affected by the procedure and all related costs regardless of who actually is responsible for the costs [16]. When looking at a specific surgical procedure, the initial total costs associated with the procedure as well as long-term total costs must be considered. The initial costs of the surgery and initial hospitalization costs will include the costs associated with the use of the operating room, surgeon and anesthesiologist fees, surgical implant costs such as those for spinal instrumentation, and other supplies used during the procedure. General costs of operating room time and associated personnel can be estimated per given time unit to allow for estimation of the cost impact of longer procedures. Postoperative hospitalization costs can also be itemized. In addition to a standard room and board cost, there will be laboratory fees, medications, supplies, radiology fees, and other ancillary services such as physical therapy.

To get a true sense of the cost profile of the procedure, the long-term costs must be evaluated in addition to initial costs. In spine procedures, there are many relevant delayed costs that may have a significant impact on the overall cost. Repeat surgical procedures, complications, and repeat hospital admissions related to the primary procedure are important components that need to be analyzed. Furthermore, the recovery time in the postoperative period can be quantified into a cost associated with the procedure. Although this is somewhat controversial, this is typically analyzed in the form of lost productivity, and there are many ways that have been described to quantify this value [17]. In several spine surgery reports, the time to return to work has been utilized as a proxy for this productivity cost.

8.3 Decreased Costs with MIS Spine Surgery

There are many theoretical reasons why a MIS approach to spine surgery should produce specific areas of cost savings. The overall concept of less tissue disruption that is the basis for MIS surgery should translate into less surgical trauma and therefore cost savings in the postoperative period as the patient is able to be mobilized more rapidly and experiences a faster recovery. As such, the cost savings are expected to be realized in the postoperative period for MIS spine surgery.

The postoperative period following MIS spine procedures has been carefully analyzed. The largest volume of data is available for MIS lumbar micro-discectomy. In lumbar micro-discectomy, muscle-splitting approaches performed through a tubular retractor have been advocated as a minimally invasive technique and have been described for initial as well as revision discectomy [11, 12]. In this procedure, a transmuscular approach is taken to the lumbar spine. This approach is considered less invasive than the subperiosteal dissection performed in the traditional "open" micro-discectomy procedure. There have been several large studies comparing the postoperative clinical outcomes with tubular approaches compared to open micro-discectomy. In a multicenter trial of 100 randomized patients, the tubular micro-discectomy group saw a slightly faster clinical recovery but only when the procedure was performed at the more experienced clinical center [18]. This effect was predominately due to early reductions in back pain scores for the tubular group at the experienced center. A randomized, single-center trial of 125 patients demonstrated equivalent clinical results for the two approaches but a decrease in postoperative analgesic use was detected in the tubular micro-discectomy group [19]. Likewise, the analysis of a single surgeon series of 66 patients indicated that patients who underwent tubular micro-discectomy had lower immediate postoperative narcotic utilization and shorter postoperative hospitalization times [20].

Despite these improvements in postoperative recovery, substantially less has been reported on the actual impact of this MIS approach on overall costs of micro-discectomy. The largest analysis to date comparing tubular to conventional micro-discectomy was performed in the Netherlands by Arts et al. [21]. This randomized controlled trial of 328 patients demonstrated slightly less favorable outcomes for tubular micro-discectomy at 1-year postsurgery and nearly identical outcomes at 2 years [21, 22]. The cost-effectiveness analysis of this trial has also recently been released where it was concluded that tubular micro-discectomy was unlikely to be cost-effective compared to conventional techniques [23]. In this cost-effectiveness analysis, it was demonstrated that the average costs for surgery, including the initial hospital admission, were higher for tubular discectomy. However, this analysis was performed outside of the USA, so it is difficult to translate these results to practice in the USA where healthcare costs are significantly different.

For more complicated MIS procedures, such as lumbar fusion, it would be expected that the MIS approach should have even greater cost savings in the postoperative recovery period. That is, most micro-discectomies are performed in the outpatient setting and have relatively rapid postoperative recovery times. Larger fusion procedures have much more significant costs associated with postoperative hospitalization, recovery time, and complications. The ability of MIS procedures to reduce the costs of these postoperative expenses may have a substantial impact on the overall cost profile of the procedure.

There is relatively limited data on the costs associated with MIS fusion compared to open fusion procedures. Wang et al. analyzed outcomes and hospital charges following open compared to MIS lumbar interbody fusion in a series of 74 patients at the University of Miami [24]. This was a retrospective evaluation of open posterior lumbar interbody fusion (PLIF) compared to MIS trans-foraminal lumbar interbody fusion (TLIF). For single-level procedures, the average length of stay for the MIS TLIF group was approximately one day shorter than the open PLIF group (3.9 vs. 4.8 days, $p=0.01$). This report also demonstrated an average hospital charge for single-level MIS TLIF procedures of $70,159 compared to $78,444 for open PLIF procedures. The data for the two-level procedures failed to reach statistical significance. This was likely attributable to the smaller sample size of 15 patients in the two-level group.

A formal cost-effectiveness analysis has also been reported for 30 nonrandomized patients with grade 1 spondylolisthesis who underwent open versus MIS TLIF [25]. Patients were assigned to treatment groups based on surgeon preference, and costs were estimated using patient-reported resource utilization and Medicare mean total diagnosis-related surgery costs. This analysis showed a shorter length of postoperative hospitalization for the MIS TLIF group (median of 3.0 days for MIS vs. 5.0 days for open TLIF, $p=0.001$), decreased postoperative narcotic utilization, and a shorter time to return to work (8.3 weeks for MIS vs. 16.3 weeks for open, $p=0.02$). However, the overall 2-year outcomes in terms of quality adjusted life years gained and the overall cost-effectiveness ratio did not demonstrate a statistically significant difference between groups. The authors did state that the study needed twice as many patients to be powered to detect a significant difference given these results.

The cost saving associated with the use of percutaneous pedicle screws has also been directly analyzed by Wang et al. [26]. This analysis utilized a large inpatient dataset containing over 6,000 patients who underwent single- and two-level lumbar fusions. Patients were classified according to the type of pedicle screw used during the fusion procedure: cannulated versus noncannulated screws. The patients that had cannulated screws implanted were classified as having "MIS" fusions while all others as "open" fusions. The study demonstrated a significant decrease in the postoperative length of hospitalization in the MIS group. The difference was of the greatest magnitude in the patients that underwent two-level procedures (3.4 days for MIS fusion vs. 4.0 days for open fusion, $p<0.001$). Additionally, total hospital costs were analyzed for the two groups. No statistically significant difference was found for single-level MIS compared to open fusion costs. However, for two-level procedures, there was an average lower total cost in the MIS group of almost 2,000 dollars (total average cost of $33,879 for MIS compared to $35,984 for open fusions, $p=0.002$).

Finally, the cost associated with the treatment of postoperative complications is another major cost that could be decreased by MIS-based procedures. In traditional, open spinal deformity surgical fusion procedures, the complication rate has been reported to range from 10 % to as high as almost 70 % of procedures [27–29]. It is expected that certain postoperative complications such as medical complications or postoperative infections should be decreased with MIS procedures. This has been evaluated for postoperative surgical site infection rates by McGirt et al. [30]. For this analysis, a hospital discharge and billing dataset was utilized to compare the surgical site infection rate for open compared to MIS lumbar interbody fusion procedures. It was demonstrated that there was no difference in the infection rate following single-level MIS compared to open procedures. However, for two-level procedures, the infection rate decreased to 4.6 % for MIS procedures compared to 7.0 % for open fusion ($p=0.03$). This translated to a cost savings of $38,400 per 100 two-level MIS fusion procedures. This finding has also been confirmed in a literature review of 362 MIS TLIF patients compared to 1,133 open TLIF patients [31]. This review found a surgical site infection rate of 0.6 % in the MIS TLIF cohort compared to 4.0 % in open TLIF cohort ($p<0.01$).

8.4 Increased Costs with MIS Spine Surgery

On the other hand, there are many reasons why the surgical costs of minimally invasive spinal procedures should be more costly than traditional open surgery. First, minimally invasive procedures rely on specialized instruments and retractors. This equipment is essential to allow procedures to be performed through incisions that are smaller and less disruptive than traditional open techniques. For example, any type of MIS decompression procedure will mandate a specialized retractor and tissue dilator system. This usually includes sequential muscle-dilating tubes. These retractors may be disposable or have disposable components that are replaced with each procedure, such as a disposable fiber-optic light source. The costs associated with these systems are likely to be greater than a traditional surgical retractor.

A specific example of a specialized retractor is the access systems developed by several vendors for lateral approaches to the thoracolumbar spine. In these procedures, a minimally invasive, transpsoas approach is taken [32]. However, given the location of the lumbosacral plexus within the psoas muscle, specialized neuro-monitoring techniques are necessary to enable the selection of a nerve-sparing trajectory through the psoas muscle. As such, not only are tissue dilators needed, but also equipment to monitor free-running and evoked EMG during the procedure is essential. These instruments are critical to the safety of the procedure. These specialized instruments are typically disposable and have a cost associated that may not be present in cases using more traditional open techniques.

Furthermore, in addition to specialized retractors and instruments, specialized spinal implants are needed for MIS fusion procedures. A well-known example is cannulated pedicle screws used in MIS instrumented fusions. These screws are capable of being placed percutaneously and are essential to MIS fusion procedures. These cannulated implants command a premium compared to traditional pedicle screw instrumentation. Furthermore, more advanced imaging techniques are typically required for safe placement of these screws. Uniplanar or biplanar fluoroscopy as well as spinal navigation systems are often employed for the placement of these screws. The combination of the premium for the implants and the imaging systems used for safe placement typically will be more costly than those used in tradition techniques.

Recent data has demonstrated the increased implant costs for MIS procedures. A recent analysis by Lucio et al. of initial hospital cost differences between open two-level PLIF and MIS two-level lateral interbody fusion demonstrated increased implant/instrumentation costs in the MIS group [33]. This analysis looked at the initial hospital costs of over 200 patients that underwent two-level open compared to MIS lumbar fusion. The implant/instrumentation costs in the MIS group were an average of $3,810 greater than the open group ($p<0.05$). However, overall initial hospital costs were lower in the MIS group as cost savings were evident in almost all other cost categories including room and board, medications, laboratory studies, physical therapy, and decreased readmission and reoperation costs.

In addition to the need for costly, specialized instruments and instrumentation, there is an important fundamental difference in MIS spine fusion surgery that is inherently more costly. Due to the limited exposure provided by muscle-splitting approaches to the spine in MIS procedures, MIS fusions primarily rely on interbody fusion techniques as opposed to posterolateral fusions. A robust discectomy can be performed through a very small skin incision allowing for the preparation of a large fusion surface on the vertebral endplates. In contrast, posterolateral fusion techniques are not readily applicable to most MIS fusion procedures as they require more extensive muscle dissection that cannot be achieved in a muscle-splitting approach. As such, interbody fusion is utilized in the majority of MIS fusion procedures. Interbody fusion procedures usually involve structural cages or other grafts that may add a several 1,000 dollars in costs to the procedure. It was recently demonstrated in Medicare patients that "complex" fusion procedures such as 360° fusions performed through a single incision had greater hospital charges and complication rates than "simple" fusion procedures such as posterolateral fusion ($80,888 mean charge for complex fusions compared to $58,511 mean charge for simple fusion procedures, $p<0.05$) [7].

Along with a greater reliance on interbody fusion, there is likely a greater reliance on fusion adjuncts such as allograft, biologics, and bone graft extenders with MIS fusion procedures. Due to the minimal exposure in MIS procedures, there may be less autologous bone removed that is available to use as local structural or morselized autograft. For example, in a MIS lateral interbody fusion, there is typically no locally harvested autologous bone graft available during the procedure. Thus, there may be a reliance on graft extenders and other commercially available products that have higher associated costs. It has been well documented that the use of bone morphogenetic proteins is associated with significantly higher initial surgical costs for spinal fusion procedures [34]. The percentage of MIS fusion procedures that utilize BMP is not known.

Finally, the surgical time of MIS procedures must be considered in the cost profile. Operating room time is extremely valuable as significant personnel and other resources are dedicated to the patient while undergoing the procedure. If the MIS procedure requires more surgical time than the open procedure, then this will translate into significantly increased costs for the MIS procedure.

Conclusions

The rate of utilization of MIS procedures in spinal surgery is unknown. However, there has been significant interest in the development of these techniques over the past two decades, and many are considered a routine part of the modern spine surgeon's armamentarium. Furthermore, there is relatively little cost data related to these procedures. As summarized above, there are many reasons why a MIS approach should increase surgical costs. These costs need to be further explored and defined relative to open procedures. Likewise, the expected cost savings produced in the postoperative period need to be further clarified and quantified. Once these cost analyses are performed, the overall cost profile of a given MIS procedure can be determined and compared to open procedures.

References

1. Carey TS, Evans AT, Hadler NM, Lieberman G, Kalsbeek WD, Jackman AM, et al. Acute severe low back pain. A population-based study of prevalence and care-seeking. Spine. 1996;21:339–44.
2. Cypress BK. Characteristics of physician visits for back symptoms: a national perspective. Am J Public Health. 1983;73:389–95.
3. Deyo RA, Cherkin D, Conrad D, Volinn E. Cost, controversy, crisis: low back pain and the health of the public. Annu Rev Public Health. 1991;12:141–56.
4. Martin BI, Deyo RA, Mirza SK, Turner JA, Comstock BA, Hollingworth W, et al. Expenditures and health status among adults with back and neck problems. JAMA. 2008;299:656–64.
5. Lipson SJ. Spinal-fusion surgery – advances and concerns. N Engl J Med. 2004;350:643–4.
6. Deyo RA, Mirza SK. Trends and variations in the use of spine surgery. Clin Orthop Relat Res. 2006;443: 139–46.
7. Deyo RA, Mirza SK, Martin BI, Kreuter W, Goodman DC, Jarvik JG. Trends, major medical complications, and charges associated with surgery for lumbar spinal stenosis in older adults. JAMA. 2010;303:1259–65.
8. Martin BI, Mirza SK, Comstock BA, Gray DT, Kreuter W, Deyo RA. Are lumbar spine reoperation rates falling with greater use of fusion surgery and new surgical technology? Spine (Phila Pa 1976). 2007;32:2119–26.
9. Patil PG, Turner DA, Pietrobon R. National trends in surgical procedures for degenerative cervical spine disease: 1990–2000. Neurosurgery. 2005;57:753–8; discussion 753–8.
10. Wang MC, Kreuter W, Wolfla CE, Maiman DJ, Deyo RA. Trends and variations in cervical spine surgery in the United States: Medicare beneficiaries, 1992 to 2005. Spine. 2009;34:955–61.
11. Perez-Cruet MJ, Foley KT, Isaacs RE, Rice-Wyllie L, Wellington R, Smith MM, et al. Microendoscopic lumbar discectomy: technical note. Neurosurgery. 2002;51:S129–36.
12. Smith JS, Ogden AT, Shafizadeh S, Fessler RG. Clinical outcomes after microendoscopic discectomy for recurrent lumbar disc herniation. J Spinal Disord Tech. 2010;23:30–4.
13. Schwender JD, Holly LT, Rouben DP, Foley KT. Minimally invasive transforaminal lumbar interbody fusion (TLIF): technical feasibility and initial results. J Spinal Disord Tech. 2005;18 Suppl:S1–6.
14. Wang MY, Anderson DG, Poelstra KA, Ludwig SC. Minimally invasive posterior fixation. Neurosurgery. 2008;63:197–203.
15. Wang MY, Mummaneni PV. Minimally invasive surgery for thoracolumbar spinal deformity: initial clinical experience with clinical and radiographic outcomes. Neurosurg Focus. 2010;28:E9.
16. Gold MR. Cost-effectiveness in health and medicine. New York: Oxford University Press; 1996.
17. Drummond MF. Drummond MFMfteeohcp: methods for the economic evaluation of health care programmes. 3rd ed. Oxford/New York: Oxford University Press; 2005.
18. Franke J, Greiner-Perth R, Boehm H, Mahlfeld K, Grasshoff H, Allam Y, et al. Comparison of a minimally invasive procedure versus standard microscopic discotomy: a prospective randomised controlled clinical trial. Eur Spine J Off Publ Eur Spine Soc Eur Spinal Deform Soc Eur Sect Cerv Spine Res Soc. 2009;18:992–1000.
19. Brock M, Kunkel P, Papavero L. Lumbar microdiscectomy: subperiosteal versus transmuscular approach and influence on the early postoperative analgesic consumption. Eur Spine J Off Publ Eur Spine Soc Eur Spinal Deform Soc Eur Sect Cerv Spine Res Soc. 2008;17:518–22.
20. Harrington JF, French P. Open versus minimally invasive lumbar microdiscectomy: comparison of operative times, length of hospital stay, narcotic use and complications. Minim Invasive Neurosurg MIN. 2008;51:30–5.
21. Arts MP, Brand R, van den Akker ME, Koes BW, Bartels RH, Peul WC. Tubular diskectomy vs conventional microdiskectomy for sciatica: a randomized controlled trial. JAMA J Am Med Assoc. 2009;302:149–58.
22. Arts MP, Brand R, van den Akker ME, Koes BW, Bartels RH, Tan W, et al. Tubular diskectomy vs

conventional microdiskectomy for the treatment of lumbar disk herniation: 2-year results of a double-blind randomized controlled trial. Neurosurgery. 2011;69: 135–44.
23. van den Akker ME, Arts MP, van den Hout WB, Brand R, Koes BW, Peul WC. Tubular diskectomy versus conventional microdiskectomy for the treatment of lumbar disk related sciatica: cost utility analysis alongside a double-blinded randomized controlled trial. Neurosurgery. 2011;69:829–35.
24. Wang MY, Cummock MD, Yu Y, Trivedi RA. An analysis of the differences in the acute hospitalization charges following minimally invasive versus open posterior lumbar interbody fusion. J Neurosurg Spine. 2010;12:694–9.
25. Parker SL, Adogwa O, Bydon A, Cheng J, McGirt MJ. Cost-effectiveness of minimally invasive versus open transforaminal lumbar interbody fusion for degenerative spondylolisthesis associated low-back and leg pain over two years. World Neurosurg. 2012;78:178–84.
26. Wang MY, Lerner J, Lesko J, McGirt MJ. Acute hospital costs after minimally invasive versus open lumbar interbody fusion: data from a US national database with 6106 patients. J Spinal Disord Tech. 2012;25:324–8.
27. Charosky S, Guigui P, Blamoutier A, Roussouly P, Chopin D. Complications and risk factors of primary adult scoliosis surgery: a multicenter study of 306 patients. Spine. 2012;37:693–700.
28. Cho KJ, Suk SI, Park SR, Kim JH, Kim SS, Choi WK, et al. Complications in posterior fusion and instrumentation for degenerative lumbar scoliosis. Spine. 2007;32:2232–7.
29. Schwab FJ, Hawkinson N, Lafage V, Smith JS, Hart R, Mundis G, et al. Risk factors for major peri-operative complications in adult spinal deformity surgery: a multi-center review of 953 consecutive patients. Eur Spine J. 2012;21: 2603–10.
30. McGirt MJ, Parker SL, Lerner J, Engelhart L, Knight T, Wang MY. Comparative analysis of perioperative surgical site infection after minimally invasive versus open posterior/transforaminal lumbar interbody fusion: analysis of hospital billing and discharge data from 5170 patients. J Neurosurg Spine. 2011;14:771–8.
31. Parker SL, Adogwa O, Witham TF, Aaronson OS, Cheng J, McGirt MJ. Post-operative infection after minimally invasive versus open transforaminal lumbar interbody fusion (TLIF): literature review and cost analysis. Minim Invasive Neurosurg MIN. 2011;54:33–7.
32. Ozgur BM, Aryan HE, Pimenta L, Taylor WR. Extreme Lateral Interbody Fusion (XLIF): a novel surgical technique for anterior lumbar interbody fusion. Spine J Off J North Am Spine Soc. 2006;6:435–43.
33. Lucio JC, Vanconia RB, Deluzio KJ, Lehmen JA, Rodgers JA, Rodgers W. Economics of less invasive spinal surgery: an analysis of hospital cost differences between open and minimally invasive instrumented spinal fusion procedures during the perioperative period. Risk Manag Healthc Policy. 2012; 5:65–74.
34. Cahill KS, Chi JH, Day A, Claus EB. Prevalence, complications, and hospital charges associated with use of bone-morphogenetic proteins in spinal fusion procedures. JAMA. 2009;302:58–66.

The MiSLAT Algorithm: Minimally Invasive Evaluation and Treatment for Adult Degenerative Deformity

9

Praveen V. Mummaneni, Michael Y. Wang, Fernando E. Silva, Lawrence G. Lenke, John E. Ziewacz, Beejal Y. Amin, and Tsung-Hsi Tu

9.1 Introduction

The goals of adult spinal deformity treatment are to reduce pain, arrest progression of the deformity, restore sagittal and coronal balance, improve neurological function, and improve cosmesis. Traditional open approaches can achieve these goals. However, surgical treatment of adult spinal deformity is associated with substantial surgical risks, especially due to the increased age and associated medical comorbidities of many patients with adult spinal deformity. Open scoliosis surgery is associated with prolonged operative times and significant blood loss. Complication rates of adult deformity surgery are as high as 41.2 % [1]. A recent International Spine Study Group (ISSG) study reviewed a total of 953 adult spinal deformity patients with minimum 2-year follow-up to identify patients with major perioperative complications. Ninety-nine major complications were observed in 72 patients (7.6 %). The most common complications were excessive blood loss (>4 L) and deep wound infection requiring reexploration of the wound and pulmonary embolism [2]. Minimally invasive approaches for adult spinal deformity surgery have been developed to address the high perioperative morbidity of traditional open approaches [3–6].

P.V. Mummaneni, MD (✉) • J.E. Ziewacz, MD, MPH
T.-H. Tu, MD
Department of Neurological Surgery,
University of California, San Francisco,
San Francisco, CA, USA
e-mail: mummanenip@neurosurg.ucsf.edu

M.Y. Wang, MD
Department of Neurological Surgery, University of Miami Miller School of Medicine, Miami, FL, USA
e-mail: mwang2@med.miami.edu

F.E. Silva, MD
North Texas Neurosurgical and Spine Center,
Fort Worth, TX 76104, USA

L.G. Lenke, MD
Washington University School of Medicine,
St. Louis, MO 63110, USA

B.Y. Amin, MD
Loyola University Health System,
Maywood, IL 60153, USA

9.2 Challenges of Minimally Invasive Deformity Surgery and Initial Results

In order to be a viable option in the treatment of adult scoliosis, MIS techniques must be able to achieve the same objectives as open techniques: (1) adequate decompression should be achieved with minimally invasive surgery, (2) implants should be accurately placed with minimally invasive approaches, (3) a solid fusion should be established, and (4) sagittal balance should be maintained/restored. Recently, several publications have addressed these issues. Anand et al. reported 28 patients treated with three or more levels of anterior and posterior deformity surgery with a mean age of 67.7 years and mean follow-up time of 22 months [7]. Mean intraoperative blood loss was 500 cc for combined anterior and

M.Y. Wang et al. (eds.), *Minimally Invasive Spinal Deformity Surgery*,
DOI 10.1007/978-3-7091-1407-0_9, © Springer-Verlag Wien 2014

posterior minimally invasive deformity surgery, and the operative times were a mean of 500 min. The visual analog scale, treatment intensity scale, 36-Item Short Form Health Survey, and Oswestry Disability Index (ODI) scores at 1 year were significantly improved compared to preoperative values. The mean coronal Cobb angles were 22° preoperatively and 7.5° postoperatively. However, the authors did not report results of sagittal balance correction. Complications were noted in 23 patients, mostly transient dysesthesia (17/23) related to the extreme lateral interbody fusion (XLIF) approach. Transient thigh dysesthesia is a known complication of lateral interbody approaches [8].

Tormenti et al. reported their retrospective review of eight cases performed with a combined anterior XLIF and posterior open pedicle screw fixation surgery and compared this cohort to 4 cases who underwent posterior-only open surgery [9]. The mean preoperative and postoperative coronal Cobb angles were 39° and 13° in the minimally invasive surgery group versus 19° and 11° in the posterior-only group. One case of cecal perforation during the anterior approach was reported in this series. However, the authors did not utilize minimally invasive percutaneous dorsal fixation and did not report sagittal balance parameters.

Dakwar et al. retrospectively reviewed 25 adult degenerative deformity patients who underwent a minimally invasive lateral approach for three or more levels with a mean follow-up of 11 months. The mean intraoperative blood loss was 53 ml per level with a mean length of stay of 6.2 days [10]. Visual analog scale scores and ODI improved significantly postoperatively. Complications included three cases of transient postoperative anterior thigh numbness, one case of rhabdomyolysis requiring temporary hemodialysis, one case of implant failure, and one case of asymptomatic subsidence. The authors concentrated on coronal curve correction rather than on sagittal plane correction, and one-third of their cases failed to demonstrate restoration of sagittal balance.

Wang and Mummaneni retrospectively reviewed 23 patients with thoracolumbar deformity treated with minimally invasive approaches [6]. The mean age was 64.4 years with a mean follow-up of 13.4 months. The mean blood loss was 477 ml. The coronal Cobb angles improved from 31.4° preoperatively to 11.5° postoperatively. Lumbar lordosis improved from 37.4 preoperatively to 47.5° postoperatively. All of the 16 patients who underwent interbody fusion at every level achieved solid fusion. However, of the seven cases without use of interbody fusion at every level, two patients had pseudarthrosis. Seven patients developed thigh dysesthesia or numbness on the side of the minimally invasive lateral approach.

These initial experiences demonstrate that MIS deformity correction can be achieved safely and effectively, with acceptable complication rates. However, challenges remain, particularly the restoration of sagittal balance.

9.3 Patient Evaluation

Leg and back pain are the principal symptoms for which adult deformity patients seek medical attention. It is important to ascertain whether the pain is radicular in nature versus purely axial. If the pain is radicular, then it is important to know whether the pain is indeed congruent with foraminal stenosis. Additionally, it is important to note if the location of the stenosis is central, paracentral (lateral recess), foraminal, or extraforaminal. Axial pain may be related to radiographic instability (spondylolisthesis) or sagittal imbalance.

To clinically assess the patient, the patient must stand with his or her knees fully extended. The degree of sagittal and coronal imbalance, including trunk shift is noted. Any degree of shoulder and/or pelvic asymmetry is also noted. Clinical assessment of the degree of flexibility of the structural curve is ascertained by bending maneuvers. Pelvic obliquity and leg length discrepancy are also evaluated and noted. A thorough neurological examination including motor strength, reflexes, sensory testing, and gait testing are performed. The trochanters and sacroiliac joints are palpated for any degree of tenderness. Hip and knee contractures are evaluated.

As with all deformity patients, full 36-in. standing posterior-anterior and lateral radiographic views are obtained. Additionally, supine long cassette radiographs are obtained; the latter are important in that they permit further evaluation of the flexibility of the curve in both planes.

This is particularly important in minimally invasive approach planning as it will help the surgeon decide whether an osteotomy is needed for fixed sagittal imbalance. Careful attention must be paid to plan correction of any fractional curves at the lumbosacral junction.

Appropriate measurements are undertaken with particular attention to the parameters of the sacropelvic region, including the lumbar lordosis/pelvic incidence mismatch. Ideally, lumbar lordosis should match the pelvic incidence ±10°. This is important in planning any degree of correction necessary to alleviate the patient's symptoms, since sagittal balance correction has been associated with improved clinical outcomes in patients undergoing scoliosis surgery [11–13]. Computed tomography and MRI images are also obtained. In patients who have cardiac pacemakers, a computed tomographic myelogram is an important adjunct to the radiographic evaluation when MRI is not possible. To further elucidate the pain generators, provocative testing such as facet and nerve root blocks can be of great value to the deformity surgeon.

9.4 Treatment Planning and Classification

Operative interventions require evaluation of the unique needs and goals of each patient. In order to guide operative decision-making, several classification schemes as well as levels of treatment have been proposed for adult spinal deformity. In 2010, Lenke et al. published a "treatment levels" guide to adult degenerative deformity management [14]. In this scheme, the patient's needed treatment is classified into six treatment levels, based on clinical and radiographic findings. Of the six Lenke-Silva treatment levels, treatment levels I–IV could be appropriately treated with current minimally invasive techniques based on recently published literature [6, 7, 10]. We have modified the Lenke-Silva paradigm to create an algorithm for minimally invasive treatment of spinal deformity, which we have termed the MiSLAT (Mummaneni, M. Wang, Silva, Lenke, Amin, Tu) algorithm (Fig. 9.1). The MiSLAT algorithm can further be simplified to guide surgeons to "small," "medium," and "big" surgery, based on clinical and radiographic parameters (Fig. 9.2).

9.5 The MiSLAT Algorithm

9.5.1 MiSLAT Treatment Level I

This patient population typically presents with symptoms consistent with neurogenic claudication due to central and/or lateral recess stenosis. These patients have no significant degree of back pain and/or any complaints consistent with their deformity. These patients do not have sagittal or coronal imbalance. The treatment goal is nerve root decompression and not deformity correction. Minimally invasive techniques are well suited for this treatment level. Typically, a tubular retractor is used to perform an ipsilateral hemilaminotomy and foraminotomy. Then, by angling the tubular retractor medially, an undercutting contralateral decompression is also possible ("ipsi-contra" decompression). This type of "ipsi-contra" minimally invasive tubular decompression may be performed at one or two contiguous levels through one small incision. However, the presence of radiographic instability precludes this approach/procedure. Patients in this treatment level cannot have subluxation of greater than 2 mm and no sagittal and/or coronal imbalance, and the curve should be less than 30°.

9.5.2 MiSLAT Treatment Level II

Typically in the MiSLAT level II cases, the decompression involves levels of the spine which are radiographically unstable and concomitant focal instrumentation at the area of decompression is recommended. This treatment level can be achieved via minimally invasive techniques as well. This level of treatment is well suited for patients who have neurogenic claudication, minimal to moderate low back pain, Cobb angles less than 30°, >2 mm subluxation, and lack of anterior bridging osteophytes at the decompression site. However, these patients should not have lumbar kyphosis or global imbalance. These patients

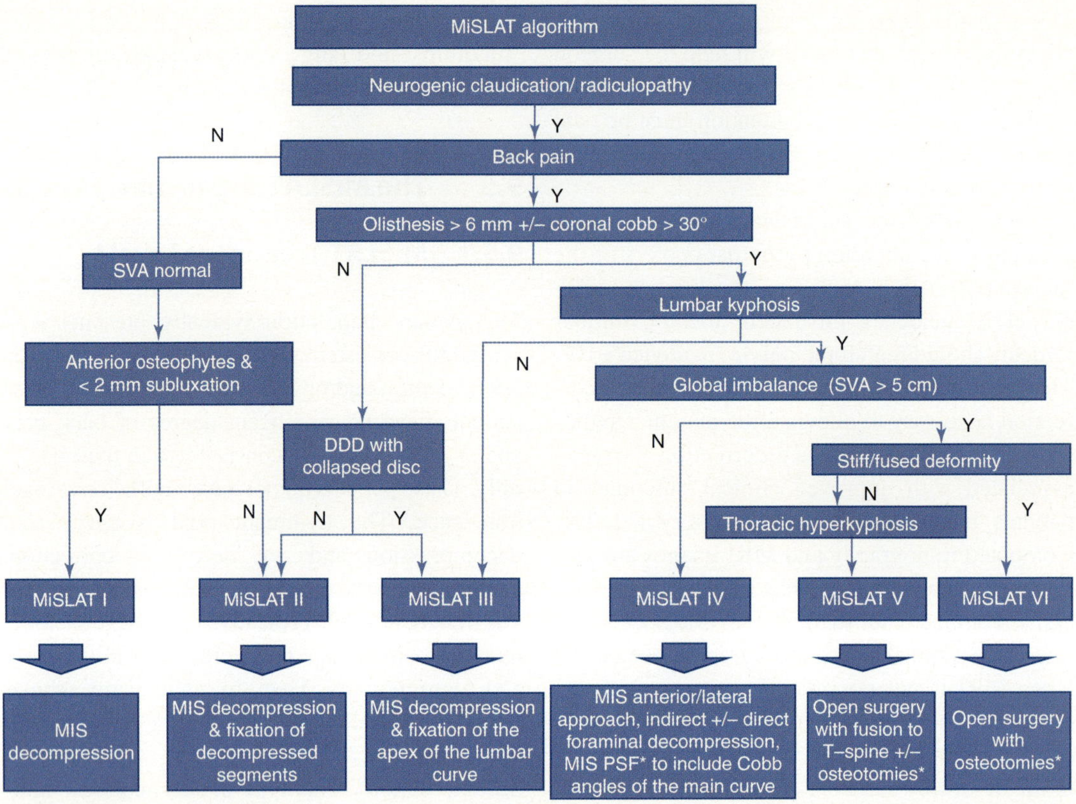

Fig. 9.1 MisLAT algorithm

benefit from focal decompression and minimally invasive fixation/fusion of the decompressed levels – typically using an expandable tubular retractor to perform a transforaminal interbody fusion with mini-open or percutaneous pedicle screw fixation at one or two contiguous levels.

MiSLAT treatment levels I and II are considered "small" surgery in the abbreviated MiSLAT algorithm (Fig. 9.2).

9.5.3 MiSLAT Treatment Level III

These patients suffer from back pain in addition to neurogenic claudication and radiculopathy. They have over 2 mm of subluxation, lack anterior bridging osteophytes, and Cobb angles greater than 30°. Besides extensive decompression and focal instrumentation at the decompressed levels of the lumbar spine, anterior or posterior interbody fusion of the apex of the lumbar curve is typically needed. Here again, minimally invasive techniques are well suited as they achieve the same goals as the open approaches. As with treatment level I, extensive decompression at multiple levels can be done through expandable tubular retractors; and, as with treatment level II, instrumentation can be performed via percutaneous or mini-open techniques, and interbody grafting achieved posteriorly via tubular retractors. Alternatively, minimally invasive lateral interbody procedures or anterior interbody fusions may be used with concomitant posterior percutaneous fixation. These anterior or lateral interbody procedures allow for indirect foraminal decompression by distracting the interbody space.

9.5.4 MiSLAT Treatment Level IV

These patients have claudication-radicular symptoms, back pain, and lumbar hypolordosis/

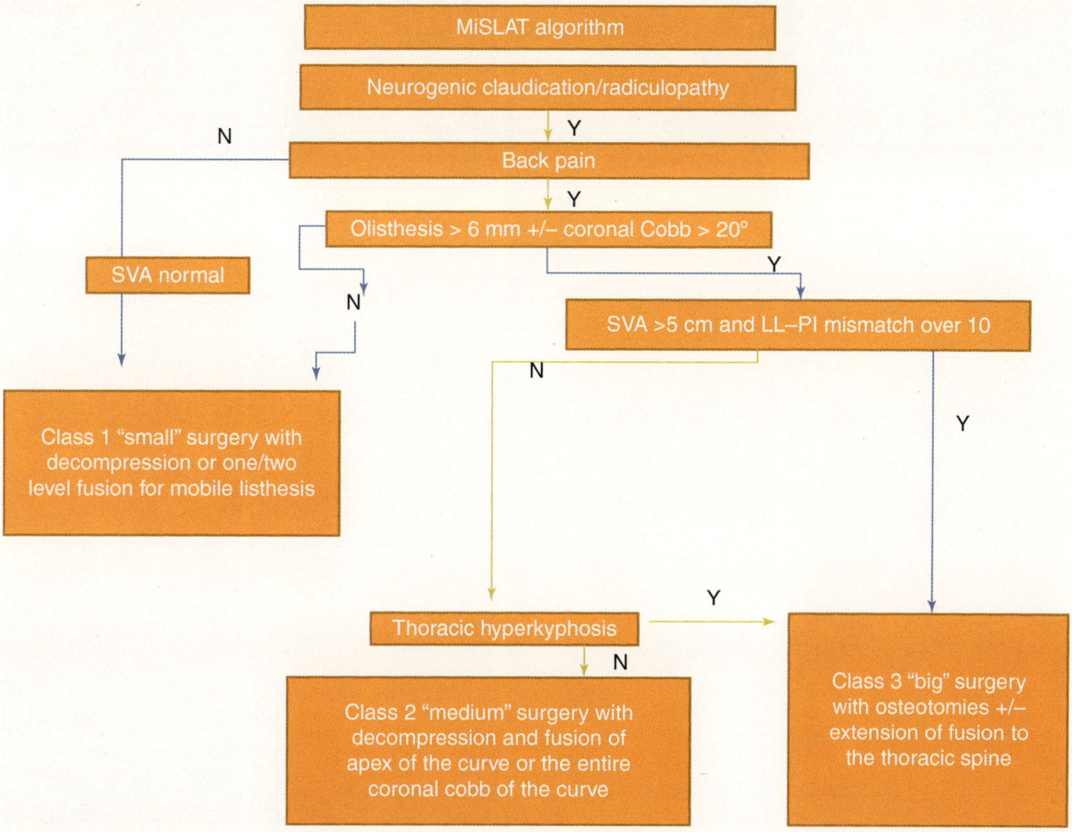

Fig. 9.2 Abbreviated MisLAT algorithm

kyphosis. The goal of the operative intervention includes decompression, instrumentation, interbody fusion, and correction of lumbar flat back or kyphosis. Radiographs of these patients demonstrate segmental instability and loss of lumbar lordosis, but no significant global imbalance (SVA<5 cm) (Fig. 9.3a–d). As already delineated, decompression, instrumentation, and interbody graft placement and arthrodesis can all be undertaken via minimally invasive techniques. Lordotic interbody grafts are typically placed from a minimally invasive lateral approach prior to posterior segmental mini-open or percutaneous pedicle screw instrumentation. The minimally invasive laterally placed interbody cages not only serve in kyphoscoliosis correction and derotation but also place the pedicles in a more "physiologic" angle, making dorsal pedicle fixation easier. Particular attention is paid to restoring normal segmental lordosis in the lower levels of correction, particularly at L4–L5 and L5–S1 (typically via TLIF), as two-thirds of lumbar lordosis comes from these two segments. Also, it is important to match the lumbar lordosis to the patient's individual pelvic incidence plus/minus ten degrees [12, 15, 16]. MiSLAT IV treatment typically involves fixation of the Cobb angles of the lumbar curve (beyond just the apex of the curve). If the curve extends to S1 or if the L5–S1 disc space is collapsed, then the instrumentation may need to extend to S1. In these cases, it may also be necessary to place iliac instrumentation in long fusions (L2 or above to sacrum) to help achieve a solid fusion at the lumbosacral junction and avoid sacral insufficiency fracture. Recent advances in minimally invasive techniques allow iliac screw fixation via percutaneous minimally invasive techniques [17]. MiSLAT III and IV levels are "medium" surgery in the simplified algorithm (Fig. 9.2).

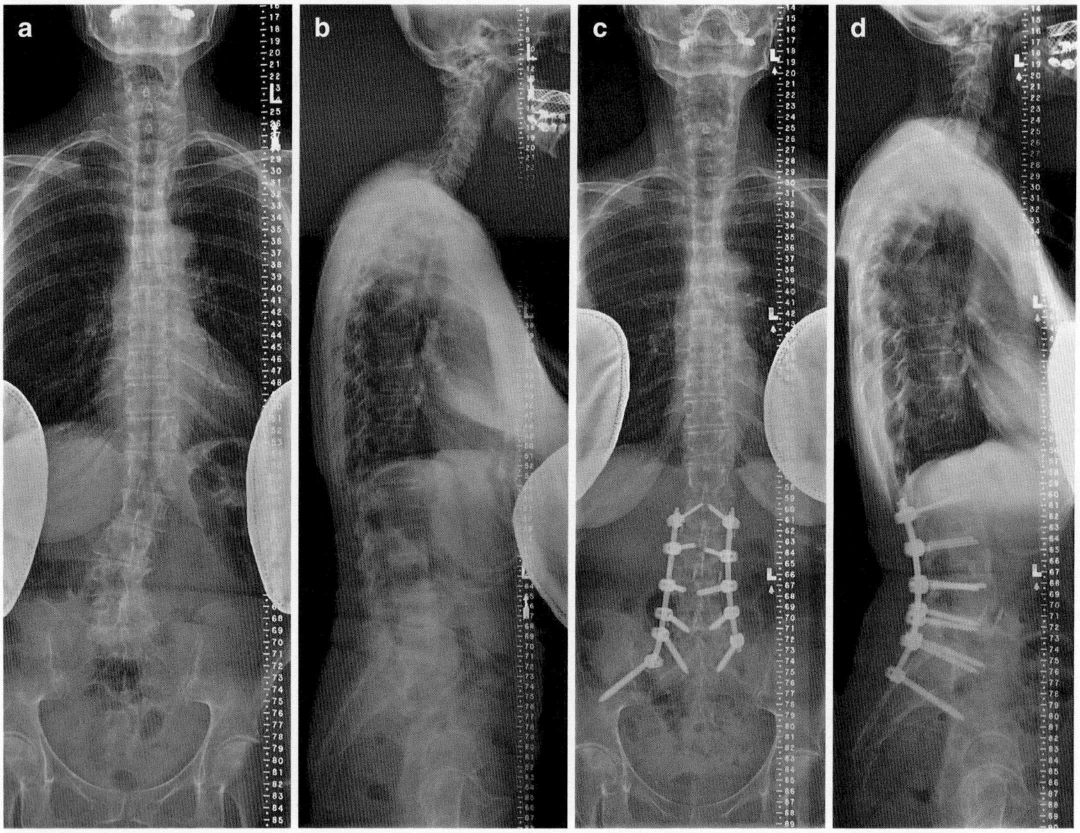

Fig. 9.3 Example of MisLAT IV patient

MiSLAT levels I–IV can now be performed using current minimally invasive techniques. Basic principles of proximal and distal fusion levels established for open surgery are also applicable to minimally invasive deformity treatment. As the soft tissue overlying the spine is preserved with minimally invasive approaches, typical cranial stopping points for multilevel lumbar instrumentation in MiSLAT IV treatments may vary from T10 to L2.

9.5.5 MiSLAT Treatment Levels V and VI

Schwab et al. recently updated the previous published SRS-Schwab classification to incorporate the spinopelvic parameters, which is highly correlated with HRQOL scores [18]. The classification is comprised of curve type, which is aimed at describing the relevant coronal aspects of the deformity and three modifiers to characterize sagittal components of the deformity. The inter- and intra-rater reliability and inter-rater agreement for the updated classification are excellent. When it comes to utilizing minimally invasive procedures to treat patients classified with SRS-Schwab classification, the patients with PI-LL modifier "B" or "C" (i.e., PI-LL value is greater than 20°) and/or global balance modifier "P" or "VP" (i.e., SVA is greater than 5 cm) are typically not suitable for a minimally invasive approach. These patients may need more extensive osteotomies to achieve sagittal vertical axis corrections [19]. These patients would fit into MiSLAT levels V or VI. This is "big" or open surgery in the simplified MiSLAT algorithm (Fig. 9.2).

In MiSLAT levels V and VI (Fig. 9.4), the need for standard open approach with

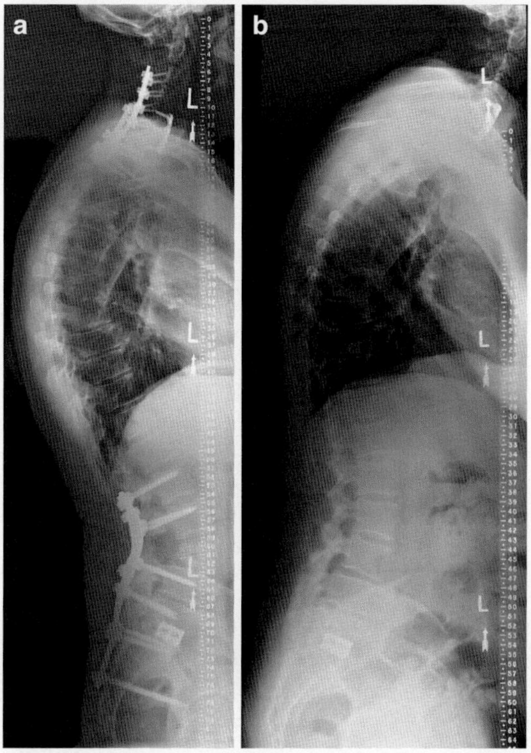

Fig. 9.4 Example of MisLAT V/VI patient

osteotomies remains as current minimally invasive techniques typically do not permit the achievement of the treatment goals (restoration of spinal balance). In the future, minimally invasive techniques may be applicable to patients in these levels. As an example, the use of a mini-open pedicle subtraction osteotomy is currently being explored. Initial laboratory investigations with cadavers demonstrated the use of bilateral tubular retractors to perform the necessary bone removal [20]. However, mini-open pedicle subtraction osteotomy has not yet gained widespread clinical use.

Conclusions

Surgery for adult spinal deformity is aimed at alleviation of neurological compression and improvement of spinal balance. The high complication rates from open surgery could potentially be avoided through a minimally invasive approach. The MiSLAT algorithm is a stepwise approach to decision-making regarding patient and procedure selection in minimally invasive deformity correction. Not all deformity cases can be appropriately treated with minimally invasive techniques. Patients with Lenke-Silva classification V and VI deformity cannot be easily corrected adequately with minimally invasive surgery in our opinion. This includes patients with curves with Cobb >30°, apical rotation >grade II, lateral olisthesis >6 mm, and sagittal imbalance requiring PSO. These cases still require traditional open surgery.

Minimally invasive deformity surgery is still in its early stages. The MiSLAT algorithm will require further validation and longer follow-up with assessment of spinal balance correction and standardized clinical outcomes are necessary to validate minimally invasive approaches for patients with Lenke-Silva 1–4 classifications. Clinically relevant issues such as pseudarthrosis, proximal junctional kyphosis, and adjacent level disease following minimally invasive surgery are topics for further study.

References

1. Yadla S, Maltenfort MG, Ratliff JK, Harrop JS. Adult scoliosis surgery outcomes: a systematic review. Neurosurg Focus. 2010;28:E3.
2. Mummaneni P, Smith J, Shaffrey C, Schwab F, Hawkinson N, Lafage V, et al. Risk factors for major perioperative complications in adult spinal deformity surgery. In 79th AANS Annual Scientific Meeting. Denver, 2011
3. Chi JH, Dhall SS, Kanter AS, Mummaneni PV. The mini-open transpedicular thoracic discectomy: surgical technique and assessment. Neurosurg Focus. 2008;25:E5.
4. Dhall SS, Wang MY, Mummaneni PV. Clinical and radiographic comparison of mini-open transforaminal lumbar interbody fusion with open transforaminal lumbar interbody fusion in 42 patients with long-term follow-up. J Neurosurg Spine. 2008;9:560–5.
5. Mummaneni PV, Wang MY, Silva FE, Lenke LG, Amin BY, Tu TH. Minimally invasive evaluation and treatment for adult degenerative deformity–using the MiSLAT algorithm. Scoliosis Research Society E-text; 2013. Available: http://etext.srs.org/book/.
6. Wang MY, Mummaneni PV. Minimally invasive surgery for thoracolumbar spinal deformity: initial

clinical experience with clinical and radiographic outcomes. Neurosurg Focus. 2010;28:E9.
7. Anand N, Rosemann R, Khalsa B, Baron EM. Mid-term to long-term clinical and functional outcomes of minimally invasive correction and fusion for adults with scoliosis. Neurosurg Focus. 2010;28:E6.
8. Cummock MD, Vanni S, Levi AD, Yu Y, Wang MY. An analysis of postoperative thigh symptoms after minimally invasive transpsoas lumbar interbody fusion. J Neurosurg Spine. 2011;15:11–8.
9. Tormenti MJ, Maserati MB, Bonfield CM, Okonkwo DO, Kanter AS. Complications and radiographic correction in adult scoliosis following combined transpsoas extreme lateral interbody fusion and posterior pedicle screw instrumentation. Neurosurg Focus. 2010;28:E7.
10. Dakwar E, Cardona RF, Smith DA, Uribe JS. Early outcomes and safety of the minimally invasive, lateral retroperitoneal transpsoas approach for adult degenerative scoliosis. Neurosurg Focus. 2010;28:E8.
11. Glassman SD, Hamill CL, Bridwell KH, Schwab FJ, Dimar JR, Lowe TG. The impact of perioperative complications on clinical outcome in adult deformity surgery. Spine (Phila Pa 1976). 2007;32:2764–70.
12. Lafage V, Schwab F, Patel A, Hawkinson N, Farcy JP. Pelvic tilt and truncal inclination: two key radiographic parameters in the setting of adults with spinal deformity. Spine (Phila Pa 1976). 2009;34:E599–606.
13. Schwab FJ, Smith VA, Biserni M, Gamez L, Farcy JP, Pagala M. Adult scoliosis: a quantitative radiographic and clinical analysis. Spine (Phila Pa 1976). 2002; 27:387–92.
14. Silva FE, Lenke LG. Adult degenerative scoliosis: evaluation and management. Neurosurg Focus. 2010;28:E1.
15. Lafage V, Ames C, Schwab F, Klineberg E, Akbarnia B, Smith J, et al. Changes in thoracic kyphosis negatively impact sagittal alignment after lumbar pedicle subtraction osteotomy: a comprehensive radiographic analysis. Spine (Phila Pa 1976). 2012;37:E180–7.
16. Schwab F, Patel A, Ungar B, Farcy JP, Lafage V. Adult spinal deformity-postoperative standing imbalance: how much can you tolerate? An overview of key parameters in assessing alignment and planning corrective surgery. Spine (Phila Pa 1976). 2010;35:2224–31.
17. Wang MY, Ludwig SC, Anderson DG, Mummaneni PV. Percutaneous iliac screw placement: description of a new minimally invasive technique. Neurosurg Focus. 2008;25:E17.
18. Schwab F, Ungar B, Blondel B, Buchowski J, Coe J, Deinlein D, et al. SRS-Schwab adult spinal deformity classification: a validation study. Spine (Phila Pa 1976). 2012;37:1077–82.
19. Mummaneni PV, Dhall SS, Ondra SL, Mummaneni VP, Berven S. Pedicle subtraction osteotomy. Neurosurgery. 2008;63:171–6.
20. Voyadzis JM, Gala VC, O'Toole JE, Eichholz KM, Fessler RG. Minimally invasive posterior osteotomies. Neurosurgery. 2008;63:204–10.

Part II

Percutaneous Segmental Fixation

10 Fluoroscopic Techniques in MIS Surgery

D. Greg Anderson

10.1 Introduction

Minimal access surgical techniques have inherently limited visualization and are therefore dependent on imaging technologies for surgical positioning. The most common, economical, and available intraoperative imaging modality is C-arm fluoroscopy. Due to the complex topography of the spine, overlapping shadows are produced on the fluoroscopic image that must be interpreted and translated to the surgeon's understanding of spinal anatomy. This chapter will focus on practical understanding and successful application of the C-arm for spinal procedures. This information is considered paramount to performing safe fluoroscopically assisted minimal access spine surgery.

10.2 The C-Arm Image Intensifier

The C-arm image intensifier is a primary source of intraoperative images available in most operating rooms. The relatively low cost, portability of the C-arm, and the rapid image acquisition make this equipment very useful during spinal procedures. Disadvantages of the C-arm include radiation exposure, the bulk of the equipment within the operative field, and the need (in most cases) for a dedicated, trained technician to operate the C-arm unit during surgery.

The C-arm image intensifier has an x-ray source which produces the x-ray beam on one side of the C. On the opposite side of the C, an image detector is mounted perpendicular to the direction of the x-ray beam (Fig. 10.1). X-rays emanate from a relative point-source and travel radially outward in all directions. The x-ray tube focuses the x-rays into a "relative" beam. The x-ray beam exits the tube and crosses the imaged tissue, where some of the x-rays are absorbed by the tissue (Fig. 10.2). The variable absorption of x-rays by various tissue structures produces the visualized fluoroscopic image. The path of x-rays emanating from the x-ray tube is not parallel but rather is slightly divergent (Fig. 10.3). X-rays at the edges of the x-ray tube have a larger divergence angle compared to x-rays in the central region of the tube. These factors produce certain imaging distortions as discussed below.

To reduce radiation exposure, the image detector utilizes a cesium iodide phosphor to enhance the raw fluoroscopic image by a factor of 10 [1]. Despite the relatively low radiation exposure of the C-arm compared to other imaging modalities, the surgeon and team are often working in close proximity to the x-ray beam and thus may be exposed to substantial radiation on a cumulative basis [2]. Therefore, the use of proper personal protective equipment (lead apron, thyroid shields, and leaded glasses) is mandatory when working with a C-arm.

D.G. Anderson
Department of Orthopaedics, Thomas Jefferson University, Philadelphia, PA, USA
e-mail: greg.anderson@rothmaninstitute.com

M.Y. Wang et al. (eds.), *Minimally Invasive Spinal Deformity Surgery*,
DOI 10.1007/978-3-7091-1407-0_10, © Springer-Verlag Wien 2014

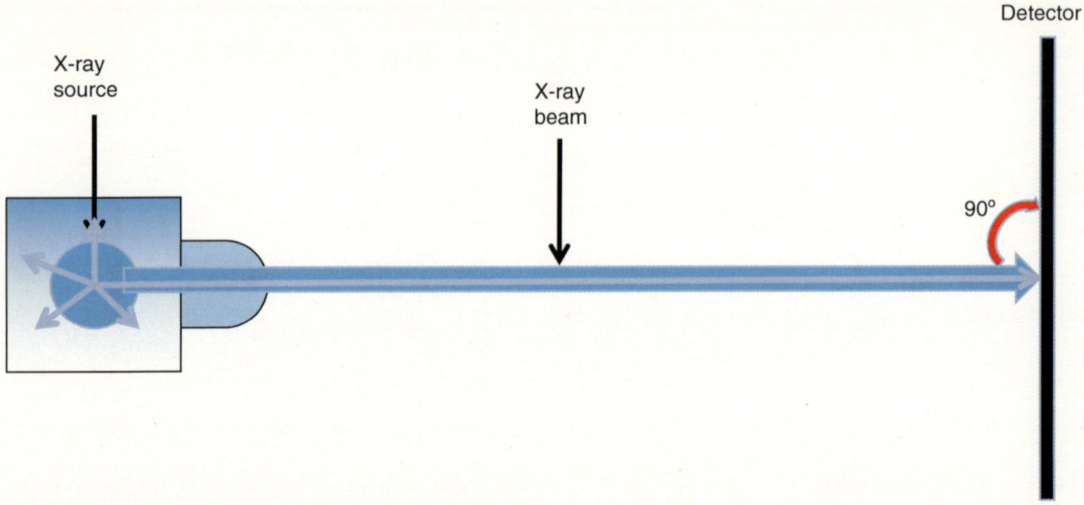

Fig. 10.1 The image detector is set perpendicular to the direction of the x-ray beam

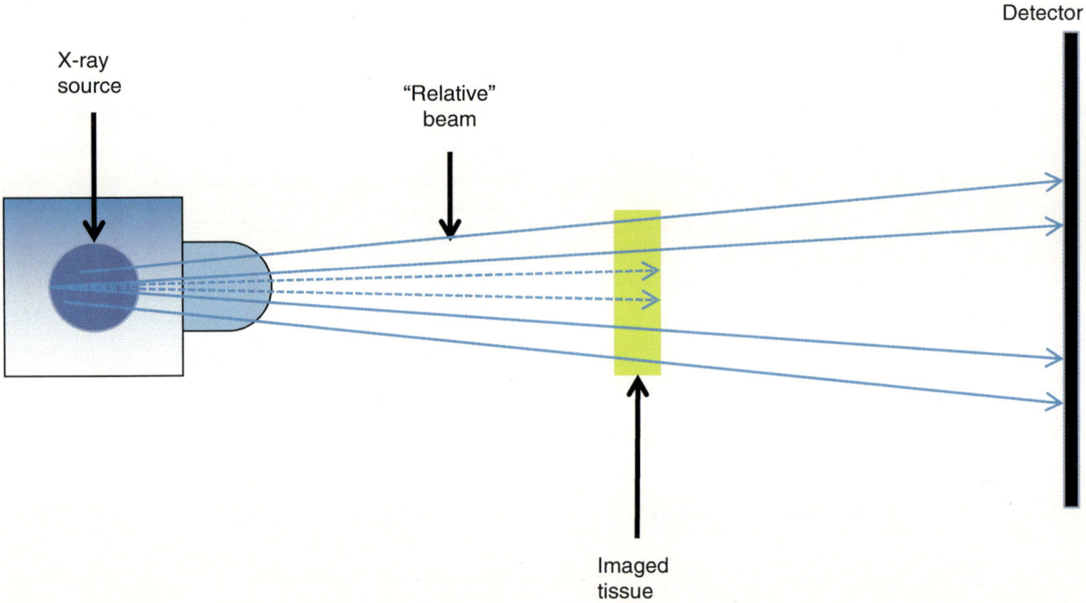

Fig. 10.2 X-ray beam exits the x-ray tube and crosses the imaged tissue, where some of the x-rays are absorbed by the tissue

10.3 Magnification, Distortion, and Parallax

To properly use the C-arm image intensifier, it is important to understand various types of image distortions which can be produced by the C-arm unit. If not understood and corrected, these imaging misrepresentations have the potential to lead a surgeon to misinterpret the images and make an error in conducting the surgery.

Magnification always occurs, to some degree, due to the divergent path of x-rays emanating from the x-ray tube. The divergent x-ray beam passes through the tissue prior to reaching the

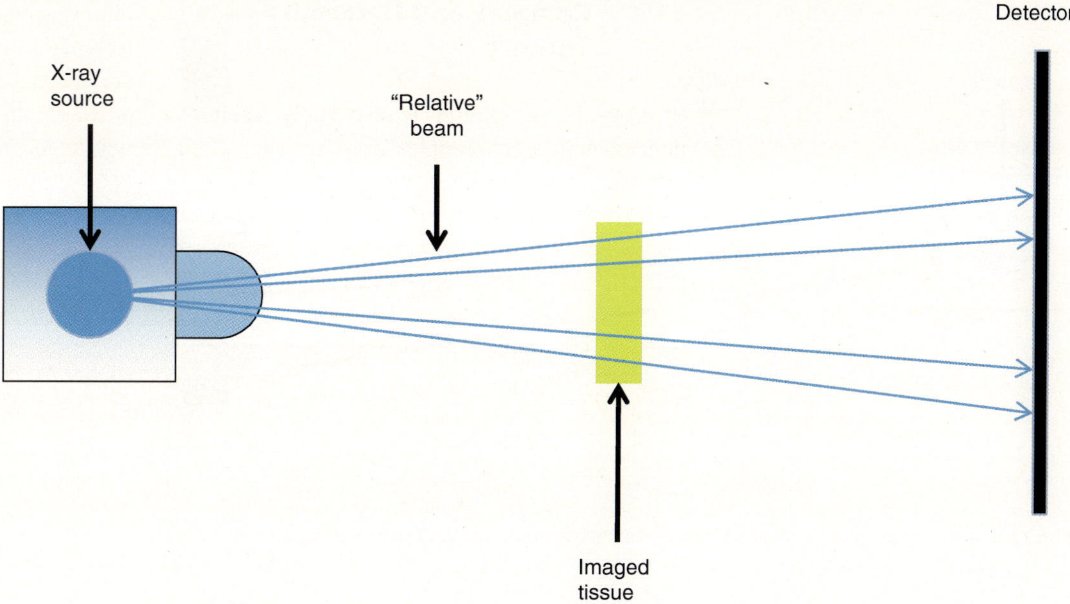

Fig. 10.3 Divergence of the x-ray beam

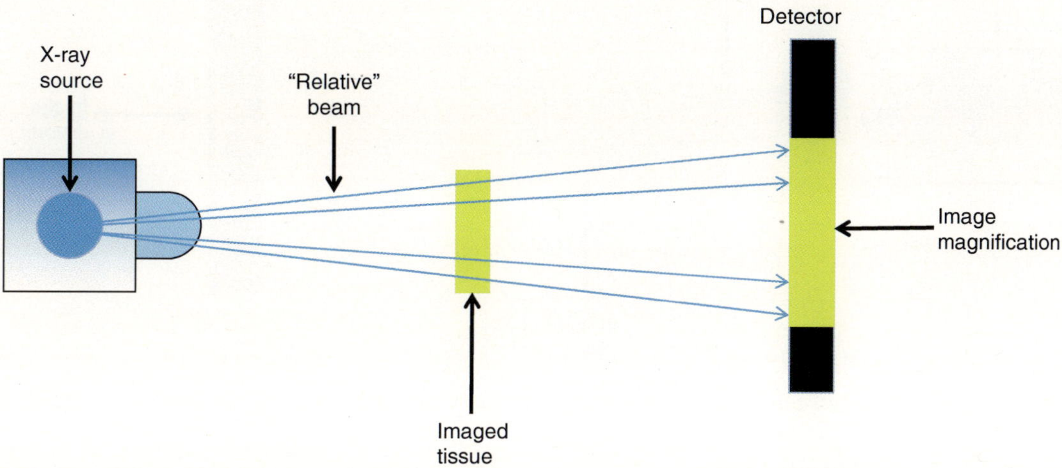

Fig. 10.4 Image magnification due to beam divergence

detector surface, producing an image that is larger than the tissue structure which was imaged (Fig. 10.4). Image magnification is greater when the imaged tissue is closer to the x-ray source (and thus farther from the image detector) (Fig. 10.5). Magnification may be useful in certain instances to enhance anatomic detail of a particular structure. To achieve greater magnification, simply reposition the C-arm x-ray source closer to the body. When it is more desirable to have a larger field of view (to image more vertebrae in a single image), the image source should be moved farther from the patient's body.

Image distortion can occur in several ways. First, distortion can occur when the x-ray beam is not generally perpendicular to the detector surface. This type of distortion does not occur with the use of the C-arm image intensifier because the x-ray beam is always perpendicular to the image detector based on the design of the unit. Another type of

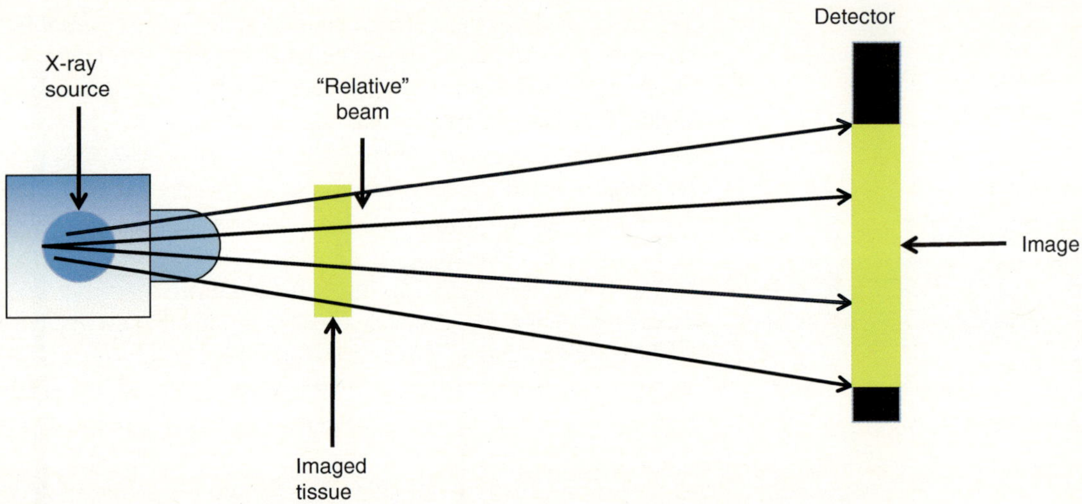

Fig. 10.5 Greater magnification is produced when the imaged object is placed closer to x-ray source

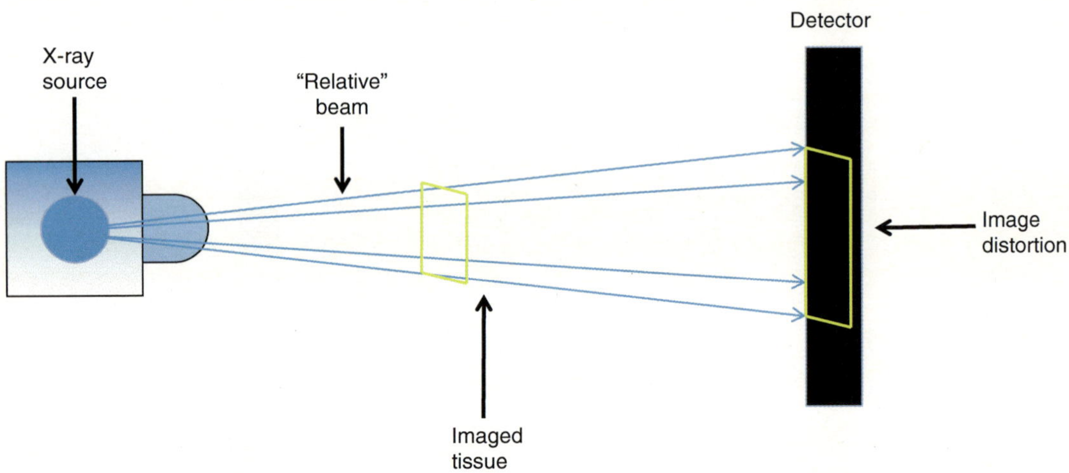

Fig. 10.6 One type of image distortion is produced by misalignment of the imaged tissue, relative to the path of the x-ray beam

distortion, which occurs commonly with the use of fluoroscopy, involves misalignment of an anatomic structure within the x-ray beam. In this fashion, the imaged structure is not aligned in an orthogonal manner to the detector surface. An example of this type of distortion would be attempting to obtain a lateral view of vertebrae when the vertebrae are misaligned (oblique) to the plane of the detector (Fig. 10.6). It is important for the surgeon to recognize this type of distortion and correct it by realigning the C-arm to provide a true image of the segment.

Parallax is the appearance of an altered relationship between objects in the foreground and background of an image, based on the vantage point of the viewer. Parallax occurs, during C-arm usage, when viewing structures along the borders of the image. The divergent x-ray beam passes obliquely through structures at the periphery of the image which distorts the optical relationship between foreground and background objects (Fig. 10.7). This effect is greatest when using a C-arm with a larger detector surface (i.e., 12 in. rather than the 8 in. detector surface). Parallax should be avoided

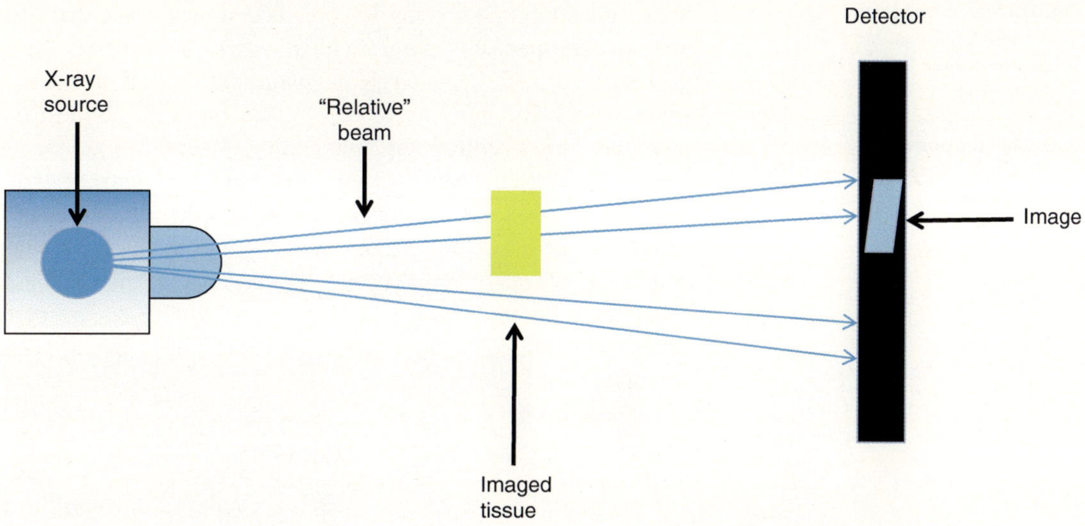

Fig. 10.7 Parallax phenomenon can lead to image distortion by placing the imaged tissue towards the periphery of the x-ray field

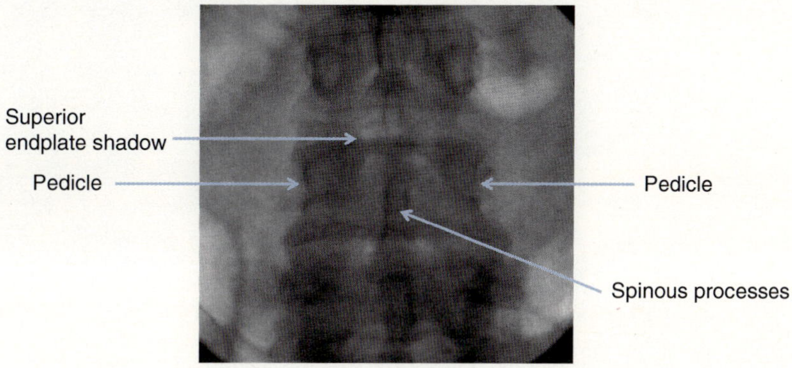

Fig. 10.8 In the true AP view, the superior endplate shadow forms a single radiopaque line with the pedicles immediately caudal to the superior endplate. The spinous process is equal distant between the pedicles

by positioning the structures of interest within the central region of the image field.

10.4 Standard Fluoroscopic Images of the Spine

The standard fluoroscopic views used during spinal surgery include the true anteroposterior (AP) view, the true lateral view (Lat), and the en face view (en face).

In a properly aligned true AP view, the superior endplate appears as a single radiopaque line and the pedicle shadows are located immediately caudal to the superior endplate. The spinous process shadow is an equal distance between the pedicle shadows. The transverse processes may sometimes be seen lateral to the pedicle shadows and are aligned parallel to the superior endplate shadow (Fig. 10.8).

In a properly aligned true lateral view, the superior cortex of the vertebral body projects as a single radiopaque line. The pedicles shadows (right and left) should be superimposed. The posterior cortex of the vertebral body (below the pedicles) will project as a single shadow, indicating that no rotation of the vertebrae exists (Fig. 10.9).

The en face is obtained by first starting with the true AP view. The C portion of the C-arm is rotated (generally 10–30° oblique to the true AP view) until the x-ray beam is aligned with the

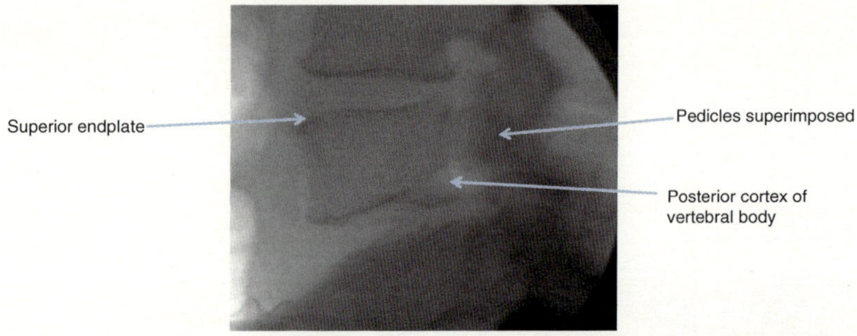

Fig. 10.9 The true lateral view should demonstrate a single radiopaque line for the superior endplate, the pedicles should be superimposed and the posterior cortex should appear as a single shadow

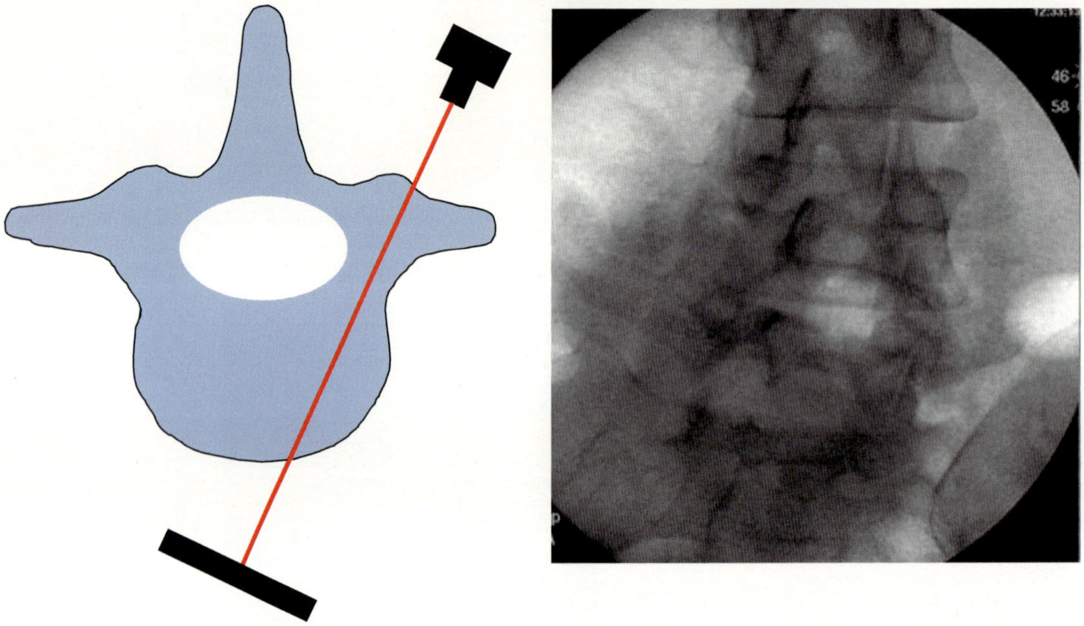

Fig. 10.10 *En face* view of the pedicle. The C-arm is aligned with the central axis of the pedicle. Notice how the medial boarder of the superior articular process is even with the medial boarder of the pedicle

central axis of the pedicle. The exact amount of rotation can be measured from the preoperative imaging study or can be estimated by rotating the image until the medial margin of the superior articular process aligns with the medical wall of the pedicle on the fluoroscopic image (Fig. 10.10).

10.5 Tips and Tricks for Successful C-Arm Usage

Prior to a fluoroscopically based case, the surgeon should discuss the surgical plan with the C-arm technician, because successful surgery depends on good choreography of movement and successful communication between these individuals throughout the operation. The surgeon should ensure that the patient is positioned on a radiolucent spinal frame with good access for the C-arm to enter and move freely about the surgical field. Any leads, wires, or tubes that may obscure the fluoroscopic images should be repositioned. Proper personal protective equipment should be donned prior to the procedure. It is a good idea to check spot images of the spine to ensure that the C-arm equipment is working correctly and image quality is acceptable prior to initiating the surgical approach.

The C-arm should be utilized at the onset of surgery to mark out the location of the surgical incisions. This principle is crucial to the success of a minimal access approach as malposition of the approach may prevent the surgeon from achieving the goals of the operation. It is generally easiest for the surgeon to stand on the opposite side of the table from the C-arm base. This limits the ergonomic challenges of working next to the most bulky portion of the equipment. **The most important aspect of using the C-arm is to ensure properly aligned images are obtained!** Each time an image is obtained, it should first be critically analyzed to be sure the alignment is acceptable before executing a surgical maneuver based on the image. Once the alignment of a particular level (e.g., L4) has been obtain for a true AP view, it should be marked out by the C-arm technician on C-arm unit. To do this, a piece of cloth or silk tape is placed along the angle indicator and a line is drawn indicating the proper alignment for the true AP image of the vertebra. Make sure to keep the field sterile during movement of the C-arm from a lateral to AP views. Various strategies may be utilized for proper sterility during C-arm movement and this should be planned out with the team in advance of surgery. To reduce radiation exposure to the team, step back 1–2 steps when possible while obtaining a fluoroscopic image. These tips should prove useful during fluoroscopically assisted procedures.

10.6 Limitations of Fluoroscopic Imaging

Although fluoroscopic images are very useful during spinal procedures, it is important to understand the limitations of two-dimensional images which involved the many superimposed tissues. Several principles should be remembered. **First, improper alignment of the fluoroscopic images will produce an inaccurate interpretation of the position of instruments and implants!** Therefore, proper alignment of the C-arm is the single most critical step for success in a fluoroscopically based procedure. Second, the most accurate fluoroscopic understanding will be obtained by reviewing orthogonal images in two perpendicular planes (e.g., AP and lateral). Third, fluoroscopic images do not provide an "axial"-type view like a CT. Therefore, small pedicle breeches may be undetected using fluoroscopy alone. Various surgical techniques, when combined with fluoroscopy, can limit the risk of a pedicle breech. Fourth, image quality can be severely degraded by various patient characteristics such as obesity, osteopenia, or obscuring structures (e.g., vascular stents). Fifth, successful use of the C-arm involves communication and understanding between the surgeon and the fluoroscopic technician. Depending on the experience of the technician, additional time to ensure accurate communication of the goals of C-arm alignment and movements may be required.

Conclusion

C-arm fluoroscopy is, by far, the most utilized technology for imaging during spinal procedures and is a necessary component of most minimal access approaches performed today. A good understanding of this technology and good fluoroscopic technique will provide the surgeon with the ability to navigate successfully during minimal access spinal approaches. The most important factor remains the ability of the surgeon to obtain and interpret standard C-arm images. Mastery of C-arm skills can be achieved with good training and surgical diligence.

References

1. Jones DP, Robertson PA, Lunt B, Jackson SA. Radiation exposure during fluoroscopically assisted pedicle screw insertion in the lumbar spine. Spine (Phila Pa 1976). 2000;25(12):1538–41. PubMed PMID: 10851103.
2. Rampersaud YR, Foley KT, Shen AC, Williams S, Solomito M. Radiation exposure to the spine surgeon during fluoroscopically assisted pedicle screw insertion. Spine (Phila Pa 1976). 2000;25(20):2637–45.

11 Image Guidance for Minimally Invasive Deformity Surgery

Roger Härtl

11.1 Introduction

There is agreement among surgeons that imaging techniques are essential for most spinal procedures regardless of the complexity of the operation, the anatomical region, and the level of training and comfort level of the individual surgeon. It is essential for localization of pathology, avoidance of wrong-level surgery, and the insertion of implants. This is even more important in minimally invasive spinal (MIS) procedures that lack the open visualization of anatomical reference points that can be used for orientation. Traditionally, this has involved the use of radiograph or image intensification guidance either as a control at the end of a procedure or for active guidance throughout surgery.

More recently, stereotactic 2-D or 3-D imaging techniques and even robotic surgery have been introduced and gained acceptance in disciplines such as cranial neurosurgery and some orthopedic trauma procedures. Computer-assisted surgery (CAS) uses navigation systems to improve visibility to the surgical field and increase the accuracy of surgery and instrumentation placement by virtually linking the operated bony anatomy with pre- or intraoperative imaging studies, usually CT scans. The use of CAS has first been described for spinal instrumentation placement in the mid-1990s [1–4]. In CAS a virtual representation of the surgeon's instruments is shown in relation to the patient's anatomy that is displayed on a separate computer screen. Pre- or intraoperative CT scans or image intensifier images are used to generate a "virtual surgical reality." This surgical "GPS" requires the attachment of a reference array with reflective beads to the patient's spinal anatomy and to the surgical instrument to be tracked. The 2-D information obtained by two infrared cameras tracking these beads is converted into a 3-D representation based on the different reflective angles. Tracking using electromagnetic instead of infrared technology is being evaluated and has shown some promising results [5, 6].

R. Härtl, MD
Weill Cornell Brain & Spine Center, Starr Building, Room 651, 525 East 68th Street, 99, New York, NY 10021, USA
e-mail: roger@hartlmd.net

11.2 Potential Advantages and Disadvantages of CAS

Supporters of CAS state that stereotactic navigation has the potential to:

- Improve accuracy of instrumentation placement and optimize the size of instrumentation used
- Reduce radiation exposure to surgeon and staff
- Enable less invasive approaches through smaller access
- Allow preoperative planning of instrumentation size and trajectories and osteotomy procedures
- Allow verification of screw accuracy intraoperatively (true intraoperative CT scanners or intraoperative portable cone beam CT systems)

M.Y. Wang et al. (eds.), *Minimally Invasive Spinal Deformity Surgery*, DOI 10.1007/978-3-7091-1407-0_11, © Springer-Verlag Wien 2014

- Minimize the risks of wrong-level surgery
- Decrease reoperation rate

Potential disadvantages of CAS include:

- The learning curve associated with the technologies for the surgeon and the OR staff could be significant.
- Upfront costs of the capital equipment.
- Interruption of surgical "flow."
- Additional equipment and footprint in the OR.
- Lack of scientific data supporting its clinical benefit.
- Limited imaging quality and field of view with mobile 3-D imaging devices currently on the market.
- Potential increase in OR time.
- Potential line-of-sight limitations for optical systems.
- Concerns about accuracy and interference with metallic instruments using electromagnetic navigation systems.

11.3 Navigation Systems Used in MIS Surgery

The goal of MIS procedures is to achieve outcomes that are comparable or superior to conventional surgery but with less postoperative pain, quicker recovery, reduced blood loss, less soft-tissue damage, smaller surgical incisions, and less scarring. MIS evolved as a logical consequence out of the advancements in at least four different surgical areas:

- Microsurgery using the microscope or endoscope
- New spinal access strategies via percutaneous or mini-open procedures
- New spinal instrumentation (hardware)
- Neuronavigation/CAS using 2- or 3-D imaging technology

Surgical 3-D navigation requires 2 components:

- An imaging system and the navigation platform. Current spinal imaging for MIS primarily works with either of the following:
  - Intraoperative portable cone beam CT systems (isocentric fluoroscopy systems such as the Siemens "Iso-C," the Medtronic "O-arm," or a system made by Ziehm) [7]
  - True intraoperative CT scanners [8, 9]
- A 3-D navigation software platform such as the ones currently provided by Brainlab, Medtronic Stealth, Stryker, etc.

These imaging systems can also be used to confirm implant placement intraoperatively. Some of the portable isocentric C-arms and portable scanners offer the advantage that they can also be used as regular C-arms; however, their imaging quality is inferior to stationary CT scans.

11.4 Integration of 3-D Navigation into the MIS Workflow

Successful integration of navigation requires meticulous planning of each case as well as training of the surgeon and the surgical staff including the X-ray technician and scrub nurse. Initial training should be obtained in a cadaver lab if possible. The layout of the operating room and footprint of the various devices used should be discussed preoperatively with the team. It is helpful to draw this out initially. Some of the newer navigation platforms allow the surgeon to control the computer screen remotely. If this is not the case the surgeon should assign and train a member of the team to run the screen.

MIS procedures typically consist of at least three distinct surgical steps:

- Decompression
- Placement of an interbody device and bone graft or bone graft substitute and
- Instrumentation

The sequence of these surgical steps is variable and based on the surgeon's preference and sometimes also on the type of implants and instrumentation used. 3-D navigation can be helpful for each of these steps. It can confirm the correct level for the decompression. Navigation has also been used to guide in the placement of interbody devices, for posterior lumbar but also for lateral transpsoas approaches. Currently, CAS is mainly used to facilitate the placement of screws in all regions of the spine, from the occiput to the iliac crest and ilio-sacral joint.

11.5 One- or Two-Level MIS TLIF

For a one- or two-level lumbar TLIF procedure, we perform the decompression first, followed by the discectomy and the placement of the interbody spacer. Navigated pedicle screw placement is performed last. The procedure is accomplished through two small incisions, each approximately 3–4 cm off the midline. Fluoroscopic imaging guides the initial incision placement; an AP view is used to mark the incision along the outer margins of the facet joint of interest. The contralateral incision is later performed using image guidance. The initial incision is typically made on the more symptomatic side since this is where a facetectomy and complete decompression is performed. A Wiltse trans-muscular approach is utilized and serial dilators (Insight Access® system, Synthes Spine, Westchester PA; or METRx® retractors, Medtronic Sofamor Danek, Memphis TN) are introduced on the side of decompression and angled towards the facet joint and lamina to be removed. A 22 mm tubular retractor is then fixed into position. The surgical microscope is introduced and a complete or partial facetectomy is undertaken with a high-speed drill. The inferior articulating process can be removed first and used as bone graft. In stenosis cases, a laminectomy is performed by angling the tube medially, tilting of the patient away from the surgeon and by undercutting the spinous process and contralateral lamina (Fig. 11.1). A discectomy is then performed and the vertebral endplates are carefully prepared for the fusion. For the interbody fusion, we use an expandable PEEK cage and morselized bone from the facetectomy or iliac crest, in some cases also BMP (Fig. 11.2).

Next, the navigation reference array (VectorVision®, Brainlab AG, Feldkirchen, Germany) is attached with 2 percutaneous Steinman pins to the posterior iliac crest. A 3-D image set is obtained using the Siremobil Iso-C3-D (Siemens AG, Munich, Germany) and imported into the navigation system. Using a navigated pointer or drill guide through a mini-open or percutaneous approach, the ideal transpedicular trajectory is determined, and the diameter and length of the planned screws are simulated on the screen (Fig. 11.3). We currently use a custom-made navigated drill tube that allows the insertion of a drill, tap, and a pedicle screw without screwhead [10]. The advantage of this system is that it avoids the use of K-wires and that it reduces the number of instruments that need to be navigated (Figs. 11.4 and 11.5).

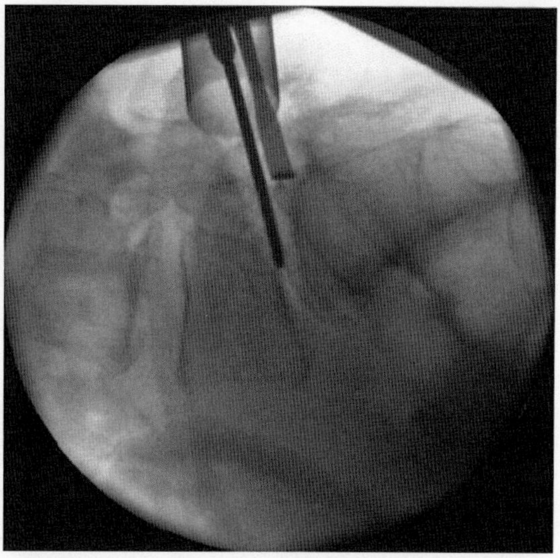

Fig. 11.1 A 55-year-old with back and radicular pain due to grade II spondylolisthesis at L5/S1. Tubular retractor in place. The decompression has been performed through a 22 mm tubular retractor and the disc space is being entered

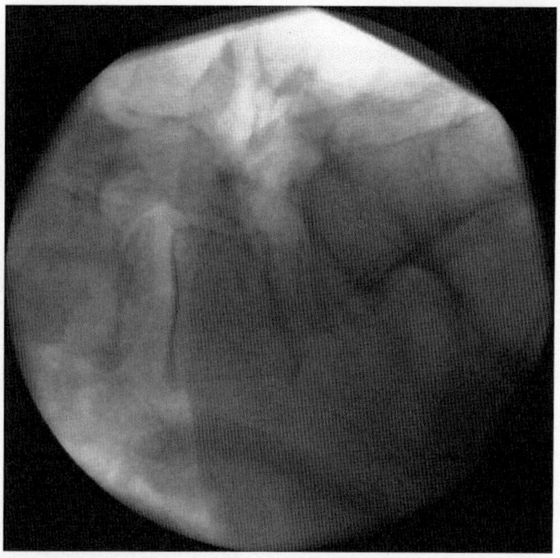

Fig. 11.2 An expandable interbody cage has been applied. The tubular retractor has been removed and the screws will be placed next

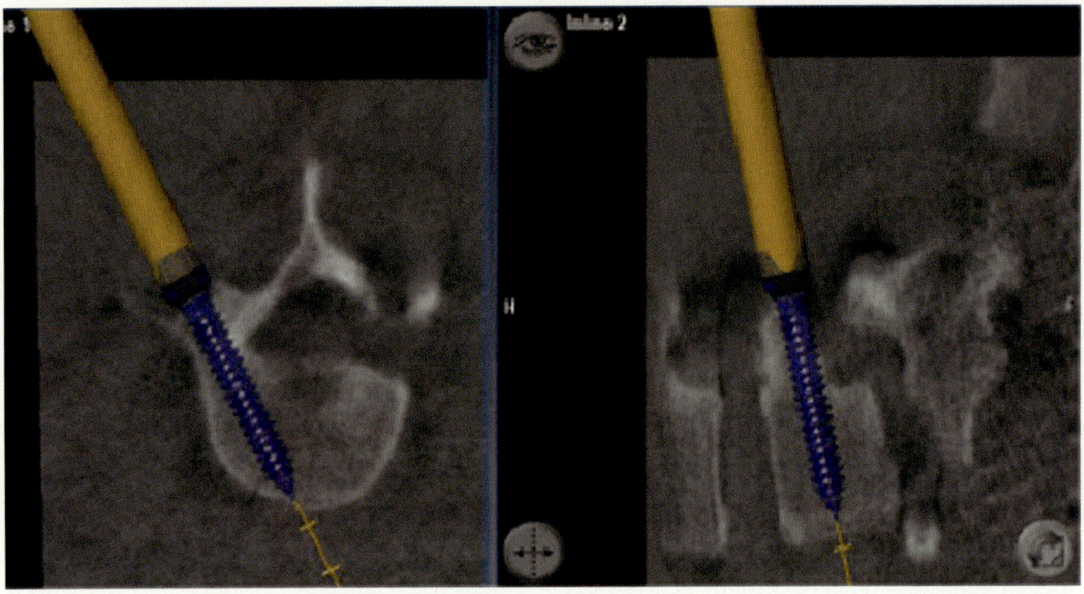

Fig. 11.3 Using a navigated pointer or drill guide through a mini-open or percutaneous approach, the ideal transpedicular trajectory is determined, and the diameter and length of the planned screws are simulated on the computer screen

Fig. 11.4 Navigated drill tube that allows the insertion of a drill, a tap, and a pedicle screw without screwhead. The advantage of this system is that it avoids the use of K-wires and that it reduces the number of instruments that need to be navigated

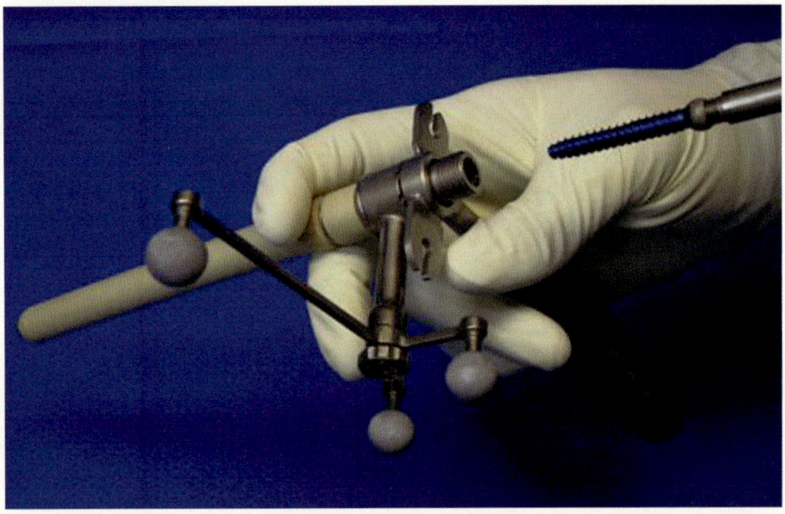

Several other options are available: A navigated drill guide can be used that allows the preparation of a starting hole with various sized drill bits into the pedicle. K-wires can then be introduced over which the tap and screws can be inserted. The advantage of this approach is that a control spin can be obtained with the K-wires in place to confirm accurate positioning. A third option involves the use of precalibrated instruments including the awl, pedicle probe, tap, and screwdriver. Many spinal instrumentation manufacturers have these now available. Nottmeier recently described how this approach can be utilized in order to implant pedicle screws without the use of K-wires [11].

Navigation can also be used to determine the ideal positioning and trajectory of the TLIF or PLIF cage and in order to determine the desired rod length by measuring the distance between the screwheads (Figs. 11.6 and 11.7).

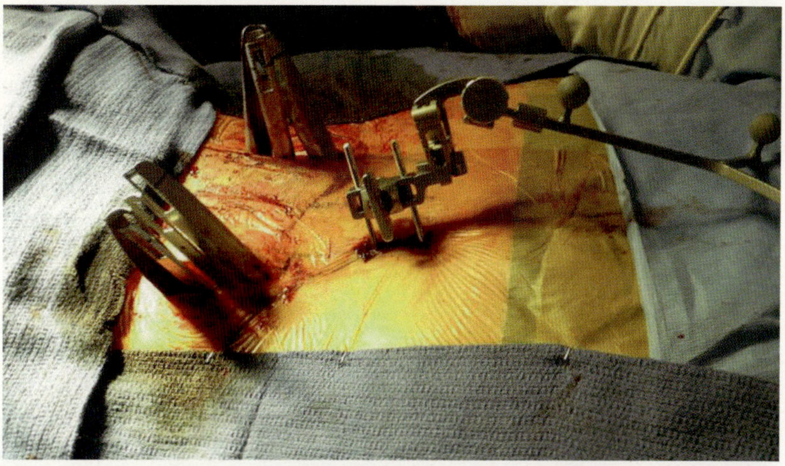

Fig. 11.5 The screw extension posts are visible through two small incisions. Steinman pins with reference array have been placed into the left iliac crest. The rods will be measured and placed next

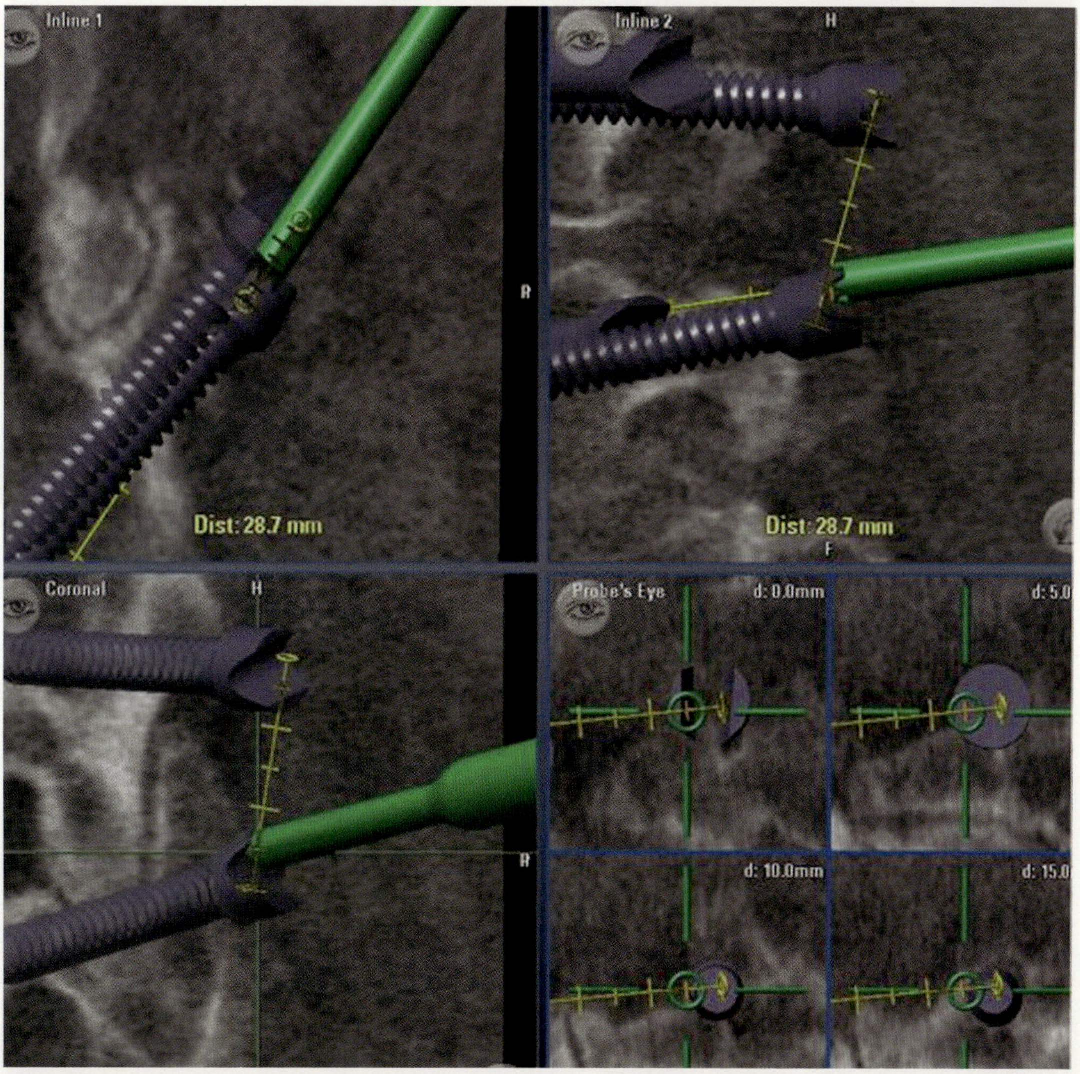

Fig. 11.6 Navigation can be used to determine the desired rod length by measuring the distance between the screwheads

11.6 Complex and Deformity Surgery

Stereotactic navigation is especially useful in patients with more complex anatomy, such as significant spondylolisthesis or degenerative scoliosis. Navigation can also be used to determine the best trajectory for intervertebral cage placement and for trans-sacral fixation [12] (Fig. 11.8). In the lumbar spine, it is used to determine the length of rods and to align screws during a multilevel fusion so that the percutaneous rod placement is facilitated. In the cervical spine, CAS facilitates the minimally invasive resection of odontoid masses via a transnasal route, which is a significant improvement when compared to conventional maximally invasive transoral surgery [13, 14].

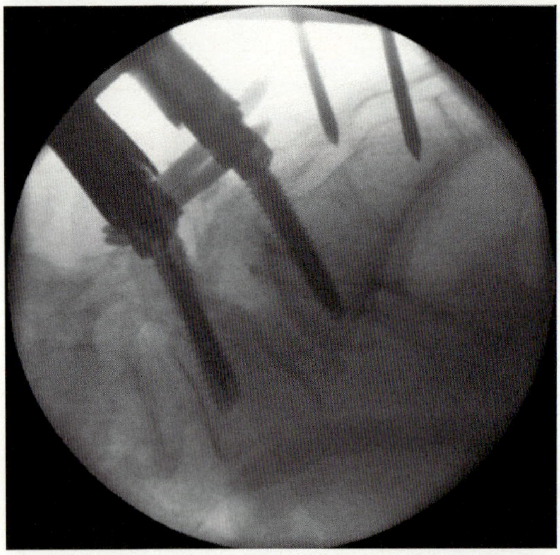

Fig. 11.7 Steinman pins with reference array have been placed into the iliac crest. Screws have been placed with a navigated drill guide. Rods have been locked in place

In more complex thoracolumbar deformity cases, the interbody part is frequently being accomplished via a separate anterior or lateral approach. This surgery may also include the placement of iliac crest screws [15]. In principle, navigation is performed in a similar fashion as described above (Fig. 11.9a, b).

A few differences or additional challenges, however, apply. Some authors have reported good accuracy with multilevel cases where the reference array was placed > 10 levels away from the surgery site [8]. We disagree and recommend placement of the reference array into the iliac crest for cases up to L3. If the fusion extends above L3, we will typically reposition the reference array more cranially using a spinous process clamp. In our experience this will maximize accuracy and safety. Another challenge is that current intraoperative portable cone beam CT systems have a limited field of view and therefore only allow the imaging of up to 3–5 vertebral bodies. This adds time, radiation

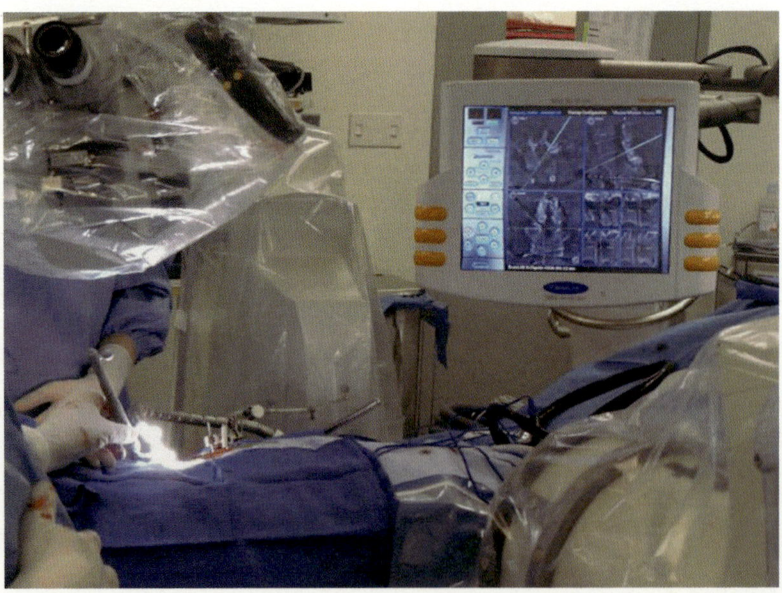

Fig. 11.8 The use of 3D navigation under the microscope to determine the optimal entry point and angle of an intervertebral cage

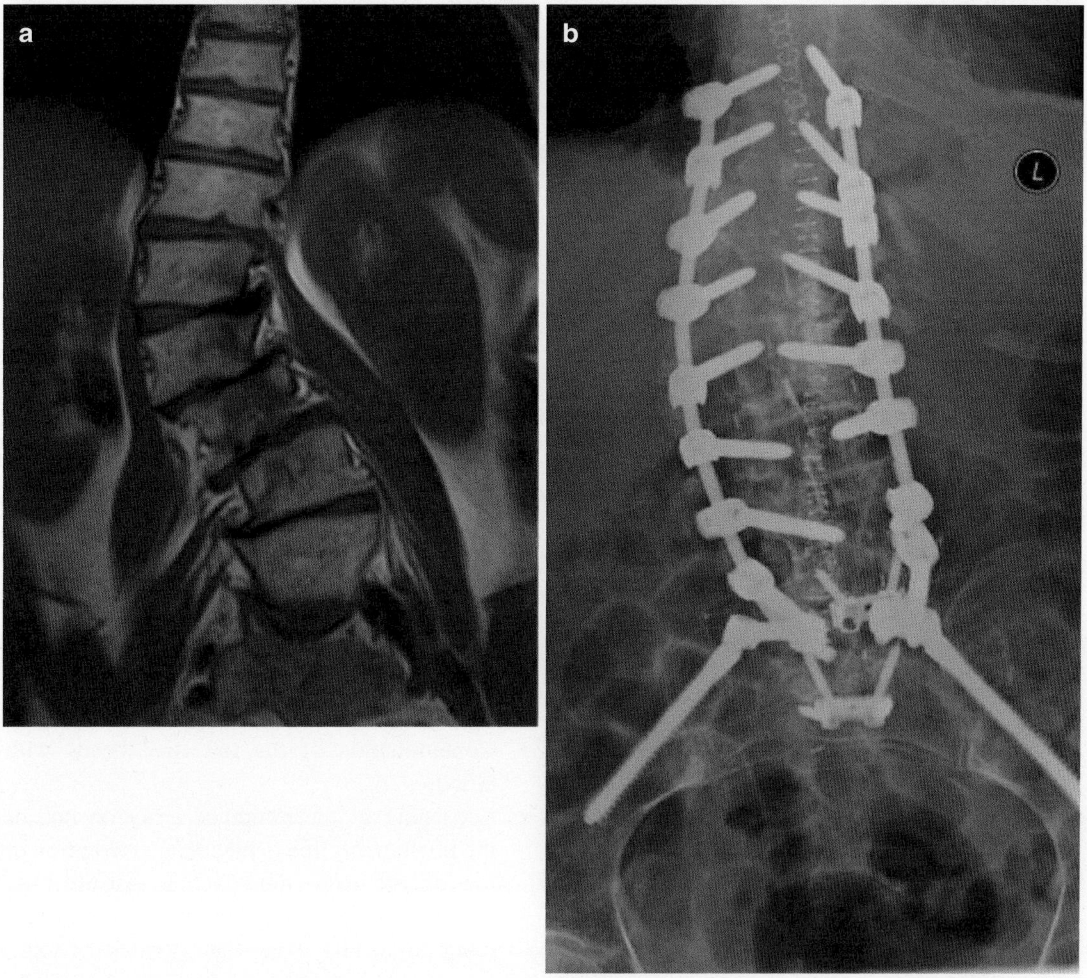

Fig. 11.9 A 75-year-old patient with back and leg pain before and after MIS deformity correction. (**a**) Preoperative MRI showing significant degenerative scoliosis. (**b**) Postoperative AP X-rays demonstrating placement of pedicle screws from T10 to L5 and iliac crest screws. Instrumentation was placed with 3D navigation

exposure, and complexity to multilevel deformity cases. The solution here is the use of a true intraoperative CT scanner.

The current advantage of using navigation in complex anatomy cases is that screw placement is clearly more accurate and technically more straightforward than with conventional AP/lateral fluoroscopy. Screw fit is maximized and there is no need to "skip" levels due to small or complex pedicle anatomy as is frequently seen in multilevel cases with conventional MIS techniques. A recent systematic literature review confirmed that navigation provided higher screw placement accuracy compared with conventional methods especially in scoliosis cases [16]. We found that CAS was associated with improved screw placement accuracy and that it was employed in cases with a higher degree of surgical complexity such as MIS cases, deformity, and revision surgery [17]. As the technology improves, it is likely that CAS will become more important in deformity surgery.

11.7 Navigation Without K-Wires

The use of K-wires can be harmful to the patient as they can break or bend during the procedure and cause visceral or vascular injury. In addition, the surgical workflow using K-wires is complex and requires the use of multiple instruments that go back and forth between the surgeon and the scrub nurse. We introduced a navigated guide tube that allows drilling, tapping, and the placement of the final screw without the need for K-wires [10]. This instrument facilitates the workflow in the operating room by reducing the number of instruments that need to be navigated and reduces the potential risks associated with current techniques for the insertion of percutaneous or mini-open pedicle screws by eliminating the need for K-wires (Fig. 11.4). Nottmeier recently described an approach to implant pedicle screws without the use of K-wires using precalibrated instruments including an awl, pedicle probe, tap, and screwdriver [15].

11.8 Radiation Exposure

When used intelligently, CAS can help make spine surgery safer for the patient as well as the surgeon and the operating room staff: The issue of radiation exposure using 2nd-generation CAS for MIS has been addressed by Nottmeier et al. [18]. In 25 MISS cases with 228 screws placed using a portable cone beam CT navigation, there was no radiation exposure to the surgeon. This requires, though, that K-wires are not used.

11.9 Learning Curve and Troubleshooting

Navigation does not replace surgical experience, judgment, meticulous preparation, and technique. For the surgeon who uses navigation for the first time, it will neither make surgery "easier" nor will it facilitate the workflow. Navigation requires careful planning and training not only for the surgeon but also for the whole team: the scrub nurse, the assistants, the X-ray technician, and others. There is a learning curve and initially some additional time will be required to successfully incorporate navigation. Many of the initial negative reports on navigation were due to the first generation systems not being user-friendly and that surgeons did not spend the time to really master this new technique. In the author's experience, one of the hardest tasks is to teach navigation to assistant surgeons who do not have the experience and understanding and who may believe that navigation enables "videogame" or "plug and play" surgery. The contrary is true: Accurate navigation requires very meticulous and gentle surgical technique and constant vigilant interpretation of what the computer screen shows versus the surgeon's tactile feedback. Subtle discrepancies may indicate a mismatch between the actual anatomy and what the screen shows and this requires immediate troubleshooting. In the majority of cases, this does *not* mean that navigation failed. Easily correctable reasons include:

- The surgeon's instrument may exert too much pressure that can lead to distortion of the anatomy. For this reason, we prefer using a battery-driven drill rather than a navigated awl or pedicle finder.
- Contamination of the reflective beads with blood.
- Loosening of the reference array on one of the instruments due to mechanical irritation or the use of a mallet to impact the instrument.
- "Skiving" of the navigated instrument off the bone, especially along the lateral facet joint. For this reason it is helpful to try and place the entry point of the instrument over a flat bone surface. The use of a battery-driven drill also minimizes slipping off the bone.

In very rare cases the navigation may truly be off and it may be required to obtain intraoperative control 3-D imaging if that is available and to repeat the navigation steps. We also recommend that screws in the lumbar spine, once placed, should be stimulated and, if possible, their accuracy should be routinely verified using intraoperative 3-D imaging if available. As a cutoff for repositioning, we use 10 mAmps for direct screw stimulation and any medial breach on intraoperative 3-D imaging. Lateral breaches, however, can also be critical if they exceed several millimeters. In experienced hands the rate of screws that need to be repositioned is very low.

11.10 Impact of Navigation on Screw Accuracy and Clinical Outcome

Computer 3-D navigation techniques in spinal instrumentation can improve screw placement accuracy compared to conventional or "freehand" placement of pedicle screws [19–25]. A meta-analysis comparing computer-navigated spine surgery and non-assisted pedicle screw insertions (4814 navigated and 3725 non-navigated) showed that there is a significantly lower risk of pedicle perforation for CAS pedicle screw insertion compared to non-navigated insertion with an overall pedicle perforation risk 6 % for CAS and 15 % for non-navigated insertion [22]. This meta-analysis did not reveal a difference in total operative time or estimated blood loss when comparing the two techniques. In reviewing our experience, we compared navigated versus non-navigated pedicle screw placement in 260 patients and 1,434 screws looking at screw accuracy, screw size, and the complexity of surgery [17]. CAS was associated with improved screw placement accuracy and was employed in cases with a higher degree of surgical complexity such as MISS cases, deformity, and revision surgery. Interestingly, we found that CAS was associated with the use of larger pedicle screws and a higher screw-to-pedicle diameter ratio. This is explained by the ability with CAS to plan and optimize the diameter of the screw used which is important especially in patients with poor bone quality or deformities (Fig. 11.3). A recent systematic literature review of a total of 43 in vitro and clinical papers confirmed that navigation provided higher screw placement accuracy compared with conventional methods [16]. In addition, the authors showed that CT-based and 3-D fluoroscopy-based navigation was more accurate than 2-D fluoroscopy-based navigation system.

Verma et al. performed a systematic review of the literature addressing functional outcome and the incidence of neurological complications between navigation and conventional surgery [26]. The comparison of neurological complications demonstrated an odds ratio in favor of using navigation for pedicle screw insertion; however, there was no statistical significance. The authors concluded that there were insufficient data in the literature to infer a conclusion in terms of fusion rate, pain relief, and health outcome scores. This is the only study so far that has attempted to correlate navigation results to clinical outcome.

11.11 Robotic Surgery

Robotic surgery uses preoperative CT scans for the placement of pedicle screws in the lumbar and thoracic spine [27–29]. For example, the RenaissanceTM is a semiactive surgical guidance robot (Mazor Robotics Ltd., Caesarea, Israel) that has been designed to direct instruments to predetermined locations along the spine. On a graphic user interface with software, the surgeon uses the preoperative CT scan to plan the trajectory of the screws. Intraoperative fluoroscopic X-rays with targeting devices are then matched with the CT-based virtual images, as well as the surgeon's plan. A clamp is attached to the spinous process or a minimally invasive frame is mounted to the iliac crest and a spinous process. The miniature robot is then attached to the clamp and/or frame. The robot aligns itself to the desired entry point and trajectory, as dictated by the surgeon's preoperative plan. Studies using robotic surgery show high levels of implant accuracy for open and percutaneous screw placement [30, 31]. Downsides of robotic surgery include that active tracking is not possible and implant accuracy can only be checked after surgery with a CT scan.

11.12 Future Developments and Outlook

Spinal navigation clearly offers advantages over conventional surgery including greater screw accuracy, reduced radiation exposure, and better planning of the size and position of implants. Therefore, it is surprising to see that CAS is not widely accepted among spine surgeons. The current viewpoint of the spine surgeon on navigation in their everyday practice is an important issue, which has not been studied. A survey-based study was therefore conducted in order to assess opinions on CAS that describe the current global attitudes of surgeons on the use of navigation in spine surgery [32]. This study showed that despite a widespread distribution of navigation systems in North America and Europe, only 11 % of surgeons use it routinely. High-volume surgeons, neurological surgeons, and surgeons with a busy MIS practice are more likely to use CAS. "Routine users" consider the accuracy, potential of facilitating complex surgery, and reduction in radiation exposure as the main advantages. The lack of equipment, inadequate training, and high costs are the main reasons why "non-users" do not use CAS.

These data send strong messages to the community of spine surgeon and their industrial partners:

1. In theory, surgeons generally see value in CAS and almost 80 % hold positive opinions about CAS.
2. In reality, current CAS systems do not meet surgeons' expectations in terms of time efficiency, ease of use, and integration into the surgical workflow.
3. CAS systems have to be affordable and cost-efficient in order to increase their availability.
4. Training has to be more readily available to overcome the demanding learning curve for CAS. This training should not only address individual surgeons but ideally should also include the surgical team in order to improve integration of CAS into the existing work flow.
5. Valid scientific data are needed to clarify the precision of CAS, radiation exposure levels, and cost-effectiveness. This will require well-designed, prospective clinical trials.

In conclusion, navigation in spine surgery is a rapidly evolving field and we are still at an early stage of the technology. More advanced and user-friendly systems that work, for example, with true intraoperative CT scanners are becoming available, and it will be interesting to see how these systems will impact the use and acceptance of navigation [8, 9]. Spinal navigation will move away from the use of K-wires which will minimize the need for intraoperative X-rays use and it will greatly facilitate the work flow. Spine surgeons will increasingly integrate the benefits of microscopic magnification, intraoperative real-time imaging, and pre- and intraoperative planning and 3-D navigation. The future of CAS will include more widespread access to better software and imaging technologies and the combination of CAS with different imaging modalities and possibly intraoperative functional monitoring, such as electrophysiology [33]. There is little doubt that navigation will in the future become a vital part of MIS procedures and a standard armamentarium for spinal surgeons.

References

1. Nolte LP, Zamorano L, Arm E, et al. Image-guided computer-assisted spine surgery: a pilot study on pedicle screw fixation. Stereotact Funct Neurosurg. 1996;66(1–3):108–17.
2. Nolte LP, Zamorano L, Visarius H, et al. Clinical evaluation of a system for precision enhancement in spine surgery. Clin Biomech. 1995;10(6):293–303.
3. Foley KT, Smith MM. Image-guided spine surgery. Neurosurg Clin N Am. 1996;7(2):171–86.
4. Kalfas IH, Kormos DW, Murphy MA, et al. Application of frameless stereotaxy to pedicle screw fixation of the spine. J Neurosurg. 1995;83(4):641–77.
5. Fraser J, Gebhard H, Irie D, Parikh K, Härtl R. Iso-C/3-dimensional neuronavigation versus conventional fluoroscopy for minimally invasive pedicle screw placement in lumbar fusion. Minim Invasive Neurosurg. 2010;53(4):184–90.
6. von Jako RA, Carrino JA, Yonemura KS, et al. Electromagnetic navigation for percutaneous guide-wire insertion: accuracy and efficiency compared to conventional fluoroscopic guidance. Neuroimage. 2009;47 Suppl 2:T127–32.
7. Hott JS, Deshmukh VR, Klopfenstein JD, et al. Intraoperative Iso-C C-arm navigation in craniospinal surgery: the first 60 cases. Neurosurgery. 2004;54(5):1131–6.
8. Scheufler KM, Franke J, Eckardt A, Dohmen H. Accuracy of image-guided pedicle screw placement using intraoperative computed tomography-based navigation with automated referencing. Part II: thoracolumbar spine. Neurosurgery. 2011;69(6):1307–16.
9. Zausinger S, Scheder B, Uhl E, Heigl T, Morhard D, Tonn JC. Intraoperative computed tomography with integrated navigation system in spinal stabilizations. Spine (Phila Pa 1976). 2009;34(26):2919–26.
10. Shin BJ, Njoku IU, Tsiouris AJ, Härtl R. Navigated guide tube for the placement of mini-open pedicle screws using stereotactic 3D navigation without the

use of K-wires: a technical note. J Neurosurg Spine. 2013;18(2):178–83.
11. Nottmeier EW, Fenton D. Three-dimensional image-guided placement of percutaneous pedicle screws without the use of biplanar fluoroscopy or Kirschner wires: technical note. Int J Med Robot. 2010;6(4): 483–8.
12. Luther N, Tomasino A, Parikh K, et al. Neuronavigation in the minimally invasive presacral approach for lumbosacral fusion. Minim Invasive Neurosurg. 2009; 52(4):196–200.
13. Leng LZ, Anand VK, Härtl R, et al. Endonasal endoscopic resection of an os odontoideum to decompress the cervicomedullary junction. Spine. 2009;34(4):E139–43.
14. Laufer I, Greenfield JP, Anand VK, et al. Endonasal endoscopic resection of the odontoid process in a nonachondroplastic dwarf with juvenile rheumatoid arthritis: feasibility of the approach and utility of the intraoperative iso-C three-dimensional navigation. J Neurosurg Spine. 2008;8(4):376–80.
15. Nottmeier EW, Pirris SM, Balseiro S, Fenton D. Three-dimensional image-guided placement of S2 alar screws to adjunct or salvage lumbosacral fixation. Spine J. 2010;10(7):595–601.
16. Tian NF, Huang QS, Zhou P, Zhou Y, Wu RK, Lou Y, Xu HZ. Pedicle screw insertion accuracy with different assisted methods: a systematic review and meta-analysis of comparative studies. Eur Spine J. 2011;20(6):846–59.
17. Iorgulescu JB, Luther N, Geannette C. Comparison of navigated versus non-navigated pedicle screw placement in 260 patients and 1434 screws: screw accuracy, screw size, and the complexity of surgery. 80th AANS Annual Scientific Meeting. Miami. 2012.
18. Nottmeier EW, Bowman C, Nelson KL. Surgeon radiation exposure in cone beam computed tomography-based, image-guided spinal surgery. Int J Med Robot. 2012;8(2):196–200.
19. Assaker R, Reyns N, Vinchon M, Demondion X, Louis E. Transpedicular screw placement: image-guided versus lateral-view fluoroscopy: in vitro simulation. Spine (Phila Pa 1976). 2001;26(19):2160–4.
20. Austin MS, Vaccaro AR, Brislin B, Nachwalter R, Hilibrand AS, Albert TJ. Image-guided spine surgery: a cadaver study comparing conventional open laminoforaminotomy and two image-guided techniques for pedicle screw placement in posterolateral fusion and nonfusion models. Spine (Phila Pa 1976). 2002;27(22):2503–8.
21. Nottmeier EW, Seemer W, Young PM. Placement of thoracolumbar pedicle screws using three-dimensional image guidance: experience in a large patient cohort. J Neurosurg Spine. 2009;10(1):33–9.
22. Shin B, James A, Njoku I, Härtl R. Pedicle screw navigation: a systematic review and meta-analysis of perforation risk for computer navigated versus free-hand insertion. J Neurosurg Spine. 2012;17(2): 113–22.
23. Parker SL, McGirt MJ, Farber SH, et al. Accuracy of free-hand pedicle screws in the thoracic and lumbar spine: analysis of 6816 consecutive screws. Neurosurgery. 2011;68(1):170–8.
24. Rajasekaran S, Vidyadhara S, Ramesh P, Shetty AP. Randomized clinical study to compare the accuracy of navigated and non-navigated thoracic pedicle screws in deformity correction surgeries. Spine (Phila Pa 1976). 2007;32(2):E56-64.
25. Richter M, Mattes T, Cakir B. Computer-assisted posterior instrumentation of the cervical and cervico-thoracic spine. Eur Spine J. 2004;13(1):50–9.
26. Verma R, Krishan S, Haendlmayer K, Mohsen A. Functional outcome of computer-assisted spinal pedicle screw placement: a systematic review and meta-analysis of 23 studies including 5,992 pedicle screws. Eur Spine J. 2010;19(3):370–5.
27. Lieberman IH, Hardenbrook MA, Wang JC, Guyer RD. Assessment of Pedicle Screw Placement Accuracy, Procedure Time, and Radiation Exposure Using a Miniature Robotic Guidance System. J Spinal Disord Tech. 2012;25(5):241–8.
28. Shoham M, Lieberman IH, Benzel EC, et al. Robotic assisted spinal surgery–from concept to clinical practice. Comput Aided Surg. 2007;12(2):105–15.
29. Thomale UW, Kneissler M, Hein A, et al. A spine frame for intra-operative fixation to increase accuracy in spinal navigation and robotics. Comput Aided Surg. 2005;10(3):151–5.
30. Devito DP, Kaplan L, Dietl R, et al. Clinical acceptance and accuracy assessment of spinal implants guided with SpineAssist surgical robot: retrospective study. Spine (Phila Pa 1976). 2010;35(24):2109–15.
31. Kantelhardt SR, Martinez R, Baerwinkel S, Burger R, Giese A, Rohde V. Perioperative course and accuracy of screw positioning in conventional, open robotic-guided and percutaneous robotic-guided, pedicle screw placement. Eur Spine J. 2011;20(6):860–8.
32. Härtl R, Lam KS, Wang J, Korge A, Kandziora F, Audige L. Worldwide survey on the use of navigation in spine surgery. World Neurosurg. 2013;79(1): 162–72.
33. Idler C, Rolfe KW, Gorek JE. Accuracy of percutaneous lumbar pedicle screw placement using the oblique or "owl's-eye" view and novel guidance technology. J Neurosurg Spine. 2010;13(4):509–15.

Nuances of Percutaneous Thoracolumbar Pedicle Screw Fixation

12

D. Greg Anderson

12.1 Introduction

Minimally invasive surgical techniques have grown in popularity in recent years due to the theoretical advantages of smaller incisions, reduced muscle stripping, and a quicker postsurgical recovery [1]. The emergence of new technologies for minimally invasive placement of percutaneous subfascial pedicle screws and rods has allowed surgeons to achieve secure spinal fixation through a limited surgical approach [2–4]. The placement of percutaneous pedicle screws relies on imaging modalities, most commonly the C-arm image intensifier, to visualize the anatomic landmarks necessary for pedicle targeting [1]. The current chapter will focus on the nuances of performing percutaneous pedicle fixation in the thoracolumbar spine using C-arm fluoroscopy.

12.2 Anatomy

12.2.1 Pedicle

The pedicle forms a cylindrical bone bridge between the dorsal spinal elements and the vertebral body. The pedicle has a strong cortical shell with a central core of cancellous bone. Pedicle size and angulation vary significantly throughout the spinal column. In general, the transverse width of the pedicle is less than the pedicle height (Fig. 12.1a). The exception is the L5 pedicle which often has a width that is greater than its height. Pedicles between T10 and L1 generally have a transverse width of at least 7 mm, while pedicles below L1 generally have a transverse width of 8 mm or more. Due to the variability between patients, the best strategy for choosing the ideal implant size is to measure the specific pedicle dimensions from the preoperative imaging studies.

Medial angulation of the pedicles increases as one descends caudally from the thoracolumbar junction through the lumbosacral region (Fig. 12.1b). The nerve roots course along the medial aspect of the pedicle and occupy the rostral portion of the neural foramen. Therefore, violation of the medial or caudal pedicle cortices places the adjacent nerve root at the greatest risk of injury [5, 6]. The precise angulation of the pedicles can best be determined by measuring this parameter on the preoperative imaging studies.

12.2.2 Thoracic Spine

In the thoracic spine, the relationship between the transverse process and the central axis of the pedicles differs compared to the lumbar region and varies by region within the thoracic spine. The pedicle is localized along the cranial portion of the transverse process in the upper thoracic region

D.G. Anderson
Thomas Jefferson University, Philadelphia, PA, USA

M.Y. Wang et al. (eds.), *Minimally Invasive Spinal Deformity Surgery*,
DOI 10.1007/978-3-7091-1407-0_12, © Springer-Verlag Wien 2014

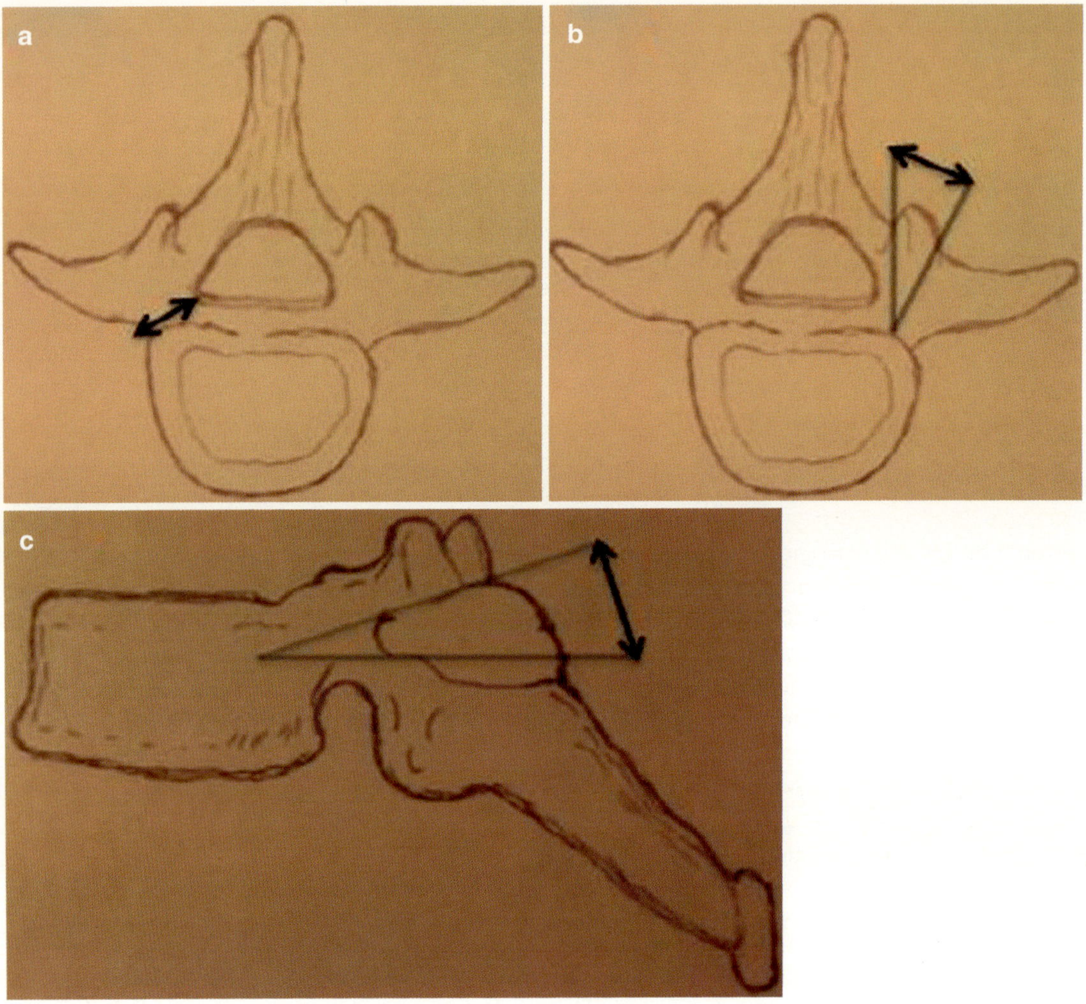

Fig. 12.1 Diagram illustrating pedicle (**a**) width, (**b**) medial angulation (axial plane), and (**c**) sagittal angulation

but is closer to the mid-transverse process in the mid and lower thoracic region. Due to variation between patients, fluoroscopic guidance with the true anterior-posterior (AP) view is helpful to define the exact pedicle location during surgery. The rib head lies along the lateral margin of the thoracic pedicles and adds to the bony corridor available for screw fixation. Both pedicle angulation and vertebral body depth must be considered more carefully in the upper thoracic region, where shorter implants are generally required [5, 6]. The great vessels are at particular risk in the thoracic region if a pedicle screw is misplaced either anteriorly or in a lateral direction on the left side where the aorta may lie along the lateral margin of the pedicle-rib complex [5, 6].

12.2.3 Lumbar Spine

The conventional entry site for pedicle screw placement in the lumbar spine is at the junction of the lateral facet (superior articular process) and mid-portion of the transverse process [5, 6]. The pars interarticularis is generally located at the medial boarder of the pedicle at the L1 to L4 levels and is at the level of the mid-pedicle at L5. Facet hypertrophy may lead to overgrowth of the superior-lateral facet joint which may overlie the pedicle starting point in many cases, particularly in the lower lumbar region. Fortunately, the true AP fluoroscopic view will precisely localize the pedicle and guide the surgeon to the correct starting point. The medial angulation of the pedicles increases from the L1 level (where it is minimal) to the L5 level (where it is generally 15° or more). In some cases, the medial angulation of the pedicles at the L5 level will make the true AP view hard to interpret; in these cases the en face view is helpful to define the pedicle boundaries.

12.3 Principles of Minimally Invasive Spinal Instrumentation

Implantation of a percutaneous pedicle screw construct in the thoracolumbar spine is achieved by following a standard sequence of surgical steps. It is important for the surgeon to adhere to the prescribed surgical steps and to verify the adequacy of each step before continuing on to the next surgical step when following the targeting strategy discussed in this chapter.

Precise localization of all surgical incisions should be done fluoroscopically prior to making the incisions. The incisions should be adequate in size to allow placement of the implants without undue trauma or stretch of the soft tissues. Light bleeding from the percutaneous incisions can generally be controlled with manual pressure at the incision site during pedicle targeting, thus limiting the need for electrocautery.

Good quality, properly aligned imaging is critical for successful targeting of the pedicles in a percutaneous fashion. The surgeon must understand how to obtain and interpret properly aligned fluoroscopic images prior to attempting percutaneous pedicle fixation using the described technique.

12.3.1 Preoperative Planning

Preoperative planning begins by careful analysis of the imaging studies to define the sites for implant placement along with the dimensions and angulation of the specific pedicles to be instrumented. The strategy for surgical incisions should be considered in light of all the surgical goals for the procedure including the need for neurologic decompression and/or posterior element fusion. In some cases, a single skin incision may be used to access separate fascial incisions that can be used to access different regions of the vertebral column [1, 7].

12.3.2 Fluoroscopic Imaging

When performing a minimally invasive surgical approach, the surgeon must obtain good quality fluoroscopic imaging of the vertebral column. The initial procedural step is to position the patient prone on a radiolucent spinal table or frame. The patient should be "squared up" or positioned to reduce trunk rotation. Next, the location of the surgical incisions should be demarcated on the skin using fluoroscopic guidance.

Prior to making any surgical incisions, C-arm images should be obtained and analyzed to verify that the quality of imaging is sufficient and that the pedicles are able to be clearly visualized on properly aligned fluoroscopic images. Severe osteopenia, morbid obesity, or intra-abdominal contrast may preclude adequate visualization of the bony landmarks and prevent safe implantation of percutaneous pedicle screws. In this situation, an alternative surgical technique should be utilized.

The key fluoroscopic views used during the placement of percutaneous thoracolumbar pedicle screws are the true AP view, the true lateral view, and the en face view (Fig. 12.2a–c). Proper alignment of the C-arm is a critical step with each of these fluoroscopic views. A properly aligned true AP image will demonstrate a "flat" superior

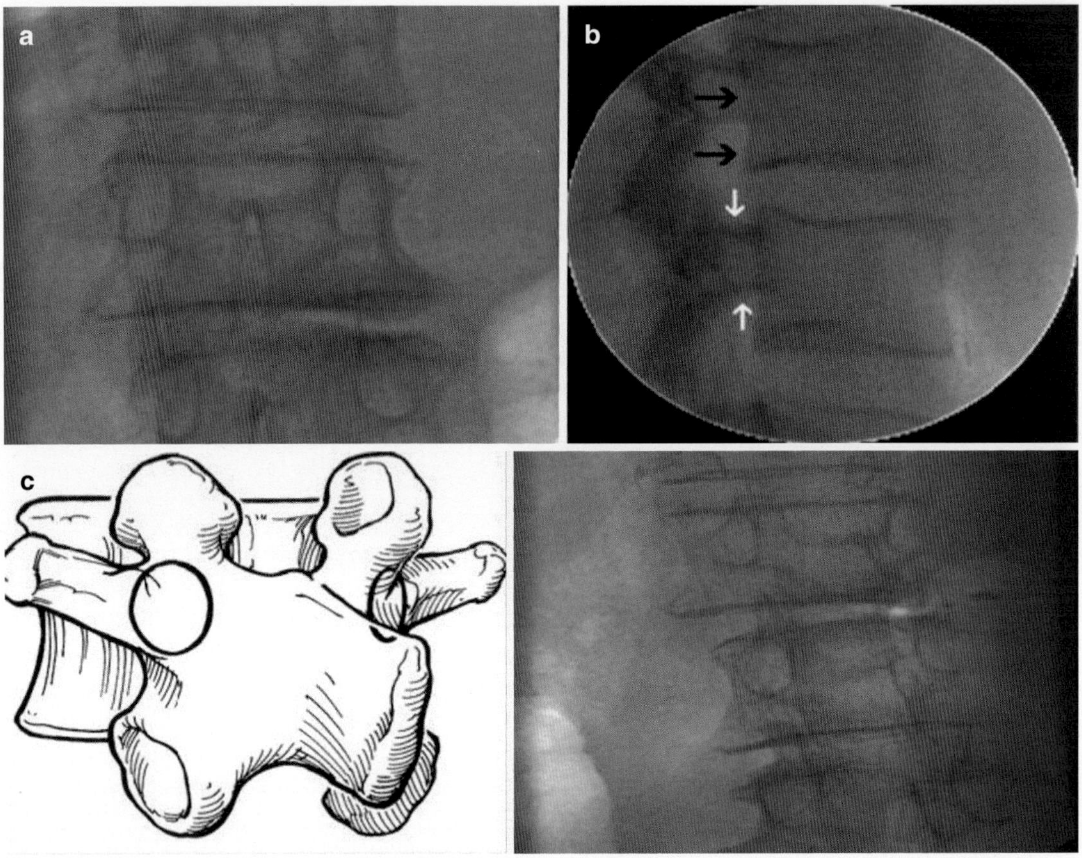

Fig. 12.2 Shows the most useful fluoroscopic views: (**a**) true AP view, (**b**) true lateral view (notice the pedicles are overlapped [*white arrows*] and the posterior cortex of the vertebral body is a single line [*black arrows*], and (**c**) en face view

end plate (only one superior end plate shadow should be seen) [Fig. 12.2a]. The pedicles should be localized just caudal to the superior end plate, and the spinous process should be centered between the pedicles. On the true lateral fluoroscopic image, the superior end plate should again appear "flat." The pedicles should be superimposed. The surgeon should also analyze the posterior cortex of the vertebral body to be sure that there is no malrotation (only a single shadow should be seen) (Fig. 12.2b). Any malrotation should be corrected prior to proceeding. The en face view is obtained by starting with the true AP view and then rotating the C-arm until the fluoroscopic beam is in line with the pedicle axis (Fig. 12.2c). When the C-arm is aligned with the pedicle axis, the greatest medial-lateral width will be seen, and the medial boarder of the superior articular process will generally align along the medial boarder of the pedicle. When targeting a pedicle with the en face view, the middle of the pedicle (not the lateral wall of the pedicle as in the AP view) is targeted. In all cases, it is important that the region of the vertebra that is being targeted is localized in the mid-portion of the fluoroscopic image to ensure that the parallax phenomenon does not lead to misinterpretation of the image.

12.3.3 Facet or Intertransverse Fusion

If fusion of the facet joints of the intertransverse process area is planned, this portion of the procedure should be performed prior to the placement of pedicle screws and rods, which may block

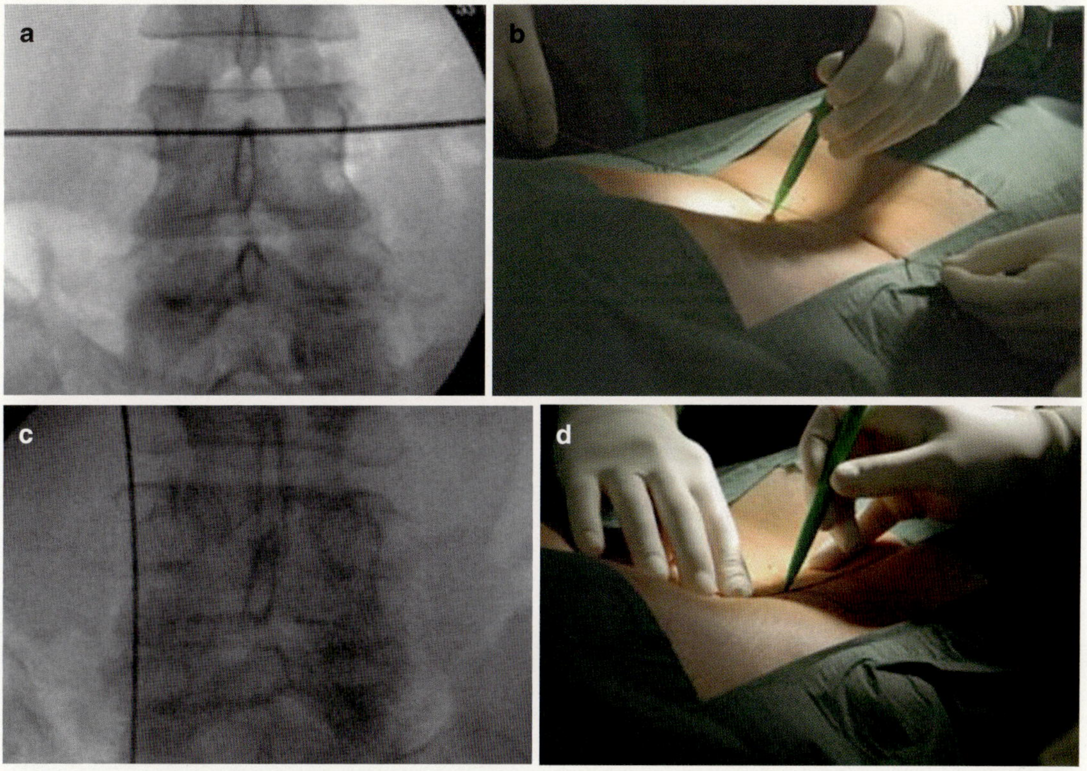

Fig. 12.3 (**a** and **b**) A K wire is placed over the patient's back and a fluoroscopic true AP view is obtained. The K wire is adjusted to demarcate the location of the center of the pedicles. A line is then drawn on the skin corresponding to the center of the pedicles for guidance in making the surgical incisions. (**c** and **d**) The K wire is then aligned over the lateral boarder of the pedicles, and a *vertical line* is demarcated on the skin. The skin incisions should be made 1.5–2 cm lateral to the intersection of the *vertical and horizontal lines* at each level

access to these regions. When performing a facet fusion, a tubular retractor may be used to provide access to the facet joint for decortications and grafting. To perform an intertransverse fusion, the intermuscular plane between the multifidus and longissimus muscles can be used to gain access to the intertransverse region for meticulously decorticated and grafting. After the grafting has been completed, the retractor can be withdrawn, and percutaneous targeting of the pedicles can be performed as described below.

12.3.4 Marking Out the Surgical Incision

Using the true AP view, a horizontal line is drawn on the skin corresponding to the mid-pedicle at each vertebral level (Fig. 12.3a, b). The sagittal plane angulation of the true AP views of each level can be recorded on the C-arm, by placing a tape next to the angle indicators and marking the angulation of the particular level (Fig. 12.4). This will facilitate rapid return to the properly angulated view for each level later in the case. In similar fashion, vertical lines are drawn along the lateral boarders of the pedicle in the construct (Fig. 12.4a, b). The skin incisions are generally positioned 1.5–2 cm lateral to the intersection of the vertical and horizontal lines for each level. In more obese patients, a slightly more lateral skin incision should be utilized.

12.3.5 Percutaneous Pedicle Targeting

After the incisions have been demarcated, the skin and fascia are sharply incised. Blunt finger dissection may be used to gently palpate the base of the transverse process as a guide to Jamshidi needle placement. A Jamshidi needle or similar instrument is "docked" against the bone at the base of the transverse process. The location of the needle tip is then evaluated using the true AP fluoroscopic view, and the needle tip is adjusted as needed to localize the needle tip at the 9 o'clock pedicle position on the left and 3 o'clock position on the right (Fig. 12.5). Once the needle tip is in the correct position, the needle is gently tapped to penetrate the cortex to a depth of about 2–3 mm (bone divot), which will prevent needle slippage. The shaft of the needle is then marked 20 mm above the skin edge (Fig. 12.7). The markings allow the surgeon to follow the depth of needle tip as it is passed through the pedicle. The needle is then held with the proper lateral to medial angulation corresponding to the central pedicle axis on the axial plane (as determined by fluoroscopic image and preoperative planning). The needle must also be aligned for the sagittal plane, which can be done by ensuring that on the true AP view, the needle shaft appears to be parallel to the superior end plate. With the needle in proper alignment, it is tapped through the pedicle until the marking on the needle shaft reaches the skin edge. When the marking on the needle shaft reaches the skin edge, the needle tip has traversed the pedicle to a depth corresponding the junction of the pedicle and vertebral body.

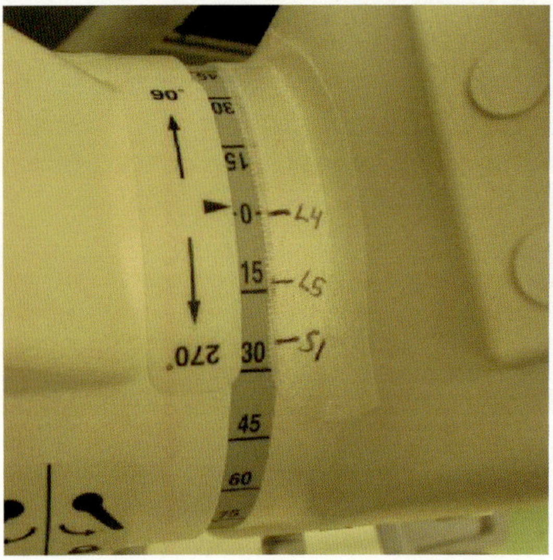

Fig. 12.4 Tape is placed along the C-arm angle indicator, and marks are made corresponding to the sagittal plane angulation of the L4, L5, and S1 levels. This will facilitate rapid return to properly oriented views of each level

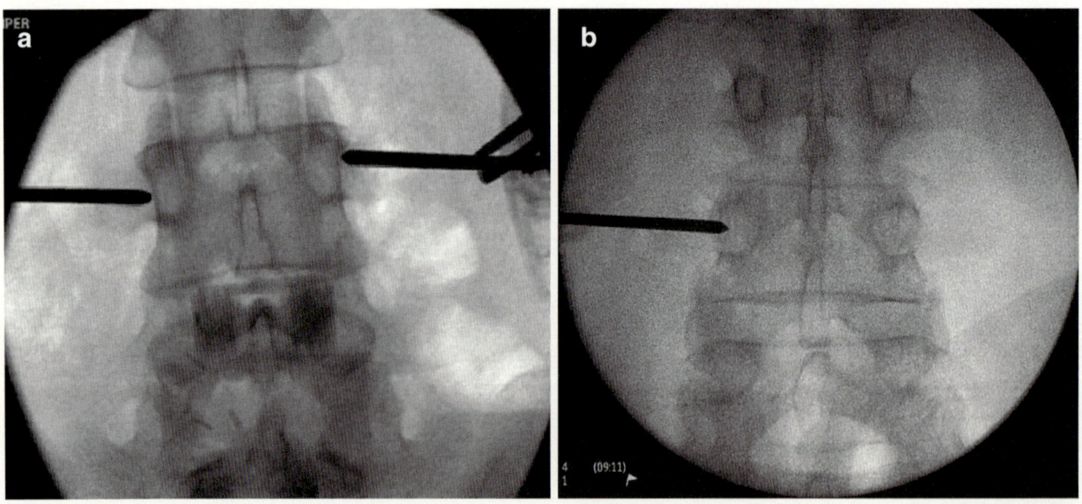

Fig. 12.5 (**a**) True AP images show docking of the Jamshidi needle over the lateral wall of the pedicle at the 9 o'clock pedicle position on the *left* and the 3 o'clock position on the *right*; notice the needle needs to be aligned in the sagittal plane prior to insertion by making the needle shaft *parallel* to the superior end plates of the vertebral body; (**b**) the needle tip is seen just inside the 9 o'clock position after it has been tapped about 2–3 mm into the cortex of the bone to prevent needle slippage, and the needle has been aligned in the sagittal plane

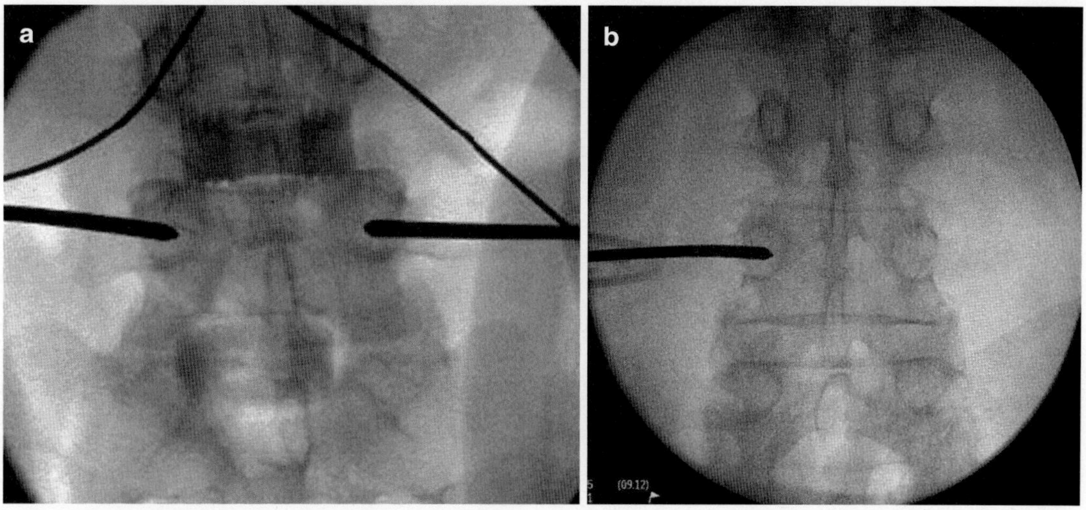

Fig. 12.6 (**a**) Jamshidi needles at approximately 20 mm depth within the pedicle. The needle tip is localized approximately at the junction of the pedicle and vertebral body. The needle tips are both between ½ and ¾ of the distance (from lateral to medial) across the pedicle and thus in an acceptable position. (**b**) Another view of a Jamshidi needle at the 20 mm depth in acceptable position

When the needle has penetrated the pedicle to a depth of approximately 20 mm, an AP fluoroscopic view is obtained, and the tip of the needle is analyzed relative to the pedicle shadow. The needle tip should appear within the pedicle shadow between ½ and ¾ of the distance across the pedicle (from lateral to medial) (Fig. 12.6). Once the needle position has been confirmed, a guide wire is introduced through the needle shaft and penetrated into the vertebral body to a depth of about 20 mm beyond the end of the needle shaft. This can often be done manually, or a clamp may be applied to the guide wire 20 mm above the top of the needle shaft, and then the clamp can be tapped until it reaches the top of the needle shaft.

Tactile feedback provides important information to the surgeon throughout the procedure. For instance, the Jamshidi needle should pass smoothly through the pedicle with light to moderate mallet taps. If excessively hard bone is encountered, it is likely that the needle tip has been misplaced medially into the facet joint and is encountering the articular surface of the superior articular process. In this situation, the needle will need to be removed and a more lateral starting point utilized. Often a thin, firm bony layer is encountered at the junction of the pedicle and vertebral body which serves as an additional clue to the needle depth. When guide wires are inserted through the needle shaft, cancellous bone should be palpated at the floor of the needle shaft. The guide wire can generally be passed through the cancellous bone of the vertebral body using manual finger pressure. The cancellous bone of the vertebral body has a characteristic "crunchy" feel during this maneuver.

12.3.6 Pedicle Screw and Rod Insertion

After each of the pedicles in the construct has been successfully targeted and guide wires have been placed, the C-arm should be adjusted to the true lateral projection, and the position of each guide wire should be confirmed on a lateral fluoroscopic image (see Fig. 12.8). Next, a cannulated pedicle preparation instrument (e.g., bone tap) is used to expand the pedicle passage. It is important for the surgeon to maintain manual control of the guide wires throughout this process to prevent inadvertent anterior migration or guide wire dislodgement (see Fig. 12.9). Once the pedicle preparation instrument has passed the base of the pedicle, stimulus-evoked electromyography can

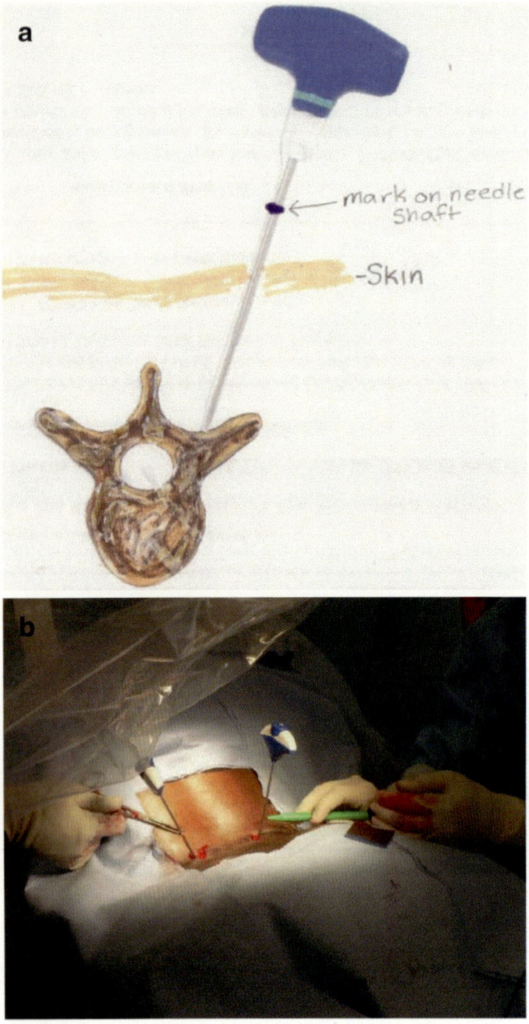

Fig. 12.7 (**a**) Diagram showing the marking of a Jamshidi needle 20 mm above the skin edge, (**b**) picture of marking of the Jamshidi needle 20 mm above the skin edge

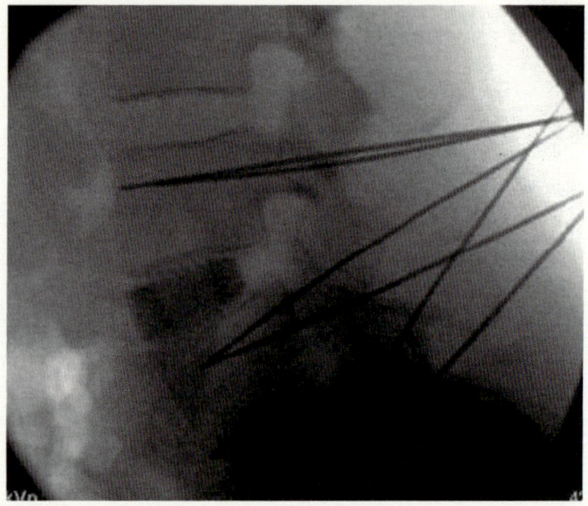

Fig. 12.8 True lateral fluoroscopic image of L4 with guide wires in place

be utilized, according to surgeon preference, to test the voltage threshold of each pedicle site (see Fig. 12.10). An absence of low-voltage activity suggests the absence of a pedicle wall breech.

Cannulated pedicle screws are then inserted over the guide wires. It is important to ensure that the pedicle screws are placed to a depth such that they form a smooth contour to facilitate rod capture (Fig. 12.11). The contour of the screws can be accessed by evaluating the height of the screw extensions. Adjustment of the screw height can be made, as necessary, to achieve a smooth contour between adjacent pedicle screws.

Rod measurement is generally performed with a measuring device provided by the pedicle screw manufacture. Once a rod of appropriate length has been selected, rod contouring should be performed. The surgeon can obtain a good estimate of the rod contour by evaluating the contour of the screw extensions (Fig. 12.12). However, in spinal deformity cases, the contour of the rod will need to accommodate the planned deformity correction.

Rod passage typically uses a rod handle. Generally speaking, the rod is passed sequentially through the screw extensions, beginning at one end of the construct. Rod passage requires some tactile awareness to "feel" the tip of the rod entering each screw extension. Once the rod has successfully passed into a screw extension, the rotation of that extension becomes fixed, and this confirms successful rod capture. Steering of the rod during rod passage is achieved by manipulation of the rod handle and in some cases by manipulation of the screw extensions. Rod passage and capture is generally more difficult in long constructs and those with significant deformity. However, with some practice most surgeons

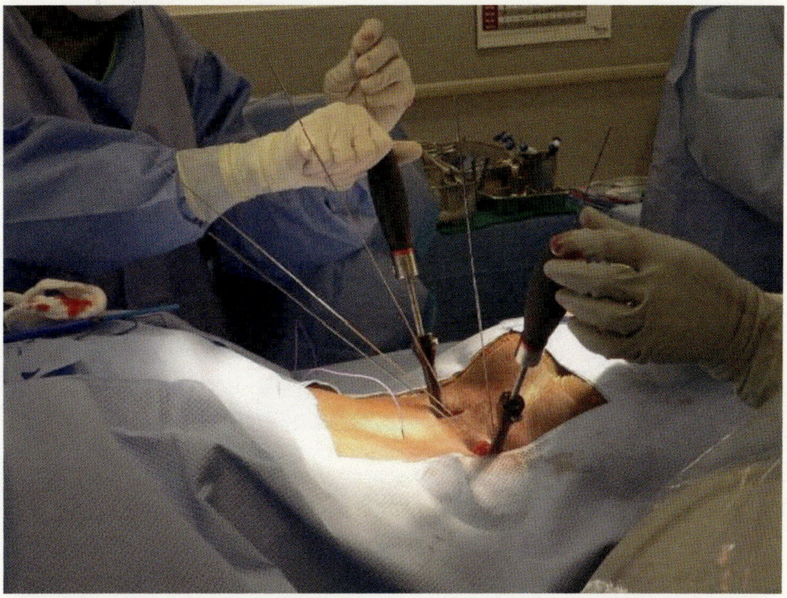

Fig. 12.9 The surgeon must manually hold the guide wire while tapping or inserting pedicle screws to prevent wire migration or dislodgement

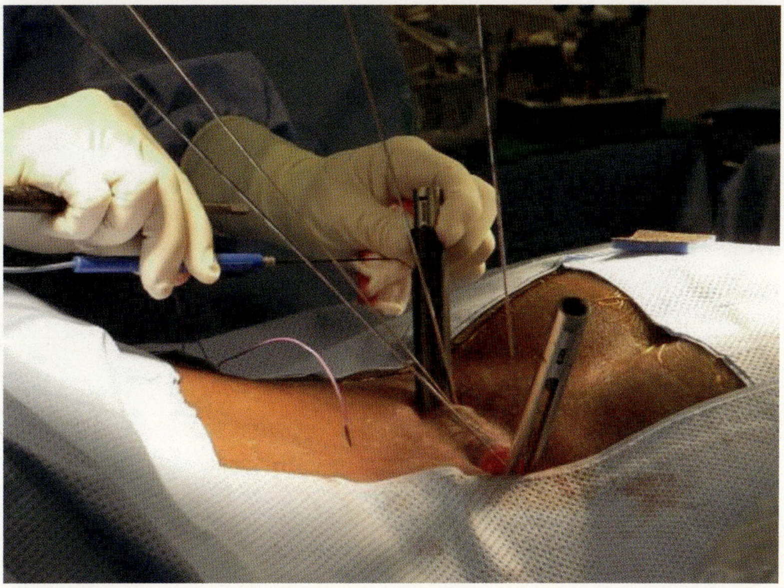

Fig. 12.10 The surgeon is using stimulus-evoked electromyography to test the integrity of the pedicle

can learn to successfully pass percutaneous rods even in multi-level deformity cases.

Once the rod has been successfully passed, the screw cap at the end of the construct (generally opposite the rod handle) is placed to prevent rod slippage, and then the rod handle can be detached. Next, the cap at the most lordotic portion of the construct should be placed. This is done to seat the rod into the screws with the proper rotational orientation to match the necessary lordosis of the construct. The remainder of the screw caps are then placed sequentially, using rod persuasion as needed to achieve reduction of the rod into the screw heads. Depending on the goals of the

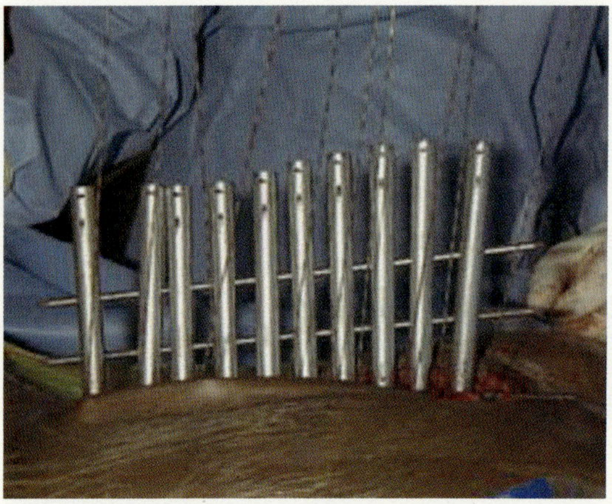

Fig. 12.11 The tops of the screw extensions form a smooth contour which will facilitate rod passage and rod/screw capture

surgical procedure, compression or distraction may be applied to the construct to achieve adjustments in the vertebral position prior to final tightening. Once the construct is in the desired position, the construct is securely tightened to lock the construct in place.

After final tightening, the screw extensions are detached, and wound closure is performed in a routine manner. The authors prefer to use subcuticular stitches with a skin sealant (e.g., Dermabond, Ethicon, Cornelia, GA). Local anesthetic agents, injected at the surgical site, are helpful to limit postoperative discomfort. Patients are generally mobilized as rapidly as possible following surgery. Rehabilitation and follow-up imaging are planned according to the nature of the surgical procedure.

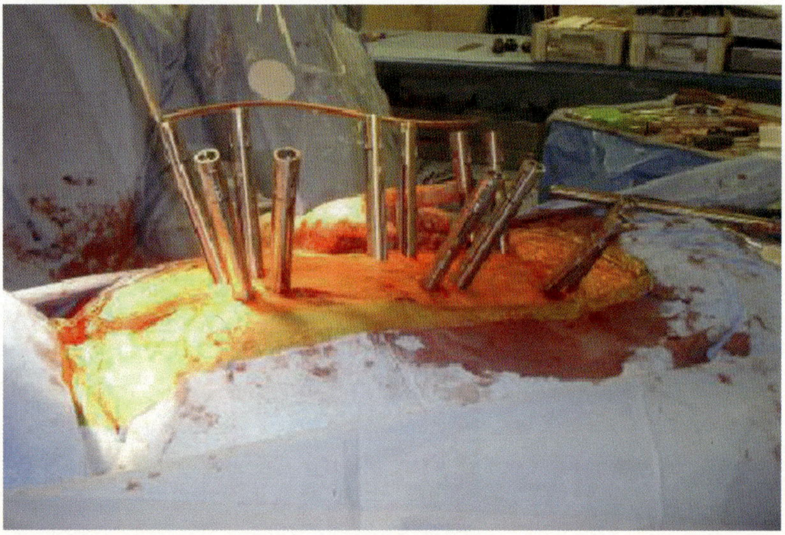

Fig. 12.12 Rod contouring is performed to match the sagittal plane alignment of the construct. Both rod length and contouring can be estimated by evaluating the screw extensions

Conclusion

Thoracolumbar percutaneous pedicle screw instrumentation and fusion can be achieved through a series of well-defined and reproducible surgical steps. To achieve good results, the surgeon must be familiar with obtaining and interpreting C-arm fluoroscopic images and have a good understanding of the three-dimensional anatomy of the spinal column. A variety of surgical nuances have been learned over time which may prove useful to the surgeons who wish to become proficient in the use of percutaneous instrumentation. Fortunately, the benefits of reduced patient morbidity and improved recovery from surgery far outweigh the efforts and learning curve associated with gaining these surgical skills.

References

1. Harris EB, Massey P, Lawrence J, Rihn J, Vaccaro A, Anderson DG. Percutaneous techniques for minimally invasive posterior lumbar fusion. Neurosurg Focus. 2008;25(2):E12.
2. Foley KT, Gupta SK. Percutaneous pedicle screw fixation of the lumbar spine: preliminary clinical results. J Neurosurg. 2002;97(1):7–12.
3. Anderson DG, Samartzis D, Shen FH, Tannoury C. Percutaneous instrumentation of the thoracic and lumbar spine. Orthop Clin North Am. 2007;38(3): 401–8.
4. Khoo LT, Palmer S, Laich DT, Fessler RG. Minimally invasive percutaneous posterior lumbar interbody fusion. Neurosurgery. 2002;51(5):S166–1.
5. Benzel EC. Spine surgery: techniques, complication avoidance, and management. New York: Churchill Livingstone; 2005. p. 1054.
6. Zindrick MR, Wiltse LL, Widell EH, Thomas JC, Holland WR, Field BT, Spencer CW. A biomechanical study of intrapedicular screw fixation in the lumbosacral spine. Clin Orthop Relat Res. 1986;203: 99–112.
7. Kim DH, Jaikumar S, Kam AC. Minimally invasive spine instrumentation. Neurosurgery. 2002;51(5):S15–25.

Rod Contouring, Passage, and Connection

13

Bernhard Meyer, Michelle Falcone, Michael Y. Wang, Yi Lu, and Steven Wu

Despite being a somewhat trite topic at first glance, most surgeons familiar with minimally invasive posterior spinal fixation know that contouring, passing, and connecting rods can be a challenging and cumbersome step in these procedures. This was particularly the case with the first generation of MIS instrumentation. Short-segment percutaneous posterior fixation (i.e., monosegmental or bisegmental) for various indications – primarily fractures – could be accomplished without special instruments or modifications of implants [1]. However, the advent of advance MIS techniques required the development of specially designed instruments to accomplish multi-level screw-rod fixation [2].

Early attempts were problematic for fixation beyond 3 segments and even more harrowing when a major deformity was present. The prerequisite for this were specially designed instruments and implants, which are now available from several medical device companies in the field. However, this required a migration away from automated rod passage systems which were very effective for connecting two or even three screw heads but had limited flexibility in connecting more fixation points. The key features with respect to the problem described in this chapter are the (a) reduction screw extenders and (b) a steerable rod inserter to allow for the passage of longer precontoured rods without direct visual feedback under fluoroscopic and tactile control. Large extender windows over the screw tulips and the possibility of gradual reduction under visual control (by means of scales on the proximal end of the extender) are more or less mandatory elements as well as a tight and robust rod/inserter interface. In addition, the use of rod entry point estimators, rod length confirmation tools, and external markers on proximal extenders to facilitate alignment has been helpful.

Between 2008 and 2010, the first meaningful series of long-segment fixation were published [3–6] describing the feasibility, safety, and limitations of this approach. Most patients in these series were primarily less complicated cases of adult degenerative deformities (i.e., those limited to the lumbar spine or shorter curves). While multiple techniques are available for achieving successful rod contouring, passage, and connection, the following is the description of my approach and strategy for meeting these challenges. One also has to keep in mind that this is a continually

B. Meyer (✉)
Department of Neurosurgery, Klinikum rechts der Isar, Technical University of Munich, Ismaningerstr. 22, 81672 Munich, Germany
e-mail: bernhard.meyer@lz.tum.de

M. Falcone • M.Y. Wang
Department of Neurological Surgery, University of Miami, Jackson Memorial Hospital, Miami, FL 33163, USA

Y. Lu, M.D., Ph.D.
Department of Neurosurgery, Brigham and Women's Hospital, Harvard Medical School, Boston, MA, USA
e-mail: ylu4@partners.org

S. Wu
Department of Neurosurgery, Brigham and Women's Hospital, Harvard Medical School, Boston, MA, USA

M.Y. Wang et al. (eds.), *Minimally Invasive Spinal Deformity Surgery*, DOI 10.1007/978-3-7091-1407-0_13, © Springer-Verlag Wien 2014 evolving field, with advances in techniques, technology, and instrumentation occurring regularly.

During preoperative planning, several key interdependent features must be assessed, which will determine the degree of difficulty to be expected during any rod maneuver:

1. Length of the construct
2. Severity of coronal and sagittal deformity
3. Desired/necessary degree of reduction
4. The number of distinct curves the rod must traverse
5. Any complicated connections, such as with iliosacral screws

These elements exist in concert with comprehensive classifications that may trigger differential treatment [7].

1. *Length of construct*: Since almost all cases are Schwab type V or IV with a preponderance of the former [8], the vast majority of constructs can be considered as short (up to L2) or intermediate (up to T10). They will thus comprise (depending on the inclusion of S1) either 4 or less segments in the former group or up to 8 in the latter.
2. *Severity of deformity*: Coronal Cobb angles >30° as well as subluxations>6 mm will increase the difficulty. Any major sagittal imbalance [9, 10], which is a major limiting factor in MIS corrections, also complicates the correction. If the construct is considered and requires extension to the construct to the upper thoracic area, then two curves must typically be traversed (thoracolumbar and lumbosacral) [10].
3. *Degree of correction*: The degree of sagittal correction can be critical to optimal outcomes. If the sagittal vertical axis (SVA) exceeds 10 cm, osteotomies will be needed for correction. This also limits the ability of the surgeon to pass a single rod, as it is not possible to pass a lordotic rod into a severely kyphotic spine. Thus a two-rod technique may have to be utilized. Non-kyphotic deformities can often be corrected through appropriate contouring with anterior releases [11, 12]. Coronal deformities even below 30° cannot be properly corrected with derotation techniques alone [13, 14] given the stiffness of the spine. In these cases appropriate anterior or intersomatic releases may be necessary using multiple MIS TLIFs or anterolateral approaches. Curves greater than 30° should be preferentially reduced below this limit by anterior asymmetric release and intersomatic fusion. A reduction of the remaining curve is then possible by derotation.
4. *The number of distinct curves the rod must traverse*: Passing a rod through both the thoracolumbar and lumbosacral junctions requires the rod to be in an "S" shape to have the proper final contour. Thus, it may not be possible to access all the screw saddles appropriately without a small opening in the muscle fascia.
5. *Any complicated connections, such as with iliosacral screws*: Since the iliac screw heads will be offset laterally and dorsally to pedicle screws, proper screw entry site planning is critical. Starting the sacral screws in a more cranial position and leaving them 3–6 mm proud, along with starting the iliac screws caudally and more ventrally, can improve the ease of connections. However, it is also often necessary to place a small lateral bend in the caudal aspect of the rods as well.

The following steps would be performed in a long-segment MIS deformity surgery:

- Once all screws and screw extenders are in place and lined up with the aid of the markers and lateral fluoroscopy, the rod measurement tool is placed on the skin next to the extenders after being bent to be in contact with the skin over the complete length.
- A rod of the corresponding length is firmly attached to the steerable rod inserter before any contouring. Compensation for any curvature is critical. The rod is then bent in the appropriate planes to achieve the desired degree of deformity correction.
- Starting on the concave side, the most cephalad extender is held perpendicular to the skin, and the rod entry point estimator is attached to mark the place for the stab incision. Rods are often inserted in a cranio-caudal direction for safety reasons. Laminar shingling minimizes the risk of unintentional rod passage into the spinal canal.
- The passage of the rod is controlled by lateral fluoroscopy to ensure that it remains below the muscle fascia. Movements should be smooth without excessive force. Once the rod is in the first window, this can be controlled with a rod confirmation tool brought into the

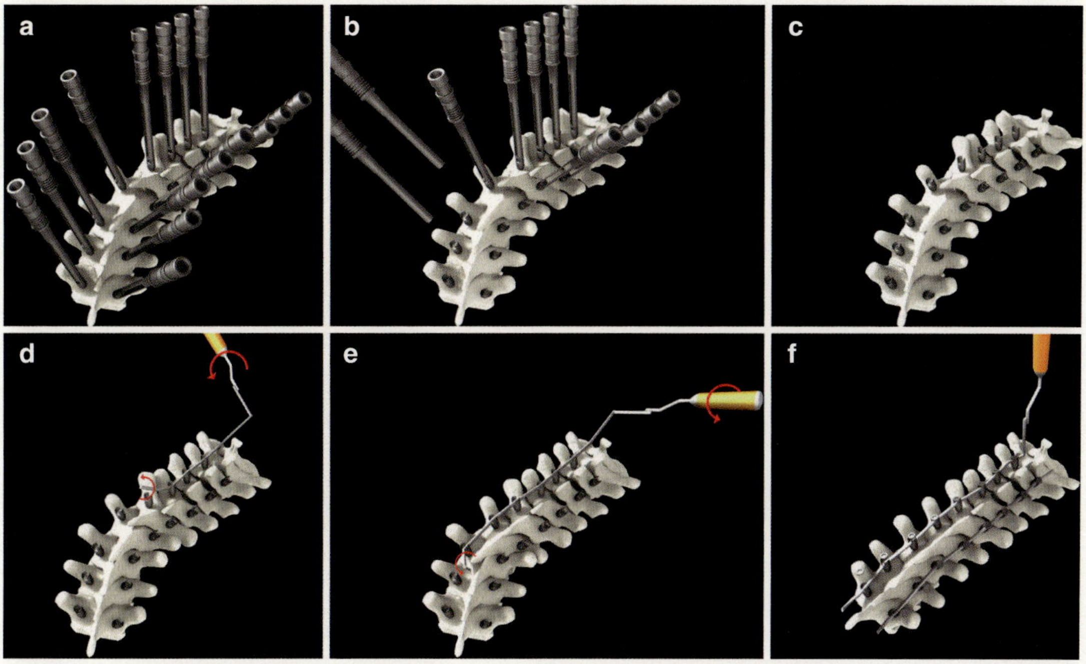

Fig. 13.1 Rod passage with rotation of the rod along its long axis to drive the rod laterally or medially to engage all the screw heads in a deformed spine. This requires a bend at the leading portion of the rod

extender shaft or by slightly twisting the extender. This is repeated for every screw.

- The complete passage requires twisting movements of the inserter up to 90° to both sides along the long axis of the rod to "steer it medially or laterally" (Fig. 13.1). A combination of tactile feedback and fluoroscopic control is used.
- From the center to periphery, the extenders are then reduced in a stepwise fashion with the aid of the reduction nuts, which are facilitated by the markers visible on the extender ends. Usually three rounds are needed until complete reduction to allow successive correction to avoid screw pullout.
- The contralateral rod is inserted after the necessary pre-contouring. The inserter is detached after all set screws are tight and final imaging control, has been performed.

References

1. Ringel F, Stoffel M, Stüer C, Meyer B. Percutaneous transmuscular pedicle screw fixation of the thoracic and lumbar spine. Neurosurgery. 2006;59(ONS Suppl 4):361–7.
2. Foley KT, Gupta SK. Percutaneous pedicle screw fixation of the lumbar spine: preliminary clinical results. J Neurosurg. 2002;97 Suppl 1:7–12.
3. Wang MY, Anderson DG, Poelstra KA, Ludwig SC. Minimally invasive posterior fixation. Neurosurgery. 2008;63 Suppl 3:197–203.
4. Anand N, Baron EM, Thaiyananthan G, Khalsa K, Goldstein TB. Minimally invasive multilevel percutaneous correction and fusion for adult lumbar degenerative scoliosis: a technique and feasibility study. J Spinal Disord Tech. 2008;21(7): 459–67.
5. Wang MY, Mummaneni PV. Minimally invasive surgery for thoracolumbar spinal deformity: initial clinical experience with clinical and radiographic outcomes. Neurosurg Focus. 2010;28(3):E9.
6. Scheufler KM, Cyron D, Dohmen H, Eckardt A. Less invasive surgical correction of adult degenerative scoliosis, part I: technique and radiographic results. Neurosurgery. 2010;67(3):696–710.
7. Silva FE, Lenke LG. Adult degenerative scoliosis: evaluation and management. Neurosurg Focus. 2010;28(3):E1.
8. Schwab F, Farcy JP, Bridwell K, et al. A clinical impact classification of scoliosis in the adult. Spine (Phila Pa 1976). 2006;31(18):2109–14.
9. Villard J, Ringel F, Meyer B. Sagittal balance: a useful tool for neurosurgeons. Adv Tech Stand Neurosurg. 2012 (in press).
10. Le Huec JC, Charosky S, Barrey C, Rigal J, Aunoble S. Sagittal imbalance cascade for simple degenerative spine and consequences: algorithm of decision for appropriate treatment. Eur Spine J. 2011;20 Suppl 5:699–703.

11. Acosta F, Liu J, Slimack N, Moller D, Fessler R, Koski T. Changes in coronal and sagittal plane alignment following minimally invasive direct lateral interbody fusion for the treatment of degenerative lumbar disease in adults: a radiographic study. J Neurosurg. 2011;15:92–6.
12. Khoo LT, Palmer S, Laich DT, Fessler RG. Minimally invasive percutaneous posterior lumbar interbody fusion. Neurosurgery. 2002;51:S166–81.
13. Cheng JS, Lebow RL, Schmidt MH, Spooner J. Rod derotation techniques for thoracolumbar spinal deformity. Neurosurgery. 2008;63 Suppl 3:149–56.
14. Lee SM, Suk SI, Chung E-R. Direct vertebral rotation: a new technique of three dimensional deformity correction with segmental pedicle screw fixation in adolescent idiopathic scoliosis. Spine. 2004;29(3): 343–9.

14 Percutaneous Sacropelvic Fixation

Michael Y. Wang

14.1 Introduction

Lumbopelvic fixation has increasingly become an important adjunct for stabilization of the lumbosacral spine. The ability to place larger diameter and longer screws anterior to the center of gravity of the body promotes stability both regionally and globally and can also reduce the likelihood of a pseudarthrosis or hardware construct failure [20]. For these reasons, the use of iliac screws and bolts has become popular since the original descriptions of the precursors to these methods by Allen and Ferguson [1].

Current indications for iliac screw fixation include situations where substantial biomechanical stabilization is required in the lumbosacral spine. This includes settings with long constructs, spinal deformity, severe osteoporosis, a previous failed fusion, or severe instability due to trauma, tumor, or infection [3, 6, 7, 10]. In addition, iliac fixation is useful in cases where no other feasible caudal fixation points are available, such as for revision fusion surgery. Because the human pelvis contains a significant cancellous bone space bordered by inner and outer cortical walls, screws or bolts of a substantial diameter and length can be placed safely for fixation. This allows the placement of screws between 65 and 120 mm in length and 7.0–10.0 mm in diameter [16].

While the placement of iliac screws has become widely accepted, there remain several methods for ensuring proper hardware placement. Manual digital palpation of the lateral iliac wing to the sciatic notch allows the surgeon to directly determine the screw trajectory and bony confines manually. More recently indirect palpation of the inner cortical walls of the pelvis using a curved pedicle finder has been advocated, minimizing the need for soft tissue disruption. In either case extensive muscular dissection over the posterior superior iliac spine is needed to expose the screw entry points.

Pain secondary to iliac screw placement may be due to several causes, including hardware prominence, disruption of the sacroiliac joint, and screw loosening [4]. However, local soft tissue destruction and muscular devitalization for surgical exposure may play a role as well. For these reasons, we have sought to develop a method for the minimally invasive placement of iliac screws.

Percutaneous pedicle screw fixation techniques have now become widely accepted as an option for lumbosacral fixation [2, 5, 8, 9, 11–14, 17]. The general principle of percutaneous pedicle screw instrumentation has been fluoroscopically guided K-wire placement followed by screw tract preparation and hardware placement using cannulated instruments and implants. The use of screw extensions then allows the surgeon to control the implant and secure and connect it to the adjacent levels.

M.Y. Wang, M.D., FACS
Departments of Neurological Surgery &
Rehab Medicine, University of Miami Miller
School of Medicine, 1095 NW 14th Terrace,
Lois Pope Life Center, D4-6, Miami, FL 33136, USA
e-mail: mwang2@med.miami.edu

M.Y. Wang et al. (eds.), *Minimally Invasive Spinal Deformity Surgery*,
DOI 10.1007/978-3-7091-1407-0_14, © Springer-Verlag Wien 2014

We have sought to extend these methods for application in sacropelvic fixation and initially described the technique in a case report [19]. We have since expanded the application of this method report here our preliminary results with image-based percutaneous iliac screw placement.

14.2 Surgical Technique for Image-Based Iliac Targeting

X-ray imaging is used to visualize the body of the ischium by angling the fluoroscope in a steep Ferguson view in the sagittal plane and in the plane of the ilium in the coronal plane. This "obturator outlet view" allowed for visualization of the inner and outer tables as well as the "teardrop" configuration of the ischial body (Figs. 14.1 and 14.2). This teardrop shape is the overlapping of the two-dimensional projection of the inner and outer tables of the ilium from medially to laterally [15]. Thus, targeting this region insures proper screw placement.

The screw entry site is located just ventral to the posterior superior iliac spine (PSIS). A drill or small osteotome is used to remove the cortical bone so that the screw head may be recessed to minimize hardware prominence. This entry site into the cancellous bone also minimizes the risk of inadvertent entry into the sacroiliac joint. A Jamshidi needle is then advanced to a depth of 80 mm under fluoroscopic guidance to keep the tip of the needle within the teardrop. This is followed by K-wire exchange and placement of a cannulated awl, tap, and instrumentation with Viper™ titanium alloy percutaneous iliac screws (Depuy Spine, Inc, Raynham, Massachusetts).

Hardware connections were made between screws and rods with the assistance of screw extensions. Subfascial rod passage was performed in a cranial to caudal direction by inserting the rod through the most cranial screw's incision. This allowed for precise control of the length of rod passed beyond the iliac screw saddle distally in an effort to minimize hardware prominence. In several cases two-plane rod bending was necessary to place the distal rod laterally to meet the iliac screw head.

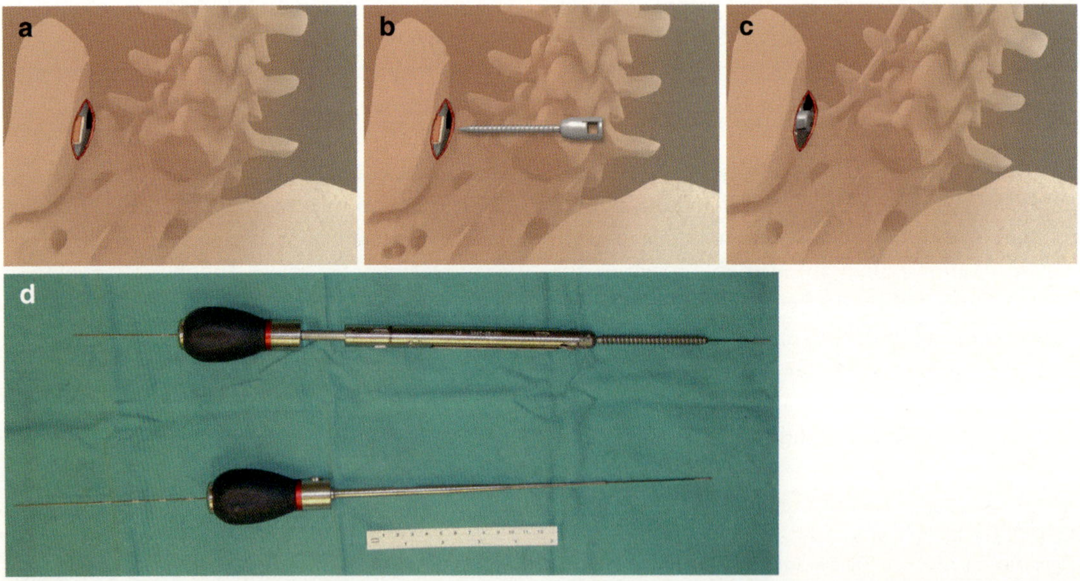

Fig. 14.1 (**a–c**) Artist's depiction of a technique for minimally invasive sacroiliac screw placement. A small skin and muscle opening is placed medial to the PSIS to allow entry into the cancellous bone. Cannulation then occurs under fluoroscopic guidance. (**d**) Percutaneous cannulated iliac screws measuring 8 mm in diameter and 65 mm long

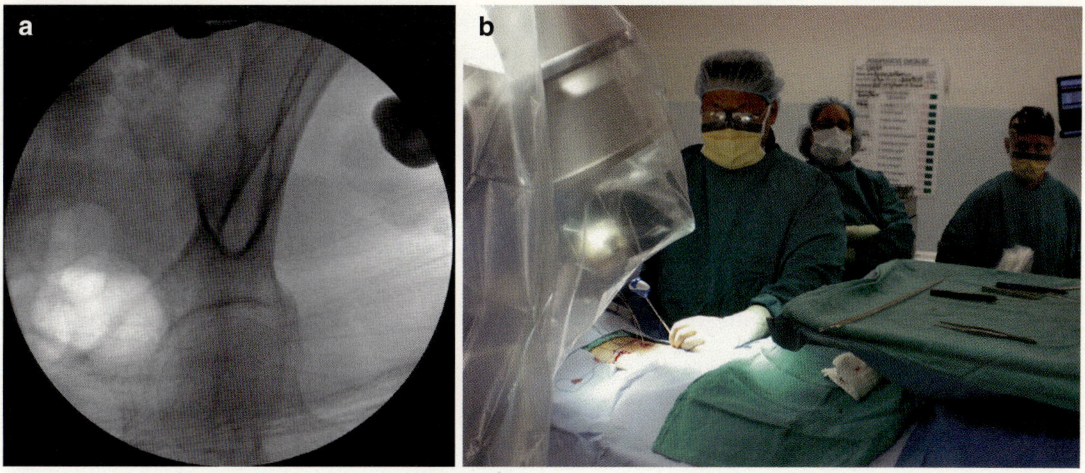

Fig. 14.2 (**a**) Obturator outlet view with fluoroscopy demonstrating the "teardrop" projection as the idealized endpoint for the screw tip. (**b**) Intraoperative view show the coronal and sagittal angulation needed to obtain the obturator outlet view to allow percutaneous screw placement over a guidewire, with screw extensions to allow for construct assembly

14.3 Clinical Applications

We have placed 61 sacropelvic screws using this technique [18]. All patients underwent CT scanning with three-dimensional reconstruction to assess screw placement and were found to have no bony breaches. This experience has increased our confidence that the targeting method innovated by Chapman and colleagues is reliable and safe. Furthermore, use of the obturator outlet view does not require special equipment, image guidance, or other advance technique.

We have applied percutaneous iliac screws in the settings of spinal infection, trauma, deformity, and neoplasia (Figs. 14.3, 14.4, and 14.5). In these settings, its use has been for the same indications and biomechanical purposes as traditional open sacroiliac fixation. It should also be noted that later explantation of screws may also be necessary given the relatively high rates of screw loosening with long-term follow-up after fusion has occurred.

One drawback of the technique may be that screw explantation is more difficult than when using an offset connector. While we have a limited experience with explantations, it would require mobilization of the rod from the screw saddle a sufficient distance to allow screw removal, as opposed to open cases where the offset connector can simply be disengaged.

One of the practical drawbacks of this minimally invasive method involves the difficulties associated with connecting complex three-dimensional constructs beneath the fascia. For example, mating S1 pedicle and iliac screws will often require a lateral offset connector or complex two-plane rod bending given the more lateral and dorsal location of the iliac screw head (Fig. 14.6). We initially avoided this problem by avoiding connections with an S1 pedicle screw, thus allowing greater length along the rod to transition dorsally and laterally to the iliac screw head. However, we recognized that this resulted in a biomechanically inferior construct when compared to open surgery. In this series three patients had concomitant S1 pedicle screws, all later in the series after we had acquired experience in planning screw placement to allow easier screw-rod connection (Fig. 14.3). In these cases careful attention must be paid to recessing the iliac screw saddles and increasing the sagittal distance between screw heads (i.e., placing the S1 screws high in the pedicle and starting the iliac screw in a more caudal position). Furthermore, keeping the screw heads in line in the coronal plane will minimize the need for two-plane rod bending. Additional problems with the minimally invasive approach in these settings include (1) inadvertent entry into the sacroiliac joint or pelvic cavity with the sharper Jamshidi needles and (2) difficulties with creating a recessed location for the screw saddles to prevent hardware prominence.

Ultimately, the safety of this technique can only be demonstrated with larger clinical series. The bony pelvis can vary in thickness and geometry, and the soft tissues, including neural and vascular structures, do not conform to a standard or reliable anatomic arrangement. Thus, minimally invasive iliac screw placement can prove more difficult due to variations in pelvic anatomy when the traditional landmarks cannot be directly palpated or visualized. However, the ability to fixate the pelvis will likely significantly expand the spectrum of pathologies that are treatable using a minimally invasive approach.

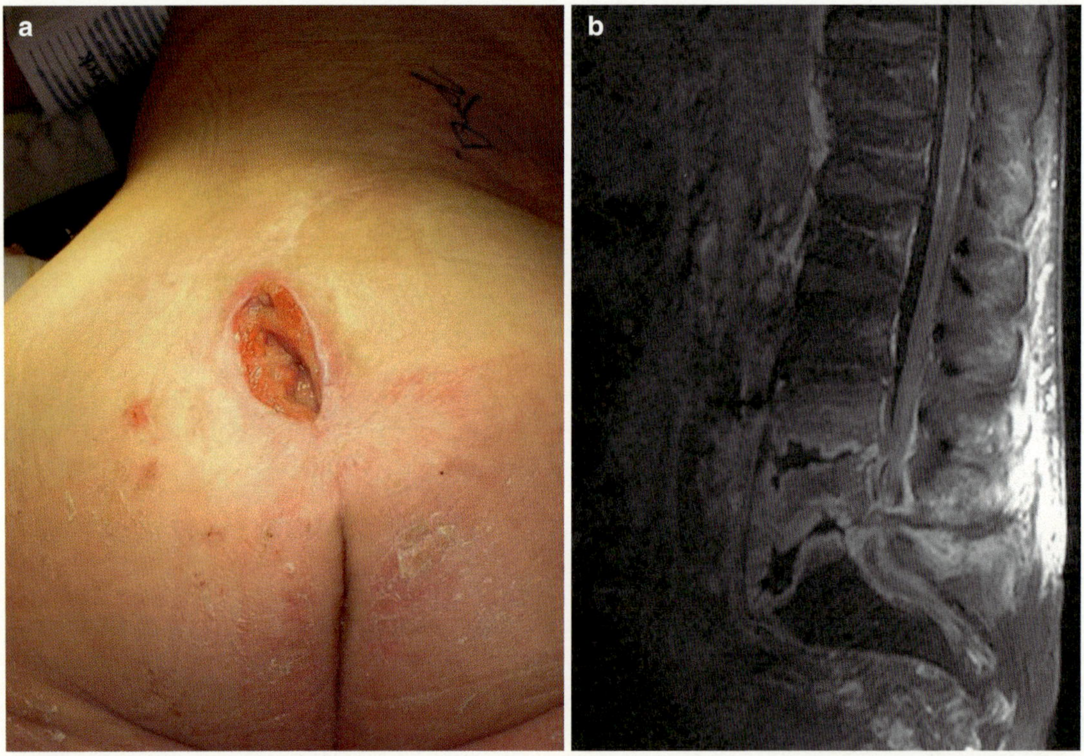

Fig. 14.3 (**a**) Case of a 46-year-old paraplegic who developed a sacral decubitus ulcer. This was treated with a local flap, which failed, and he subsequently developed osteomyelitis at the lumbosacral junction due to exposed bone. (**b** and **c**) The patient failed 6 months of intravenous antibiotic treatment with progression of osteomyelitis and back pain with deformity and bony destruction as demonstrated on MRI and CT imaging. (**d**) The patient was treated with an anterior debridement of L4–S1 with iliac crest autograft reconstruction and (**e**) percutaneous instrumentation from L4 to the ilium. (**f**) Proper iliac screw placement was confirmed with CT scanning. (**g**) The surgical incisions avoided the infected and affected soft tissues. (**h**) Fixation, debridement, and antibiotic treatment resulted in resolution of the open wound without need for another soft tissue flap to promote healing

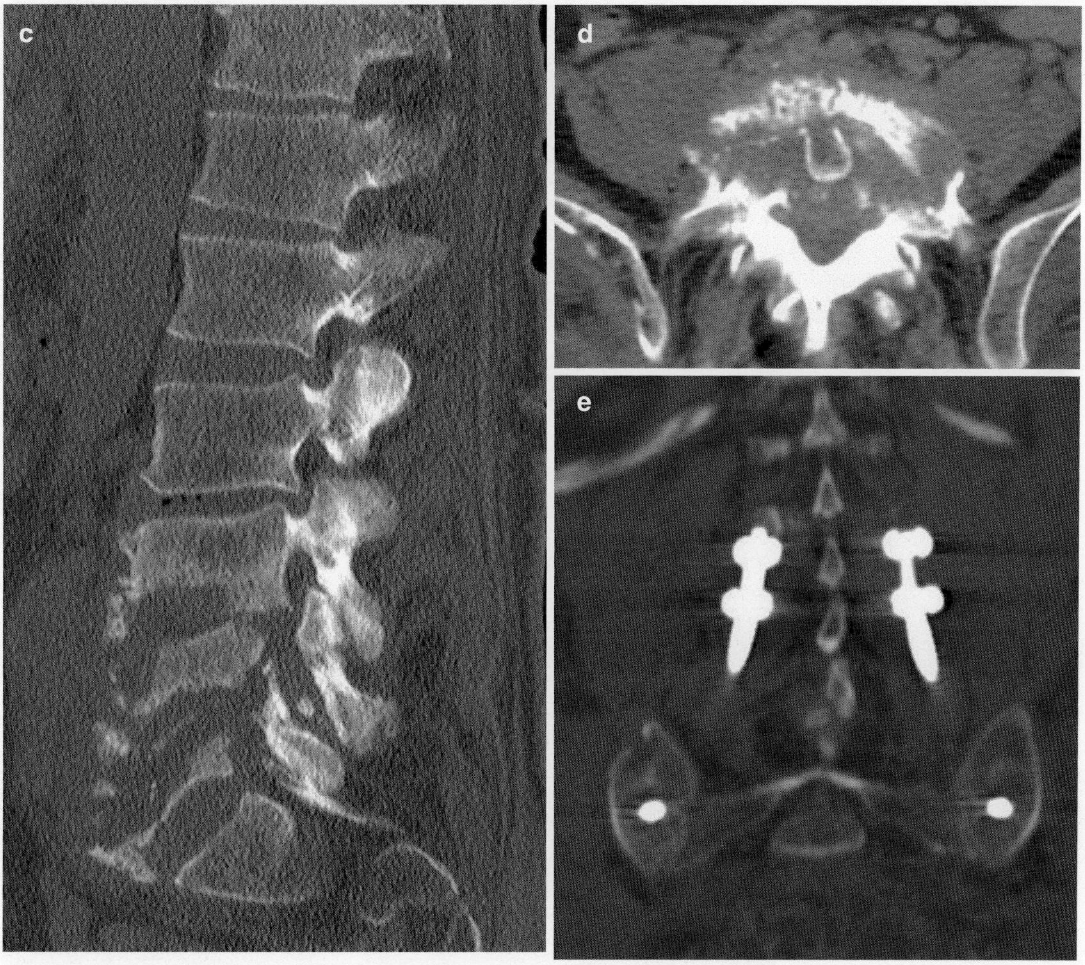

Fig. 14.3 (continued)

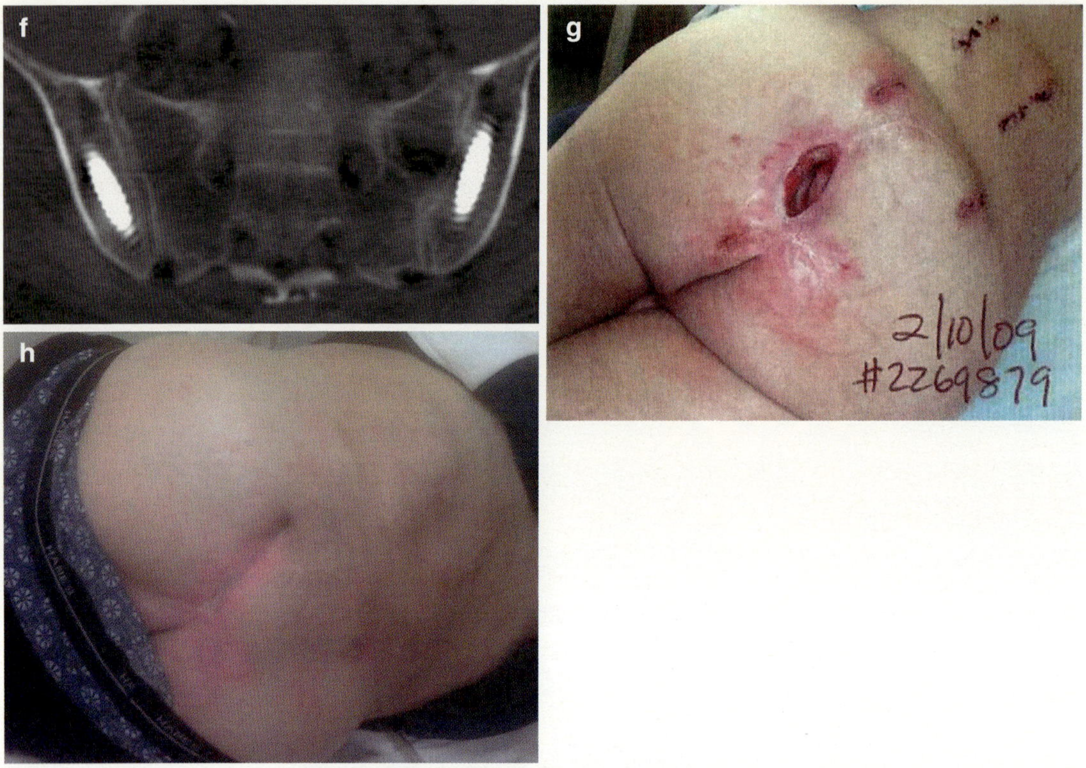

Fig. 14.3 (continued)

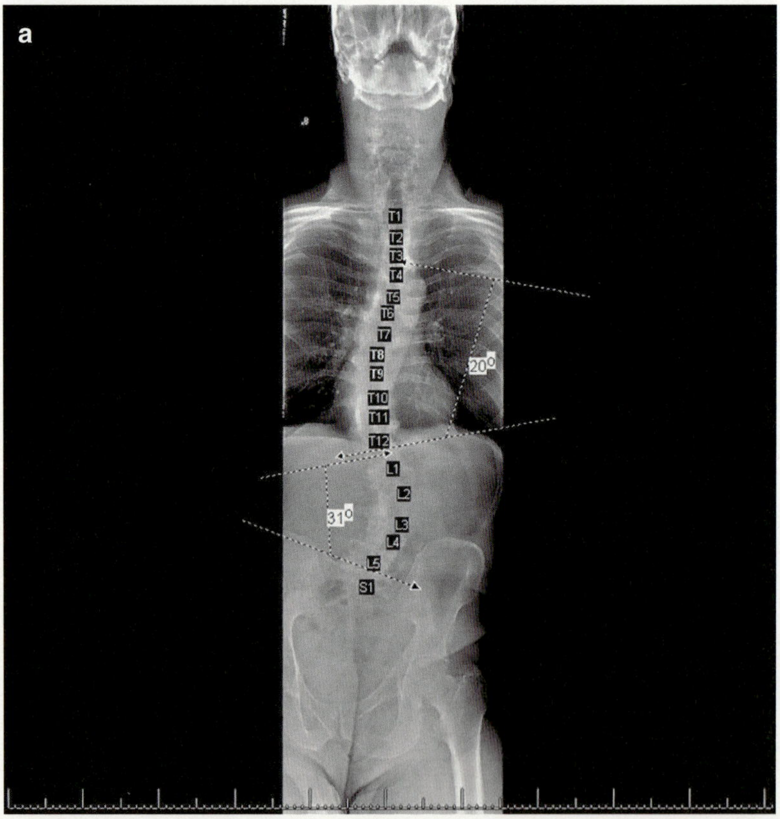

Fig. 14.4 (**a–d**) AP and lateral imaging of a patient with lumbar degenerative scoliosis and positive sagittal balance which was treated with minimally invasive interbody fusion and percutaneous instrumentation demonstrating the use of percutaneous iliac screws in correction with S1 pedicle screws. (**e**) CT scanning demonstrates proper recession of screw saddles to minimize hardware prominence

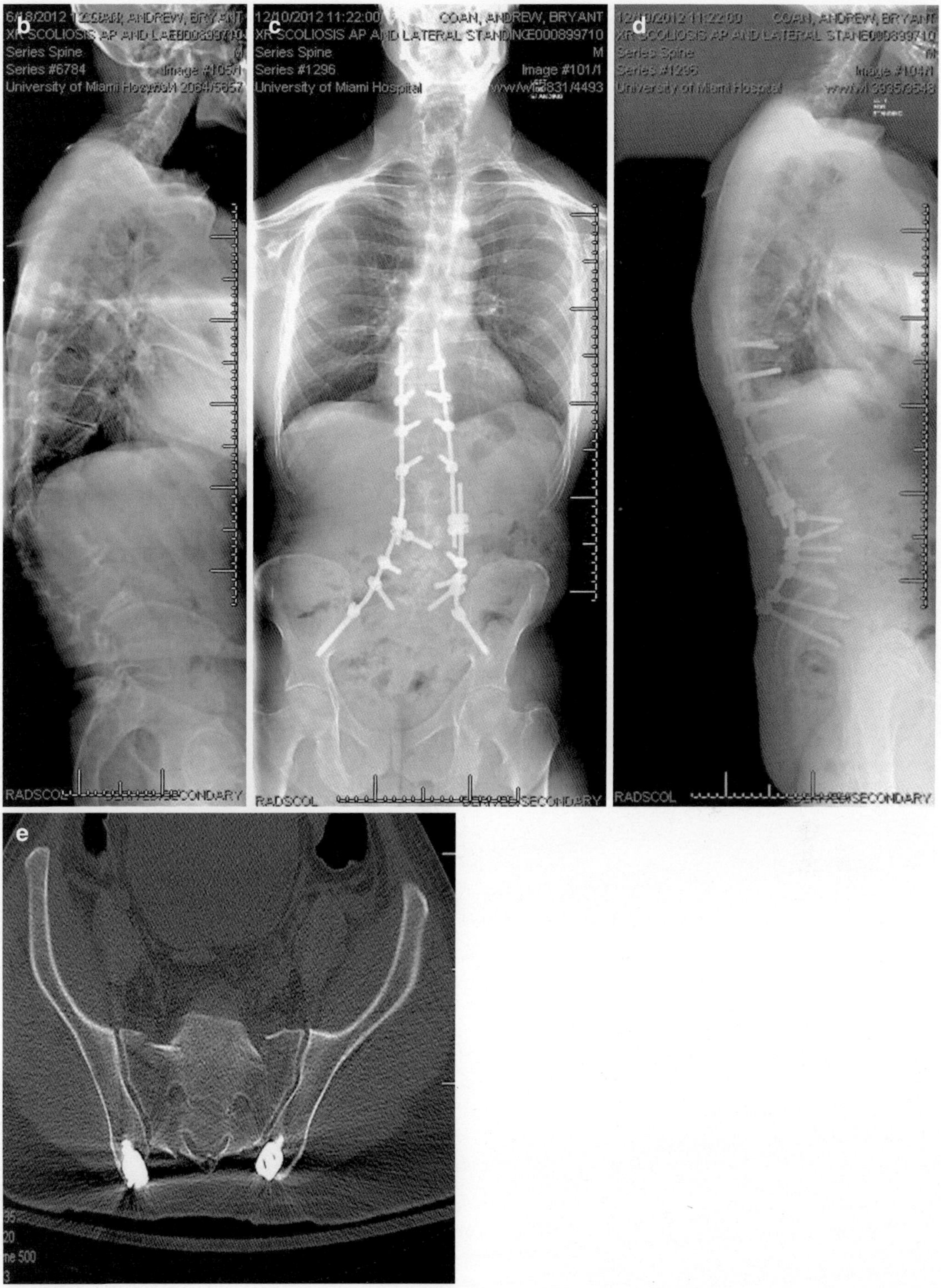

Fig. 14.4 (continued)

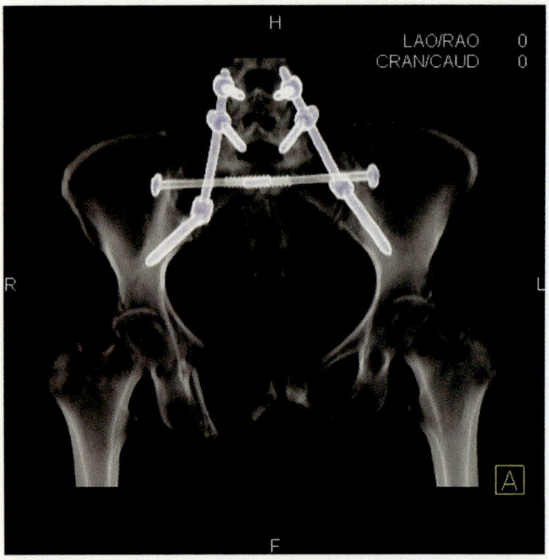

Fig. 14.5 Postoperative imaging demonstrating application of iliac screws in concert with an iliosacral pin to treat a complex sacropelvic fracture

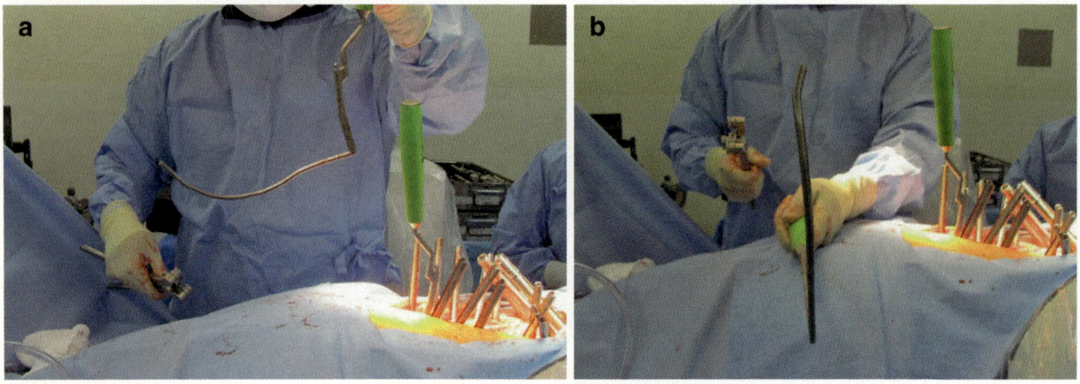

Fig. 14.6 (**a** and **b**) Two-plane rod bending at the caudal end of the construct ensures proper S1 iliac hookup. The rod must be bent to rise dorsally as it spans laterally to meet the iliac screw saddle

References

1. Allen B, Ferguson R. The Galveston technique for L-rod instrumentation of the scoliotic spine. Spine. 1982;7:276–84.
2. Anand N, Baron E, Thaiyananthan G, Khalsa K, Goldstein T. Minimally invasive multilevel percutaneous correction and fusion for adult lumbar degenerative scoliosis: a technique and feasibility study. J Spinal Disord Tech. 2008;21:459–67.
3. Bellabarba C, Schildhauer T, Vaccaro A, Chapman J. Complications associated with surgical stabilization of high-grade sacral fracture dislocations with sacropelvic instability. Spine. 2006;31:S80–8.
4. Emami A, Deviren V, Berven S, Smith J, Hu S, Bradford D. Outcome and complications of long fusions to the sacrum in adult spinal deformity. Spine. 2002;27:776–86.
5. Foley K, Gupta S. Percutaneous pedicle screw fixation in the lumbar spine: preliminary clinical results. J Neurosurg Spine. 2002;97:7–12.
6. Fujibayashi S, Neo M, Nakamura T. Palliative dual iliac screw fixation for lumbosacral metastasis. J Neurosurg Spine. 2007;7:99–102.
7. Gilelman A, Joseph S, Carrion W, Stephen M. Results and morbidity in a consecutive series of patients undergoing spinal fusion with iliac screws for neuromuscular scoliosis. Orthopedics. 2008;31:329.
8. Jaikumar S, Mik D, Kam A. History of minimally invasive surgery. Neurosurgery. 2002;S2:1–14.
9. König B, Stöckle U, Sati M, Nolte L, Haas N. Virtual fluoroscopy: safe zones for pelvic screw fixations. In Medical Image Computing and Computer-Assisted Intervention – MICCAI 2000. Heidelberg: Springer, 2000. pp. 287–319
10. Lippman C, Salehi S, Liu J, Ondra S. Salvage technique of posterior iliac bolt placement in long-segment spinal constructs with a previous posterior iliac crest harvest: technical note. Neurosurgery. 2006;58:ONS178–9.
11. Lonner B. Emerging minimally invasive technologies for the management of scoliosis. Orthop Clin North Am. 2007;38:431–40.
12. Lowery G, Kulkarni S. Percutaneous posterior spine instrumentation. Eur Spine J. 2000;9:S126–30.
13. Magerl F. Verletzungen der Brust- und Lendenwirbelsaule. Langenbecks Arch Chir. 1980;352:428–33.
14. Orchowski J, Polly D, Kuklo T, Klemme W, Schroeder T. Use of fluoroscopy to evaluate iliac screw position. Am J Orthop. 2006;35:144–6.
15. Schildhauer T, McCulloch P, Chapman J, Mann F. Anatomic and radiographic considerations for placement of transiliac screws in lumbopelvic fixation. J Spinal Disord. 2002;15:199–205.
16. Tumialan L, Mummaneni P. Long-segment spinal fixation using pelvic screws. Neurosurgery. 2008;63 Suppl 3:183–90.
17. Wang M, Anderson D, Poelstra K, Ludwig S. Minimally invasive posterior fixation for spinal deformities. Neurosurgery. 2008;63:A197–204.
18. Wang M, Williams S, Mummaneni P, Sherman J. Minimally invasive percutaneous iliac screws: initial 24 case experience with CT confirmation. J Spinal Disord. 2012. p. 5.
19. Wang MY, Ludwig SC, Anderson DG, Mummaneni PV. Percutaneous iliac screw placement: description of a new minimally invasive technique. Neurosurg Focus. 2008;25:E17.
20. Zheng Z, Yu B, Chen H, Aladin D, Zhang K, Zhang J, Liu H, Luk K, Lu W. Effect of iliac screw insertion depth on the stability and strength of lumbo-iliac fixation constructs: an anatomical and biomechanical study. Spine. 2009;34:E565–72.

15 Management of Osteoporotic Bone

John E. Ziewacz, Darryl Lau, Sigurd H. Berven, Armed J. Awad, and Praveen V. Mummaneni

15.1 Introduction

As the population ages and life span increases, the prevalence of osteoporosis, defined as a dual-energy X-ray absorptiometry scan (DEXA) value <−2.5, is increasing [12, 59]. Concomitant with this increase is an increase in spinal fractures and deformity associated with osteoporosis [19, 60]. As techniques for spinal instrumentation improve, spinal surgery is being considered in older patients, many of whom have osteoporosis [9, 12, 17, 19, 30, 33, 35, 36, 38, 45, 52, 57, 59, 64, 66, 70, 72, 74, 76]. It is estimated that in patients over the age of 50 who undergo spine surgery, 51.3 % of females and 14.5 % of males have osteoporosis [12]. Of women who undergo surgery for scoliosis correction, it is estimated that 10 % have osteoporosis [83]. Osteoporosis is a significant independent predictor of complications, particularly hardware related, in spine surgery [17, 64]. As a result, particular attention must be paid when instrumenting the osteoporotic spine [30]. With the advancement and expansion of minimally invasive techniques [18, 36, 37, 45, 51, 58, 66, 69] including for deformity correction [1, 2, 4, 15, 54, 77], it is important for the spine surgeon to carefully follow patients with osteoporosis undergoing spinal fusions to ensure they do not develop pseudoarthrosis and/or implant loosening.

J.E. Ziewacz • D. Lau • P.V. Mummaneni (✉)
Department of Neurological Surgery, University of California, San Francisco, San Francisco, CA, USA
e-mail: mummanenip@neurosurg.ucsf.edu

S.H. Berven
Department of Orthopedic Surgery, University of California, San Francisco, San Francisco, CA, USA

A.J. Awad
University of Miami, Miami, FL, USA

15.2 Complications of Osteoporosis

Osteoporosis significantly increases the risk of complications of spinal surgery, particularly in multilevel fusions [17, 64]. One study of elderly patients (mean age 68.7 year.) who underwent multilevel fusion noted that 35/80 patients (43.8 %) experienced implant loosening and adjacent segment degeneration occurred in 26 patients (32.5 %) [64]. Of these, 8 (22.8 %) and 17 (65.3 %), respectively, required reoperation [64]. The authors concluded as a result that osteoporosis should be considered preoperatively and that osteoporosis should be corrected prior to surgical treatment [64]. Another study of patients over the age of 65 who underwent fusions at greater than 5 levels noted that early complications included pedicle fractures and compression fractures and occurred in 13 % of patients. Late complications included pseudoarthroses, adjacent level degeneration, compression fractures, and junctional kyphosis, which occurred in 26 % of patients [17]. A study of 66 patients over the age of 70 who underwent minimally invasive lumbar interbody fusions (XLIF and TLIF) noted five major complications (7.4 %) [36]. The major complications

M.Y. Wang et al. (eds.), *Minimally Invasive Spinal Deformity Surgery*,
DOI 10.1007/978-3-7091-1407-0_15, © Springer-Verlag Wien 2014

Table 15.1 Complications of osteoporosis in spine surgery

Complications of osteoporosis in spine surgery
Subsidence
Pedicle fracture
Proximal junctional kyphosis
Compression fracture
Pseudoarthrosis
Implant loosening/haloing

included four patients who experienced graft subsidence after undergoing stand-alone XLIF procedures and one patient experienced adjacent segment degeneration (Table 15.1).

15.3 Preoperative Evaluation and Medical Management

Preoperative evaluation of the patient with suspected osteoporosis includes a DEXA scan and metabolic labs (vitamin D, parathyroid hormone, and calcium). These tests are important in determining the extent of osteopenia or osteoporosis and therefore aid in preoperative planning. Currently, a dual-energy X-ray absorptiometry scan (DEXA) for bone mineral density measurement is considered the gold standard for osteoporosis diagnosis. A DEXA value of <-1 to >-2.5 is considered osteopenic, and a level <-2.5 is considered osteoporotic. Some surgeons advocate not operating on severely osteoporotic patients due to the increased risk, though set cutoffs for avoiding surgery have not been determined [17]. Despite the importance of the osteoporotic spine on results of spinal fusion, only 44 % of surgeons in one study ordered preoperative DEXA scan and 12 % ordered vitamin D and calcium levels prior to considering instrumented fusion [19].

Before we discuss medical treatment of osteoporosis, we need to understand the normal bone growth. Typical bone mainly consists of osteoblasts, osteocytes, and osteoclasts. Osteoblasts cells are bone-forming cells, while osteoclasts are responsible for bone resorption. In normal bone, remodeling of bone is a continuous constant process [63]. Osteoporosis develops when there is an imbalance between bone resorption and bone formation. This imbalance can be caused by three mechanisms: inadequate peak in bone mass during skeleton growth, excessive osteoclastic bone resorption, and insufficient new bone formation response during bone remodeling [63].

Two types of osseous tissue form bone: trabecular bone and cortical bone. Trabecular bone (cancellous bone) is the soft, spongelike bone in the periphery of long bones and vertebrae. Cortical bone (compact bone) is the dense, hard outer layer of bones and the middle of long bones. Trabecular bone has a greater surface area for metabolic activity than cortical bone; therefore, it is more affected in osteoporosis. This explains why wrist, hip, and spine (bones with relatively high trabecular bone) are common sites of osteoporotic fractures.

Several pharmacologic treatments are used in treatment of osteoporosis or low bone density. American College of Physicians (ACP) recommends that clinicians choose among drugs on the basis of risks, benefits, and adverse effects in individual patients [62]. Secondary causes of osteoporosis must be excluded before commencement of medical treatment. Alcoholism, multiple myeloma, osteomalacia, use of glucocorticoids, and medical illnesses such as rheumatoid arthritis need to be first excluded as these conditions would require specialized management in addition to standard medical management of osteoporosis [17].

Bisphosphonates act through osteoclast inhibition, reducing bone turnover. They are synthetic analogs of pyrophosphate which bind to hydroxyapatite in bone remodeling, hence reducing bone resorption activity of osteoclasts. Bisphosphonates drug class includes alendronate, etidronate, ibandronate, pamidronate, risedronate, and zoledronic acid. All of them, except etidronate and pamidronate, are approved by Food and Drug Administration (FDA) for osteoporosis treatment. Because of the strong evidence of bisphosphonates in effectively reducing the risk for vertebral, nonvertebral, and hip fractures, they are considered as first-line treatment of osteoporosis [62]. Alendronate and risedronate have been studied more than drugs in the class. Alendronate (70 mg once weekly or 10 mg daily) is the first-line option in treatment of osteoporosis.

Table 15.2 Initial diagnostic evaluation of osteoporosis

Initial diagnostic evaluation of osteoporosis
Dual-Energy X-Ray Absorptiometry (DEXA) Scan (T-score <−2.5 = osteoporosis)
Calcium level
25-hydroxy vitamin-D
Comprehensive metabolic panel
Complete blood count

Risedronate (35 mg once weekly or 5 mg daily) is an alternative choice in case of alendronate intolerance. Zoledronic acid, with alendronate and risedronate, lies in the first-line in osteoporosis treatment [79]. Alendronate is also considered the first-line in the treatment of steroid-induced osteoporosis. However, it is not FDA approved in prevention of steroid-induced osteoporosis. Risedronate is considered the first-line in prevention of steroid-induced osteoporosis.

Parathyroid hormone (PTH) is another strategy for osteoporosis treatment. The mechanism of action of PTH in producing net bone formation is complex and not completely elucidated. The extent to which these drugs impact fusion is largely unknown. Animal studies have demonstrated that bisphosphonates appear to impede fusion mass, but human studies demonstrate increased fusion mass radiographically, though clinical outcome was not affected [31]. To date, PTH has not been studied in humans regarding its potential to improve fusion (Table 15.2). In animal studies, however, it has been shown to improve the fusion rate and fusion mass [31]. In light of the complications associated with osteoporosis and fusion, it may be prudent to consider delaying surgery in patients with osteoporosis when possible and allowing for treatment in order to improve bone quality. However, the absolute cutoff for avoiding surgery has not been defined, and there is no definitive evidence that treatment of osteoporosis prior to spine surgery improves outcomes [17, 32].

More recently, two agents have been introduced for the treatment of osteoporosis: denosumab, which is a monoclonal antibody that inhibits the activation and differentiation of osteoclasts, resulting in less bone resorption, and teriparatide (recombinant parathyroid hormone 1–34), which in contrast directly stimulates bone growth [46]. Both have been found to reduce vertebral fracture risk in postmenopausal women with osteoporosis [46]. However, their effects on patients undergoing spinal deformity correction are unknown. A recent prospective cohort study found that teriparatide was more effective than combined vertebroplasty and anti-resorper agent for treating post-vertebroplasty new-onset adjacent vertebral compression fractures [73].

Denosumab is a new drug recently approved by FDA in 2010. It is fully human monoclonal antibody that targets the receptor activator of nuclear factor-κB ligand (RANKL) that blocks its binding to RANK, inhibiting the differentiation and activity of osteoclasts. Denosumab is considered as first-line agent in osteoporosis treatment [79].

FREEDOM, a randomized clinical trial, included 7,868 postmenopausal women with osteoporosis found that denosumab (60 mg once every 6 months) for 36 months was associated with a reduction in the risk of vertebral, nonvertebral, and hip fractures [14]. The FREEDOM trial was extended for up to 10 years. First 2 years results (represents 5 years since FREEDOM study commencement) showed further increase in bone density at the lumbar spine and total hip [56].

The DECIDE trial compared the efficacy and safety of denosumab with alendronate in 1,189 postmenopausal women with low bone mass. Denosumab achieved better results in both bone density and bone turnover reduction compared with alendronate and similar safety profile [8]. Another trial showed more adherence and compliance of patients receiving denosumab than those taking alendronate [27].

Mixed treatment comparison in a recent meta-analysis showed that denosumab is more effective than alendronate, risedronate, and other drugs in preventing new vertebral fractures [26].

Teriparatide is the only FDA-approved anabolic drug for osteoporosis treatment. Preotact, a new anabolic agent, is pending FDA approval. Teriparatide (20 μg/day) has been proved to decrease both spine and vertebral fractures but hip fractures in postmenopausal women with history of previous vertebral fractures [55, 61]. The manufacturers of teriparatide, Eli Lilly and

Company, state in the insert package that teriparatide treatment should not exceed 2 years [20]. This is based on osteosarcoma cases developed in rats treated with teriparatide for 2 years [75, 78]. However, osteosarcoma was not reported in clinical studies of humans taking teriparatide. The Osteosarcoma Surveillance Study group have recently published the findings of the first 7 years of that ongoing 15 years study evaluating the potential association between teriparatide and the development of osteosarcoma in humans [3]. Interestingly, there were no osteosarcoma patients who had a prior history of teriparatide treatment.

Teriparatide increases bone density at most sites and decreases nonvertebral fractures compared to alendronat [6]. Additionally, teriparatide is superior to alendronate for treating glucocorticoid-induced osteoporosis [67]. Moreover, case reports show that teriparatide is effective in treatment of alendronate-associated osteonecrosis of the jaw [11, 29, 41, 43]. However, cost considerations and lack of studies showing hip fracture reduction prevent using teriparatide as a first-line agent.

Combination of teriparatide and alendronate is not recommended. Combination treatment is not more effective than either agent alone [5, 22]. Moreover, alendronate decreases the effect of teriparatide to increase bone density and turnover in both men and women [23, 24].

Calcitonin, which had previously been employed, is no longer considered appropriate therapy for osteoporosis [46].

In 2010, the American Association of Clinical Endocrinologists (AACE) published guidelines and recommendations for diagnosis and treatment of osteoporosis [79]. Based on level of evidence, they generated the following recommendations for choosing drugs in osteoporosis treatment:

- First-line agents: alendronate, risedronate, zoledronic acid, denosumab
- Second-line agent: ibandronate
- Second- or third-line agent: raloxifene
- Last-line agent: calcitonin
- Treatment for patients with very high fracture risk or in whom bisphosphonate therapy has failed: teriparatide
- Recommendation against the use of combination therapy.

Table 15.3 Summary of surgical techniques for managing the osteoporotic spine

Surgical strategies for managing osteoporosis
Expandable pedicle screws
Polymethylmethacrylate (PMMA) augmentation
Cannulated screws filled with PMMA
Increased levels of fixation (including pelvic fixation)
Bicortical screw purchase
Dual-threaded pedicle screws
Less-rigid implants

15.4 Surgical Strategies for the Osteoporotic Spine

In light of the significant challenges in the surgical management of osteoporotic bone, multiple surgical strategies aimed at improving pullout strength, augmenting fusion, and reducing complications have been employed. Among these are expandable pedicle screws, polymethyl methacrylate (PMMA) augmentation, cannulated screws filled with PMMA, increased levels of fixation, bicortical screw purchase, dual threaded screws, and less rigid implants, among others (Table 15.3).

Biomechanical data suggests that pedicle screws that expand within the pedicle may substantially improve pullout strength in bone compromised by osteoporosis [13, 48]. Early work by Cook et al. reported that 86 % of patients with osteoporosis who underwent expandable pedicle screw placement experienced fusion, with no instances of screw pullout or loosening [13]. In a preliminary study, Wu et al. described 125 consecutive patients with severe osteoporosis who underwent placement of expandable pedicle screws. They also noted no instances of screw loosening or pullout, and patients experienced significantly improved outcomes as measured by Japanese Orthopedic Association (JOA) scores and visual analog scale (VAS) scores [80]. In another comparison of expandable pedicle screws with conventional pedicle screw constructs in the treatment of patients with osteoporosis who underwent lumbar spine fusion demonstrated that in 80 patients who received expandable screws, there was a 92.5 % fusion rate compared to 77 patients who underwent conventional pedicle screw placement who demonstrated an 80.5 % fusion rate.

This result was statistically significant [81]. Furthermore, in the same study, screw loosening occurred in a significantly lower percentage (4.1 %) of screws placed in the expandable group compared to 12.9 % of screws placed in the conventional group [81]. Furthermore, JOA and Oswestry Disability Index (ODI) scores were significantly better compared to preoperative scores in the expandable pedicle screw group [81]. A biomechanical comparison of expandable pedicle screws and PMMA-augmented pedicle screws in osteoporotic cadavers suggested that both expandable screws and PMMA-augmented screws exhibited significantly enhanced stability as compared with conventionally placed screws [48]. The problem with expandable pedicle screws, however, is revision surgery. Typically, these implants destroy the pedicle if removal is necessary for any reason.

Polymethyl methacrylate has been used with increasing frequency to augment the fusion constructs in osteoporotic patients. Several studies have demonstrated the utility of PMMA in increasing pullout strength and improving fixation [16, 38, 48, 52, 59, 68, 84]. Biomechanical data in cadavers suggests that PMMA-augmented pedicle screws provide superior screw stability as compared to conventional pedicle screws, and this fixation is comparable to that of expandable pedicle screws [48]. In one cadaver study, as bone mineral density decreased, PMMA-augmented screws demonstrated significantly stronger pullout strength as compared to bicortically placed conventional pedicle screws at S1 [84]. In a 3-year follow-up study of 37 osteoporotic patients undergoing pedicle screw placement with PMMA augmentation, Moon et al. found that VAS scores for back and leg pain were significantly reduced from 7.87 to 2.30 and 8.82 to 1.42 ($p=0.006$), respectively [54]. Further demonstrating the clinical utility of PMMA-augmented pedicle screws, Sawakami et al. showed a significant decrease in haloing around PMMA-augmented screws (29.4 % vs. 71.4 %) and a significantly higher fusion rate (94.1 % vs. 76.1 %) [68]. Additionally, PMMA augmentation has been found to be useful in anterior approaches as well [38]. A study of 62 osteoporotic patients who underwent ALIF with or without PMMA augmentation and were followed for over 2 years demonstrated that those who had PMMA augmentation demonstrated significantly less graft subsidence (5.2 % vs. 19.6 %, $p=0.001$). Furthermore, the vertebral body height at the index level was significantly higher in the PMMA group (10.7 % vs. 3.9 %, $p=0.001$) [38]. Another option for PMMA-augmented fusion for minimally invasive surgery is pedicle screw placement with cannulated screws through which PMMA is injected. A prospective study of this technology in osteoporotic patients over the age of 70 with a mean follow-up of 20–49 months demonstrated that no radiographic or clinical cases of nonunion were observed and that pain and function were improved at 6 months and maintained at final follow-up [59]. Additionally, there was no evidence of cement leakage, a known complication of PMMA-augmented screws [17, 59]. However, a comparison of standard screws with PMMA augmentation and screws with cannulated PMMA augmentation in a synthetic vertebral body revealed greater pullout strength in the standard screw group [10]. This has not been corroborated clinically, however. One concern with PMMA screw augmentation is that vertebrectomy may be necessary if the PMMA becomes infected postoperatively.

In addition to expandable pedicle screws and PMMA-augmented screws, other surgical techniques for the osteoporotic spine have been advocated to reduce the complications associated with osteoporotic bone in spinal fusion. One such technique includes the application of Nesplon tape in either the sublaminar or sub-pars space connected to a rod. One study of this technique demonstrated that tape applied in this manner in cadaver specimen resulted in significantly stronger fixation and a stiffer construct when compared to pedicle screw constructs alone [28]. This may be due to the higher regional bone density concentration in the lamina as compared to the pedicle. Evidence suggests that the insertional torque required to place a pedicle screw is positively correlated with the patient's bone mineral density [42]. Because of this, knowing the bone density prior to surgery may influence the number of levels needed for fusion in osteoporotic patients [42]. Some authors advocated adding

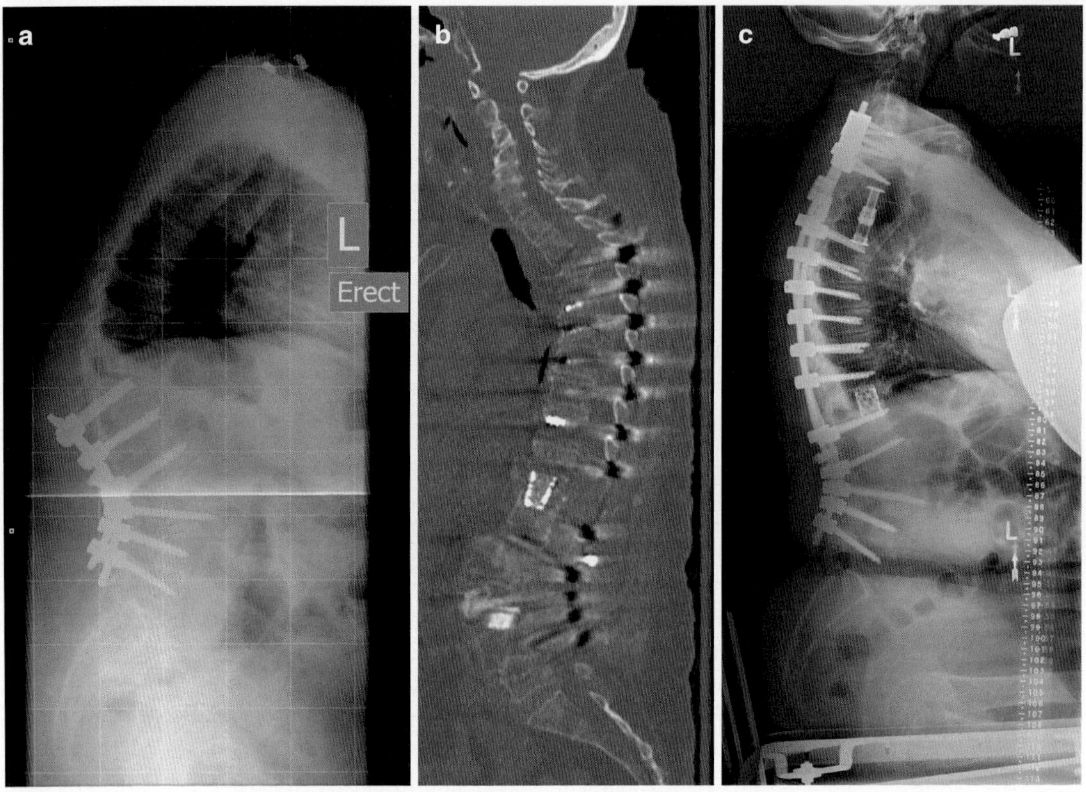

Fig. 15.1 (**a**) Lateral X-Ray demonstrating a T11 fracture and kyphotic deformity following L2 pedicle subtraction osteotomy in a 59 yo woman with a history of chronic steroid use for Lupus and osteoporosis. (**b**) Sagittal CT reconstruction in the same patient demonstrating a T3-4 compression fracture with resultant kyphosis and progressive paraparesis following T11 vertebral column resection and extension of fusion to T3. (**c**) Lateral scoliosis X-Ray in the same patient following T3-4 vertebral column resection and extension of fusion to C7

multiple levels of fusion in the osteoporotic spine, with routine extension to the pelvis for lumbosacral fixation in patients with osteoporosis [17]. Also, same-diameter tapping prior to pedicle screw placement was shown to result in decreased insertional torque and thus pullout strength, and therefore, undertapping or not tapping prior to pedicle screw insertion has been advocated [17] (Fig. 15.1).

15.5 Vertebroplasty/Kyphoplasty for Osteoporotic Fractures

Osteoporotic vertebral fracture is a significant cause of pain and disability in the elderly [50, 65]. The incidence of osteoporotic vertebral fracture is likely to increase as the population ages. Recently, vertebroplasty and kyphoplasty have been employed to treat both the pain and deformity associated with these fractures [40, 50, 65]. Their use has been increasing at a rapid rate [40]. Vertebroplasty is meant to reduce the pain of fractured vertebrae and prevent worsening of vertebral body height loss by direct pedicular injection of PMMA. Kyphoplasty, on the other hand, uses an expandable balloon to try to reverse the kyphosis caused by the fracture and create space for PMMA to be injected in order to address both the pain and deformity associated with vertebral compression fractures. A recent study questioned the efficacy of vertebroplasty in the management of osteoporotic compression fractures [34]. In a randomized trial of 131 patients with one to three levels of vertebral body fracture, 68 patients underwent vertebroplasty and 63 underwent sham injections of local anesthetic. At 1 month and 3 months, there was no significant difference in outcomes between the vertebroplasty and control group [34]. However, there was a significant trend toward a clinically meaningful result (defined as a 30 % reduction in pain) in the vertebroplasty group ($p = 0.06$). Also, there was no control group who received only medical management, and there was significant crossover from the control group to the vertebroplasty group at 3 months (51 % vs. 13 %) [34]. In contrast, a randomized controlled trial of 80 patients comparing vertebroplasty vs. optimal medical management of vertebral compression fractures in osteoporosis noted that the vertebroplasty group experienced significantly improved VAS scores at 1 week that persisted over 36 months as well as improved quality-of-life (QoL) scores that persisted at 36 months compared to the control group [21]. Similarly in another randomized controlled trial of vertebroplasty and maximal medical therapy that included 202 patients, there was a significant decrease in VAS pain scores at 1 month that persisted at 1 year [39]. These prospective studies suggested that vertebroplasty is effective and durable in the treatment of osteoporotic vertebral fractures. Further work has demonstrated that this may be the case in the very elderly as well. DePalma et al. prospectively studied vertebroplasty for osteoporotic vertebral compression fractures in 123 consecutive nonagenarians and found that mean VAS scores decreased significantly from 7.6 preprocedure to 3.1 at 30 min following the procedure, 1.2 at 1 month, and 0.5 at 2 years, respectively [16].

Kyphoplasty has not been studied to the same degree as vertebroplasty. However, studies demonstrated its potential value [25, 49, 71, 82]. A study of 26 patients undergoing kyphoplasty for osteoporotic vertebral compression fractures demonstrated a statistically significant reduction in VAS scores from 7.7 to 3.1 and 2.9 at 1 day and 3 months following the procedure [49]. Additionally, sagittal Cobb angle was significantly reduced from 18.5 degrees before the procedure to 9.2 degrees after ($p < 0.001$) [49]. Mirroring this result, a study of kyphoplasty in 27 fractured vertebrae in 25 patients noted a significant reduction in Cobb angle (17.18 degrees to 9.35 degrees, $p < 0.05$). Furthermore, anterior and medial vertebral body heights were increased by 33 and 50 %, respectively [82]. Evidence suggested this improvement in vertebral body height and Cobb angle was sustained at 12 months [25]. In a prospective study of 40 kyphoplasty patients with 1-year follow-up, anterior and medial vertebral body height were increased by 51.25 % and 52.29 %, respectively, with no loss at 1 year [25]. Additionally, scores on the VAS, North American Spine Society scale, and Short Form (SF)-36 scores improved significantly at 1 year [25].

Direct comparison of vertebroplasty and kyphoplasty in a randomized controlled fashion has not occurred. However, a review of the literature on these treatments demonstrated that both were more efficacious at reducing pain and improving mobility in the short-term compared to conservative therapy alone [7].

Despite the relative safety of vertebroplasty and kyphoplasty, complications have been reported. The main complications include cement leakage, cement embolism, and adjacent level fracture [25, 44, 47]. One analysis of patients who experienced vertebral fracture after kyphoplasty noted that 12/14 (86 %) occurred within 6 months of the vertebroplasty and that 10/14 (71 %) of the fractures occurred at the adjacent level, raising the question of the effect of vertebroplasty on fractures at adjacent levels [47]. However, other studies have noted low levels of adjacent fractures and that many of the fractures would have occurred anyway and were related to the degree of osteoporosis [53]. In some studies, the adjacent fracture rate was lower in those treated with vertebroplasty [21]. A meta-analysis of complications associated with vertebroplasty and kyphoplasty concluded that when analyzing all studies as well as only prospective studies, vertebroplasty was found to have increased procedure-related complications including symptomatic and asymptomatic cement leakage [44]. Future prospective studies are necessary to corroborate this analysis.

Conclusions

Osteoporosis significantly affects the outcome of spinal surgery. Patients with osteoporosis are more likely to experience fractures and surgical complications, particularly hardware-related complications including junctional kyphosis and screw pullout. Spine surgeons must be aware of these factors and understand approaches to mitigating the consequences of osteoporosis in surgical patients. A thorough preoperative workup can identify osteoporosis and may allow for delaying surgery in order to treat the osteoporosis prior to intervention. Newer agents such as teriparatide or denosumab may prove useful in the medical management of osteoporosis prior to surgery. When this is not possible, multiple surgical techniques can be useful in managing the osteoporotic spine including adding fusion segments, undertapping, using expandable pedicle screws, and/or augmentation with PMMA, either prior to pedicle screw insertion or through cannulated screws, among other techniques. Finally, for osteoporotic vertebral fractures, vertebroplasty and kyphoplasty are safe and effective strategies for reducing pain and disability associated with these fractures.

References

1. Anand N, Baron EM. Minimally invasive approaches for the correction of adult spinal deformity. Eur Spine J. 2012;22:S232–41.
2. Anand N, Baron EM, Thaiyananthan G, Khalsa K, Goldstein TB. Minimally invasive multilevel percutaneous correction and fusion for adult lumbar degenerative scoliosis: a technique and feasibility study. J Spinal Disord Tech. 2008;21:459–67.
3. Andrews EB, Gilsenan AW, Midkiff K, Sherrill B, Wu Y, Mann BH, et al. The US postmarketing surveillance study of adult osteosarcoma and teriparatide: study design and findings from the first 7 years. J Bone Miner Res. 2012;27:2429–37.
4. Benglis DM, Elhammady MS, Levi AD, Vanni S. Minimally invasive anterolateral approaches for the treatment of back pain and adult degenerative deformity. Neurosurgery. 2008;63:191–6.
5. Black DM, Greenspan SL, Ensrud KE, Palermo L, McGowan JA, Lang TF, et al. The effects of parathyroid hormone and alendronate alone or in combination in postmenopausal osteoporosis. N Engl J Med. 2003;349:1207–15.
6. Body JJ, Gaich GA, Scheele WH, Kulkarni PM, Miller PD, Peretz A, et al. A randomized double-blind trial to compare the efficacy of teriparatide [recombinant human parathyroid hormone (1–34)] with alendronate in postmenopausal women with osteoporosis. J Clin Endocrinol Metab. 2002;87:4528–35.
7. Boonen S, Wahl DA, Nauroy L, Brandi ML, Bouxsein ML, Goldhahn J, et al. Balloon kyphoplasty and vertebroplasty in the management of vertebral compression fractures. Osteoporos Int. 2011;22:2915–34.
8. Brown JP, Prince RL, Deal C, Recker RR, Kiel DP, de Gregorio LH, et al. Comparison of the effect of denosumab and alendronate on BMD and biochemical markers of bone turnover in postmenopausal women with low bone mass: a randomized, blinded, phase 3 trial. J Bone Miner Res. 2009;24:153–61.
9. Cavagna R, Tournier C, Aunoble S, Bouler JM, Antonietti P, Ronai M, et al. Lumbar decompression and fusion in elderly osteoporotic patients: a prospective study using less rigid titanium rod fixation. J Spinal Disord Tech. 2008;21:86–91.
10. Chen LH, Tai CL, Lee DM, Lai PL, Lee YC, Niu CC, et al. Pullout strength of pedicle screws with cement augmentation in severe osteoporosis: a comparative study between cannulated screws with cement injection and solid screws with cement pre-filling. BMC Musculoskelet Disord. 2011;12:33.
11. Cheung A, Seeman E. Teriparatide therapy for alendronate-associated osteonecrosis of the jaw. N Engl J Med. 2010;363:2473–4.
12. Chin DK, Park JY, Yoon YS, Kuh SU, Jin BH, Kim KS, et al. Prevalence of osteoporosis in patients requiring spine surgery: incidence and significance of osteoporosis in spine disease. Osteoporos Int. 2007;18:1219–24.
13. Cook SD, Barbera J, Rubi M, Salkeld SL, Whitecloud 3rd TS. Lumbosacral fixation using expandable pedicle screws. An alternative in reoperation and osteoporosis. Spine J. 2001;1:109–14.
14. Cummings SR, San Martin J, McClung MR, Siris ES, Eastell R, Reid IR, et al. Denosumab for prevention of fractures in postmenopausal women with osteoporosis. N Engl J Med. 2009;361:756–65.
15. Dakwar E, Cardona RF, Smith DA, Uribe JS. Early outcomes and safety of the minimally invasive, lateral retroperitoneal transpsoas approach for adult degenerative scoliosis. Neurosurg Focus. 2010;28:E8.
16. DePalma MJ, Ketchum JM, Frankel BM, Frey ME. Percutaneous vertebroplasty for osteoporotic vertebral compression fractures in the nonagenarians: a prospective study evaluating pain reduction and new symptomatic fracture rate. Spine (Phila Pa 1976). 2011;36:277–82.
17. DeWald CJ, Stanley T. Instrumentation-related complications of multilevel fusions for adult spinal deformity patients over age 65: surgical considerations and treatment options in patients with poor bone quality. Spine (Phila Pa 1976). 2006;31:S144–51.
18. Dhall SS, Wang MY, Mummaneni PV. Clinical and radiographic comparison of mini-open transforaminal lumbar interbody fusion with open transforaminal lumbar interbody fusion in 42 patients with long-term follow-up. J Neurosurg Spine. 2008;9:560–5.
19. Dipaola CP, Bible JE, Biswas D, Dipaola M, Grauer JN, Rechtine GR. Survey of spine surgeons on attitudes regarding osteoporosis and osteomalacia screening and treatment for fractures, fusion surgery, and pseudoarthrosis. Spine J. 2009;9:537–44.

20. Eli Lilly and Company. US Forteo prescribing information. Indianapolis: Eli Lilly and Company; 2004.
21. Farrokhi MR, Alibai E, Maghami Z. Randomized controlled trial of percutaneous vertebroplasty versus optimal medical management for the relief of pain and disability in acute osteoporotic vertebral compression fractures. J Neurosurg Spine. 2011;14:561–9.
22. Finkelstein JS, Hayes A, Hunzelman JL, Wyland JJ, Lee H, Neer RM. The effects of parathyroid hormone, alendronate, or both in men with osteoporosis. N Engl J Med. 2003;349:1216–26.
23. Finkelstein JS, Leder BZ, Burnett SM, Wyland JJ, Lee H, de la Paz AV, et al. Effects of teriparatide, alendronate, or both on bone turnover in osteoporotic men. J Clin Endocrinol Metab. 2006;91:2882–7.
24. Finkelstein JS, Wyland JJ, Lee H, Neer RM. Effects of teriparatide, alendronate, or both in women with postmenopausal osteoporosis. J Clin Endocrinol Metab. 2010;95:1838–45.
25. Foo LS, Yeo W, Fook S, Guo CM, Chen JL, Yue WM, et al. Results, experience and technical points learnt with use of the SKy Bone Expander kyphoplasty system for osteoporotic vertebral compression fractures: a prospective study of 40 patients with a minimum of 12 months of follow-up. Eur Spine J. 2007;16:1944–50.
26. Freemantle N, Cooper C, Diez-Perez A, Gitlin M, Radcliffe H, Shepherd S, et al. Results of indirect and mixed treatment comparison of fracture efficacy for osteoporosis treatments: a meta-analysis. Osteoporos Int. 2013;24:209–17.
27. Freemantle N, Satram-Hoang S, Tang ET, Kaur P, Macarios D, Siddhanti S, et al. Final results of the DAPS (Denosumab Adherence Preference Satisfaction) study: a 24-month, randomized, crossover comparison with alendronate in postmenopausal women. Osteoporos Int. 2012;23:317–26.
28. Hamasaki T, Tanaka N, Kim J, Okada M, Ochi M, Hutton WC. Pedicle screw augmentation with polyethylene tape: a biomechanical study in the osteoporotic thoracolumbar spine. J Spinal Disord Tech. 2010;23:127–32.
29. Harper RP, Fung E. Resolution of bisphosphonate-associated osteonecrosis of the mandible: possible application for intermittent low-dose parathyroid hormone [rhPTH(1–34)]. J Oral Maxillofac Surg. 2007;65:573–80.
30. Hart RA, Prendergast MA. Spine surgery for lumbar degenerative disease in elderly and osteoporotic patients. Instr Course Lect. 2007;56:257–72.
31. Hirsch BP, Unnanuntana A, Cunningham ME, Lane JM. The effect of therapies for osteoporosis on spine fusion: a systematic review. Spine J. 2012;13:190–9.
32. Hu SS, Berven SH. Preparing the adult deformity patient for spinal surgery. Spine (Phila Pa 1976). 2006;31:S126–31.
33. Jo DJ, Seo EM, Kim KT, Kim SM, Lee SH. Lumbosacral spondyloptosis treated using partial reduction and pedicular transvertebral screw fixation in an osteoporotic elderly patient. J Neurosurg Spine. 2012;16:206–9.
34. Kallmes DF, Comstock BA, Heagerty PJ, Turner JA, Wilson DJ, Diamond TH, et al. A randomized trial of vertebroplasty for osteoporotic spinal fractures. N Engl J Med. 2009;361:569–79.
35. Kanayama M, Ishida T, Hashimoto T, Shigenobu K, Togawa D, Oha F, et al. Role of major spine surgery using Kaneda anterior instrumentation for osteoporotic vertebral collapse. J Spinal Disord Tech. 2010;23:53–6.
36. Karikari IO, Grossi PM, Nimjee SM, Hardin C, Hodges TR, Hughes BD, et al. Minimally invasive lumbar interbody fusion in patients older than 70 years of age: analysis of peri- and postoperative complications. Neurosurgery. 2011;68:897–902. discussion 902.
37. Kim DH, Jaikumar S, Kam AC. Minimally invasive spine instrumentation. Neurosurgery. 2002;51:S15–25.
38. Kim KH, Lee SH, Lee DY, Shim CS, Maeng DH. Anterior bone cement augmentation in anterior lumbar interbody fusion and percutaneous pedicle screw fixation in patients with osteoporosis. J Neurosurg Spine. 2010;12:525–32.
39. Klazen CA, Lohle PN, de Vries J, Jansen FH, Tielbeek AV, Blonk MC, et al. Vertebroplasty versus conservative treatment in acute osteoporotic vertebral compression fractures (vertos II): an open-label randomised trial. Lancet. 2010;376:1085–92.
40. Lad SP, Patil CG, Lad EM, Hayden MG, Boakye M. National trends in vertebral augmentation procedures for the treatment of vertebral compression fractures. Surg Neurol. 2009;71:580–4. discussion 584–585.
41. Lau AN, Adachi JD. Resolution of osteonecrosis of the jaw after teriparatide [recombinant human PTH-(1–34)] therapy. J Rheumatol. 2009;36:1835–7.
42. Lee JH, Park JW, Shin YH. The insertional torque of a pedicle screw has a positive correlation with bone mineral density in posterior lumbar pedicle screw fixation. J Bone Joint Surg Br. 2012;94:93–7.
43. Lee JJ, Cheng SJ, Jeng JH, Chiang CP, Lau HP, Kok SH. Successful treatment of advanced bisphosphonate-related osteonecrosis of the mandible with adjunctive teriparatide therapy. Head Neck. 2011;33:1366–71.
44. Lee MJ, Dumonski M, Cahill P, Stanley T, Park D, Singh K. Percutaneous treatment of vertebral compression fractures: a meta-analysis of complications. Spine (Phila Pa 1976). 2009;34:1228–32.
45. Lee P, Fessler RG. Perioperative and postoperative complications of single-level minimally invasive transforaminal lumbar interbody fusion in elderly adults. J Clin Neurosci. 2012;19:111–4.
46. Levis S, Theodore G. Summary of AHRQ's comparative effectiveness review of treatment to prevent fractures in men and women with low bone density or osteoporosis: update of the 2007 report. J Manag Care Pharm. 2012;18:S1–15. discussion S13.

47. Lin H, Bao LH, Zhu XF, Qian C, Chen X, Han ZB. Analysis of recurrent fracture of a new vertebral body after percutaneous vertebroplasty in patients with osteoporosis. Orthop Surg. 2010;2:119–23.
48. Liu D, Wu ZX, Pan XM, Fu SC, Gao MX, Shi L, et al. Biomechanical comparison of different techniques in primary spinal surgery in osteoporotic cadaveric lumbar vertebrae: expansive pedicle screw versus polymethylmethacrylate-augmented pedicle screw. Arch Orthop Trauma Surg. 2011;131:1227–32.
49. Liu JB, Tang XM, Xu NW, Bao HT. Preliminary results for the treatment of a pain-causing osteoporotic vertebral compression fracture with a Sky Bone Expander. Korean J Radiol. 2008;9:420–5.
50. Manson NA, Phillips FM. Minimally invasive techniques for the treatment of osteoporotic vertebral fractures. Instr Course Lect. 2007;56:273–85.
51. Mobbs RJ, Sivabalan P, Li J. Minimally invasive surgery compared to open spinal fusion for the treatment of degenerative lumbar spine pathologies. J Clin Neurosci. 2012;19:829–35.
52. Moon BJ, Cho BY, Choi EY, Zhang HY. Polymethylmethacrylate-augmented screw fixation for stabilization of the osteoporotic spine : a three-year follow-up of 37 patients. J Korean Neurosurg Soc. 2009;46:305–11.
53. Movrin I, Vengust R, Komadina R. Adjacent vertebral fractures after percutaneous vertebral augmentation of osteoporotic vertebral compression fracture: a comparison of balloon kyphoplasty and vertebroplasty. Arch Orthop Trauma Surg. 2010;130: 1157–66.
54. Mundis GM, Akbarnia BA, Phillips FM. Adult deformity correction through minimally invasive lateral approach techniques. Spine (Phila Pa 1976). 2010;35:S312–21.
55. Neer RM, Arnaud CD, Zanchetta JR, Prince R, Gaich GA, Reginster JY, et al. Effect of parathyroid hormone (1–34) on fractures and bone mineral density in postmenopausal women with osteoporosis. N Engl J Med. 2001;344:1434–41.
56. Papapoulos S, Chapurlat R, Libanati C, Brandi ML, Brown JP, Czerwinski E, et al. Five years of denosumab exposure in women with postmenopausal osteoporosis: results from the first two years of the FREEDOM extension. J Bone Miner Res. 2012;27: 694–701.
57. Park SB, Chung CK. Strategies of spinal fusion on osteoporotic spine. J Korean Neurosurg Soc. 2011;49: 317–22.
58. Park SH, Park WM, Park CW, Kang KS, Lee YK, Lim SR. Minimally invasive anterior lumbar interbody fusion followed by percutaneous translaminar facet screw fixation in elderly patients. J Neurosurg Spine. 2009;10:610–6.
59. Pinera AR, Duran C, Lopez B, Saez I, Correia E, Alvarez L. Instrumented lumbar arthrodesis in elderly patients: prospective study using cannulated cemented pedicle screw instrumentation. Eur Spine J. 2011; 20(3):408–14.
60. Ponnusamy KE, Iyer S, Gupta G, Khanna AJ. Instrumentation of the osteoporotic spine: biomechanical and clinical considerations. Spine J. 2011;11: 54–63.
61. Prevrhal S, Krege JH, Chen P, Genant H, Black DM. Teriparatide vertebral fracture risk reduction determined by quantitative and qualitative radiographic assessment. Curr Med Res Opin. 2009;25:921–8.
62. Qaseem A, Snow V, Shekelle P, Hopkins Jr R, Forciea MA, Owens DK. Pharmacologic treatment of low bone density or osteoporosis to prevent fractures: a clinical practice guideline from the American College of Physicians. Ann Intern Med. 2008;149:404–15.
63. Raisz LG. Pathogenesis of osteoporosis: concepts, conflicts, and prospects. J Clin Invest. 2005;115: 3318–25.
64. Rollinghoff M, Zarghooni K, Groos D, Siewe J, Eysel P, Sobottke R. Multilevel spinal fusion in the aged: not a panacea. Acta Orthop Belg. 2011;77:97–102.
65. Rollinghoff M, Zarghooni K, Schluter-Brust K, Sobottke R, Schlegel U, Eysel P, et al. Indications and contraindications for vertebroplasty and kyphoplasty. Arch Orthop Trauma Surg. 2010;130:765–74.
66. Rosen DS, O'Toole JE, Eichholz KM, Hrubes M, Huo D, Sandhu FA, et al. Minimally invasive lumbar spinal decompression in the elderly: outcomes of 50 patients aged 75 years and older. Neurosurgery. 2007;60:503–9. discussion 509–510.
67. Saag KG, Zanchetta JR, Devogelaer JP, Adler RA, Eastell R, See K, et al. Effects of teriparatide versus alendronate for treating glucocorticoid-induced osteoporosis: thirty-six-month results of a randomized, double-blind, controlled trial. Arthritis Rheum. 2009;60:3346–55.
68. Sawakami K, Yamazaki A, Ishikawa S, Ito T, Watanabe K, Endo N. Polymethylmethacrylate augmentation of pedicle screws increases the initial fixation in osteoporotic spine patients. J Spinal Disord Tech. 2012;25:E28–35.
69. Smith ZA, Fessler RG. Paradigm changes in spine surgery: evolution of minimally invasive techniques. Nat Rev Neurol. 2012;8:443–50.
70. Sudo H, Ito M, Abumi K, Kotani Y, Takahata M, Hojo Y, et al. One-stage posterior instrumentation surgery for the treatment of osteoporotic vertebral collapse with neurological deficits. Eur Spine J. 2010;19: 907–15.
71. Tang H, Zhao JD, Li Y, Chen H, Jia P, Chan KM, et al. Efficacy of percutaneous kyphoplasty in treating osteoporotic multithoracolumbar vertebral compression fractures. Orthopedics. 2010;33:885.
72. Tokuhashi Y, Ajiro Y, Umezawa N. Outcomes of posterior fusion using pedicle screw fixation in patients>or=70 years with lumbar spinal canal stenosis. Orthopedics. 2008;31:1096.
73. Tseng YY, Su CH, Lui TN, Yeh YS, Yeh SH. Prospective comparison of the therapeutic effect of teriparatide with that of combined vertebroplasty with antiresorptive agents for the treatment of new-onset adjacent vertebral compression fracture after

percutaneous vertebroplasty. Osteoporos Int. 2012;23: 1613–22.
74. Uchida K, Nakajima H, Yayama T, Miyazaki T, Hirai T, Kobayashi S, et al. Vertebroplasty-augmented short-segment posterior fixation of osteoporotic vertebral collapse with neurological deficit in the thoracolumbar spine: comparisons with posterior surgery without vertebroplasty and anterior surgery. J Neurosurg Spine. 2010;13:612–21.
75. Vahle JL, Sato M, Long GG, Young JK, Francis PC, Engelhardt JA, et al. Skeletal changes in rats given daily subcutaneous injections of recombinant human parathyroid hormone (1–34) for 2 years and relevance to human safety. Toxicol Pathol. 2002;30: 312–21.
76. Vougioukas V, Hubbe U, Kogias E, Psarras N, Halatsch ME. Vertebroplasty combined with image-guided percutaneous cement augmented transpedicular fixation for the treatment of complex vertebral fractures in osteoporotic patients. J Neurosurg Sci. 2010;54:135–41.
77. Wang MY, Mummaneni PV. Minimally invasive surgery for thoracolumbar spinal deformity: initial clinical experience with clinical and radiographic outcomes. Neurosurg Focus. 2010; 28:E9.
78. Watanabe A, Yoneyama S, Nakajima M, Sato N, Takao-Kawabata R, Isogai Y, et al. Osteosarcoma in Sprague–Dawley rats after long-term treatment with teriparatide (human parathyroid hormone (1–34)). J Toxicol Sci. 2012;37:617–29.
79. Watts NB, Bilezikian JP, Camacho PM, Greenspan SL, Harris ST, Hodgson SF, et al. American Association of Clinical Endocrinologists Medical Guidelines for Clinical Practice for the diagnosis and treatment of postmenopausal osteoporosis. Endocr Pract. 2010;16(3):1–37.
80. Wu ZX, Cui G, Lei W, Fan Y, Wan SY, Ma ZS, et al. Application of an expandable pedicle screw in the severe osteoporotic spine: a preliminary study. Clin Invest Med. 2010;33:E368–74.
81. Wu ZX, Gong FT, Liu L, Ma ZS, Zhang Y, Zhao X, et al. A comparative study on screw loosening in osteoporotic lumbar spine fusion between expandable and conventional pedicle screws. Arch Orthop Trauma Surg. 2012;132:471–6.
82. Xiong J, Dang Y, Jiang BG, Fu ZG, Zhang DY. Treatment of osteoporotic compression fracture of thoracic/lumbar vertebrae by kyphoplasty with SKY bone expander system. Chin J Traumatol. 2010;13: 270–4.
83. Yagi M, King AB, Boachie-Adjei O. Characterization of osteopenia/osteoporosis in adult scoliosis: does bone density affect surgical outcome? Spine (Phila Pa 1976). 2011;36:1652–7.
84. Zhuang XM, Yu BS, Zheng ZM, Zhang JF, Lu WW. Effect of the degree of osteoporosis on the biomechanical anchoring strength of the sacral pedicle screws: an in vitro comparison between unaugmented bicortical screws and polymethylmethacrylate augmented unicortical screws. Spine (Phila Pa 1976). 2010;35:E925–31.

16 Minimally Invasive Cement-Augmented Pedicle Screw Fixation

Brian Hood and Steven Vanni

Osteoporosis is a major health threat. In the United States alone, 10 million people have osteoporosis already, and 18 million have low bone mass placing them at increased risk for the development of osteoporosis [1]. Once thought to be a natural part of aging among women, it is not longer considered age or sex dependant.

Osteoporosis is defined as a skeletal disorder characterized by compromised bone strength predisposing a person to increase risk of fractures [1]. Bone density is expressed as grams of mineral per area of volume (cm^2). Bone quality refers to architecture, turnover, damage accumulation, and mineralization. Currently, there is no accurate measure of overall bone strength [1]. Bone mineral density (BMD) is frequently used as a proxy measure and accounts for around 70 % of bone strength.

The World Health Organization defines osteoporosis as bone density 2.5 standard deviations below the mean for young healthy people [2]. Osteoporosis can either be classified as primary or secondary. Primary osteoporosis can occur in both sexes at all ages but often follows menopause in women and occurs later in life in men [1]. In contrast, secondary osteoporosis is a result of medications (glucocorticoids), other conditions (hypogonadism), or disease (celiac disease). The prevalence of osteoporosis vary by sex and ethnicity [1]. Both men and women experience an age-related decline in BMD starting in midlife. Women experience more rapid bone loss in the early years following menopause. In men, hypogonadism is an important risk factor. African-American women have higher BMD than white non-Hispanic women [1]. Mexican-American women have BMDs between those of white non-Hispanic women and African-American women (Table 16.1 and 16.2).

For men, 30–60 % of osteoporosis cases are associated with secondary causes [1], the most common causes being hypogonadism, glucocorticoids, and alcoholism. In perimenopausal

Table 16.1 Risk factors for osteoporosis

Risk factors (predictors of low bone mass)	Inconsistent predictors of low bone mass
Female sex	Levels of exercise in childhood and adolescence
Increased age	Use of alcohol- and caffeine-containing beverages
Estrogen deficiency	Late menarche
White race	Early menopause
Low weight and body mass index (BMI)	Low endogenous estrogen levels
Family history of osteoporosis	
Smoking	
History of prior fracture (hip, vertebral) [1]	

B. Hood, M.D.
Department of Neurosurgery, Brooke Army Medical Center, San Antonio, TX 78234, USA

S. Vanni, DO, DC (✉)
Department of Neurological Surgery, University of Miami, Miami, FL, USA
e-mail: svanni@med.miami.edu

M.Y. Wang et al. (eds.), *Minimally Invasive Spinal Deformity Surgery*,
DOI 10.1007/978-3-7091-1407-0_16, © Springer-Verlag Wien 2014

women, the most common causes are hypoestrogenemia, glucocorticoids, thyroid hormone excess, and anticonvulsant therapy [1].

Glucocorticoids are the most common cause of drug-related osteoporosis especially long-term administration for rheumatoid arthritis (RA) and chronic obstructive pulmonary disease (COPD). In a prospective study, a group of patients was treated with 10 mg of prednisone/day for 20 weeks and experienced an 8 % loss of BMD in the spine. In addition, other secondary causes including organ transplantation, cystic fibrosis, celiac disease, and inflammatory bowel disease are conditions associated with malabsorption and resultant osteoporosis [1].

Table 16.2 Secondary osteoporosis

Secondary osteoporosis
Genetic
Hypogonadal states
Endocrine disorders
GI disease
Hematologic disorder
Connective tissue disease
Nutritional deficiency
Drugs
Congestive heart failure (CHF)
End-stage renal disease (ESRD)
Alcoholism

The WHO has selected BMD measurements to establish criteria for the diagnosis of osteoporosis. T-score is defined as the number of standard deviations (SD) above or below the average BMD value for a young healthy white woman. T-score is to be distinguished from a Z-score which is defined as the number of SDs above or below the average BMD for age- and sex-matched controls. According to the WHO, osteoporosis is present when the T-score is below 2.5 standard deviations. T-scores were based originally on BMD obtained by dual-energy x-ray absorptiometry (DEXA) [1] (Fig. 16.1).

On the basis of simple lateral lumbar vertebral plain films, the authors proposed a grading scale to categorize the severity of osteoporosis. The classification consists of five grades: normal, initial stage, Grade 1, Grade 2, and Grade 3 (Table 16.3).

Osteoporosis plays a significant role in the progression of adult spinal instability and deformity. It has become a growing concern among the medical community as both a primary cause of musculoskeletal dysfunction and a comorbidity among patients requiring surgical intervention.

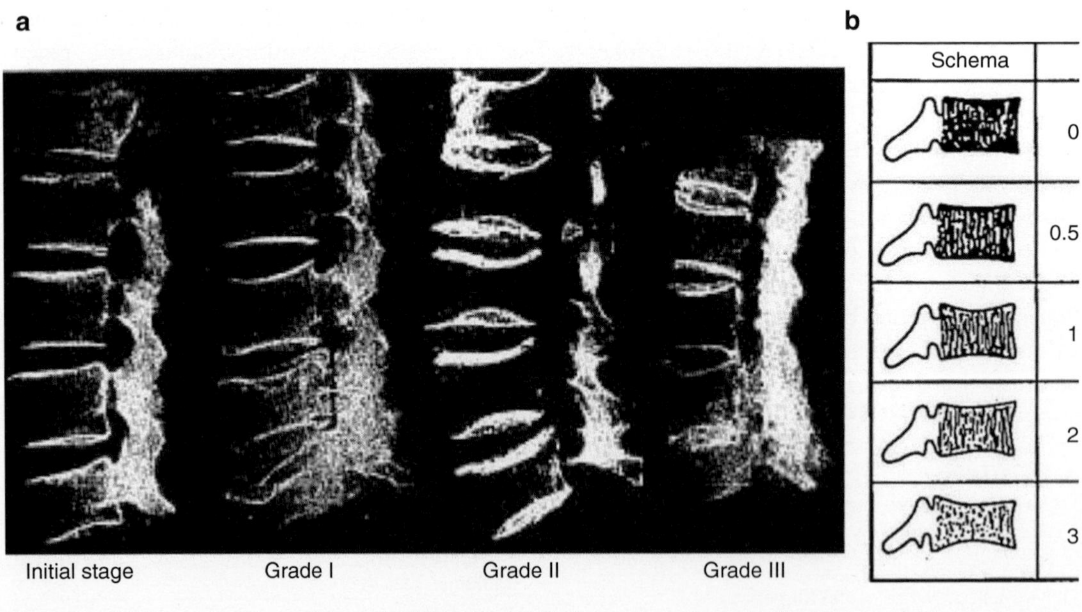

Fig. 16.1 Jikei osteoporosis grading scale. (**a**) Radiographic image in each grade. (**b**) Schema of Jikei osteoporosis grading

Table 16.3 Jikei osteoporosis grading scale

Jikei osteoporosis grading scale	
0	Normal trabecular pattern
0.5	Number of trabecula normal, bone density decreased, trabecula thin
1	Transverse trabecula decreased, vertical trabecula, and end plate prominent
2	Transverse trabecula more decrease, vertical trabecula decreased
3	Transverse trabecula almost disappear, vertical trabecula more like a ground glass image

An increased elderly population in industrial countries is a well-know problem to society and health services. In 2050, 54 % of the population will be older than 65 years in countries with a human development index of >0.9 [3]. Scoliotic deformities are prevalent in 36–48 % of osteoporotic women and worsened by osteoporotic vertebral fractures [4]. Osteoporotic patients requiring spinal instrumentation for instability or deformity are of significant concern. Not long ago, patients with osteoporosis and progressive deformity (scoliosis) or fracture, even with neurological manifestations, were considered inoperable. With advances in surgical technique and instrumentation and growing expectations of patients, surgeons are taking on greater reconstructive challenges.

16.1 Instrumenting the Osteoporotic Spine

Failure of pedicle screw fixation can result from screw loosening or pullout. As posterior pedicle screw systems increase in strength and rigidity, greater demands are placed on the bone-screw interface [5]. Interface strength can be affected by surgical insertion technique, type of implant used, augmentation with bone or bone cement, and bone density [5–10] (Table 16.4).

In the osteoporotic spine or in revision surgery, the bone-screw interface strength may be severely compromised. Previous biomechanical studies have demonstrated that pedicle screw fixation is highly correlated to BMD [7] and that increasing in screw pullout strength is possible

Table 16.4 Factors affecting bone-screw interface strength

Interface strength
Insertion technique
Type of implant
Bone density
Augmentation

using a variety of methods [5, 7–9]. An expandable pedicle screw design has been shown to markedly increase the pullout strength of the bone-screw interface [11]. Statistically significant increase in pullout strength was found when an expandable screw was compared with standard pedicle screws in both high and low BMD specimens [11, 12]. Although available, (Omega-21, Biomet Spine) expandable screws have fallen out of favor because of concerns for revision surgery. Alternative methods such as augmenting conventional screws with polymethyl methacrylate (PMMA) bone cement and calcium phosphate bone cements have also been shown to increase the strength of the bone-screw interface. However, fixation in the severely osteoporotic spine represents a challenge regardless of techniques.

The key to fixation lies in the strength of the purchase obtained by the screws in the pedicle and the trabecular bone of the vertebral body [13]. Osteoporosis is implicated as the cause of hardware failure at an unknown rate. Loss of purchase and screw loosening in older patients with degenerative spondylosis has been reported to occur intraoperatively at a rate of 1.7 % and postoperatively at a rate of 3.8 % [14]. The common problems are screw bending, breakage, and lucency at the bone-screw interface. A selected survey of the American Back Society showed the rate of screw loosening, and breakage was observed in 0.81 % and 2.9 % of 617 cases and ranged from 0.6 % to 11 % and 0.6 % to 25 % in a literature review [15].

The bone-screw interface is the main determinant of the stability of the screw. Screw loosening is mainly caused by cyclic caudocephalad toggling at the bone-screw interface when an axial compressive load is transmitted through the rod to the screw [16, 17]. If a screw is inadequately anchored into the vertebral body through the

Table 16.5 Techniques for augmenting the bone-screw interface

Techniques for augmenting the bone-screw interface
Bicortical purchase
Undertapping
Offset laminar hooks
Expandable pedicle screws
Resorbable polymers
Rib grafts
Milled bone
Matchstick bone
Bone cement (PMMA, calcium phosphate, hydroxyapatite)
Instrumentation without tapping

pedicle, loosening of the screw could lead to loss of correction and nonunion. To predict the development of screw loosening, objective assessment of the stability of the bone-screw interface is a critical issue. If surgeons could forecast which patients are likely to develop screw loosening with the potential for loss of correction and nonunion, they may choose to use supplementary augmentation.

Bone mineral density affects the stability of pedicle screws in vivo [18, 19]. Wittenberg demonstrated that loosening occurs in cadaveric spine with BMD below 0.74+−0.17 g/cc under physiological loading [8]. However, specified thresholds of BMD have rarely been identified below which screw loosening and nonunion develop in clinical practice. Based on in vivo studies, Wittenberg concluded that early loosening of pedicle screw may be expected at BMD measure by quantitative CT (QCT) less than 0.9 g/cm^2 [8]. Okuyama suggested that patients with a mean BMD less than 0.674 g/cm^2 could indicate the need for supplementation [19] (Table 16.5).

Although Pfeifer demonstrated an increase in pullout strength of 50–70 % [9] with milled and matchstick bone, this technique and several others mentioned above do not readily lend themselves to minimally invasive surgery. Previous experience with screw fixation for severe osteoporosis indicates that it is often necessary to increase the number of vertebra fused in order to avoid instrumentation failure. However, this requires longer incisions, more screws, increased operating time, and patient morbidity.

16.2 Augmentation Techniques

Cook et al. performed an evaluation of expansile pedicle screws in vivo and in vitro [11, 12] (Fig. 16.2).

In cadaver specimens with poor BMD (0.62+−0.44 g/cm^2), the mean axial pullout strength was increased 30 % [11] with the expansile screws. The specimens were further divided into very low BMD (0.28+−0.12 g/cm^2) and high (0.95+−0.34 g/cm^2). In the very low group, the axial pullout strength was increased by approximately 50 % with the expansile design as compared to a conventional self-tapping screw [11]. In the high BMD group, the pullout strength of the expansile screw was increased approximately 200 % compared to a conventional self-tapping screw [11]. In his clinical series of 14 implanted patients, 93 % obtained relief of preoperative symptoms and 13/14 (93 %) demonstrated radiographic criteria for fusion [11]. There were no reports of screw loosening or back out. This novel technology, however, has no MIS application, and it has fallen out of favor in open surgery.

16.3 Screw Geometry/Insertion

As previously mentioned, screw effectiveness is critically dependant on its interface with bone. The principle factors that determine the magnitude of screw interface are (1) the geometry of the screw, (2) bone elastic modulus (i.e., BMD), and (3) quality of fit. Components of screw geometry that increase bone-screw interface purchase are increased major thread diameter, increased thread depth, and increased length of engagement. Screw design can be optimized for a particular site, and this approach to screw performance has been well described in the literature [20].

Screw fit can be influenced by the method of hole preparation. Based on a review of the literature, hole preparation appears to be very important in osteoporotic vertebra. Tapping pilot holes into osteoporotic bone decreases the pullout strength of screws [21, 22]. Regarding screw diameter, mean axial pullout force was increased from 459+−183 N to 994+−349 N just by increasing the diameter by 1 mm [8]. Zindrick

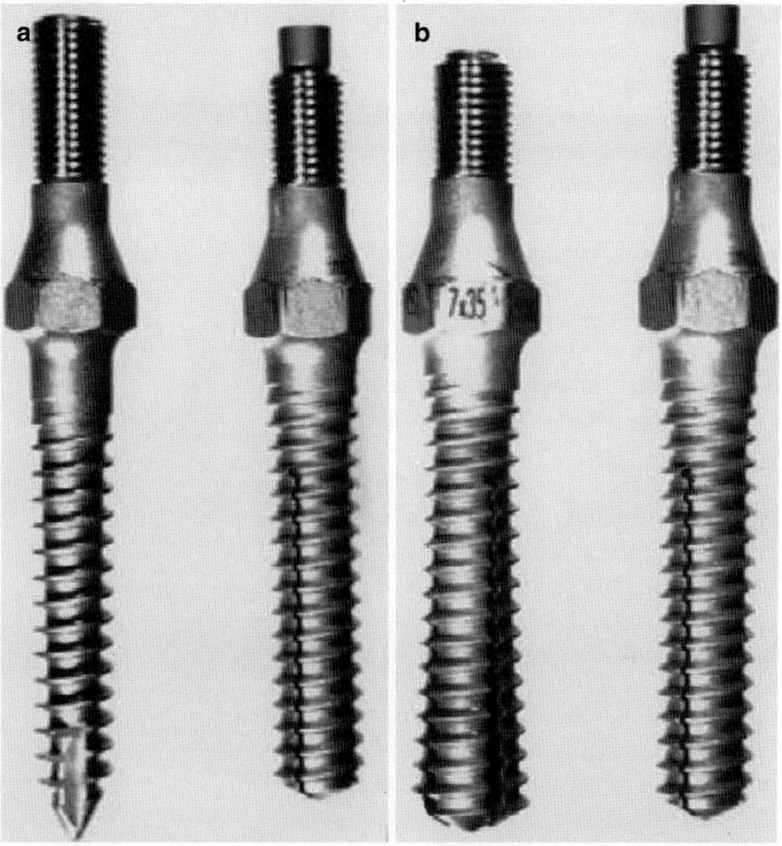

Fig. 16.2 Expansile pedicle screws

evaluated the effect of the insertion depth on the number of cycles to failure. He found an increase of approximately 430 % when comparing screws inserted to 50 % of the depth of the vertebral body as compared to those inserted through the opposite cortex [23].

Screw profile and insertion are very important components to ensuring a solid bone-screw interface. Choosing a screw that will ensure good fit, has an appropriate tread pattern (cortical to engage the pedicle wall), and is inserted to the appropriate depth to reduce the likelihood of toggle-related failure are all concepts that MIS surgeons are aware of and need to be mindful of when instrumenting osteoporotic patients.

16.4 Cement Augmentation

In early evaluation of augmenting pedicle screws, Wittenberg demonstrated a 50 % increase in bending stiffness in screws augmented with PMMA and a 20 % increase in bending stiffness with their biodegradable polymer [8]. Since their report, there have been numerous studies with augmentation materials and techniques which we will review to determine the best application for MIS surgery.

There is no question that bone cement augmentation enhances the bone-screw interface strength. PMMA was used initially for pelvic surgery, and the use of bone cement in orthopedic procedures involving joint prostheses fixation has been used with consistent demonstration of an improved bone prosthesis interface [24, 25]. Today's PMMA are radiopaque and have reduced exothermic polymerization to reduce tissue necrosis and nerve damage in case of leakage. Two cementing techniques for stabilization of a vertebra are currently in clinical use, vertebroplasty, and balloon kyphoplasty. Vertebroplasty has considerable risks regarding cement leakage and a slightly higher perioperative morbidity than balloon kyphoplasty [26].

Becker et al. [27] conducted an in vivo study on osteoporotic cadaver spines comparing augmentation techniques with PMMA. They evaluated non-augmented solid (non-cannulated) screws, perforated screw with vertebroplasty augmentation, solid screw with balloon kyphoplasty augmentation, and solid screws with vertebroplasty augmentation. They found that vertebroplasty-augmented screws, augmentation of perforated screws, and balloon kyphoplasty-augmented screws all show higher pullout resistance than non-augmented screws, but significantly higher pullout forces were only seen in the vertebroplasty-augmented group [27].

The pertinent technical comments from their study include the observation that the perforated screw had significant handling advantages. It is technically easier to inject cement directly through the screw. In addition, the screw can be positioned and verified then changed if need be, characteristics that are impossible when using a non-perforated screw. It is possible to first place screws over multiple segments then augment. They noted that a simultaneous multisegmental approach is challenging in the vertebroplasty group and nearly impossible in the balloon kyphoplasty group [27] (Fig. 16.3).

Frankel et al. also conducted a biomechanical cadaveric analysis of PMMA-augmented screws in both primary and salvage procedures [28]. They demonstrated an increase in pullout strength of 119 % in primary and 162 % in salvage procedures. This is similar to the work of Sarzier, who demonstrated an increase in pullout force of 181 % for Jikei Grade I, 206 % for Jikei Grade II, and 213 % for Jikei Grade III [10]. Importantly, Sarzier demonstrated that with augmentation, a Jikei Grade II and III vertebra exhibited pullout strength similar to levels found in non-augmented vertebrae with low-normal BMD and non-augmented Grade I vertebra, respectively [10].

Frankel also studied the effect of the volume of cement. Two groups were investigated, a low-cement group (less than 2.8 ml/pedicle) and a high-cement group (greater than 5.5 ml/pedicle). He found that cement injection less than 2.8 ml/pedicle is as effective as one that is greater than 5.5 ml/pedicle [28]. Therefore, they recommend using a lower volume of cement to reduce the likelihood of cement toxicity.

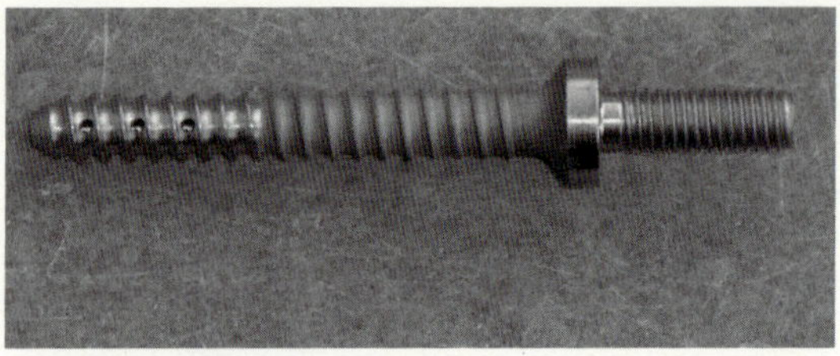

Fig. 16.3 Perforated screws

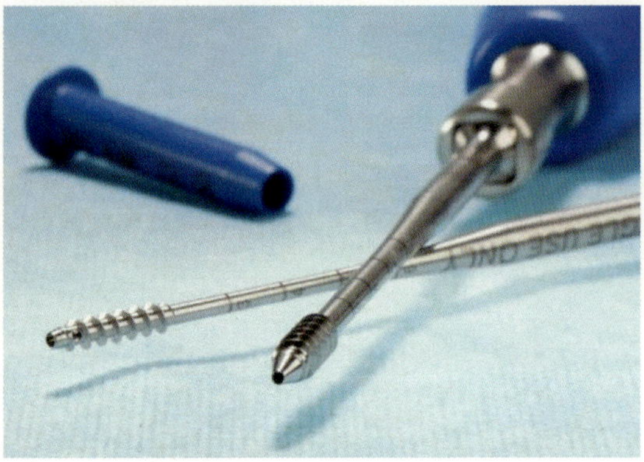

Fig. 16.4 Fenestrated tap

Frankel also proposed a new mechanism of introducing the cement to reduce the risk of posterior migration of cement along the injection track toward the neural elements. To overcome the availability of fenestrated screws, he designed a fenestrated tap that is commercially available (Pedestal, Abbot Spine). They first cannulated the pedicle with a Jamshidi needle then introduced a K-wire and removed the targeting needle. The bone tap was placed over the K-wire and threaded into the anterior third of the vertebral body. The tap was then flushed with 3–5 ml of saline, and cement was then injected through the tap under lateral fluoroscopy. The tap was left in place for approximately 1 min to allow partial consolidation of the cement then removed, and an appropriate screw was placed over the K-wire (Fig. 16.4).

In a clinical series, Frankel employed his method of cement augmentation in 23 consecutive patients who all had bone softening secondary to osteoporosis and/or metastatic spinal tumor involvement [29]. Through the placement of 158 PMMA-augmented screws, asymptomatic anterior cement extravasation was observed in 39 % of patients which is consistent with what the literature reports [30–35]. They did not observe any posterior migration of cement toward the neural elements that is associated with radiculopathy that pull out strength increased by nearly 70 % when the screw was augmented with CBC [20]. Augmentation also increased stiffness by 50 % and increased the energy absorbed by cyclic loading by more than 70 % [20] Renner et al. [36] evaluated calcium phosphate cement augmentation of pedicle screws as a function and/or myelopathy. They reported one asymptomatic PMMA pulmonary embolism and one superficial wound infection. They also reported having no construct failures in their cement-augmented cases.

PMMA is not biodegradable and persists within the trabecular bone and is likely to influence bone remodeling by affecting metabolism and changing the environment. The monomer itself is toxic and can cause a large immunologic response and can cause giant cell reaction [37]. These undesirable properties have lead to the investigation of biocompatible bone cements for screw augmentation.

Lotz et al. [20] studied an injectable biocompatible carbonated apatite cancellous bone cement (CBC) that is practically non-exothermic (Norian, SRS, Skeletal Repair System, Norian Corporation Cupertino, CA). They found in vivo of injection timing and method. Using calcium phosphate cement (CaP) BoneSource (Howmedica Osteonics, Rutherford, NJ), they augmented pedicle screws and compared them to non-augmented screws and screws augmented with PMMA. BoneSource is biocompatible, osteoconductive, and resorbable and has a high 24-h wet compressive strength. PMMA was injected such that only the distal screw was augmented. CaP was injected in two different fashions. One fashion involved only the tip of the screw as in the PMMA group. The second group involved injection of CaP distally in the vertebral body as well as along the pedicle completely encasing the screw. Comparison of CaP injection by both methods to PMMA showed that PMMA produced significantly higher pullout strength in both revision and augmentation cases [36].

Yazu et al. [38] evaluated augmentation with calcium phosphate via a fenestrated screw. Their technique lends some important technical considerations to the procedure of augmentation. Using a fenestrated screw, they first injected contrast to see if there was any extravasation into the epidural venous plexus prior to injecting cement. After augmented with CPC cement, they found pullout strength to be increased by nearly 250 % [38]. They concluded that the pullout strength was similar to PMMA even though the compressive strength was not [38]. Although they demonstrated increased strength of the bone-screw interface, in vivo studies need to be conducted to determine the long-term biocompatibility, rate of resorption, as well as the long-term biomechanical behavior of the cement. In addition, calcium phosphate cement has relatively low fracture strength, is brittle, and has high susceptibility to fatigue failure [39].

Ignatius et al. [40] designed an injectable bioresorbable polymer based on alkylene bis(dilactoyl) methycrylate that has demonstrated appropriate degradation characteristics. Augmentation with the new polymer increased pullout force by 88 % in bovine vertebra and 118 % in human vertebrae [40]. In their testing, they found the mechanical efficacy comparable to PMMA, but the biodegradable properties potentially allow osteosynthesis in osteoporotic patients. However, ongoing studies to investigate in vitro and in vivo biocompatibility are needed.

Technically, the best way to cement augmenting a screw is to first place the screw and confirms the position fluoroscopically prior to augmenting. Using a fenestrated cannulated screw, this lends itself to an MIS application and is the most logical way augment screws. This also allows multiple levels to be addressed simultaneously and maximizes augmentation in regard to cement working time. McKoy and An [41] demonstrated that a cannulated fenestrated screw had a 278 % greater pullout strength than a solid screw after augmentation.

The use of PMMA is not without risk. Systemic complications of PMMA have been extensively documented in the literature and range from pulmonary embolism [42], hypoxia [43], hypotension [44], myocardial infarction [45, 46], and sudden death [47, 48]. Although its in vivo properties of strengthening the bone-screw interface are not in question and it has been used as a salvage procedure for years, Frankel has demonstrated that through meticulous application, it can be safely used in a frail patient population.

16.5 Conclusion

PMMA is regarded as the best method to enhance screw strength significantly in osteoporotic bone [8–10, 23, 29, 49]. PMMA augmentation has been shown to provide higher strength than all alternative techniques [9, 23, 28]. Cementing enhances the fixation of the screw within the vertebral body transferring the load from the pedicle to the body. The application of cement-augmented screws can enhance the strength of anterior implants [50]. Screw supplementation with PMMA is indicated in osteoporotic patients (T-score of −2.5 by DEXA or BMD of 0.80 g/cm^2) requiring instrumentation for instability or degenerative scoliosis. The application of PMMA allows instrumentation to be applied in this complex patient population. It also allows a shorter fusion segment compared to the one without augmentation.

The use of calcium phosphate and hydroxyapatite bone cement is fascinating concepts. However, clinically, it has not been adequately tested and currently is not FDA approved for application in the spine.

Regarding the method of cement delivery, the ideal system is a cannulated fenestrated screw with cortical thread pitch. However, currently this is only available to our European colleagues. As we eagerly await its US release, we will describe below our current technique for cement augmentation.

16.6 Technique

When utilizing cement, an additional time constraint of the high viscosity cement working time is added for the surgeon. For most cements, the high viscosity working time is around 8–10 min at 68 F/20 C. In order to place instrumentation within the time constraints imposed by the varying cements, efficient work room flow is imperative. Every aspect of the case must be considered and rehearsed with the OR staff prior to mixing the cement.

The first step is planning what length and diameter screw is appropriate for the levels to be fixated. A general sense of pedicle diameter and size of the vertebral body can be gained from preoperative CT scans with sagittal and coronal reconstruction which are obtained in all of our preoperative patients (Fig. 16.5). Using this as a guide, the surgical technologist can begin to load up appropriate-sized screws prior to the placement of cement. Adjustments can be made later after the pedicles are cannulated based on intraoperative imaging. Preoperative images are clearly visible in the OR at all times, and preoperative measurements are recorded by an assistant for easy access at the time of screw placement.

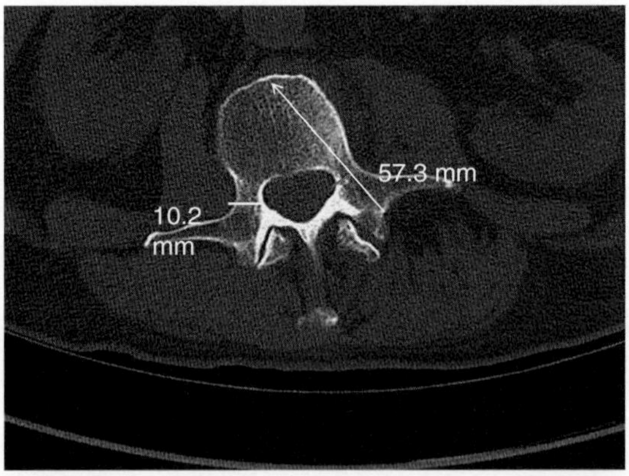

Fig. 16.5 Preoperative axial view of L3 (The preoperative measurements have been made in a standard iSite Radiology Suite. The pedicle diameter and the depth of the vertebral body are recorded, and an appropriate-sized screw is planned based on these measurements. Also note the approximately 15° of rotation. This can be accounted for perioperatively by "airplaning" the bed or rolling the arc of the image intensifier)

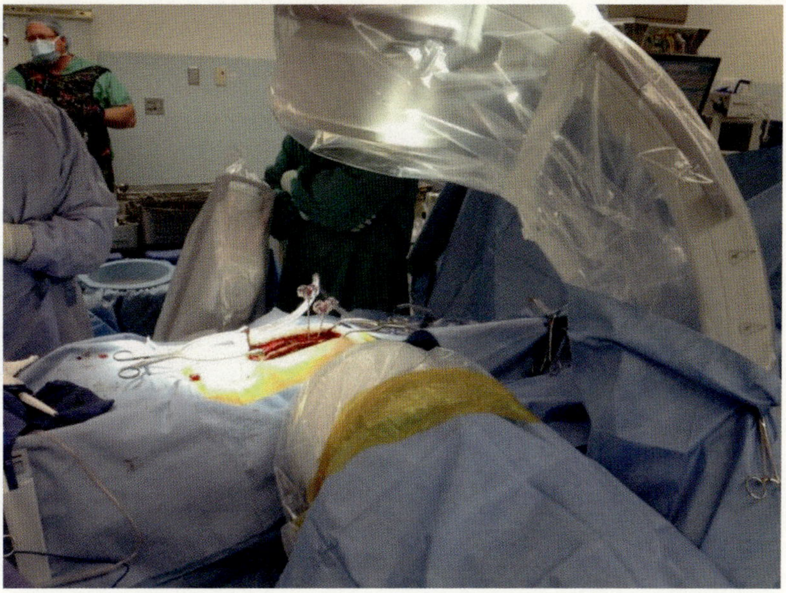

Fig. 16.6 Biplanar fluoroscopy (Intraoperative view of biplanar fluoroscopy set up. Utilization of biplanar fluoroscopy allows adequate visualization of cement during injection to avoid extravasation and saves working time during multilevel procedures)

Prior to the prep, we introduce biplanar fluoroscopy and visualize the appropriate levels under A/P and lateral fluoroscopy (Fig. 16.6). As the rotation and cranial/caudal orientation can vary tremendously in patients with significant deformity, making note of the appropriate cranial caudal orientation and arc of the A/P image intensifier for quick reference will help ensure the appropriate views are found quickly during the placement of instrumentation. Osteoporotic bone is often difficult to visualize on C-arm fluoroscopy, so the addition of an experienced radiology technician is invaluable in these cases.

After the patient is prepped and draped, the two C-arm image intensifiers are introduced sterilely into the field, and the appropriate images are obtained. Starting points are marked on the skin, and we plan our stab incisions such that they are completely aligned for cosmetic reasons postoperatively. The skin is infiltrated with 0.25 % Marcaine with epinephrine 1:200,000 prior to skin incision. The skin is scored with a 15 blade then opened with monopolar cautery. The fascia will be cut later prior to dilating. This decreases the intraoperative oozing in multilevel cases. Under A/P fluoroscopy, a Jamshidi needle is advanced 20 mm into the pedicle. Under lateral fluoroscopy, the needle is then advanced into the vertebral body. It is imperative not to violate the anterior wall of the vertebral body or the pedicle walls to reduce the chance of cement migration. At this point, the surgeon had the option to place all the Jamshidi needs or focus on several segments initially and "stage" the placement of the instrumentation. We found that within the working time of cement, four cement-augmented screws can be placed comfortably during the 8–10-min working time of the cement (Fig. 16.7).

The K-wires are then placed. In severely osteoporotic patients, we have modified our technique and have begun to use a Y-wire instead of standard Kirschner wire (Fig. 16.8). The Y-wires forked tip allows us to proceed at pace without inadvertently placing the wire through the anterior aspect of the vertebral body. Once all the K-wires or Y-wires are placed, the fascia is cut with a ten blade, and the dilators are placed through the fascia and docked onto bone. Final changes to screw length are made prior to proceeding, and the appropriate instrumentation is prepared and is made readily accessible. At this point, the surgical technologist can begin preparing the cement (Fig. 16.9). Once the levels have been tapped, the Jamshidi needle is reintroduced and the wire removed and placed aside.

At this point, work flow is crucial. The appropriate-sized screws are set aside and ready for insertion. A/P and lateral images are

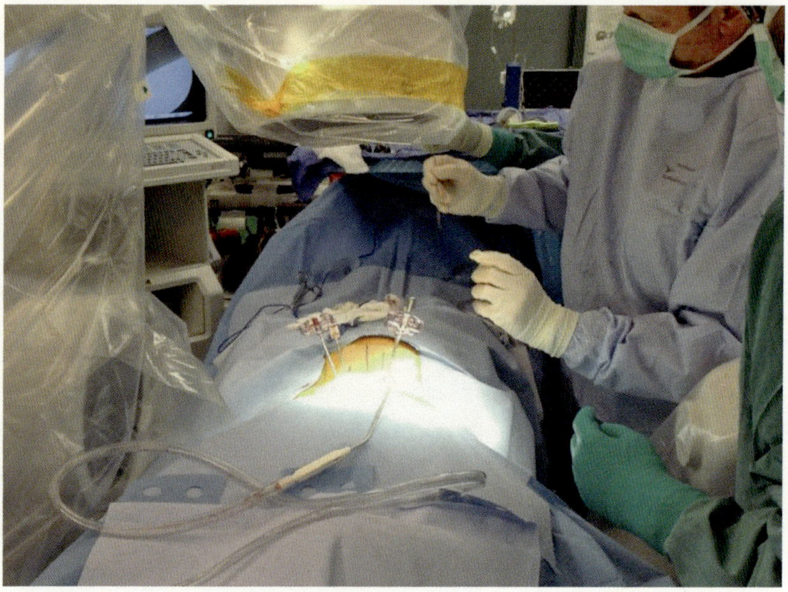

Fig. 16.7 Placement of Jamshidi needles (In this procedure, the first four pedicles have been cannulated under biplanar fluoroscopy. At this point, we remove the Jamshidi needles and place our K-wires)

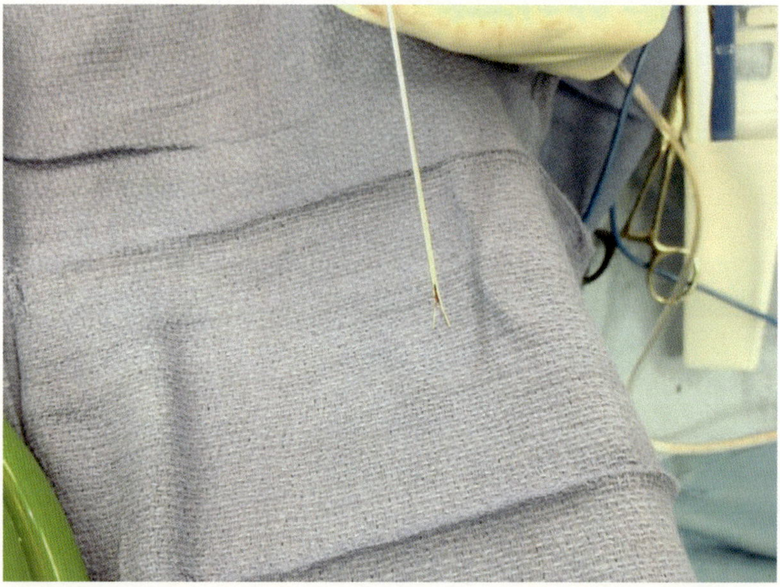

Fig. 16.8 Y-wire (The forked end of the Y-wire is extremely helpful in osteoporotic patients to prevent the wire from advancing inadvertently beyond the vertebral body)

verified, and the cement injection system is connected to the Jamshidi (Fig. 16.10). Cement is slowly injected into the vertebral body periodically checking the lateral image. Once the "blush" of cement is seen, we allow additional cement to fill without actively pumping it into the vertebral body (Fig. 16.11). The pressure injector is then disconnected, and the cannula is reintroduced into the Jamshidi needle plunging the remaining cement into the vertebral body (Fig. 16.12). This is a very important step in that it can introduce up to an additional 1 cc of cement depending on the diameter and the length of the Jamshidi needle being used. It also frees the cannula to allow the K-wire to be reintroduced smoothly (Fig. 16.13). Once

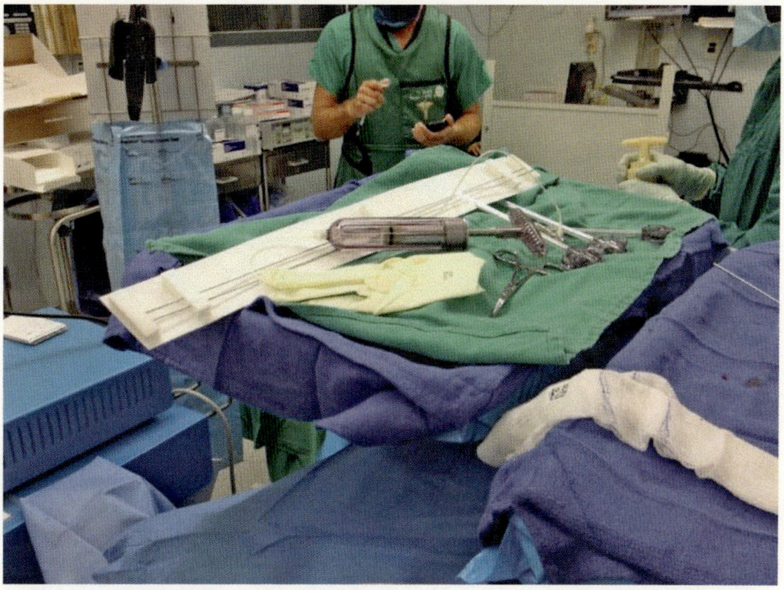

Fig. 16.9 Preparing the cement (The cement is being mixed. Mixing time is around 40–60 s, total prep time is around 3–5 min to prepare the assembly. Seen at the forefront is the pressure injector)

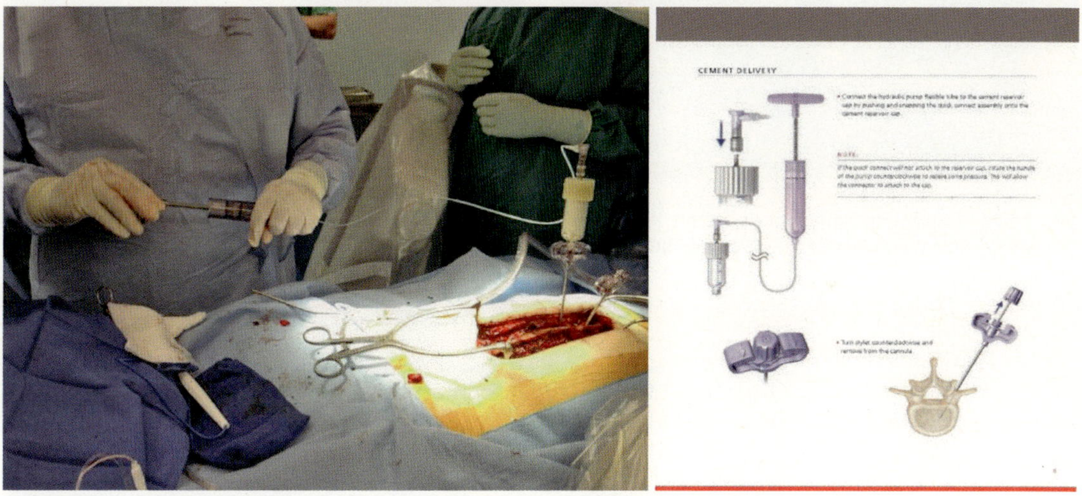

Fig. 16.10 Injecting cement (The pressure injecting system is connected and the pump twisted. The length of tubing allows the operator to stand an additional 2 ft from the image intensifiers to decrease radiation exposure)

the K-wire is reinserted, the screw is then placed over the wire in the standard fashion (Fig. 16.14). It is imperative to ensure that the height of the screw head is in alignment with the rest of the construct. Once the cement hardens, there is no way to adjust the head for rod placement (Table 16.6).

We began our cement augmentation with open procedures and have since modified it for MIS delivery of cement and placement of screws. We eagerly await the introduction of cannulated fenestrated screws in North America, as this will greatly simplify our work flow. However, the basic concepts and tenants remain very similar. It is imperative to have exceptional work flow, as cement will not wait for errors in loading equipment or having equipment available in a timely fashion.

Below are CT images postoperatively from a cement-augmented correction of deformity. The patient was previously treated with a combination of open and MIS kyphoplasty for thoracic compression fractures and developed a progressive deformity. We chose to perform open surgery as facet excision allowed additional correction of deformity (Figs. 16.15 and 16.16).

Cannulated fenestrated pedicle screws – the future of cement-augmented minimally invasive procedures (Fig. 16.17)

16.6.1 Technique

Once again, successful placement of cement-augmented screws required meticulous planning from measurements made on preoperative imaging, rehearsing steps with the OR staff to maximize work flow and obtaining adequate visualization in two planes.

The first step once again involves preparing the spine and cannulating the pedicles with Jamshidi needles, placing guide wires and dilating the

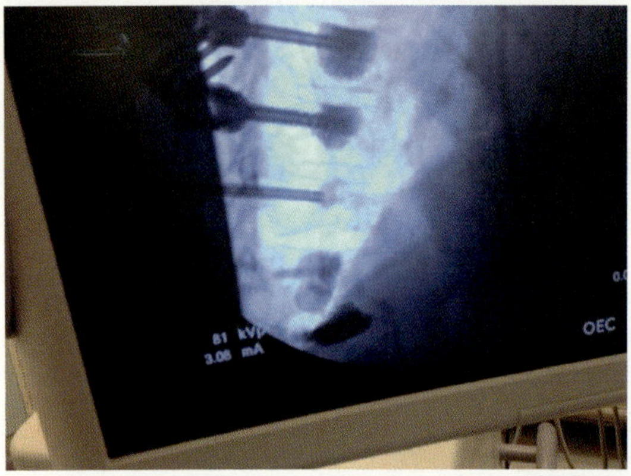

Fig. 16.11 Cement injection under lateral fluoroscopy (We inject cement until we begin to see the blush. At this point, we slow the injection and allow some "passive" filling)

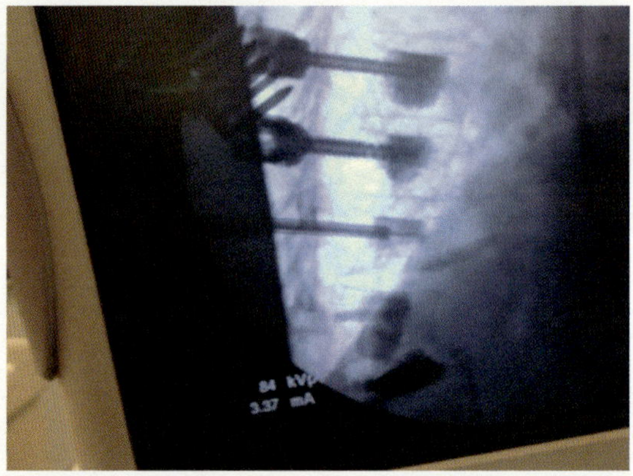

Fig. 16.13 Reintroducing the K-wire (The two levels above have been injected and instrumented. We were able to place four screws comfortably within the 8–10-min high viscosity working window of our cement)

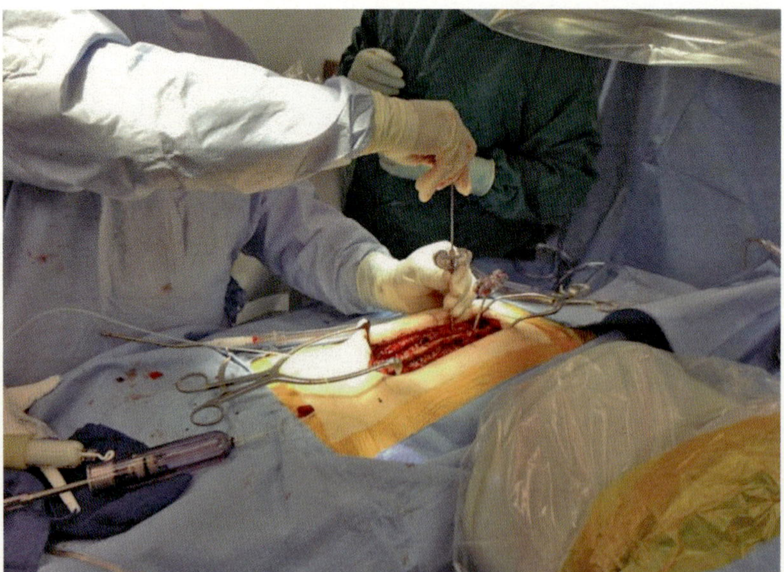

Fig. 16.12 Plunging the cannula (The pressure injector is disconnected, and the cannula is reinserted plunging the remaining cement in the cannula into the vertebral body. Depending on the diameter of the cannula selected, this can be up to an additional 1 cc of cement)

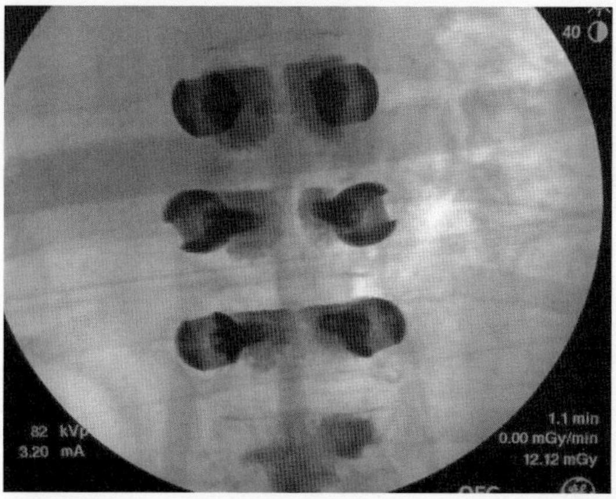

Fig. 16.14 A/P image post-instrumentation placement (Good filling of the vertebral bodies without any extravasation after placement of instrumentation)

Table 16.6 Technique pearls and pitfalls for inserting cement-augmented screws

Pearls	Pitfalls
8–10-min working time, ensure that all instrumentation is appropriately sized, loaded correctly, and easily accessible prior to injecting cement	Overly aggressive pressure injection of cement. Remember, up to 1 cc cement remains in the cannula
Plunging the cannula prior to reinsertion of K-wire allows additional cement delivery and easy passage of K-wire	Not properly aligning screw head heights. Once the cement sets, there is no way to adjust head height
Biplanar fluoroscopy allows assessment of cement and instrumentation in two planes simultaneously and saves critical time while working with cement	Do not breach the anterior wall of the vertebral body or the pedicles during cannulation

fascia. The next step involves placement of the screws after preparing the pedicle with awls and taps (Fig. 16.18). Fenestrated screws should not be placed bicortically. It is also very important not to breach the pedicle wall or the anterior cortex of the vertebral body.

Alignment guides are then placed over the screw heads, and the cement is prepared according to the manufacturer's instructions. When augmenting multiple levels, attention must be paid not to exceed the working time of the cement prior to the completion of cement delivery through the screw. When the working time

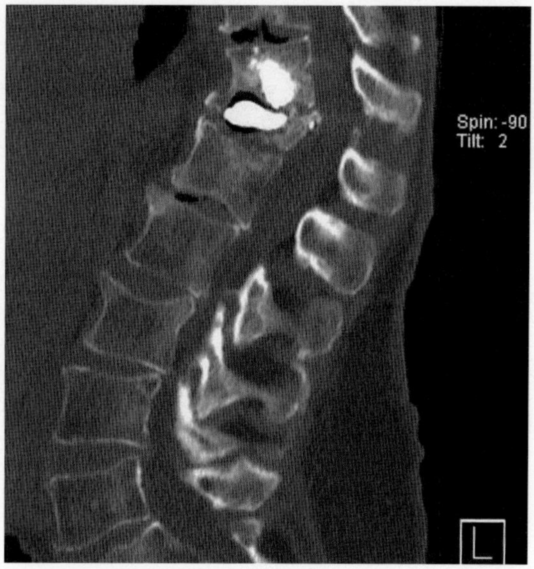

Fig. 16.15 Preoperative CT (Status post T11, T12 kyphoplasty)

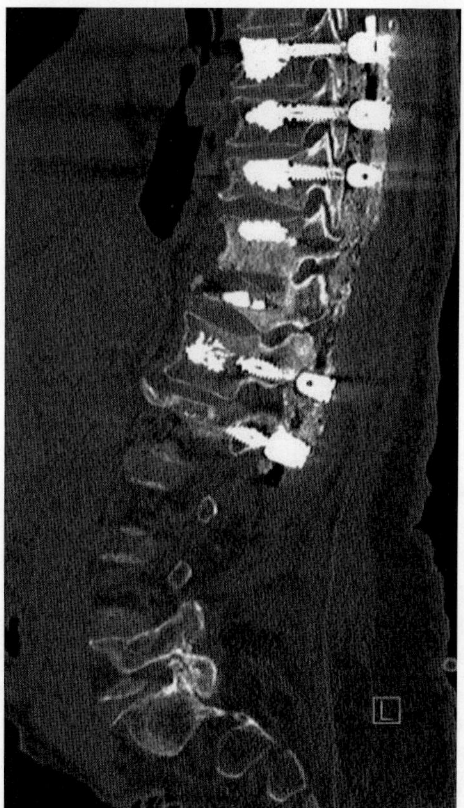

Fig. 16.16 Post op (Cement-augmented pedicle fixation three levels above and two levels below)

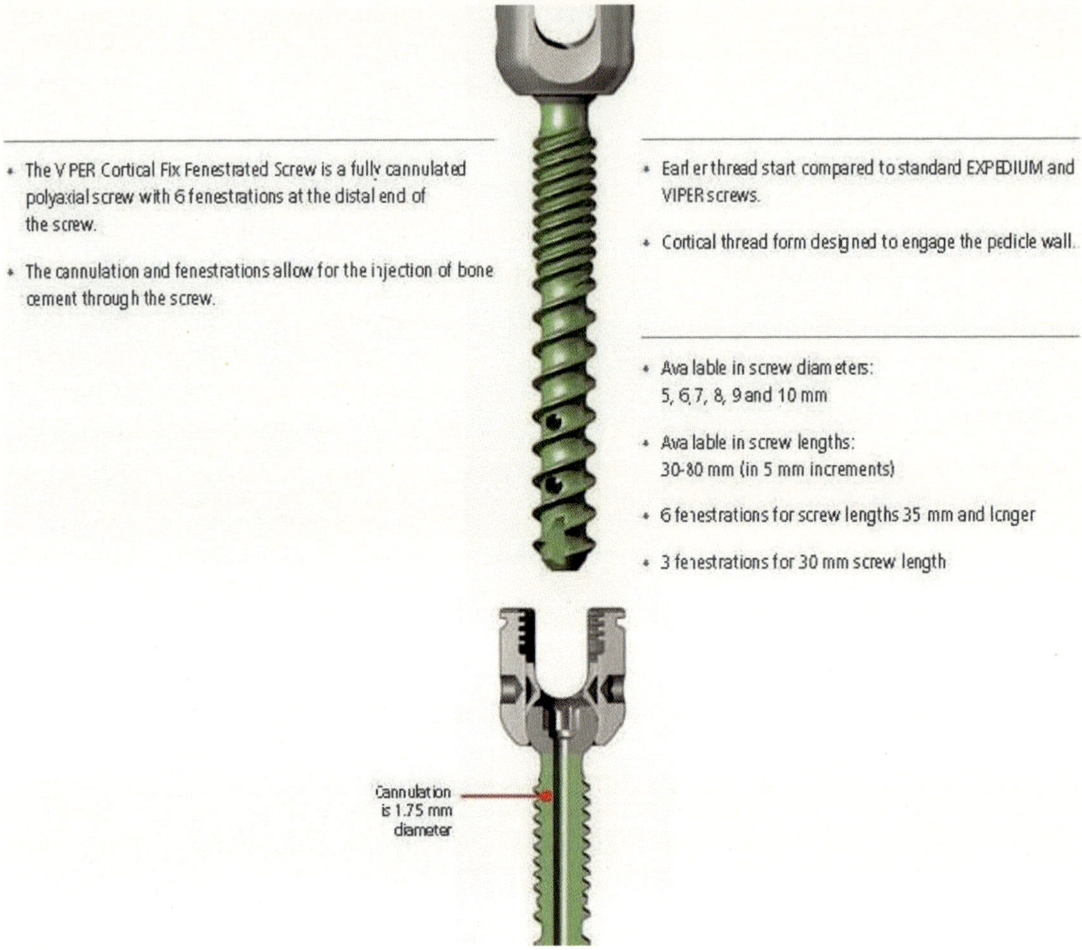

Fig. 16.17 Cannulated fenestrated pedicle screws

is close to completion, new cement should be prepared and the cannula changed for additional levels (Fig. 16.19). The cement cannula is connected to the cannula, and the cannula then placed into the alignment guide. The cement is then advanced under lateral fluoroscopic imaging. Controlled delivery is essential, and overly aggressive injection may result in extravasation and complications associated with cement extravasation. If extravasation is detected, immediately stop the injection. If desired, additional cement in the cannula can be passed into the screw using the plunger. The cannula is then removed, and subsequent levels can be augmented. Once the cement has been injected into all the desired levels, the alignment guides are removed, and the rod can be passed.

16.6.2 Case Example Number 2

A 70-year-old female with stage IV non-small cell adenocarcinoma of the lung was noted to have a lesion involving the L1 vertebral body and was treated appropriately with fractionated radiotherapy. On follow-up imaging, she was noted to have progression of the lesion with compression of the conus medullaris and was

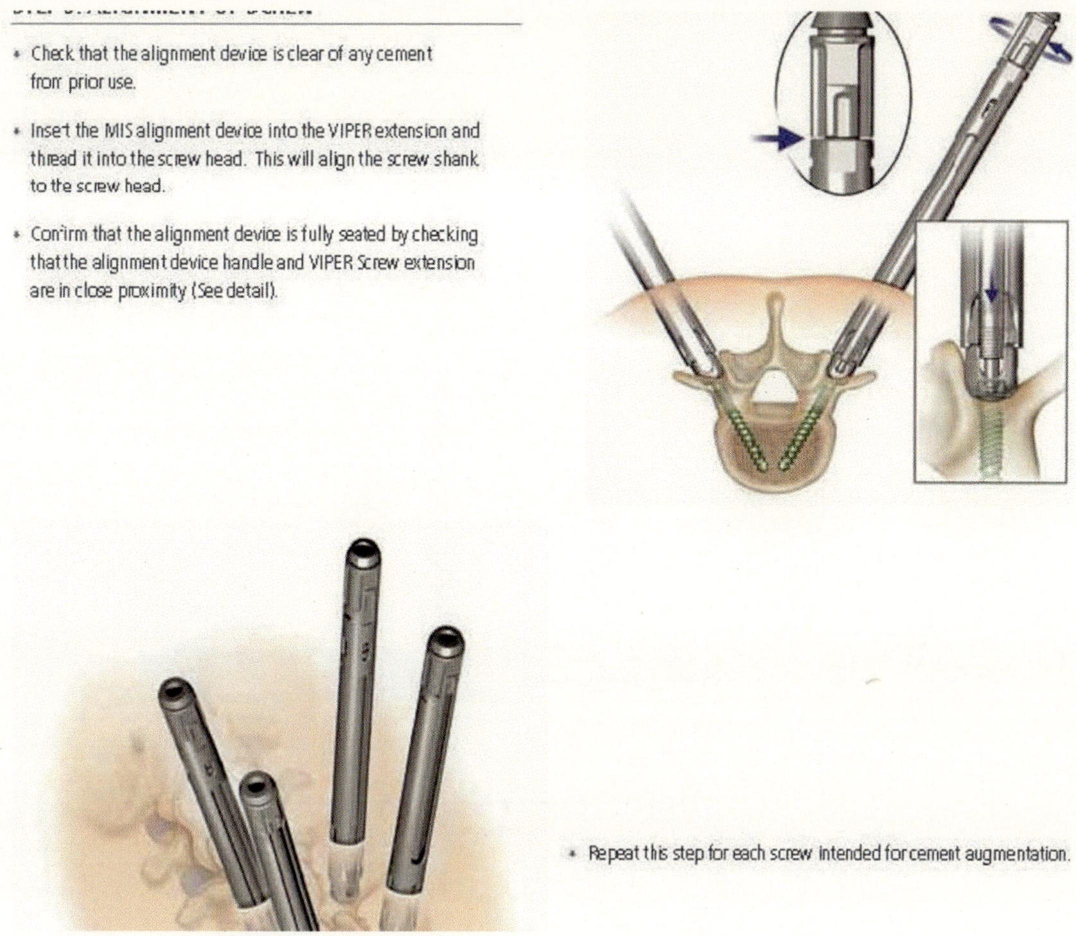

Fig. 16.18 Placement of fenestrated screws

incapacitated by pain (Figs. 16.20, 16.21 and 16.22). She was also noted to have postradiation changes as well as preexisting osteoporosis (Figs. 16.23 and 16.24). We elected to perform a minimally invasive decompression and instrumented fusion, and based on our preoperative assessment of bone quality, planning screw cement augmentation allowed us to perform a shorter construct saving operative time and morbidity.

The first stage was decompression of the neural elements accomplished via right-sided transthoracic retroperitoneal corpectomy using the Nuvasive Max Access Retractor system (Nuvasive, San Diego, California). After the decompression, reconstruction was accomplished with an expandable cage packed with autologous rib harvested during the approach.

The patient was then turned to a four post-Jackson table, and biplanar fluoroscopy was brought into the field. Under biplanar fluoroscopy, the pedicles of T12–L2 were targeted and cannulated with Jamshidi needles (Fig. 16.25). Cement was prepared and connected to the Jamshidi needles. We injected the cement under A/P and lateral fluoroscopy until a cement blush was visualized (Fig. 16.26). At this point, we back off half of a turn on the injector, disconnect the apparatus, and, using the inner stylet, plunge the remaining cement into the vertebral body.

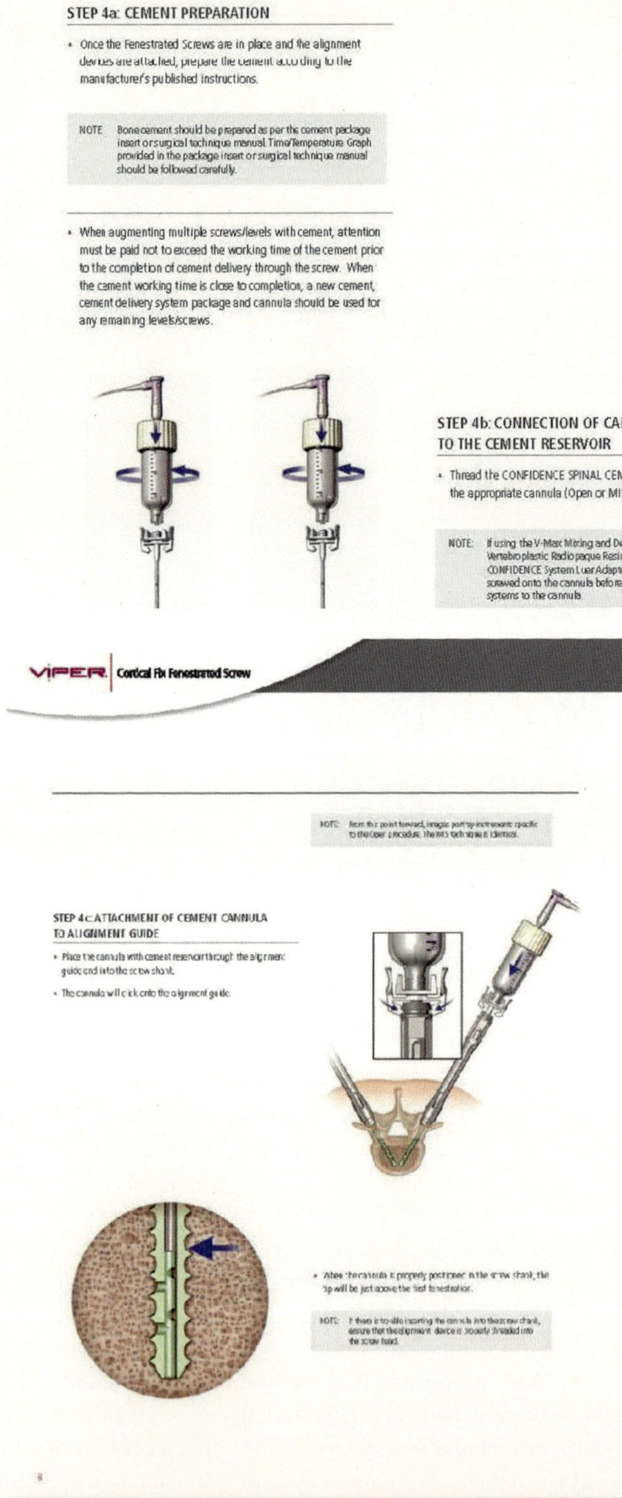

Fig. 16.19 Injection of cement

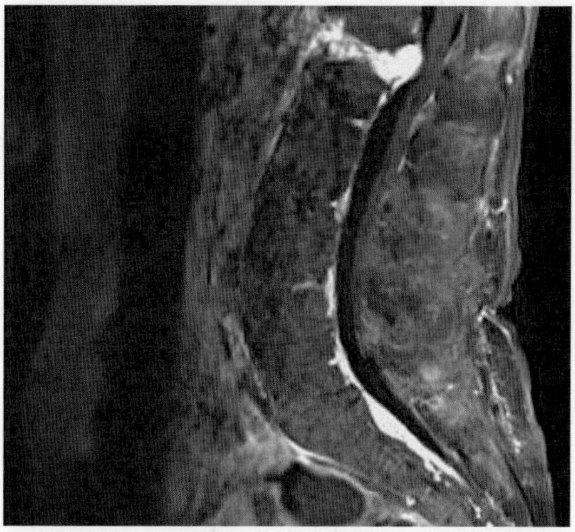

Fig. 16.20 Pre-op sagittal T1 postcontrast (Metastatic NSCC previously irradiated)

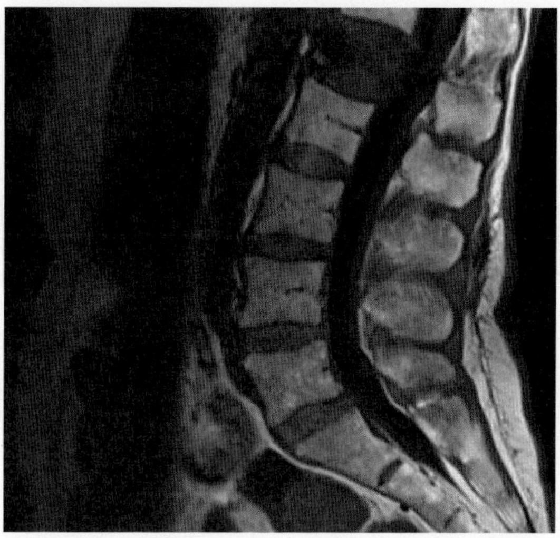

Fig. 16.21 Pre-op T1 noncontrast (Metastatic NSCC previously irradiated)

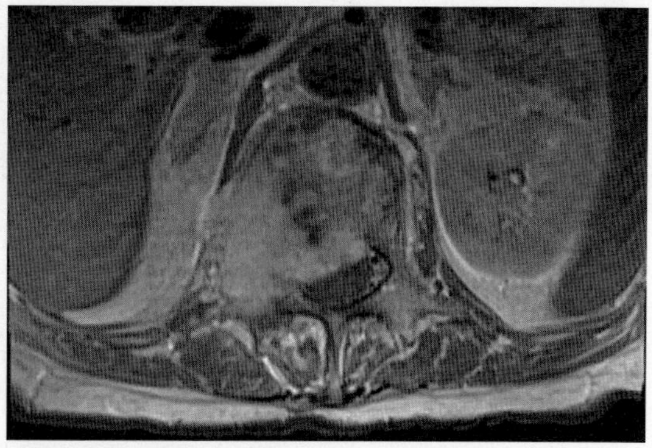

Fig. 16.22 Pre-op axial T1 with contrast

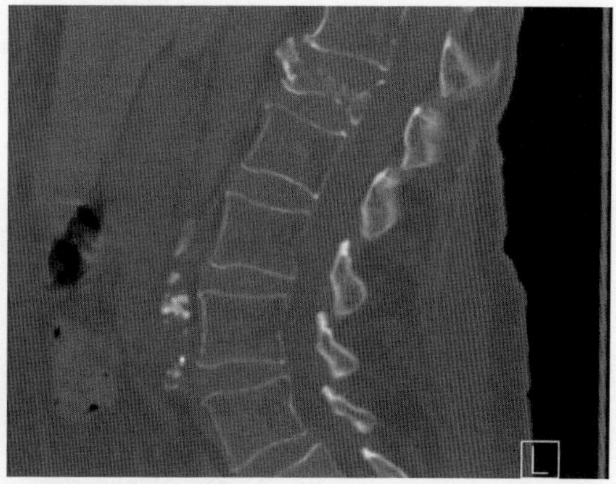

Fig. 16.23 Pre-op midsagittal CT

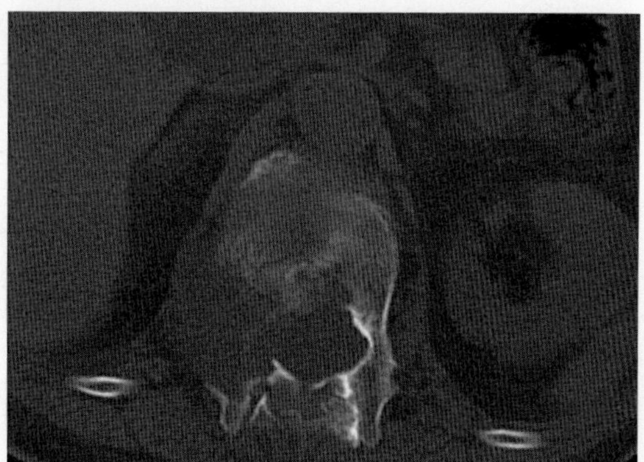

Fig. 16.24 Pre-op axial CT through L1

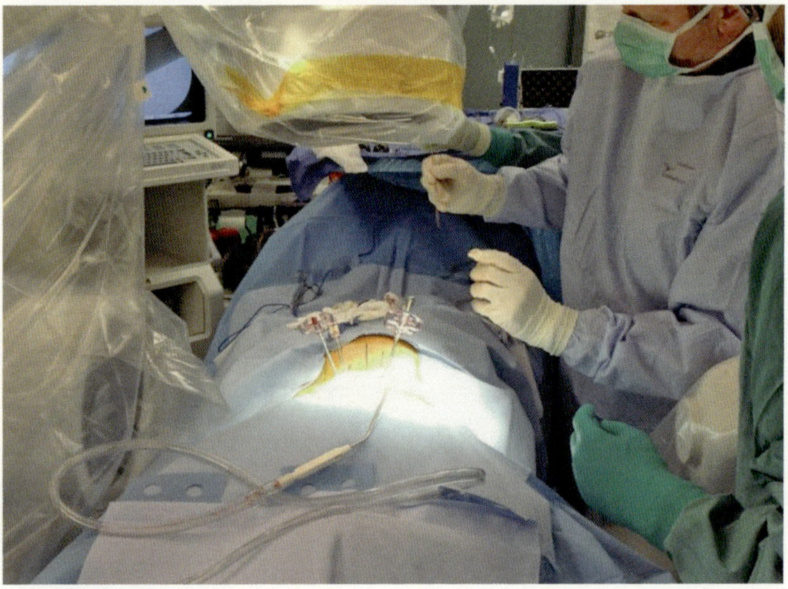

Fig. 16.25 Cannulating the pedicles (After the pedicles are cannulated under biplanar fluoroscopy, the cement is prepared. The pedicles and vertebral bodies are not tapped)

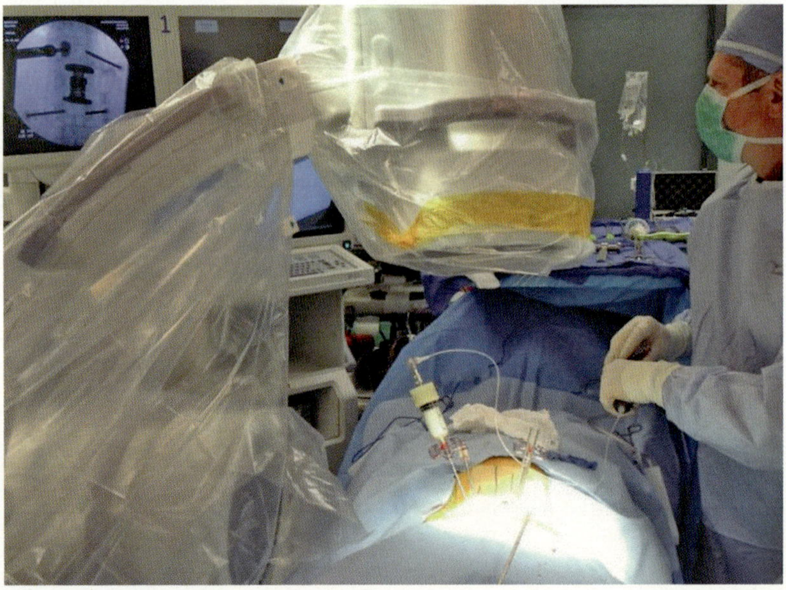

Fig. 16.26 Cement injection

A Y-wire is then introduced and the Jamshidi removed. The pedicle and vertebral body are not tapped. An appropriate screw is then introduced over the wire.

After all the screws are placed, rods are subfascially passed and secured into the polyaxial screw heads (Fig. 16.27). The construct is final tightened, and the wounds are irrigated and closed in layers (Fig. 16.28).

Postoperative CT scan with sagittal reconstruction (Fig. 16.29), axial image of upper screws (Fig. 16.30), axial image of lower screws (Fig. 16.31)

Photograph of lateral incision at 2-week follow-up visit (Fig. 16.32)

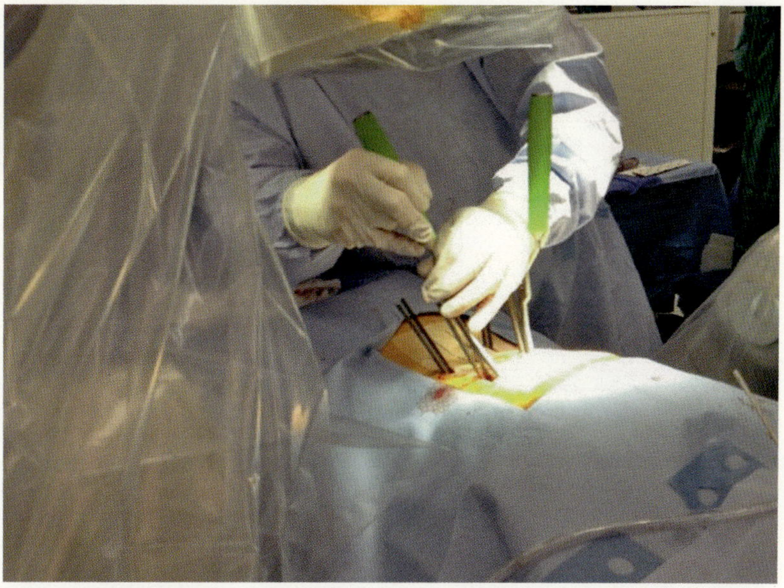

Fig. 16.27 Passing the rods (The rods are subfascially passed and set screws are placed)

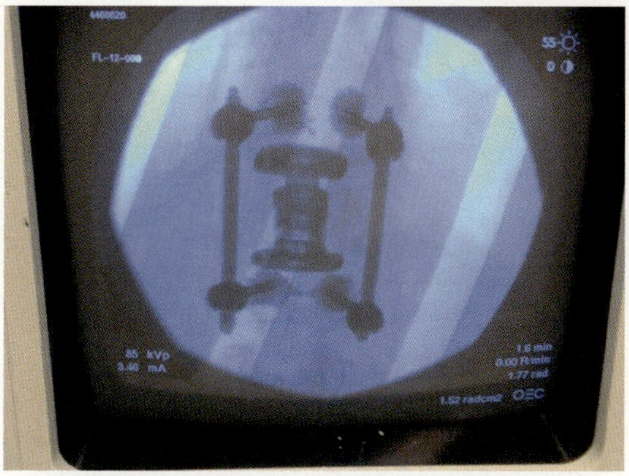

Fig. 16.28 Final intraoperative image

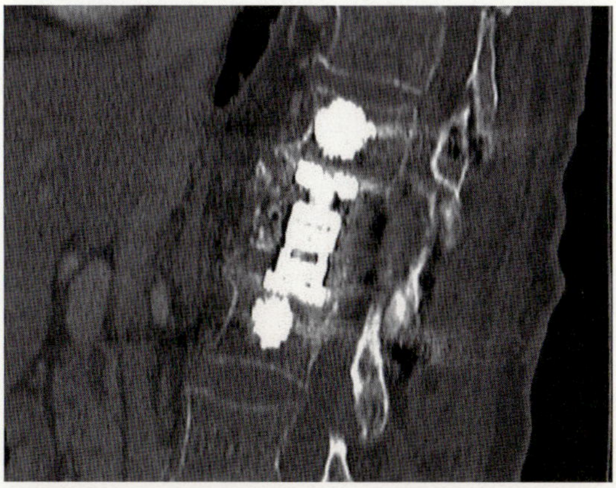

Fig. 16.29 Postoperative sagittal reconstructed CT scan

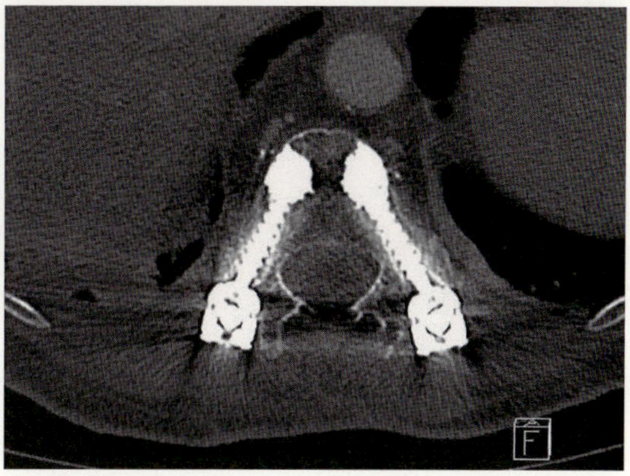

Fig. 16.30 Postoperative axial image of upper screws (Despite our meticulous technique of cement injection, note the small amount of extravasated cement)

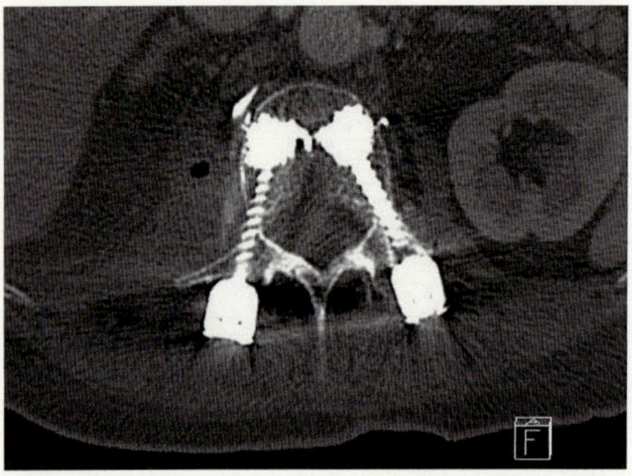

Fig. 16.31 Postoperative axial CT scan of lower screws (Again, note the small amount of extravasated cement. The patient was completely asymptomatic from cement extravasation. No extravasation was noted during intraoperative imaging with biplanar fluoroscopy)

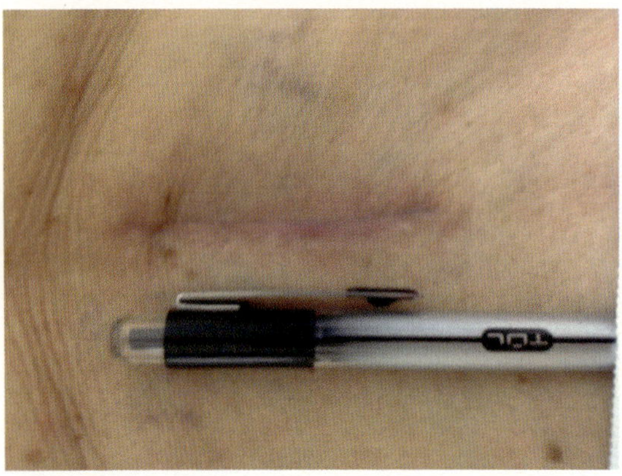

Fig. 16.32 Photograph of lateral incision at 2-week follow-up visit

References

1. NIH Consensus Development Panel on Osteoporosis Prevention, Diagnosis, and Therapy. JAMA: the journal of the American Medical Association. 2001;285(6):785–795.
2. Osteoporosis: review of the evidence for prevention, diagnosis and treatment and cost-effectiveness analysis. Introduction. Osteoporosis international : a journal established as result of cooperation between the European Foundation for Osteoporosis and the National Osteoporosis Foundation of the USA. 1998;8(Suppl 4):S7–80.
3. Crafts N. The human development index and changes in standards of living: some historical comparisons. Eur Rev Econ Hist. 1997;1:299–322.
4. Healey JH, Vigorita VJ, Lane JM. The coexistence and characteristics of osteoarthritis and osteoporosis. J Bone Joint Surg Am. 1985;67(4):586–92.
5. Cook SD, Salkeld SL, Stanley T, Faciane A, Miller SD. Biomechanical study of pedicle screw fixation in severely osteoporotic bone. Spine J. 2004;4(4):402–8. official journal of the North American Spine Society.
6. Yerby SA, Toh E, McLain RF. Revision of failed pedicle screws using hydroxyapatite cement. A biomechanical analysis. Spine. 1998;23(15):1657–61.
7. Halvorson TL, Kelley LA, Thomas KA, Whitecloud 3rd TS, Cook SD. Effects of bone mineral density on pedicle screw fixation. Spine. 1994;19(21):2415–20.
8. Wittenberg RH, Lee KS, Shea M, White 3rd AA, Hayes WC. Effect of screw diameter, insertion technique, and bone cement augmentation of pedicular screw fixation strength. Clin Orthop Relat Res. 1993;296:278–87.
9. Pfeifer BA, Krag MH, Johnson C. Repair of failed transpedicle screw fixation. A biomechanical study comparing polymethylmethacrylate, milled bone, and matchstick bone reconstruction. Spine. 1994; 19(3):350–3.
10. Sarzier JS, Evans AJ, Cahill DW. Increased pedicle screw pullout strength with vertebroplasty augmentation in osteoporotic spines. J Neurosurg. 2002;96(3):309–12.
11. Cook SD, Salkeld SL, Whitecloud 3rd TS, Barbera J. Biomechanical evaluation and preliminary clinical experience with an expansive pedicle screw design. J Spinal Disord. 2000;13(3):230–6.
12. Cook SD, Salkeld SL, Whitecloud 3rd TS, Barbera J. Biomechanical testing and clinical experience with the OMEGA-21 spinal fixation system. Am J Orthop (Belle Mead NJ). 2001;30(5):387–94.
13. Moore DC, Maitra RS, Farjo LA, Graziano GP, Goldstein SA. Restoration of pedicle screw fixation with an in situ setting calcium phosphate cement. Spine. 1997;22(15):1696–705.
14. Yuan HA, Garfin SR, Dickman CA, Mardjetko SM. A historical cohort study of pedicle screw fixation in thoracic, lumbar, and sacral spinal fusions. Spine. 1994;19(20):2279S–96.
15. Esses SI, Sachs BL, Dreyzin V. Complications associated with the technique of pedicle screw fixation. A selected survey of ABS members. Spine. 1993;18(15):2231–8. discussion 2238–2239.
16. Law M, Tencer AF, Anderson PA. Caudo-cephalad loading of pedicle screws: mechanisms of loosening and methods of augmentation. Spine. 1993;18(16): 2438–43.
17. Ashman RB, Galpin RD, Corin JD, Johnston 2nd CE. Biomechanical analysis of pedicle screw instrumentation systems in a corpectomy model. Spine. 1989; 14(12):1398–405.

18. Soshi S, Shiba R, Kondo H, Murota K. An experimental study on transpedicular screw fixation in relation to osteoporosis of the lumbar spine. Spine. 1991;16(11):1335–41.
19. Okuyama K, Abe E, Suzuki T, Tamura Y, Chiba M, Sato K. Influence of bone mineral density on pedicle screw fixation: a study of pedicle screw fixation augmenting posterior lumbar interbody fusion in elderly patients. Spine J. 2001;1(6):402–7. official journal of the North American Spine Society.
20. Lotz JC, Hu SS, Chiu DF, Yu M, Colliou O, Poser RD. Carbonated apatite cement augmentation of pedicle screw fixation in the lumbar spine. Spine. 1997;22(23):2716–23.
21. Chapman JR, Harrington RM, Lee KM, Anderson PA, Tencer AF, Kowalski D. Factors affecting the pullout strength of cancellous bone screws. J Biomech Eng. 1996;118(3):391–8.
22. Pfeiffer FM, Abernathie DL, Smith DE. A comparison of pullout strength for pedicle screws of different designs: a study using tapped and untapped pilot holes. Spine. 2006;31(23):E867–70.
23. Zindrick MR, Wiltse LL, Widell EH, et al. A biomechanical study of intrapeduncular screw fixation in the lumbosacral spine. Clin Orthop Relat Res. 1986;203:99–112.
24. Urist MR. Acrylic cement stabilized joint replacements. Curr Probl Surg. 1975;12:1–54.
25. Cameron HU, Jacob R, Macnab I, Pilliar RM. Use of polymethylmethacrylate to enhance screw fixation in bone. J Bone Joint Surg Am. 1975;57(5):655–6.
26. Taylor RS, Taylor RJ, Fritzell P. Balloon kyphoplasty and vertebroplasty for vertebral compression fractures: a comparative systematic review of efficacy and safety. Spine. 2006;31(23):2747–55.
27. Becker S, Chavanne A, Spitaler R, et al. Assessment of different screw augmentation techniques and screw designs in osteoporotic spines. Eur Spine J. 2008;17(11):1462–9. official publication of the European Spine Society, the European Spinal Deformity Society, and the European Section of the Cervical Spine Research Society.
28. Frankel BM, D'Agostino S, Wang C. A biomechanical cadaveric analysis of polymethylmethacrylate-augmented pedicle screw fixation. J Neurosurg Spine. 2007;7(1):47–53.
29. Frankel BM, Jones T, Wang C. Segmental polymethylmethacrylate-augmented pedicle screw fixation in patients with bone softening caused by osteoporosis and metastatic tumor involvement: a clinical evaluation. Neurosurgery. 2007;61(3):531–7. discussion 537–538.
30. Cortet B, Cotten A, Boutry N, et al. Percutaneous vertebroplasty in the treatment of osteoporotic vertebral compression fractures: an open prospective study. J Rheumatol. 1999;26(10):2222–8.
31. Gaughen Jr JR, Jensen ME, Schweickert PA, Kaufmann TJ, Marx WF, Kallmes DF. Relevance of antecedent venography in percutaneous vertebroplasty for the treatment of osteoporotic compression fractures. AJNR Am J Neuroradiol. 2002;23(4):594–600.
32. Jensen ME, Evans AJ, Mathis JM, Kallmes DF, Cloft HJ, Dion JE. Percutaneous polymethylmethacrylate vertebroplasty in the treatment of osteoporotic vertebral body compression fractures: technical aspects. AJNR Am J Neuroradiol. 1997;18(10):1897–904.
33. Peh WC, Gilula LA, Peck DD. Percutaneous vertebroplasty for severe osteoporotic vertebral body compression fractures. Radiology. 2002;223(1):121–6.
34. Perez-Higueras A, Alvarez L, Rossi RE, Quinones D, Al-Assir I. Percutaneous vertebroplasty: long-term clinical and radiological outcome. Neuroradiology. 2002;44(11):950–4.
35. Ryu KS, Park CK, Kim MC, Kang JK. Dose-dependent epidural leakage of polymethylmethacrylate after percutaneous vertebroplasty in patients with osteoporotic vertebral compression fractures. J Neurosurg. 2002;96(1):56–61.
36. Renner SM, Lim TH, Kim WJ, Katolik L, An HS, Andersson GB. Augmentation of pedicle screw fixation strength using an injectable calcium phosphate cement as a function of injection timing and method. Spine. 2004;29(11):E212–6.
37. Wilkes RA, Mackinnon JG, Thomas WG. Neurological deterioration after cement injection into a vertebral body. J Bone Joint Surg Br. 1994;76(1):155.
38. Yazu M, Kin A, Kosaka R, Kinoshita M, Abe M. Efficacy of novel-concept pedicle screw fixation augmented with calcium phosphate cement in the osteoporotic spine. J Orthop Sci. 2005;10(1):56–61. official journal of the Japanese Orthopaedic Association.
39. Noro T, Itoh K. Biomechanical behavior of hydroxyapatite as bone substitute material in a loaded implant model. On the surface strain measurement and the maximum compression strength determination of material crash. Bio-med Mater Eng. 1999;9(5–6):319–24.
40. Ignatius AA, Augat P, Ohnmacht M, Pokinskyj P, Kock HJ, Claes LE. A new bioresorbable polymer for screw augmentation in the osteosynthesis of osteoporotic cancellous bone: a biomechanical evaluation. J Biomed Mater Res. 2001;58(3):254–60.
41. McKoy BE, An YH. An injectable cementing screw for fixation in osteoporotic bone. J Biomed Mater Res. 2000;53(3):216–20.
42. Amar AP, Larsen DW, Esnaashari N, Albuquerque FC, Lavine SD, Teitelbaum GP. Percutaneous transpedicular polymethylmethacrylate vertebroplasty for the treatment of spinal compression fractures. Neurosurgery. 2001;49(5):1105–14. discussion 1114–1105.
43. Garfin SR, Yuan HA, Reiley MA. New technologies in spine: kyphoplasty and vertebroplasty for the treatment of painful osteoporotic compression fractures. Spine. 2001;26(14):1511–5.
44. Pinto PW. Cardiovascular collapse associated with the use of methylmethacrylate. AANA J. 1993;61(6): 613–6.

45. Patterson BM, Healey JH, Cornell CN, Sharrock NE. Cardiac arrest during hip arthroplasty with a cemented long-stem component. A report of seven cases. J Bone Joint Surg Am. 1991;73(2):271–7.
46. Nicholson MJ. Cardiac arrest following acrylic-cement implants. Anesth Analg. 1973;52(2):298–302.
47. Lamade WR, Friedl W, Schmid B, Meeder PJ. Bone cement implantation syndrome. A prospective randomised trial for use of antihistamine blockade. Arch Orthop Trauma Surg. 1995;114(6):335–9.
48. Jenkins K, Wake PJ. Cement implantation syndrome. Anaesthesia. 2002;57(4):416. author reply 416.
49. Lonstein JE, Denis F, Perra JH, Pinto MR, Smith MD, Winter RB. Complications associated with pedicle screws. J Bone Joint Surg Am. 1999;81(11):1519–28.
50. Tan JS, Bailey CS, Dvorak MF, Fisher CG, Cripton PA, Oxland TR. Cement augmentation of vertebral screws enhances the interface strength between interbody device and vertebral body. Spine. 2007;32(3):334–41.

Part III

Posterior Approaches

Interbody Cage Options

17

Asdrubal Falavigna

Interbody fusion techniques have been developed to preserve the load-bearing capacity of the spine, reestablish disc space, restore sagittal plane alignment, allow neural decompression, and facilitate compressive loading onto bone [50, 51, 53, 68]. The interbody space is an ideal location for fusion due to the broad and well-vascularized corticocancellous surface on which bone graft is placed under compression during healing [22].

Interbody cage placement can be performed in minimally invasive spine surgery since basic surgical steps including disc removal, adequate manipulation of the vertebral end plate, bone placement in the disc space, and subsequent proper placement of the interbody device were not influenced by a small operation window [21, 27, 56, 60, 78]. However, the casual placement of bone, dowels, struts, or cages into a disc space does not ensure fusion. Fusion must obey the basic principles of osteosynthesis. Therefore, meticulous preparation of the disc space and the careful selection of the interbody cages are essential for successful fusion.

The posterior lumbar approach for interbody fusion (PLIF) was introduced by Cloward to treat painful intervertebral discs damaged by degeneration [16, 17]. Since then, less invasive techniques have been developed to minimize approach-related morbidities of PLIF, such as extensive muscle dissection that produces significant pain and subsequent extended hospital stays as well as inflated costs. The development of newer interbody devices allowed using them in minimally invasive surgery (MIS) such as minimally invasive transforaminal lumbar interbody fusion (TLIF) [32] (Fig. 17.1).

Interbody cages available on the market are made of various materials and in different shapes. The design of the interbody cage is tailored to each patient's needs and depends on the surgical variables including type of approach, open or MIS; type of access, such as PLIF or TLIF; level of planned surgery; presence of scar tissue; pathology; and nerve root anatomy.

17.1 Material Options

Structural autograft or allograft bone has been used for quite some time, with less frequency since the increased use of synthetic cages [12, 23, 33]. Regardless of additional posterior fixation, tricortical iliac crest allografts without mechanical support in anterior or posterior lumbar interbody fusion tend to collapse, become displaced, or be extruded over time [20, 47, 55, 65]. This occurs because fusion is not instantaneous, so interbody constructs must be able to resist the load for some time. Pedicle screw stabilization usually alleviates this problem (Fig. 17.2). The properties of the material used to fashion interbody constructs must

A. Falavigna, M.D., Ph.D.
Professor of Neurosurgery,
University of Caxias do Sul, Brazil
e-mail: asdrubalmd@gmail.com

M.Y. Wang et al. (eds.), *Minimally Invasive Spinal Deformity Surgery*,
DOI 10.1007/978-3-7091-1407-0_17, © Springer-Verlag Wien 2014

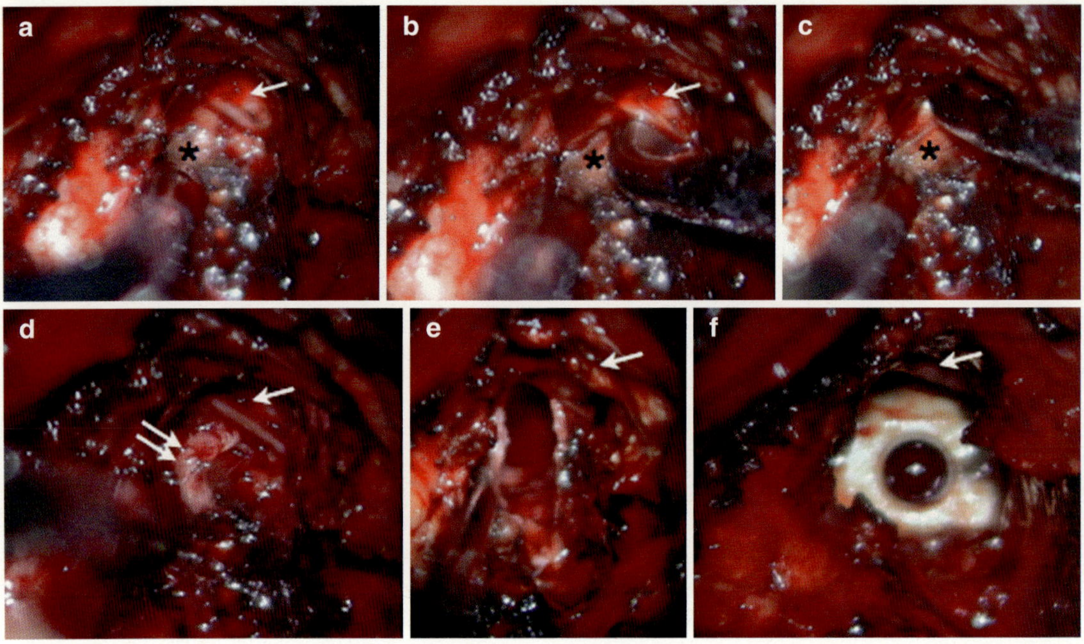

Fig. 17.1 The cage was placed using a TLIF technique in the intervertebral space. The intervertebral disc (*asterisk*) and the nerve root (*arrow*) were dissected (**a**), the nerve root was retracted medially (**b** and **c**), and the disc herniation (*double arrow*) was removed (**d**). The intervertebral space was prepared by removing the cartilaginous plate, and the disc (**e**) and the cage were placed (**f**)

be balanced to fulfill mechanical, biological, and radiological requirements such as providing structural support, resisting compressive loads, exhibiting osteoconductive-inductive proprieties to allow ingrowth of vital host bone, and being radiolucent [7, 25, 53, 66].

A variety of materials are available for use as posterior interbody cages, the most common being metals, polymers with or without carbon fiber reinforcement, and biodegradable materials (Fig. 17.3). The surgeon must decide on the best material, device configuration, and size to optimize endplate realignment, stability, and ultimately fusion. While the cages must be rigid to support the load, they cannot be too rigid because the load may be transferred to the cortical vertebral body and consequently break it. In addition, the difference in the modulus of elasticity between the cage material and the actual vertebral body leads to stress shielding and therefore delays fusion and causes pseudarthrosis [74]. According to Wolff's law, bone grows in response to stress to better accommodate that stress. Therefore, bone grafts must experience stress to promote fusion. Carbon fiber cages are closest to the modulus of elasticity of the vertebral bone, but some complications related to the carbon fiber debris have been reported [54]. Titanium implants offer a radio-opaque alternative to carbon fiber materials and provide great biomechanical strength; however, their modulus of elasticity is much greater than the cortical vertebral body so using them poses the greatest chances of subsidence [43, 58]. Polyether-ether-ketone (PEEK) cages are expected to result in lower subsidence rates than metal cages because PEEK has a modulus of elasticity similar to bone [77].

17.1.1 Metallic Devices

The most common metallic interbody devices are titanium cages [23, 33, 34]. Titanium interbody devices have become available in nearly every configuration, shape (circular, oval, rectangular,

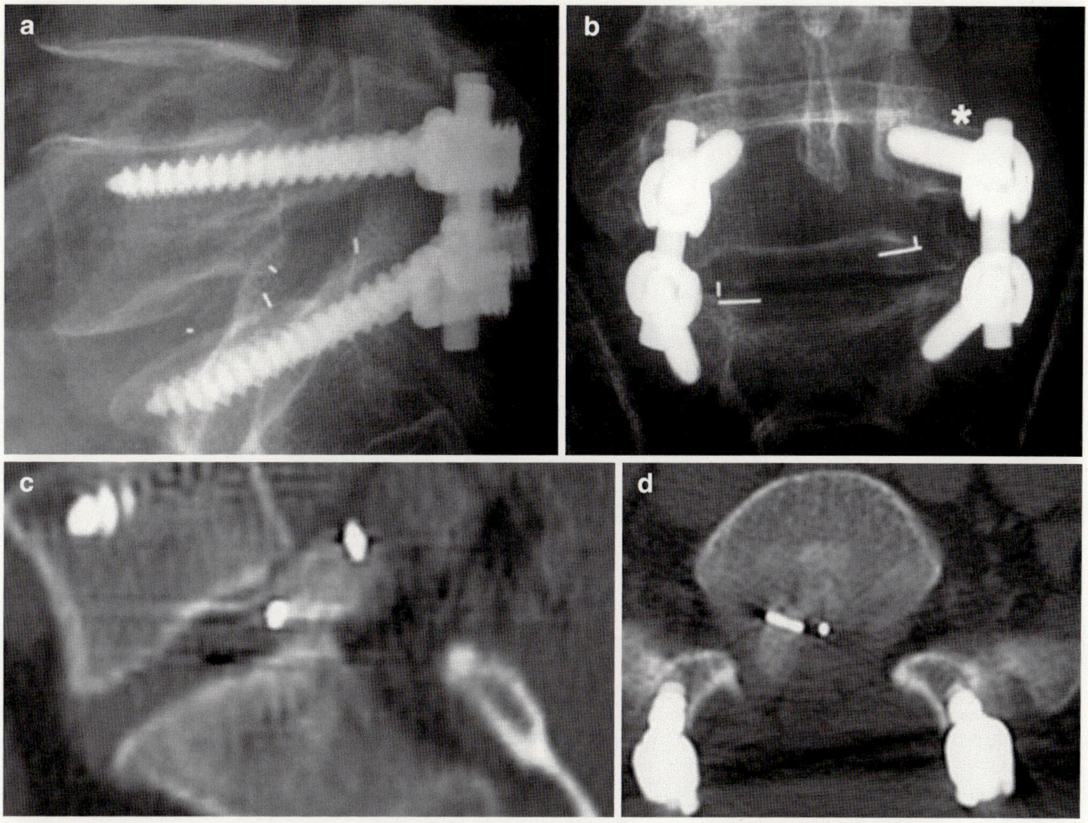

Fig. 17.2 Despite cage compression before the final screw is tightened in this case, the superior L5 right screw (*asterisk*) is loosened, and cage retropulsion occurs on the same side as observed in lateral (**a**) and anteroposterior (**b**) radiographs and lateral (**c**) and horizontal (**d**) computer tomography views of the lumbar spine

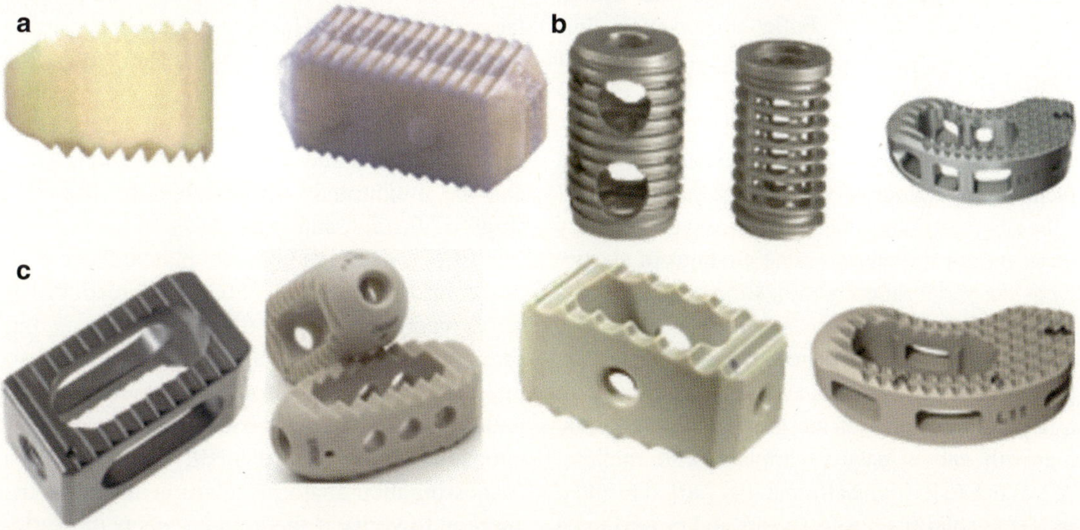

Fig. 17.3 A variety of materials are available for use as posterior interbody cages such as bone (**a**), titanium (**b**), and polymer (**c**)

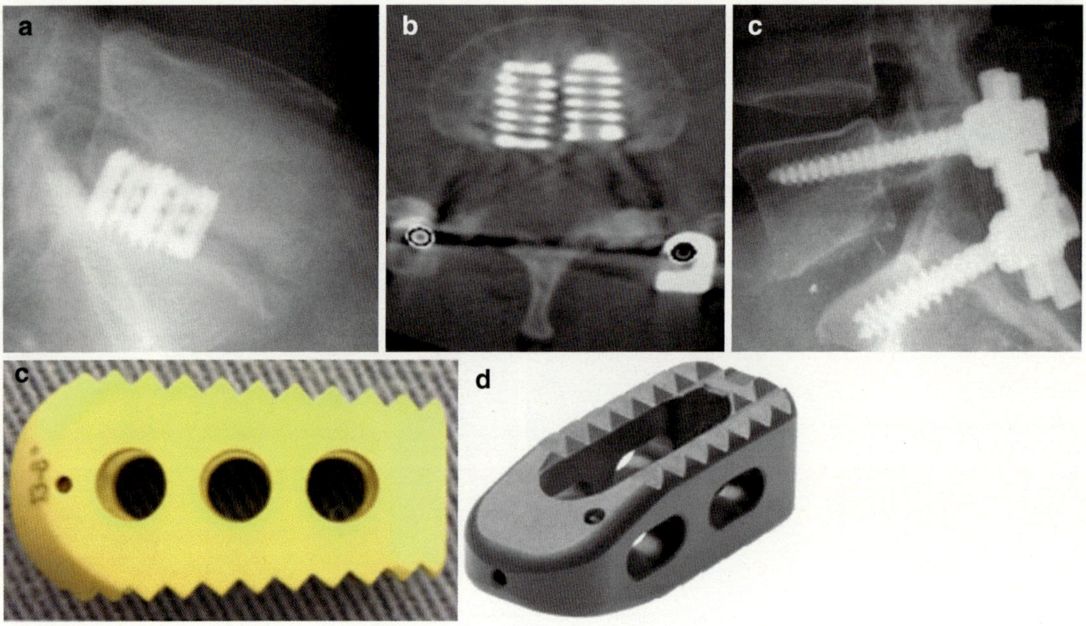

Fig. 17.4 Lateral radiograph of the lumbar spine (**a**) and a computed tomography (**b**) show a cylindrical threaded titanium cage placed in the disc space of L5/S1. A polyether-ether-ketone rectangular cage (**c**) was placed in the intervertebral space L5/S as shown in the lateral radiograph. The rectangular cage (AVS PL, Stryker) (**d**) and the Concord-type bullet-shaped cage, DePuy Synthes (**e**), have teeth on the superior and inferior surfaces to provide immediate stability and resistance to migration (**e**)

octagonal, and boomerang shapes), and size (Figs. 17.3, 17.4, and 17.5). These cages were designed to be used for TLIFs and PLIFs, either through open procedures or minimally invasive applications through tubes. Common design characteristics include bullet-shaped tips, lordotic contouring, hollow portions for insertion of bone graft or biological substitutes, and capacity to support compressive strengths.

Kok et al. [40] published their experience with a memory metal minimal access cage that is a horseshoe-shaped implant constructed from the memory metal nitinol and has the same modulus of elasticity as the vertebral body [59]. Biomechanical testing revealed an adequate subsidence resistance, comparable to or even better than the Harms cage [59]. The device combines axial support with a large contact area of the graft facilitating bony ingrowth and is easy to implant with minimal access due to its high deformability [40]. It resulted in 100 % solid fusions in 2 years and proved to be safe, although two patients required revision surgery [40].

17.1.2 Polymer Devices

Cages can be made from polymers, typically PEEK, because it is a biocompatible thermoplastic solution for in vivo applications and particularly suitable as an implant material due to its resistance to chemicals, heat, steam, radiation, and wear. This polymer combines superior strength, stiffness, and elastic modulus. Bone graft maturation and fusion within these devices can be monitored radiographically [42, 58] (Figs. 17.3, 17.4, and 17.6).

PEEK is a hard radiolucent plastic that can be non-reinforced or carbon fiber reinforced. PEEK reinforced with carbon fiber has greater compression strength while allowing excellent postoperative imaging. Most manufacturers use tantalum radio marker beads placed in the corners and at the ends of the PEEK cages to assist in locating their anatomic position and allow the surgeon to verify if the implant meets the vertebral body end plate and determines its depth (Figs. 17.2, 17.4, and 17.5). One example is the

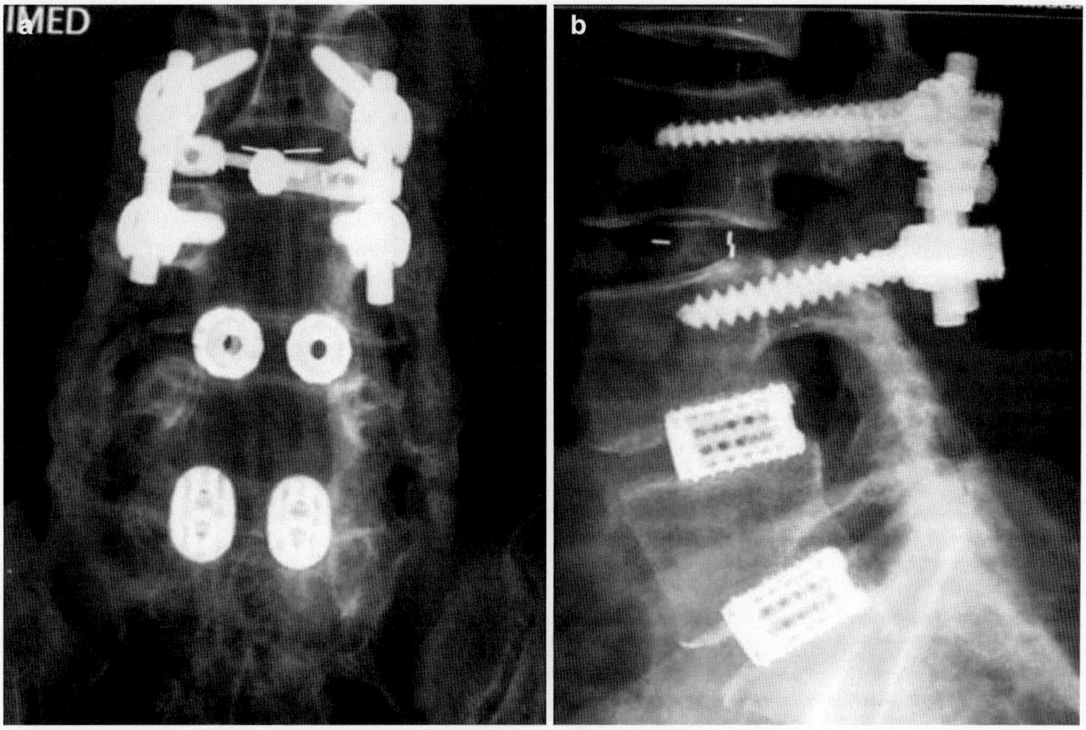

Fig. 17.5 Anteroposterior (**a**) and lateral view (**b**) radiographs of a female patient with surgery at L4/L5 and L5/S1 using stand-alone titanium circular cages. Six years after surgery she developed a symptomatic and refractory L3–L4 adjacent degenerative disc disease and had a PLIF approach using a rectangular cage combined with pedicle screw system

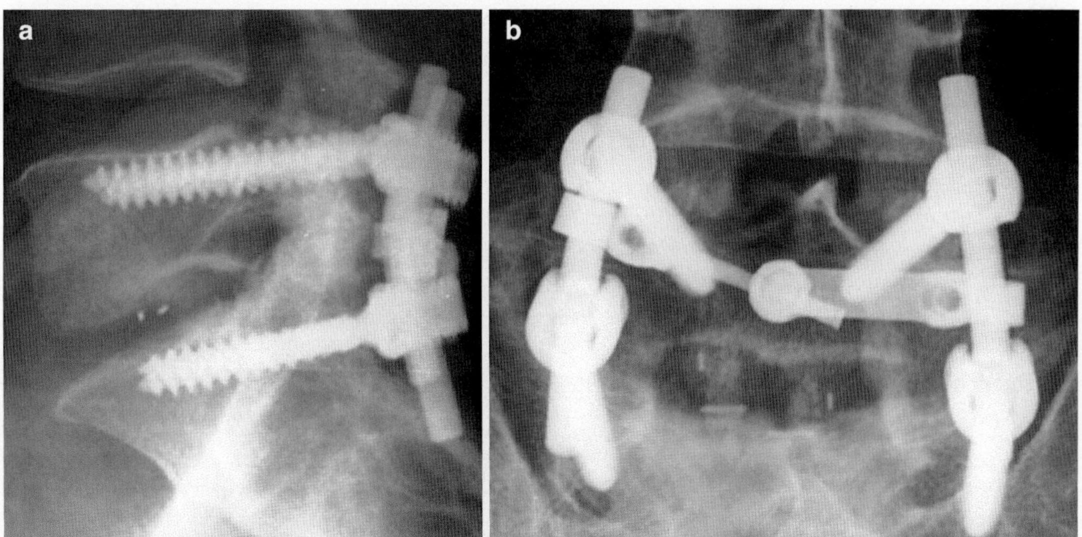

Fig. 17.6 Radiological diagnosis of bone fusion 2 years after L5–S1 surgery using a radiolucent plastic polyether-ether-ketone cages into the intervertebral space in anteroposterior (**a**) and lateral (**b**) view

PEEK-OPTIMA™ polymer which is reinforced with 30 % of carbon fiber and has an elasticity modulus of 3.6Gpa, which is very close to that of cortical bone. This material can provide load transfer between the cage and the adjacent vertebral bodies, thus promoting bony fusion, reducing the stress shielding on the cortical vertebral body, and consequently reducing subsidence [75].

17.1.3 Biodegradable

Optimizing degradable spine interbody fusion cages to meet the initial and intermediate load bearing while at the same time providing directed delivery of biofactor like human bone morphogenetic protein enables superior bone fusion. Recent advances in the field of spinal implants have led to the production of the biodegradable interbody spacer. The most commonly used implant is made of a 70/30 mixture of poly (L-lactide-co-d,L-lactide) (PLDLA) [18, 48, 71]. In vivo, these lactides are metabolized slowly to carbon dioxide and water over a 12–18-month period leaving behind newly formed bone [18, 48, 71].

The radiolucent property of PLDLA cages affords optimal postoperative assessment of bony fusion on plain radiographs, and there are no particulate debris and retained foreign body responses after they have been metabolized. Because of their slow rate of degradation, the weight-bearing load transmitted through the implant is progressively transferred to the newly forming bone, avoiding graft migration, decreasing stress shielding, and increasing the rate of arthrodesis [18, 48, 71].

Some problems, however, such as time-dependent failure have been reported regarding PLDLA cages. When statically loaded at 75 % and 25 % of their strength, the implants failed at 5 min and 3 months, respectively [63]. Moreover, diminished implant strength occurs at increased humidity and ambient temperature at physiological values [63]. In these situations, PLDLA behaves as a polymer and "stimulates dynamic rearrangement of molecular segments, resulting in a plastic flow" that can lead to graft failure after rotational and torsional forces along with the compressive forces [63, 64].

Smith et al. [64] conducted a prospective cohort study to compare fusion and complication rates in patients undergoing TLIF with carbon fiber cages versus biodegradable cages made from 70/30 PLDLA. The authors observed a statistically significant increased incidence of nonunion (18.2 %) and postsurgical cage migration (18.2 %) in patients undergoing TLIF with biodegradable cages versus carbon fiber implants (0 %).

New experimental bioabsorbable devices are currently being studied for use as spinal implants. The bioabsorbable technology continues to evolve, and its application in spine surgery will continue to expand combined with a better understanding of implant stiffness and optimization of the mechanical characteristics of implant materials.

17.2 Design Options

Immediate three-dimensional stability depends on the cage design. Most investigators agree that interbody cages provide good stability in flexion and lateral bending but little or no stability in extension and axial rotation [49, 52, 57, 72, 73]. The loss of stability in extension and axial rotation may be related to the insufficient distraction of the anterior annulus and facet joint damage, respectively.

The design of the interbody device needs to conform to the anatomic pathway in which the device is placed as well as the overall anatomy of the end plate to provide optimal structural integrity. Additionally, the cages must have a maximized open design allowing bone graft placement and fusion.

17.2.1 Shapes: Circular Versus Rectangular

The immediate stability of a rectangular porous titanium cage (contact cage), a rectangular carbon fiber cage (Brantigan cage), and a cylindrical

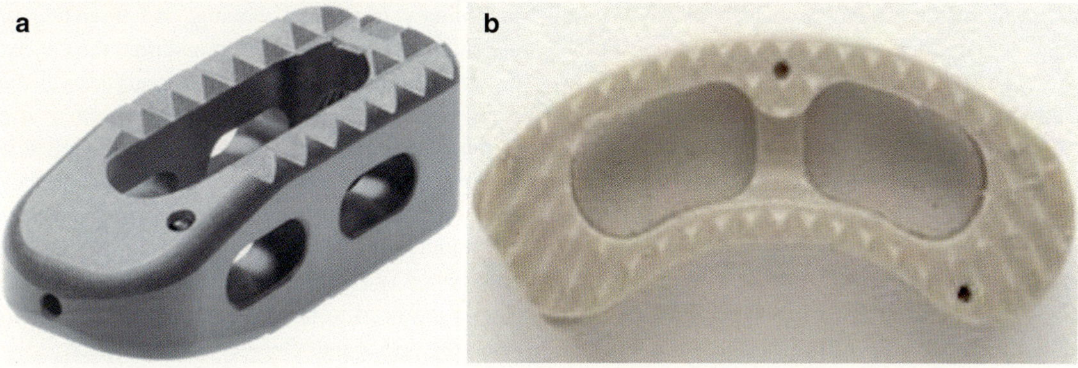

Fig. 17.7 Concord-type bullet-shaped cage, DePuy Synthes (**a**), AVS TL boomerang cage, Stryker (**b**)

threaded titanium cage (Ray TFC) was evaluated in a one-level cadaver spine inserted from a PLIF followed by titanium transpedicular fixation [49]. Before insertion, the medial portion of the articular facets was removed, and the cages were filled with autogenous bone. No significant differences were found in the three-dimensional stabilization provided by the different cage designs when combined with posterior screw fixation; however, the cylindrical cage provided greater stability against axial rotation related to the screw threads engaging the end plate than the rectangular cages [49]. Wang et al. [76] found similar results using a posterior approach in multiple lumbar levels in the cadaveric spine.

The rectangular implants can be manufactured with a smooth surface or with teeth on the superior and inferior surfaces of the cage (Figs. 17.3 and 17.4). The rectangular cage design with endplate pyramidal teeth has the advantage of providing immediate stability and resistance to migration in any direction similar to the threaded cylindrical cage [49, 57, 61, 73]. This type of cage usually has a convex surface for anatomic fit and is available in several footprints and heights.

The problem with most cages is the small contact surface of the bone graft leading to a high rate of pseudarthrosis. A rectangular cage usually has a larger axial central cavity than a cylindrical cage allowing adequate space for packing large amounts of cancellous bone graft inside the cage and exposing it to a greater graft surface area to facilitate good bony ingrowth (Fig. 17.7).

17.2.2 Size of Cages: Just Fit into Versus Distraction of the Intervertebral Space

The interbody implant sets need to be of different heights in order to choose specifically in which case the size is large enough to tension the annulus. This is essential for initial stability in extension [26]. When it is necessary to place an interbody cage with a diameter of more than 15 mm using the PLIF procedure, it is impossible to spare the facet joints at any level above L5–S1, because the mean interpeduncular distance is 17 mm at L5–S1, 14.5 mm at L4–L5, 13.5 mm at L3–L4, 12.7 mm at L2–L3, and 12.5 mm at L1–L2 [1, 2, 11]. The lumbar articular facets support 18 % of the vertical load and provide rotational stability. Instability is related to the amount of facet removal, which is directly proportional to and dictated by the size of cage. The size for cylindrical cages is their diameter and for rectangular in situ rotating cages, the cage height [4, 24, 30, 37].

17.2.3 Number of Cages: One Versus Two

Usually the TLIF implants are parallelipipedic semilunar or straight in design, and only one is implanted unless the surgeons have a preference for bilateral TLIF access. Those used for PLIF are cubic or cylindrical in shape and are placed in pairs (Figs. 17.3 and 17.5).

Some of the efficacy expected of any type of cage actually depends on the access used, before the cage has been chosen or placed in the interbody space. This explains why there are no significant differences in construct stiffness and failure loads between a unilaterally inserted cage versus bilaterally inserted cages, and that cage shape and positioning do not significantly affect the in vitro biomechanical properties of the interbody cage across the vertebral end plate if bone mineral density is within normal limits [36, 37, 44, 45, 49]. Furthermore, the biomechanical testing performed shows more favorable stiffness using a single, unilaterally fixated, obliquely oriented interbody device than the bilateral construct placed by a standard PLIF approach [79].

The intensity of load bearing at the interbody devices depends on supplementation with posterior pedicle screws and the integrity of the facet joints, ligaments, and muscles. Medial facetectomy during PLIF access usually damages the facet joints on both sides partially or completely and leads to greater instability in rotation, increasing the load bearing to the interbody device. This means that before a stabilizing procedure, there was a highly destabilizing removal of the facet joints [6]. Usually there is less instability in TLIF cases because the interbody access is unilateral, and it can be performed lateral to the foramen, preserving at least the facet on one side and a large part on the other side. As a result, despite the addition of pedicle screw fixation and a greater area for bone fusion, there are still similar or lower fusion rates when comparing PLIF with TLIF [6, 26, 49].

17.2.4 TLIF Cages Types: Single (Bullet) Versus Dual Type (Boomerang)

There are two types of devices for TLIF implants: single or dual type (Fig. 17.7). Single devices are usually straight and designed with a bullet-shaped nose to facilitate insertion and to be self-distracting. These types of cage allow extremely straight MIS exposure and implantation. The facet joints can be preserved, and there is minimal destruction of the posterior ligaments and bony end plates because no preliminary trimming, shaving, and threading of the end plates are required. In addition, the convex design of the superior and inferior surfaces of the cages and the presence of self-retaining teeth to grip the end plates make cage subsidence fairly unlikely. The dual-type devices come in the form of a kidney bean or boomerang and allow filling the anterior and middle aspects of the disc, creating greater lordosis when using the wedge cages. The disadvantage is the need to have a larger work window to insert the device into the intervertebral space [23].

17.2.5 Lordotic Versus Non-lordotic Cages

One of the goals of this surgery is to maintain or obtain lumbar lordosis. This can be achieved when interbody devices with some type of lordotic contour are placed anteriorly and posterior compression forces are applied at the pedicle screws fixation [6, 10, 39] (Fig. 17.8). In addition, the wedged cages are able to avoid cage retropulsion compared with nonwedged cages [3, 38].

Previous studies reported that parallel-sided cages used as stand-alone supports cause loss of lumbar lordosis [6, 9, 29, 39]. Takahashi et al. [69] compared the sagittal alignment of the lumbar spine after one-segment PLIF using the titanium alloy horizontal cylinder or open box-type cage with a 3° lordotic angle. There was no significant difference between the two groups in terms of changes in lumbar lordosis. The surgical procedure and the insufficient 3° cage lordotic angle are possible explanations because the lumbar intervertebral body angles increase with descending lumbar levels. The angles of L4 to L5 and L5 to S1 are normally ≥10° [29, 67, 69].

17.2.6 Cage Insertion Methods: Impaction Versus Self-Tapping Versus Rotation Versus Expandable

Impaction cages are an important category among interbody cages. These cages, having a

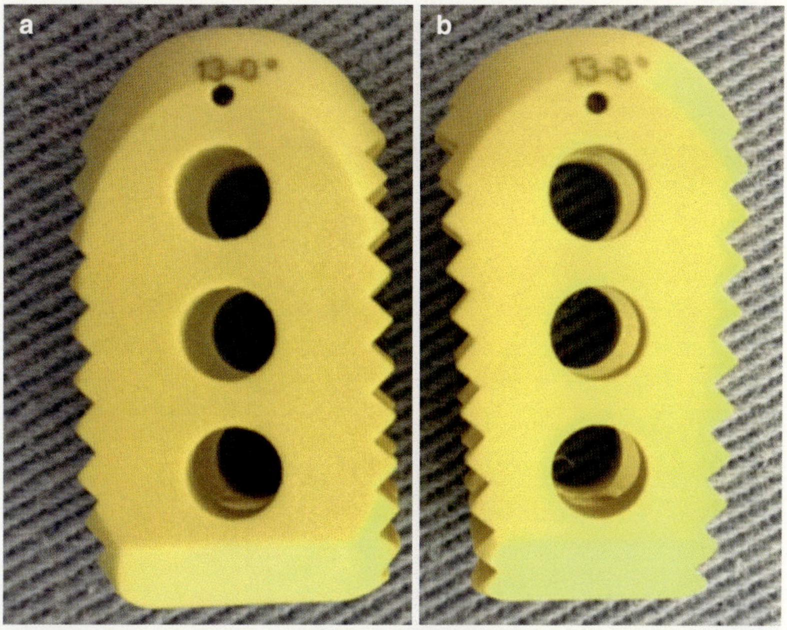

Fig. 17.8 The cage can have different morphologies according to the need for lumbar lordosis: non-lordotic cages (**a**) and 8° lordotic contouring cages (**b**) AVS PL, Stryker

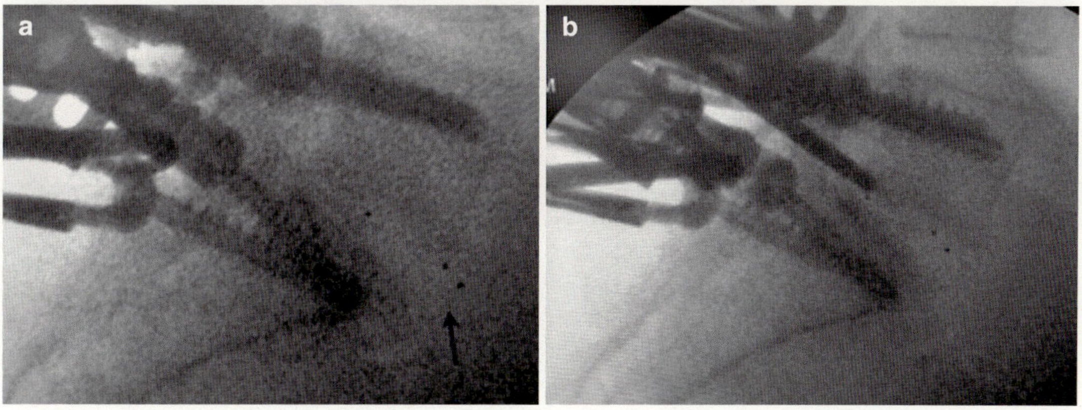

Fig. 17.9 The cage was impacted beyond the anterior border of the vertebrae (**a**), repositioned afterwards (**b**) and kept in position by screw compression and tightened

parallelipipedic shape, are inserted between the vertebrae by impaction. The downside of these cages is that they are difficult to insert into the intervertebral space either through PLIF or TLIF approaches, especially when pyramidal teeth are present (Fig. 17.9).

Costa et al. [19] reported a self-positioning, self-threading stand-alone titanium circular bullet cage. The cage was designed to be inserted by PLIF through MIS techniques. It has a blunt and tapered head allowing it to be used as a spreader and a small core facilitating self-positioning. The cage has an internal cavity and apertures in the superior and inferior surfaces, which permit packing autologous bone and facilitating bone fusion, respectively. The use of these cages as a stand-alone device was recommended only for discs that do not exceed 10 mm in height. In cases where the disc exceeds 10 mm in height, there is a need for pedicle screw fixation due to the facet joint resection in order to create a space to insert the cage. The choice of threaded circular fusion cages to restore disc height instead of rectangular cages means it is necessary to have a 50 % larger

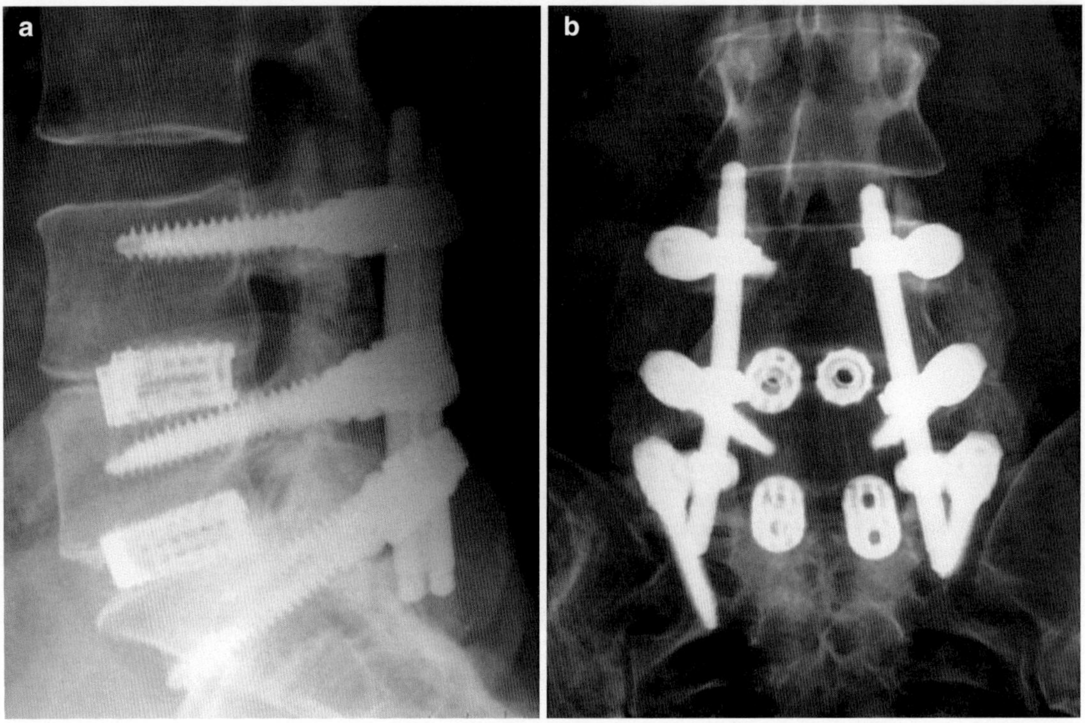

Fig. 17.10 Subsidence of the L4–L5 cages into the superior and inferior vertebrae end plate on the lateral (**a**) and anteroposterior (**b**) radiological view

diameter of the threaded fusion cage and, therefore, more extensive facetectomy [73]. Likewise, the amount of facetectomy used in the cages which were rotated inside the intervertebral space depended on cage height [73].

Expandable cages may enable easy insertion, a controlled restoration of disc height, and may require a less posterior bony removal and nerve root retraction to insert the cage [26]. Bhatia et al. [6] placed a bilateral expandable cage using a standard PLIF technique on the L4–L5 specimen after a 50 % medial facetectomy. Testing was done on the cage-alone condition and after pedicle screw fixation. Insertion of the expandable cage with retensioning of the annulus increased stability in all directions but less than the intact levels. Using the expandable cage as a stand-alone device decreased lordosis because of the geometric shape of the cage, which can be reversed after posterior pedicle fixation and posterior compression [6, 39].

17.3 Consequences of the Material Types: Subsidence

Cage subsidence is usually defined as a superior or inferior migration into the vertebral end plate ≥ 2 mm [5, 13, 14, 31, 41] (Fig. 17.10). Cage subsidence after lumbar interbody fusion has been reported in a wide range of situations, leading to a significant loss of disc space height, foraminal narrowing, and the potential for nerve root compression even using pedicle screw stabilization [7, 43, 58, 65].

Cage materials are expected to affect the incidence of subsidence caused by the difference between the modulus of elasticity of the device and the bone [77]. The rate of PEEK cages subsidence of >2 mm is considerably lower than that reported for metal cages and other interbody fusion techniques [13, 46, 70].

Besides the cage properties, the other risk factors associated with interbody fusion cage subsidence are lower bone mineral density, covering less than 30 % of the endplate area, applied excessive compressive load, endplate fracture during manipulation, and stand-alone interbody device [5, 15, 35] (Figs. 17.2 and 17.5). The idea of stand-alone interbody fusion devices was used after PLIF, but despite the surgical and technical evolution, the use of these devices as stand-alone cages is still viewed with skepticism [8, 11, 17, 58, 62].

The periphery of the vertebra end plate is the strongest bone whereas the most central portion of the bony end plates can be quite weak, especially in older patients with some degree of osteoporosis. Thus, resting an interbody device on the peripheral endplate bone is advantageous for maintaining disc height and sagittal alignment and avoiding subsidence. For this reason, there are some cages with a larger medial lateral width to ensure that the cage sits on the cortical bone at the edge of the vertebral body and to prevent implant sinkage.

To limit the risk of cage subsidence, a “sandwich” design was developed for cages. This design consists of an inner polymeric, stiff core covered with two layers made in a softer material in the areas in contact with the end plates. The soft layers are expected to create a more uniform pressure distribution at the cage-endplate interface and adapt to the geometric irregularities of the bony end plate after the surgical preparation, thus maximizing the contact area and reducing the risk of subsidence [28].

17.4 Ideal Interbody Cage

When ideal interbody cage designs are considered, some characteristics must be present, such as (1) placing it in a small window preserving the muscle, facet, and ligaments, best if percutaneously; (2) with a variable bone-like elastic modulus; (3) introducing it into the interbody space without need for impaction and thereafter rotating or expanding it inside the interbody space to reproduce an angle between the two vertebrae; (4) with a lordotic angle capable of maintaining or achieving lumbar lordosis; (5) allowing space for bone grafts outside the cages; (6) with an open design cage having a central cavity that allows space for packing large amounts of cancellous bone graft; and (7) with a convex design and some points to be fixed into the vertebra to avoid subsidence.

References

1. Amonoo-Kuofi HS. Maximum and minimum lumbar interpedicular distances in normal adult Nigerians. J Anat. 1982;135(Pt 2):225–33.
2. Amonoo-Kuofi HS, Patel PJ, Fatani JA. Transverse diameter of the lumbar spinal canal in normal adult Saudis. Acta Anat. 1990;137(2):124–8.
3. Aoki Y, Yamagata M, Nakajima F, Ikeda Y, Shimizu K, Yoshihara M, Iwasaki J, Toyone T, Nakagawa K, Nakajima A, Takahashi K, Ohtori S. Examining risk factors for posterior migration of fusion cages following transforaminal lumbar interbody fusion: a possible limitation of unilateral pedicle screw fixation. J Neurosurg Spine. 2010;13(3):381–7. doi:10.3171/2010.3.SPINE09590.
4. Bernhardt M, Bridwell KH. Segmental analysis of the sagittal plane alignment of the normal thoracic and lumbar spines and thoracolumbar junction. Spine. 1989;14(7):717–21.
5. Beutler WJ, Peppelman Jr WC. Anterior lumbar fusion with paired BAK standard and paired BAK Proximity cages: subsidence incidence, subsidence factors, and clinical outcome. Spine J Off J North Am Spine Soc. 2003;3(4):289–93.
6. Bhatia NN, Lee KH, Bui CN, Luna M, Wahba GM, Lee TQ. Biomechanical evaluation of an expandable cage in single-segment posterior lumbar interbody fusion. Spine. 2012;37(2):E79–85. doi:10.1097/BRS.0b013e3182226ba6.
7. Boucher HH. A method of spinal fusion. J Bone Joint Surg Br. 1959;41-B(2):248–59.
8. Branch CL, Branch Jr CL. Posterior lumbar interbody fusion with the keystone graft: technique and results. Surg Neurol. 1987;27(5):449–54.
9. Brantigan JW, Neidre A. Achievement of normal sagittal plane alignment using a wedged carbon fiber reinforced polymer fusion cage in treatment of spondylolisthesis. Spine J Off J North Am Spine Soc. 2003;3(3):186–96.
10. Brantigan JW, Steffee AD. A carbon fiber implant to aid interbody lumbar fusion. Two-year clinical results in the first 26 patients. Spine. 1993;18(14):2106–7.
11. Brantigan JW, Steffee AD, Geiger JM. A carbon fiber implant to aid interbody lumbar fusion. Mechanical testing. Spine. 1991;16 Suppl 6:S277–82.
12. Bridwell KH, Lenke LG, McEnery KW, Baldus C, Blanke K. Anterior fresh frozen structural allografts in the thoracic and lumbar spine. Do they work if combined with posterior fusion and instrumentation in adult patients with kyphosis or anterior column defects? Spine. 1995;20(12):1410–8.

13. Chen L, Yang H, Tang T. Cage migration in spondylolisthesis treated with posterior lumbar interbody fusion using BAK cages. Spine. 2005;30(19):2171–5.
14. Choi JY, Sung KH. Subsidence after anterior lumbar interbody fusion using paired stand-alone rectangular cages. Eur Spine J. 2006;15(1):16–22. doi:10.1007/s00586-004-0817-y. official publication of the European Spine Society, the European Spinal Deformity Society, and the European Section of the Cervical Spine Research Society.
15. Closkey RF, Parsons JR, Lee CK, Blacksin MF, Zimmerman MC. Mechanics of interbody spinal fusion. Analysis of critical bone graft area. Spine. 1993;18(8):1011–5.
16. Cloward RB. The treatment of ruptured lumbar intervertebral disc by vertebral body fusion. III. Method of use of banked bone. Ann Surg. 1952;136(6):987–92.
17. Cloward RB. The treatment of ruptured lumbar intervertebral discs by vertebral body fusion. I. Indications, operative technique, after care. J Neurosurg. 1953;10(2):154–68. doi:10.3171/jns.1953.10.2.0154.
18. Coe JD, Vaccaro AR. Instrumented transforaminal lumbar interbody fusion with bioresorbable polymer implants and iliac crest autograft. Spine. 2005;30 Suppl 17:S76–83.
19. Costa F, Sassi M, Ortolina A, Cardia A, Assietti R, Zerbi A, Lorenzetti M, Galbusera F, Fornari M. Stand-alone cage for posterior lumbar interbody fusion in the treatment of high-degree degenerative disc disease: design of a new device for an "old" technique. A prospective study on a series of 116 patients. Eur Spine J. 2011;20 Suppl 1:S46–56. doi:10.1007/s00586-011-1755-0. official publication of the European Spine Society, the European Spinal Deformity Society, and the European Section of the Cervical Spine Research Society.
20. Dennis S, Watkins R, Landaker S, Dillin W, Springer D. Comparison of disc space heights after anterior lumbar interbody fusion. Spine. 1989;14(8):876–8.
21. Dhall SS, Wang MY, Mummaneni PV. Clinical and radiographic comparison of mini-open transforaminal lumbar interbody fusion with open transforaminal lumbar interbody fusion in 42 patients with long-term follow-up. J Neurosurg Spine. 2008;9(6):560–5. doi:10.3171/SPI.2008.9.08142.
22. DiPaola CP, Molinari RW. Posterior lumbar interbody fusion. J Am Acad Orthop Surg. 2008;16(3):130–9.
23. Eck KR, Bridwell KH, Ungacta FF, Lapp MA, Lenke LG, Riew KD. Analysis of titanium mesh cages in adults with minimum two-year follow-up. Spine. 2000;25(18):2407–15.
24. Elias WJ, Simmons NE, Kaptain GJ, Chadduck JB, Whitehill R. Complications of posterior lumbar interbody fusion when using a titanium threaded cage device. J Neurosurg. 2000;93 Suppl 1:45–52.
25. Evans JH. Biomechanics of lumbar fusion. Clin Orthop Relat Res. 1985;193:38–46.
26. Folman Y, Lee SH, Silvera JR, Gepstein R. Posterior lumbar interbody fusion for degenerative disc disease using a minimally invasive B-twin expandable spinal spacer: a multicenter study. J Spinal Disord Tech. 2003;16(5):455–60.
27. Freedman BA, Rhee JM, Jackson KL. Preparing the lumbar intervertebral disk space for interbody procedures: a comparison between the traditional method and a new automated method. J Spinal Disord Tech. 2012;25(1):E1–6. doi:10.1097/BSD.0b013e318227ecfb.
28. Galbusera F, Schmidt H, Wilke HJ. Lumbar interbody fusion: a parametric investigation of a novel cage design with and without posterior instrumentation. Eur Spine J. 2012;21(3):455–62. doi:10.1007/s00586-011-2014-0. official publication of the European Spine Society, the European Spinal Deformity Society, and the European Section of the Cervical Spine Research Society.
29. Godde S, Fritsch E, Dienst M, Kohn D. Influence of cage geometry on sagittal alignment in instrumented posterior lumbar interbody fusion. Spine. 2003;28(15):1693–9. doi:10.1097/01.BRS.0000083167.78853.D5.
30. Goh JC, Wong HK, Thambyah A, Yu CS. Influence of PLIF cage size on lumbar spine stability. Spine 2000;25(1):35–9; discussion 40
31. Ha SK, Park JY, Kim SH, Lim DJ, Kim SD, Lee SK. Radiologic Assessment of Subsidence in Stand-Alone Cervical Polyetheretherketone (PEEK) Cage. J Korean Neurosurg Soc. 2008;44(6):370–4. doi:10.3340/jkns.2008.44.6.370.
32. Harms J, Rolinger H. A one-stager procedure in operative treatment of spondylolistheses: dorsal traction-reposition and anterior fusion (author's transl). Zeitschrift fur Orthopadie und ihre Grenzgebiete. 1982;120(3):343–7. doi:10.1055/s-2008-1051624.
33. Hasegawa K, Abe M, Washio T, Hara T. An experimental study on the interface strength between titanium mesh cage and vertebra in reference to vertebral bone mineral density. Spine. 2001;26(8):957–63.
34. Hoshijima K, Nightingale RW, Yu JR, Richardson WJ, Harper KD, Yamamoto H, Myers BS. Strength and stability of posterior lumbar interbody fusion. Comparison of titanium fiber mesh implant and tricortical bone graft. Spine. 1997;22(11):1181–8.
35. Javernick MA, Kuklo TR, Polly DW, Jr. Transforaminal lumbar interbody fusion: unilateral versus bilateral disk removal – an in vivo study. Am J Orthop (Belle Mead NJ). 2003;32(7):344–8; discussion 348.
36. Jost B, Cripton PA, Lund T, Oxland TR, Lippuner K, Jaeger P, Nolte LP. Compressive strength of interbody cages in the lumbar spine: the effect of cage shape, posterior instrumentation and bone density. Eur Spine J. 1998;7(2):132–41. official publication of the European Spine Society, the European Spinal Deformity Society, and the European Section of the Cervical Spine Research Society.
37. Kettler A, Schmoelz W, Kast E, Gottwald M, Claes L, Wilke HJ. In vitro stabilizing effect of a transforaminal compared with two posterior lumbar interbody fusion cages. Spine. 2005;30(22):E665–70.
38. Kimura H, Shikata J, Odate S, Soeda T, Yamamura S. Risk factors for cage retropulsion after posterior

lumbar interbody fusion: analysis of 1070 cases. Spine. 2012;37(13):1164–9. doi:10.1097/BRS.0b013e318257f12a.
39. Klemme WR, Owens BD, Dhawan A, Zeidman S, Polly Jr DW. Lumbar sagittal contour after posterior interbody fusion: threaded devices alone versus vertical cages plus posterior instrumentation. Spine. 2001;26(5):534–7.
40. Kok D, Donk RD, Wapstra FH, Veldhuizen AG. The memory metal minimal access cage: a new concept in lumbar interbody fusion-a prospective, noncomparative study to evaluate the safety and performance. Adv Orthop. 2012;2012:898606. doi:10.1155/2012/898606.
41. Kulkarni AG, Hee HT, Wong HK. Solis cage (PEEK) for anterior cervical fusion: preliminary radiological results with emphasis on fusion and subsidence. Spine J Off J North Am Spine Soc. 2007;7(2):205–9. doi:10.1016/j.spinee.2006.03.002.
42. Kurtz SM, Devine JN. PEEK biomaterials in trauma, orthopedic, and spinal implants. Biomaterials. 2007;28(32):4845–69. doi:10.1016/j.biomaterials.2007.07.013.
43. Kuslich SD, Ulstrom CL, Griffith SL, Ahern JW, Dowdle JD. The Bagby and Kuslich method of lumbar interbody fusion. History, techniques, and 2-year follow-up results of a United States prospective, multicenter trial. Spine 1998;23(11):1267–78; discussion 1279.
44. Labrom RD, Tan JS, Reilly CW, Tredwell SJ, Fisher CG, Oxland TR. The effect of interbody cage positioning on lumbosacral vertebral endplate failure in compression. Spine. 2005;30(19):E556–61.
45. Lam FC, Alkalay R, Groff MW. The effects of design and positioning of carbon fiber lumbar interbody cages and their subsidence in vertebral bodies. J Spinal Disord Tech. 2012;25(2):116–22. doi:10.1097/BSD.0b013e31820ef778.
46. Lee JH, Jeon DW, Lee SJ, Chang BS, Lee CK. Fusion rates and subsidence of morselized local bone grafted in titanium cages in posterior lumbar interbody fusion using quantitative three-dimensional computed tomography scans. Spine. 2010;35(15):1460–5. doi:10.1097/BRS.0b013e3181c4baf5.
47. Loguidice VA, Johnson RG, Guyer RD, Stith WJ, Ohnmeiss DD, Hochschuler SH, Rashbaum RF. Anterior lumbar interbody fusion. Spine. 1988; 13(3):366–9.
48. Lowe TG, Coe JD. Resorbable polymer implants in unilateral transforaminal lumbar interbody fusion. J Neurosurg. 2002;97 Suppl 4:464–7.
49. Lund T, Oxland TR, Jost B, Cripton P, Grassmann S, Etter C, Nolte LP. Interbody cage stabilisation in the lumbar spine: biomechanical evaluation of cage design, posterior instrumentation and bone density. J Bone Joint Surg Br. 1998;80(2):351–9.
50. McLaughlin MR, Haid Jr RW, Rodts Jr GE, Subach BR. Posterior lumbar interbody fusion: indications, techniques, and results. Clin Neurosurg. 2000;47: 514–27.
51. Mummaneni PV, Haid RW, Rodts GE. Lumbar interbody fusion: state-of-the-art technical advances. Invited submission from the Joint Section Meeting on Disorders of the Spine and Peripheral Nerves, March 2004. J Neurosurg Spine. 2004;1(1):24–30. doi:10.3171/spi.2004.1.1.0024.
52. Oxland TR, Hoffer Z, Nydegger T, Rathonyi GC, Nolte LP. A comparative biomechanical investigation of anterior lumbar interbody cages: central and bilateral approaches. J Bone Joint Surg Am. 2000; 82(3):383–93.
53. Panjabi MM. Biomechanical evaluation of spinal fixation devices: I. A conceptual framework. Spine. 1988;13(10):1129–34.
54. Parsons JR, Bhayani S, Alexander H, Weiss AB. Carbon fiber debris within the synovial joint. A time-dependent mechanical and histologic study. Clin Orthop Relat Res. 1985;196:69–76.
55. Pfeiffer M, Griss P, Haake M, Kienapfel H, Billion M. Standardized evaluation of long-term results after anterior lumbar interbody fusion. Eur Spine J. 1996;5(5):299–307. official publication of the European Spine Society, the European Spinal Deformity Society, and the European Section of the Cervical Spine Research Society.
56. Polikeit A, Ferguson SJ, Nolte LP, Orr TE. The importance of the endplate for interbody cages in the lumbar spine. Eur Spine J. 2003;12(6):556–61. doi:10.1007/s00586-003-0556-5. official publication of the European Spine Society, the European Spinal Deformity Society, and the European Section of the Cervical Spine Research Society.
57. Rathonyi GC, Oxland TR, Gerich U, Grassmann S, Nolte LP. The role of supplemental translaminar screws in anterior lumbar interbody fixation: a biomechanical study. Eur Spine J. 1998;7(5):400–7. official publication of the European Spine Society, the European Spinal Deformity Society, and the European Section of the Cervical Spine Research Society.
58. Ray CD. Threaded titanium cages for lumbar interbody fusions. Spine 1997;22(6):667–79; discussion 679–80.
59. Rish BL. A critique of posterior lumbar interbody fusion: 12 years' experience with 250 patients. Surg Neurol. 1989;31(4):281–9.
60. Schizas C, Tzinieris N, Tsiridis E, Kosmopoulos V. Minimally invasive versus open transforaminal lumbar interbody fusion: evaluating initial experience. Int Orthop. 2009;33(6):1683–8. doi:10.1007/s00264-008-0687-8.
61. Sengupta DK, Mehdian SM, Mulholland RC, Webb JK, Ohnmeiss DD. Biomechanical evaluation of immediate stability with rectangular versus cylindrical interbody cages in stabilization of the lumbar spine. BMC Musculoskelet Disord. 2002;3:23.
62. Simmons JW. Posterior lumbar interbody fusion with posterior elements as chip grafts. Clin Orthop Relat Res. 1985;193:85–9.
63. Smit TH, Engels TA, Wuisman PI, Govaert LE. Time-dependent mechanical strength of 70/30 Poly(L,

DL-lactide): shedding light on the premature failure of degradable spinal cages. Spine. 2008;33(1):14–8. doi:10.1097/BRS.0b013e31815e39df.
64. Smith AJ, Arginteanu M, Moore F, Steinberger A, Camins M. Increased incidence of cage migration and nonunion in instrumented transforaminal lumbar interbody fusion with bioabsorbable cages. J Neurosurg Spine. 2010;13(3):388–93. doi:10.3171/2010.3.SPINE09587.
65. Soini J. Lumbar disc space heights after external fixation and anterior interbody fusion: a prospective 2-year follow-up of clinical and radiographic results. J Spinal Disord. 1994;7(6):487–94.
66. Steffen T, Tsantrizos A, Fruth I, Aebi M. Cages: designs and concepts. Eur Spine J. 2000;9 Suppl 1:S89–94. official publication of the European Spine Society, the European Spinal Deformity Society, and the European Section of the Cervical Spine Research Society.
67. Stephens GC, Yoo JU, Wilbur G. Comparison of lumbar sagittal alignment produced by different operative positions. Spine 1996;21(15):1802–06; discussion 1807.
68. Sudo H, Oda I, Abumi K, Ito M, Kotani Y, Hojo Y, Minami A. In vitro biomechanical effects of reconstruction on adjacent motion segment: comparison of aligned/kyphotic posterolateral fusion with aligned posterior lumbar interbody fusion/posterolateral fusion. J Neurosurg. 2003;99 Suppl 2:221–8.
69. Takahashi H, Suguro T, Yokoyama Y, Iida Y, Terashima F, Wada A. Effect of cage geometry on sagittal alignment after posterior lumbar interbody fusion for degenerative disc disease. J Orthop Surg (Hong Kong). 2010;18(2):139–42.
70. Tokuhashi Y, Ajiro Y, Umezawa N. Subsidence of metal interbody cage after posterior lumbar interbody fusion with pedicle screw fixation. Orthopedics. 2009;32(4):259.
71. Toth JM, Estes BT, Wang M, Seim 3rd HB, Scifert JL, Turner AS, Cornwall GB. Evaluation of 70/30 poly (L-lactide-co-D, L-lactide) for use as a resorbable interbody fusion cage. J Neurosurg. 2002;97 Suppl 4:423–32.
72. Tsantrizos A, Andreou A, Aebi M, Steffen T. Biomechanical stability of five stand-alone anterior lumbar interbody fusion constructs. Eur Spine J. 2000;9(1):14–22. official publication of the European Spine Society, the European Spinal Deformity Society, and the European Section of the Cervical Spine Research Society.
73. Tsantrizos A, Baramki HG, Zeidman S, Steffen T. Segmental stability and compressive strength of posterior lumbar interbody fusion implants. Spine. 2000; 25(15):1899–907.
74. Tullberg T. Failure of a carbon fiber implant. A case report. Spine. 1998;23(16):1804–6.
75. Vadapalli S, Sairyo K, Goel VK, Robon M, Biyani A, Khandha A, Ebraheim NA. Biomechanical rationale for using polyetheretherketone (PEEK) spacers for lumbar interbody fusion-A finite element study. Spine. 2006;31(26):E992–8. doi:10.1097/01.brs.0000250177.84168.ba.
76. Wang ST, Goel VK, Fu CY, Kubo S, Choi W, Liu CL, Chen TH. Comparison of two interbody fusion cages for posterior lumbar interbody fusion in a cadaveric model. Int Orthop. 2006;30(4):299–304. doi:10.1007/s00264-006-0076-0.
77. Wenz LM, Merritt K, Brown SA, Moet A, Steffee AD. In vitro biocompatibility of polyetheretherketone and polysulfone composites. J Biomed Mater Res. 1990;24(2):207–15. doi:10.1002/jbm.820240207.
78. Wu RH, Fraser JF, Hartl R. Minimal access versus open transforaminal lumbar interbody fusion: meta-analysis of fusion rates. Spine. 2010;35(26):2273–81. doi:10.1097/BRS.0b013e3181cd42cc.
79. Zhao J, Hai Y, Ordway NR, Park CK, Yuan HA. Posterior lumbar interbody fusion using posterolateral placement of a single cylindrical threaded cage. Spine. 2000;25(4):425–30.

18 Multilevel TLIF for Spinal Deformity

Yi Lu, Michelle M. Falcone, Michael Y. Wang, and Steven Wu

18.1 Introduction

Adult spinal deformity (ASD) refers to an abnormal spinal curvature in the coronal, axial, and sagittal plane in adult patients. Most ASDs are de novo degenerative deformities that are caused by asymmetric disc and facet degeneration or osteoporotic spine insufficiency fracture [20]. Recent publications have indicated that the prevalence of any radiographic evidence of ASD can be as high as 60 % in adults older than 60 years of age [19, 24] and symptomatic scoliosis is seen in 6–30 % of the elderly population. Patients with ASD most commonly seek treatment due to pain and disability from the deformity and its associated disc degeneration, spinal stenosis, nerve roots compression, lateral listhesis, spondylolisthesis, and the overall loss of spinopelvic balance. Most symptomatic ASD patients are initially treated with conservative measures such as physical therapy, nonsteroidal anti-inflammatory medication, and narcotic analgesics. When conservative treatment fails, operative procedures aiming to decompress lumbar nerve roots and the thecal sac stabilize unstable motion segments, reestablish global spinal balance in all planes, and prevent deformity progression are indicated.

ASD Surgery can be very rewarding for patients, yielding significant improvements in back and leg pain. This has been proven in previous studies utilizing objective quality-of-life (QOL) measures like the Scoliosis Research Society 22 questionnaire (SRS-22) and Oswestry Disability Index (ODI) [5, 32, 33]. Nevertheless, adult deformity surgeries are highly complex and require prolonged anesthesia, a long recovery period, and extended hospital stay. Traditional open deformity surgeries are associated with high rate of serious complications, and it has been reported that open deformity surgeries have major complication rates as high as 40 %. In a series of 361 patients who underwent open deformity surgery, Pateder and colleagues reported that the 30-day mortality rate was 2.4 % [23]. In 2011, Smith et al. analyzed data from the Spinal Deformity Study Group and reported that 26.2 % of their 206 patients suffered a minor complication and 15.5 % suffered a major complication [31]. Staged procedures or combined anterior-posterior approaches have also been found to be associated with higher complication rates [26]. Interestingly, despite the fact that elderly patients were found to have higher perioperative complication rates as high as 71 %, they had the greatest improvement in pain and disability with surgery [34].

Y. Lu, M.D., Ph.D. (✉)
Department of Neurosurgery,
Brigham and Women's Hospital,
Harvard Medical School, Boston, MA, USA
e-mail: ylu4@partners.org

M.M. Falcone, ASD • M.Y. Wang, M.D., FACS
Department of Neurological Surgery,
University of Miami, Jackson Memorial Hospital,
Miami, FL, USA

S. Wu
Department of Neurosurgery,
Brigham and Women's Hospital,
Harvard Medical School, Boston, MA, USA

M.Y. Wang et al. (eds.), *Minimally Invasive Spinal Deformity Surgery*,
DOI 10.1007/978-3-7091-1407-0_18, © Springer-Verlag Wien 2014

One of the major goals of deformity surgery is to restore the coronal and sagittal balance of the spine. Traditionally, deformity surgery has been focused on correcting coronal imbalance. However, global sagittal balance has more recently been found to be more relevant in patient's symptom and surgical outcome. Glassman et al. reviewed a prospective adult spinal deformity case series with correlated radiographic measures and found that sagittal balance was the most reliable predictor of clinical symptoms [11]. Patients with positive sagittal balance and inadequate lumbar lordosis have worse physical and social function and pain. In these patients, restoration of global sagittal alignment is necessary for significant symptom improvement and pseudoarthrosis avoidance [4, 25].

In traditional open deformity surgery, a variety of techniques have been used to enhance lumbar lordosis and restore sagittal balance. Multilevel anterior lumbar interbody fusion (ALIF) has been demonstrated to be an effective method to achieve normal lumbar alignment [9, 15, 36]. Placement of an anterior graft allows distraction of the anterior disc space, increases disc space height, and improves lumbar lordosis. The large graft size used with an anterior approach also enhances construct stability. The drawback of using ALIF for lumbar alignment is the need for a two-stage surgery, which subjects patients to increased anesthesia time, higher complication rates, and additional approaches.

Rigid sagittal imbalance corrections are most often achieved with pedicle subtraction osteotomy (PSO) in adult deformity surgery [13, 18, 21, 27]. However, PSO is frequently associated with high volume of blood loss and high surgical morbidity and complications [6]. The amount of bony and soft tissue resection required in pedicle subtraction osteotomy also limits its use in minimally invasive surgery (MIS) [39].

The recently developed MIS lateral transpsoas interbody technique has been adopted with much enthusiasm in less invasive deformity surgery. This technique has been shown to be excellent in treating local degenerative arthritis, restoring foraminal height, achieving indirect neural decompression, and correcting coronal deformity [22, 29]. However, the lateral transpsoas approach has been shown to be less effective in treating sagittal imbalance and restoring lumbar lordosis. In a recently reported series of 35 patients by Acosta et al., the lateral transpsoas approach allowed a coronal Cobb angle correction from 21.4° preoperatively to 9.7° postoperatively, a statistically significant improvement. However, lumbar lordosis only changed from 42.1° to 46.2°, despite improvement in interbody height. Overall, the global sagittal alignment was unchanged [1]. These results are similar to the 5° improvement in global lordosis noted by Karikari et al [17]. Modification of the technique by adding the resection of the anterior longitudinal ligament (ALL) has been proposed to enhance sagittal correction allowed with the lateral approach [2, 7, 8, 37]. However, resecting the ALL blindly has the inherent risk of seriously injuring the great vessels. Furthermore, in adult degenerative patient hypertrophied facet joints and stiff posterior elements limited the amount of sagittal correction that can be achieved with the release of anterior elements. More importantly, the majority of physiological lumbar lordosis is found at the L5–S1 and L4–L5 levels, which are problematic to access or with the direct lateral approach.

18.2 Use of Open Multilevel TLIF for Coronal and Sagittal Deformity Correction

Jagannathan et al. published a report in 2009 demonstrating the efficacy of using multilevel TLIF to restore lumbar sagittal alignment [16]. In this retrospective study, 80 patients who had received short-segment (1, 2, or 3 level) transforaminal lumbar interbody fusion (TLIF) procedures for lumbar degenerative disorders were studied. Bilateral facetectomies with interspinous distraction were used so that a large-size boomerang-shaped graft could be placed at the anterior part of the disc space. After insertion of the interbody graft and placement of the pedicle screws, the construct was compressed. At follow-up, radiographic studies demonstrated effective increase of focal lordosis at each of the surgical levels performed. L5–S1 and L4–L5 TLIFs were most effective in restoring segmental lumbar lordosis. An average of 22.2° of segmental lordosis improvement was achieved with a L5–S1 TLIF, and L4–5 TLIF was associated with an average of 11.3° improvement. Multilevel TLIF was more effective in correcting overall lumbar lordosis than single-level surgery (27.3° +/– 3.4° vs. 17.4° +/4.4°). For the majority of patients with a preoperative sagittal imbalance of less than 10 cm, short-segment TLIF procedures were able to improve sagittal alignment. However, only 30 % of the patients with a sagittal imbalance of more than 10 cm achieved acceptable restoration, indicating the need for a more extensive surgery such as osteotomy procedures with long-segment fusion. Yson et al. also published a similar series using multilevel TLIF with bilateral facet resection for segmental lumbar sagittal correction. Similar methods of bilateral facet resection and the use of an interbody spacer placed as anterior as possible were applied demonstrating that significant lordosis restoration can be achieved using multilevel TLIF [40].

The position and the geometry of the cage significantly influence the effect of the sagittal correction after TLIF [10, 12]. In the past several publications had described the TLIF as a procedure that could reduce lumbar lordosis [9, 15]. This was likely due to the specific surgical techniques used. In both series by Jagannathan and Yson, the use of large anteriorly placed spacers helped restore of the lumbar lordosis, similar to the cantilever TLIF procedure described by Anand et al [3]. More importantly, the bilateral facetectomies, the radical discectomy to allow sufficient segmental mobilization, and final compression of the pedicle screws allowed significant restoration of lumbar lordosis.

Heary and Karimi described using unilateral placed TLIF cage for coronal balance correction [14]. In their series of four patients, TLIF cages were placed unilaterally on the concave side, and bilateral facetectomies were used to release the rigid curve. The selective applications of the increased compressive forces were used on the convex side of the construct. Mean correction of the coronal curve of 17.9° was achieved in the small series.

18.3 The Use of MIS Multilevel MIS TLIF in Adult Deformity Surgery

MIS TLIF has been widely used over the past decade to address degenerative lumbar disc disease, spondylolisthesis, and recurrent lumbar disc herniations [28]. Since open multilevel TLIF has been shown to correct sagittal imbalance efficiently, it stands to reason that multilevel MIS TLIF could be a promising approach for MIS deformity surgery, without subjecting patients to multiple stage surgeries since the whole surgery is performed with the patient in prone position. Wang published his experience using multilevel MIS TLIF with expandable cages in a series of 25 adult spinal deformity patients [38]. This case series utilized expandable interbody cages to restore anterior column height combined with percutaneous pedicle screw fixation. An average of 3.2 interbody levels were treated in these patients. The mean preoperative Cobb angle was 29.2°, improving to 9.0° postoperatively; the mean preoperative global lumbar lordosis was 27.8°, improving to 42.6° postoperatively; and the mean preoperative SVA improved from 7.4 cm to 4.3 cm postoperatively. Clinically, at 1-year follow-up, the NPS for leg pain improved from 5.1 to 1.8 after surgery, and the NPS for back pain improved from 7.6 to 3.4. The ODI score improved from 44.9 to 24.1 after surgery.

18.4 Surgical Technique

1. *Positioning*: The surgery is performed after induction of general anesthesia with the patient lying prone. Positioning on the Jackson table is critical to allow the belly to hang and to increase lordosis, as it has been shown that the use of Jackson table enhances postoperative lumbar lordosis [35].
2. *Skin Incision*: For long-segment minimally invasive deformity surgery, it is more cosmetically pleasing to use a single midline incision. The principle of minimally invasive surgery is not the size of the skin incision but the minimal disruption of normal soft tissues and bony structures to achieve the desired

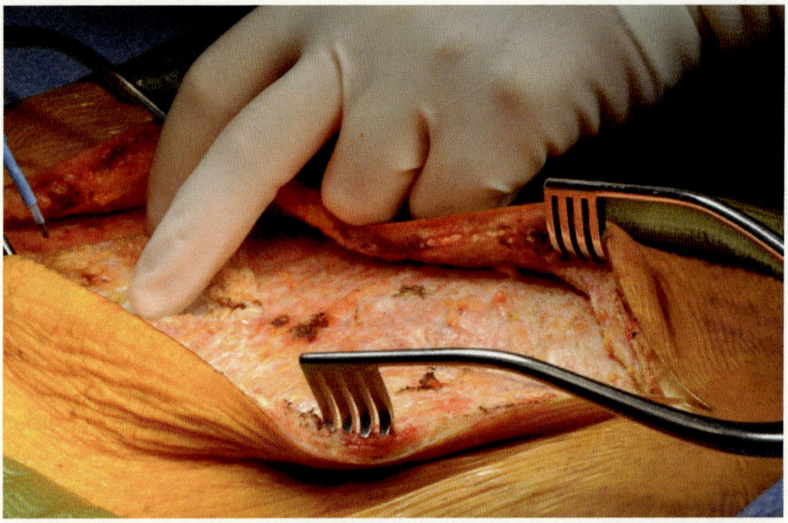

Fig. 18.1 Single midline incision and the development of the subskin fascia plane

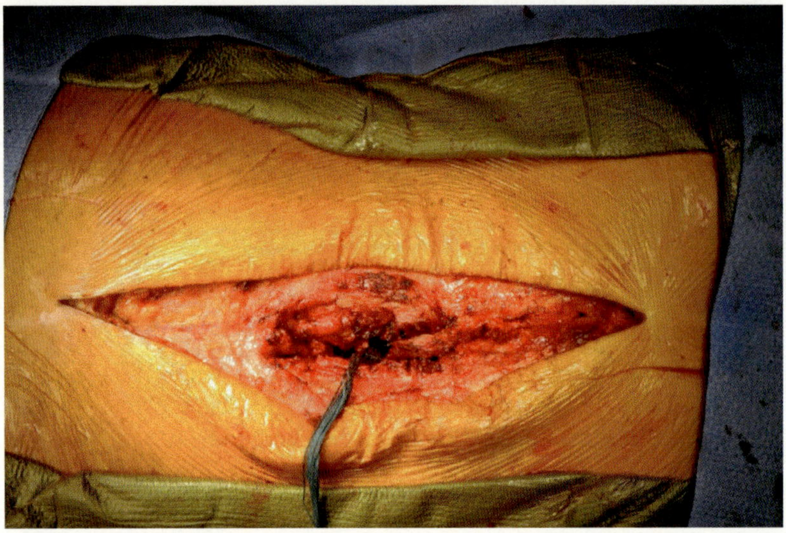

Fig. 18.2 The amount of tissue dissection for mini-open deformity surgery

outcome. A single midline incision with preservation of the fascia plane is minimally disruptive and cosmetically pleasing with better wound healing than multiple bilateral stab incisions. Furthermore, many patients already have had a previous surgery with a midline lumbar scar.

3. *Development of the Suprafascial Plane*: After making the skin incision with meticulous hemostasis, a plane is developed above the superficial fascia so that percutaneous screws can be placed and the TLIF corridor can be accessed with minimal disruption of the soft tissue envelope (Fig. 18.1).
4. *Access Corridor:* At this time, traditional MIS TLIF with fixed or expandable tubes can be used for performing the TLIF procedures. We often elect to perform multilevel TLIF in a mini-open fashion by performing subperiosteal dissection only on the side of the interbody access. Only one side of the spine is accessed to allow for facetectomies and interbody cage placement. With the preservation of muscle attachments to the spine on the contralateral side, patients generally have a much faster recovery time and less postoperative pain than traditional bilateral open procedures (Fig. 18.2). The unilateral subperiosteal

dissection is taken to the lateral facet joints, and a retractor is used to maintain the opening.

5. *Side of Approach*: The side of approach for multilevel TLIF in minimally invasive deformity surgery is very important since most ASD patients also have a coronal deformity that needs to be corrected simultaneously. The choice of which side to approach depends on the type of deformity, clinical symptoms, and the goals of the surgery. We have learned that it is more effective to access the spine from the concavity of the fractional curve (which is the convexity side of the major curve typically at the midlumbar spine) to correct coronal imbalance (Fig. 18.3). A lumbosacral fractional curve creates an uneven foundation for the entire spine, and a small lumbosacral fractional curve can lead to a significant coronal imbalance, if not compensated. By placing the interbody spacers at the lumbosacral junction ipsilateral to the side of access in the disc space, it elevates the concave side and corrects the fractional curve. When approaching from the concave side of the fractional curve, surgeons face the convexity of the midlumbar major curve. Since the spine is rotated toward the convexity of the curve, it is easier for cages to be placed across the midline to the contralateral side (which is the concave side of the major curve) further straightening up the curved lumbar spine.
6. *Facetectomy*: Following the exposure and confirmation of spinal levels, partial or complete facetectomies are performed at the level of interest. The inferior facet is generally resected using an osteotome and used as autograft fusion material. The superior facet of the inferior level is drilled to allow enough opening for the ipsilateral interbody graft placement, up to the superior edge of the pedicle. While placing the ipsilateral cage at the concave side, the required exposure of the disc space could be smaller than that of routine TLIF, especially if an expandable cage is used. When approaching the major curves from the convex side, since the axial rotation can be as great as 35° and the preferential cage insertion is toward the contralateral side of the disc space, it is frequently advantageous to approach the disc space lateral to the

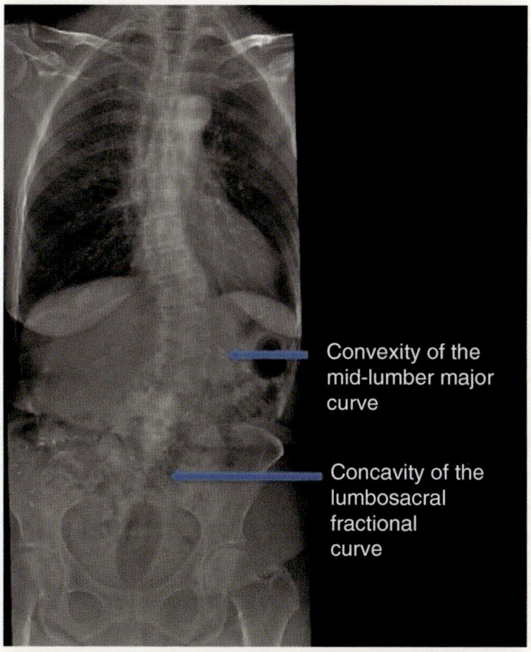

Fig. 18.3 Concavity of the lumbosacral fractional curve is on the same side of the convexity of the mid-lumbar major curve

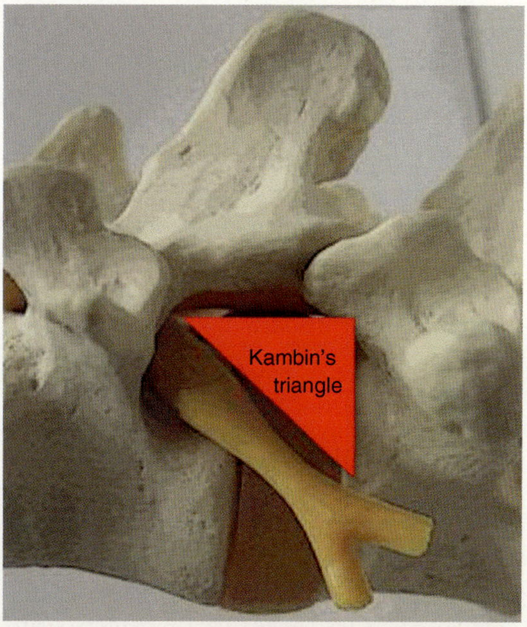

Fig. 18.4 Anatomy of Kambin's triangle

facet joint in Kambin's triangle (Fig. 18.4). In this circumstance, a true transforaminal interbody graft placement can be performed with little need for facet resection. However, a facetectomy is still beneficial as it increases the flexibility of the rigid spine and allows for the compression on the convexity of the lumbar major curve, using the contralateral interbody graft as a fulcum to correct coronal imbalance.

A midline laminectomy is typically not performed. When central, lateral recess, or foraminal decompression is needed (which is frequently a necessity in ASD patients, depending on patient's symptoms), an ipsi-contra lumbar decompression can be carried out to decompress the central canal, lateral recess on both sides, and the neural foramen on both sides.

7. *Discectomy*: At this time, a microscope is usually brought into the field for better visualization of the critical structures. Bone and soft tissue are removed to expose the disc space just rostral to the pedicle and up to the lateral border of the ligamentum flavum. The surgeon must be extra vigilant about the locations of the exiting and traversing nerve roots. The surrounding veins are secured using bipolar cautery. An incision is then made through the annulus, and insert-and-rotate shaver dilators are used to remove the intervertebral disc with great care taken to preserve the cortical vertebral endplates. This is particularly important in the setting of osteoporosis. The preparation of the interbody space for bony fusion is also contingent on adequate removal of the cartilaginous disc endplate. In addition, the medial angulation of the approach is critical and will differ by level. In surgeries in which the approach is on the side of the concavity (simple curves without a fractional component), disc removal will be predominantly ipsilateral to distract the interspace that has been closed down. In surgeries in which the approach is on the side of the convexity of the major curve (i.e., when approaching from the concavity of the fractional curve), a steep approach is taken so that the contralateral disc is assessed and removed to restore interspace height on the collapsed portion of the major curve.

8. *Graft Insertion and Interbody Fusion*: Once complete disc removal has been achieved, fusion adjuvants are placed into the disc space as far anterior in the disc space as possible. Generally, rhBMP-2 (InFuse, Medtronic Sofamor Danek) at a dose up to 1.05 mg/level is used to promote fusion across the disc space. It is particularly useful in MIS deformity surgery since less bony surface is exposed to allow for posterolateral fusion; as a result, successful interbody fusion is key to the success of the procedure. It is important to keep the BMP anteriorly in the disc space to reduce the risk of heterotopic bone growth near the neural elements. After the BMP, the autograft bone harvested from the facetectomy is packed into the disc space.

The surgeon's interbody spacer of choice can then be inserted into the disc space, with special attention paid to place the spacer in the desired location. An expandable cage is particularly useful to minimize the amount of tissue dissection required and to distract the disc space on the side of the graft placement. We have been using a 25-mm OptiMesh cage (Spineology) for this purpose. OptiMesh is a three-dimensional deployable mesh pouch that is filled with allograft granular matrix (Fig. 18.5) [41]. The device is delivered through a 7-mm diameter portal; therefore, only a very small opening in the annulus is needed to access the disc space and place the graft material (Fig. 18.6) [30]. The OptiMesh is then inflated with the granular allograft matrix within the disc space, restoring intervertebral height (Figs. 18.7 and 18.8). It should be noted

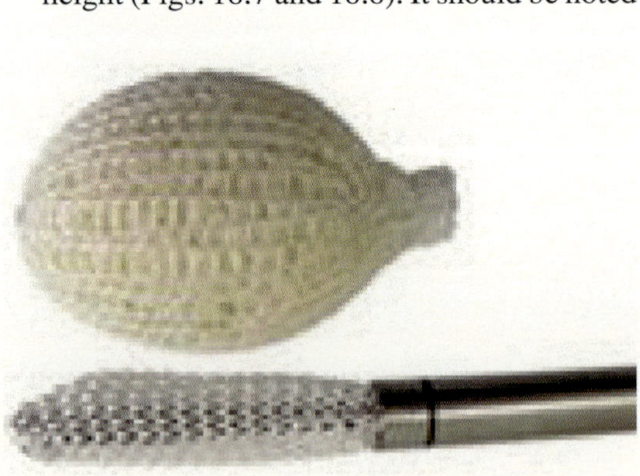

Fig. 18.5 OptiMesh Deployable Grafting System

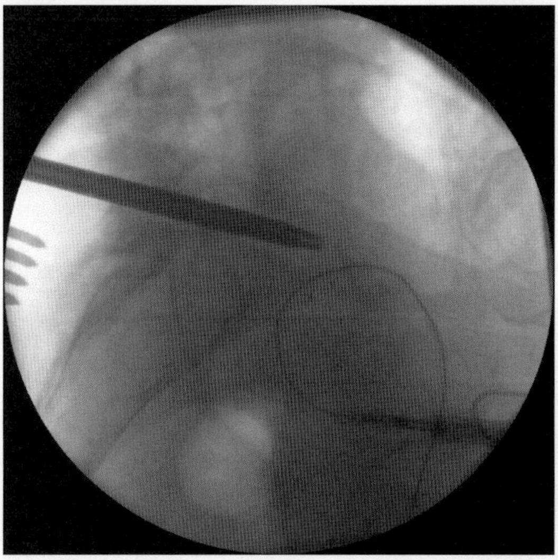

Fig. 18.6 Placement of the OptiMesh delivery portal into the L5–S1 disc space

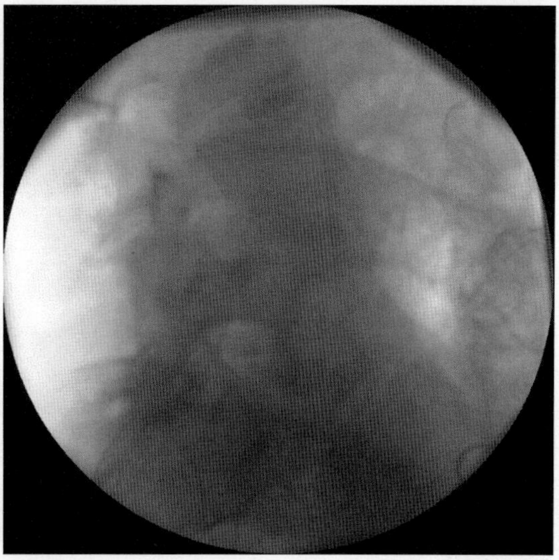

Fig. 18.8 L3–4, L4–5, and L5–S1 three-level TLIFs are performed with OptiMesh

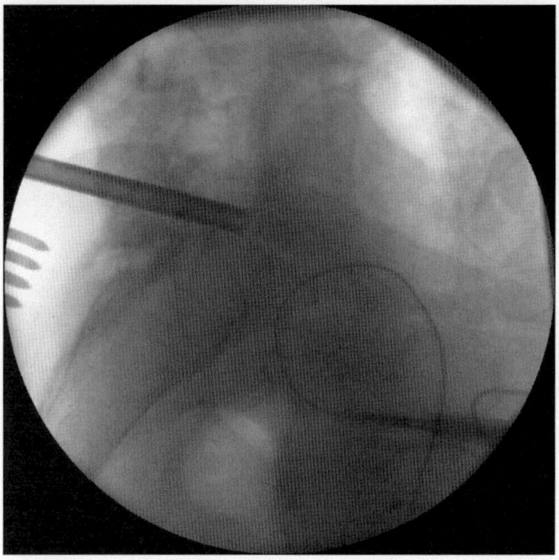

Fig. 18.7 Deliver the OptiMesh pouch into the L5–S1 disc space

that the FDA also considers this an off-label use. Because the expandable cage does not need strong impact for insertion, it is likely to be placed in the desired spot within the disc space, allowing more distraction for deformity correction upon cage expansion.

9. *Percutaneous Pedicle Screws*: Percutaneous screws are then placed in a standard fashion. We use an AP-based fluoroscopic technique for placing the percutaneous pedicle screws as it allows for compensation of any axial rotation or other spinal deformity. Using this method, the Jamshidi needle is initially docked at the junction of the transverse process and lateral facet joint. Due to the axial rotation of the ASD patient's spine, a straight AP fluoroscopic image needs to be obtained at each level. The needle is then advanced 2 cm into the bone without passing the medial wall of the pedicle on AP imaging (Fig. 18.9). Each needle is then exchanged for a K wire. An insulating sheath protects the soft tissues, while an awl and tap create the path for subsequent pedicle screw (Viper 3-D, DePuy Spine) placement under lateral fluoroscope (Fig. 18.10).
10. *Rod Insertion*: Rods are then placed subfascially by passing through the screw extensions. For details about rod contouring, passage, and connection, please see the corresponding chapter (Chap. 13) in this book. Persuasion of the screw heads to an ideally bent rod further enhances lordosis and deformity correction. Compression of the screw heads on the curve convexity (open side) also allows for lordosis enhancement and scoliosis correction.
11. *Closure:* The fascia and skin are then closed in standard fashion with a suction drain. Tacking of the skin that was elevated

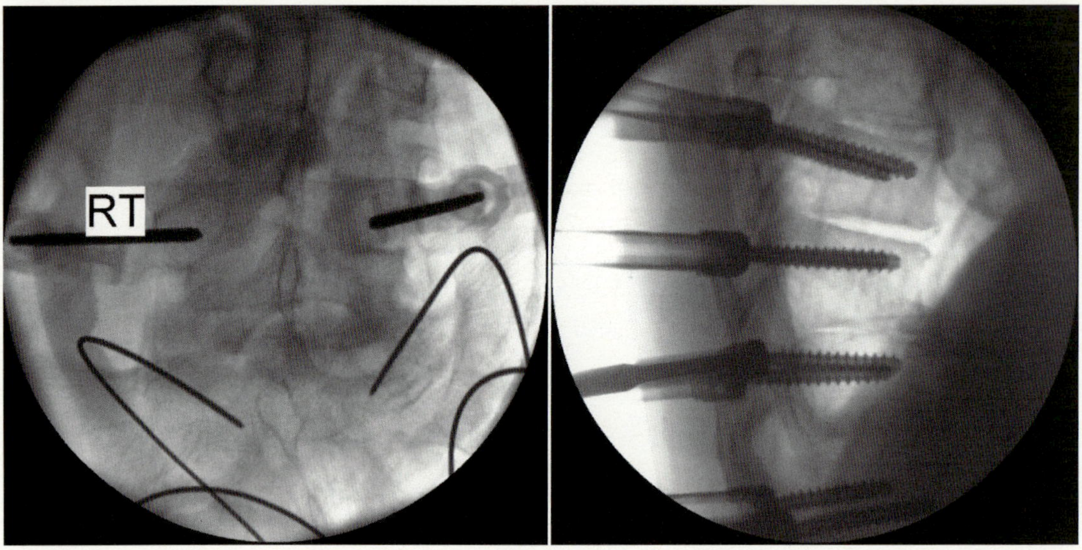

Fig. 18.9 Percutaneous screw placement

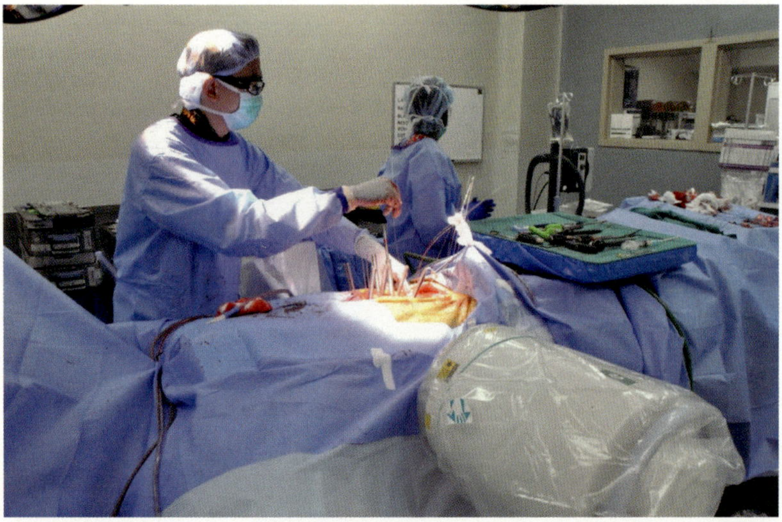

Fig. 18.10 Percutaneous pedicle screws are exchanged over K-wire and inserted under lateral fluoroscope

suprafascially is important to prevent the accumulation of a subcutaneous seroma after surgery.

18.5 Future Advances

The essential steps of MIS TLIF may in the future be made less invasive and more effective with improvements in technology. The step requiring the most exposure currently is the facetectomy. Less invasive approaches for this are being innovated with the use of a Gigli saw technique for complete removal of the posterior elements (Baxano, San Jose, California). Efficient complete facetectomies may pave the way for an MIS Smith-Petersen osteotomy (SPO) technique (Fig. 18.11).

Multilevel MIS TLIF is an easily adopted method for spinal deformity correction. The use of expandable cages and percutaneous screws renders this a less invasive approach than the traditional open TLIF technique. For coronal curves under 30° with minimal to moderate sagittal imbalance, this is an efficient technique with minimal morbidity.

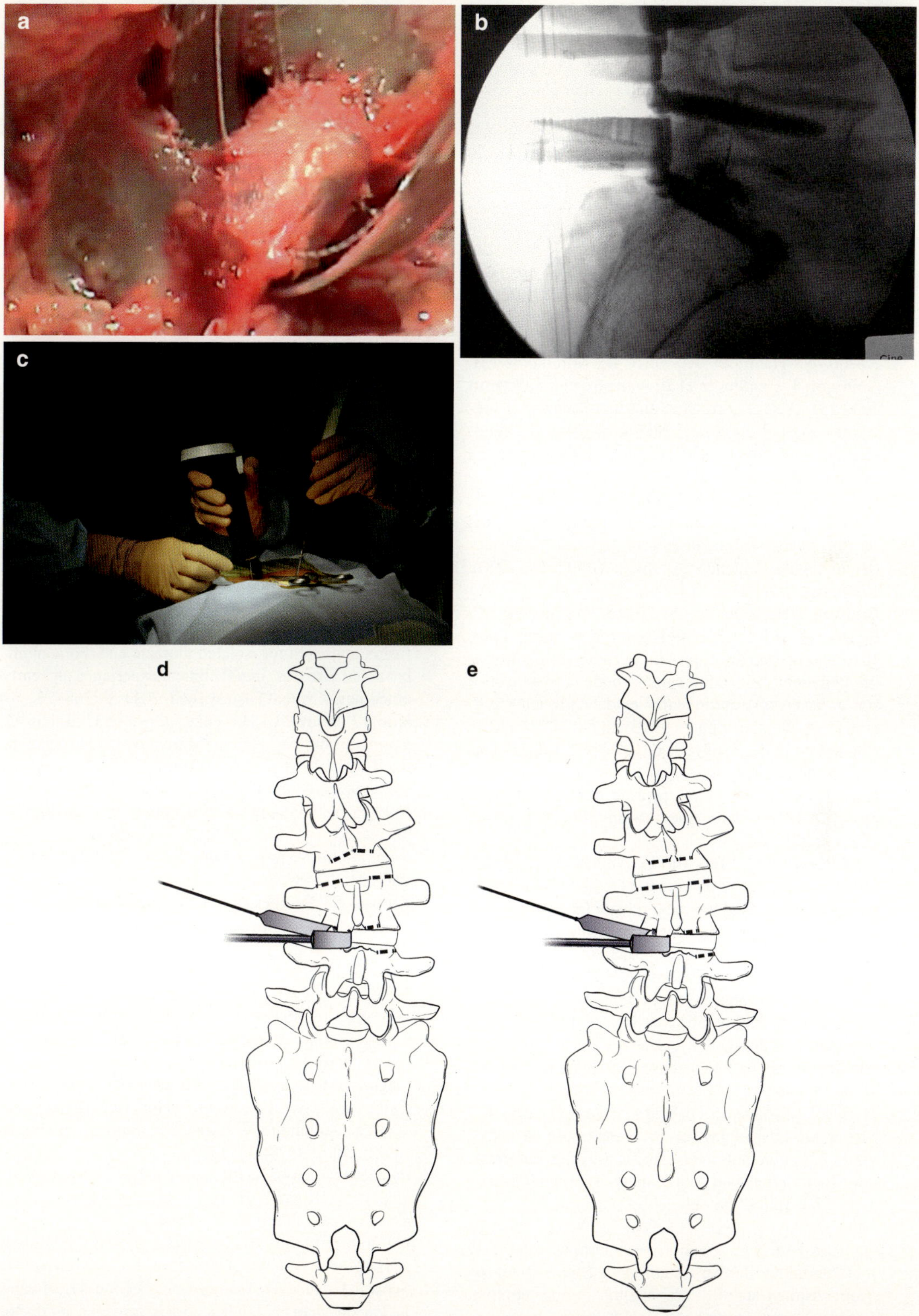

Fig. 18.11 (**a**) Use of the Baxano device to remove facet bone in a cadaver. (**b**) Lateral X-ray imaging showing the saw removing the facet joints between the pedicle screws. (**c**) External view of the reciprocating saw handles used to cut the facet joints. (**d**) Artists depiction of the removal of facets using the reciprocating saw blades. (**e**) View after the joints have been removed to allow for deformity correction

References

1. Acosta FL, Liu J, Slimack N, Moller D, Fessler R, Koski T. Changes in coronal and sagittal plane alignment following minimally invasive direct lateral interbody fusion for the treatment of degenerative lumbar disease in adults: a radiographic study. J Neurosurg Spine. 2011;15:92–6.
2. Akbarnia BA, Mundis GM, Jr., Moazzaz P, Kabirian N, Bagheri R, Eastlack RK, et al. Anterior Column Realignment (ACR) for focal kyphotic spinal deformity using a lateral transpsoas approach and ALL release. J Spinal Disord Tech. Available at: http://www.ncbi.nlm.nih.gov/pubmed/?term=akbarnia%2C+mundis%2C+eastlack; Accessed 19 Feb 2013. [Epub ahead of print].
3. Anand N, Hamilton JF, Perri B, Miraliakbar H, Goldstein T. Cantilever TLIF with structural allograft and RhBMP2 for correction and maintenance of segmental sagittal lordosis: long-term clinical, radiographic, and functional outcome. Spine (Phila Pa 1976). 2006;31:E748–53.
4. Booth KC, Bridwell KH, Lenke LG, Baldus CR, Blanke KM. Complications and predictive factors for the successful treatment of flatback deformity (fixed sagittal imbalance). Spine (Phila Pa 1976). 1999;24:1712–20.
5. Bridwell KH, Glassman S, Horton W, Shaffrey C, Schwab F, Zebala LP, et al. Does treatment (nonoperative and operative) improve the two-year quality of life in patients with adult symptomatic lumbar scoliosis: a prospective multicenter evidence-based medicine study. Spine (Phila Pa 1976). 2009;34:2171–8.
6. Buchowski JM, Bridwell KH, Lenke LG, Kuhns CA, Lehman RA, Jr., Kim YJ, et al. Neurologic complications of lumbar pedicle subtraction osteotomy: a 10-year assessment. Spine (Phila Pa 1976). 2007;32:2245–52.
7. Deukmedjian AR, Dakwar E, Ahmadian A, Smith DA, Uribe JS. Early outcomes of minimally invasive anterior longitudinal ligament release for correction of sagittal imbalance in patients with adult spinal deformity. ScientificWorldJournal. 2012;2012:789698.
8. Deukmedjian AR, Le TV, Baaj AA, Dakwar E, Smith DA, Uribe JS. Anterior longitudinal ligament release using the minimally invasive lateral retroperitoneal transpsoas approach: a cadaveric feasibility study and report of 4 clinical cases. J Neurosurg Spine. 2012;17:530–9.
9. Dorward IG, Lenke LG, Bridwell KH, O'Leary PT, Stoker GE, Pahys JM, et al. Transforaminal versus anterior lumbar interbody fusion in long deformity constructs: a matched cohort analysis. Spine (Phila Pa 1976). 2013;38:E755–62.
10. Faundez AA, Mehbod AA, Wu C, Wu W, Ploumis A, Transfeldt EE. Position of interbody spacer in transforaminal lumbar interbody fusion: effect on 3-dimensional stability and sagittal lumbar contour. J Spinal Disord Tech. 2008;21:175–80.
11. Glassman SD, Bridwell K, Dimar JR, Horton W, Berven S, Schwab F. The impact of positive sagittal balance in adult spinal deformity. Spine (Phila Pa 1976). 2005;30:2024–9.
12. Godde S, Fritsch E, Dienst M, Kohn D. Influence of cage geometry on sagittal alignment in instrumented posterior lumbar interbody fusion. Spine (Phila Pa 1976). 2003;28:1693–9.
13. Hassanzadeh H, Jain A, El Dafrawy MH, Ain MC, Mesfin A, Skolasky RL, et al. Three-column osteotomies in the treatment of spinal deformity in adult patients 60 years old and older: outcome and complications. Spine (Phila Pa 1976). 2012;38:726–31
14. Heary RF, Karimi RJ. Correction of lumbar coronal plane deformity using unilateral cage placement. Neurosurg Focus. 2010;28:E10.
15. Hsieh PC, Koski TR, O'Shaughnessy BA, Sugrue P, Salehi S, Ondra S, et al. Anterior lumbar interbody fusion in comparison with transforaminal lumbar interbody fusion: implications for the restoration of foraminal height, local disc angle, lumbar lordosis, and sagittal balance. J Neurosurg Spine. 2007;7:379–86.
16. Jagannathan J, Sansur CA, Oskouian RJ, Jr., Fu KM, Shaffrey CI. Radiographic restoration of lumbar alignment after transforaminal lumbar interbody fusion. Neurosurgery. 2009;64:955–63; discussion 963–54.
17. Karikari IO, Nimjee SM, Hardin CA, Hughes BD, Hodges TR, Mehta AI, et al. Extreme lateral interbody fusion approach for isolated thoracic and thoracolumbar spine diseases: initial clinical experience and early outcomes. J Spinal Disord Tech. 2011;24:368–75.
18. Kim YJ, Bridwell KH, Lenke LG, Cheh G, Baldus C. Results of lumbar pedicle subtraction osteotomies for fixed sagittal imbalance: a minimum 5-year follow-up study. Spine (Phila Pa 1976). 2007;32:2189–97.
19. Kobayashi T, Atsuta Y, Takemitsu M, Matsuno T, Takeda N. A prospective study of de novo scoliosis in a community based cohort. Spine (Phila Pa 1976). 2006;31:178–82.
20. Kotwal S, Pumberger M, Hughes A, Girardi F. Degenerative scoliosis: a review. HSS J. 2011;7:257–64.
21. Lee MJ, Wiater B, Bransford RJ, Bellabarba C, Chapman JR. Lordosis restoration after Smith-Petersen osteotomies and interbody strut placement: a radiographic study in cadavers. Spine (Phila Pa 1976). 2010;35:E1487–91.
22. Ozgur BM, Aryan HE, Pimenta L, Taylor WR. Extreme Lateral Interbody Fusion (XLIF): a novel surgical technique for anterior lumbar interbody fusion. Spine J. 2006;6:435–43.
23. Pateder DB, Gonzales RA, Kebaish KM, Cohen DB, Chang JY, Kostuik JP. Short-term mortality and its association with independent risk factors in adult spinal deformity surgery. Spine (Phila Pa 1976). 2008; 33:1224–8.
24. Schwab F, Dubey A, Gamez L, El Fegoun AB, Hwang K, Pagala M, et al. Adult scoliosis: prevalence, SF-36, and nutritional parameters in an elderly volunteer population. Spine (Phila Pa 1976). 2005;30:1082–5.

25. Schwab F, Patel A, Ungar B, Farcy JP, Lafage V. Adult spinal deformity-postoperative standing imbalance: how much can you tolerate? An overview of key parameters in assessing alignment and planning corrective surgery. Spine (Phila Pa 1976). 2010;35:2224–31.
26. Schwab FJ, Hawkinson N, Lafage V, Smith JS, Hart R, Mundis G, et al. Risk factors for major peri-operative complications in adult spinal deformity surgery: a multi-center review of 953 consecutive patients. Eur Spine J. 2012;21:2603–10.
27. Schwab FJ, Patel A, Shaffrey CI, Smith JS, Farcy JP, Boachie-Adjei O, et al. Sagittal realignment failures following pedicle subtraction osteotomy surgery: are we doing enough? Clinical article. J Neurosurg Spine. 2012;16:539–46.
28. Schwender JD, Holly LT, Rouben DP, Foley KT. Minimally invasive transforaminal lumbar interbody fusion (TLIF): technical feasibility and initial results. J Spinal Disord Tech. 2005;18:S1–6.
29. Sharma AK, Kepler CK, Girardi FP, Cammisa FP, Huang RC, Sama AA. Lateral lumbar interbody fusion: clinical and radiographic outcomes at 1 year: a preliminary report. J Spinal Disord Tech. 2011;24:242–50.
30. Shau DN, Parker SL, Mendenhall SK, Zuckerman SL, Godil SS, Devin CJ, McGirt MJ. Transforaminal lumbar interbody graft placement via an articulating delivery arm facilitates increased segmental lordosis with superior anterior and midline graft placement. J Spinal Disord Tech. Available at: http://www.ncbi.nlm.nih.gov/pubmed/23059702; Accessed 10 Oct 2012. [Epub ahead of print].
31. Smith JS, Sansur CA, Donaldson WF, 3rd, Perra JH, Mudiyam R, Choma TJ, et al. Short-term morbidity and mortality associated with correction of thoracolumbar fixed sagittal plane deformity: a report from the Scoliosis Research Society Morbidity and Mortality Committee. Spine (Phila Pa 1976). 2011;36:958–64.
32. Smith JS, Shaffrey CI, Berven S, Glassman S, Hamill C, Horton W, et al. Improvement of back pain with operative and nonoperative treatment in adults with scoliosis. Neurosurgery 2009;65:86–93; discussion 93–84.
33. Smith JS, Shaffrey CI, Berven S, Glassman S, Hamill C, Horton W, et al. Operative versus nonoperative treatment of leg pain in adults with scoliosis: a retrospective review of a prospective multicenter database with two-year follow-up. Spine (Phila Pa 1976). 2009;34:1693–8.
34. Smith JS, Shaffrey CI, Glassman SD, Berven SH, Schwab FJ, Hamill CL, et al. Risk-benefit assessment of surgery for adult scoliosis: an analysis based on patient age. Spine (Phila Pa 1976). 2011;36:817–24.
35. Stephens GC, Yoo JU, Wilbur G. Comparison of lumbar sagittal alignment produced by different operative positions. Spine (Phila Pa 1976). 1996;21:1802–6; discussion 1807.
36. Suh LR, Jo DJ, Kim SM, Lim YJ. A surgical option for multilevel anterior lumbar interbody fusion with ponte osteotomy to achieve optimal lumbar lordosis and sagittal balance. J Korean Neurosurg Soc. 2012;52:365–71.
37. Uribe JS, Smith DA, Dakwar E, Baaj AA, Mundis GM, Turner AW, et al. Lordosis restoration after anterior longitudinal ligament release and placement of lateral hyperlordotic interbody cages during the minimally invasive lateral transpsoas approach: a radiographic study in cadavers. J Neurosurg Spine. 2012;17:476–85.
38. Wang MY. Improvement of sagittal balance and lumbar lordosis following less invasive adult spinal deformity surgery with expandable cages and percutaneous instrumentation. J Neurosurg Spine. 2013;18:4–12.
39. Wang MY, Madhavan K. Mini-open pedicle subtraction osteotomy: surgical technique. World Neurosurg. 2012.
40. Yson SC, Santos ER, Sembrano JN, Polly Jr DW. Segmental lumbar sagittal correction after bilateral transforaminal lumbar interbody fusion. J Neurosurg Spine. 2012;17:37–42.
41. Zheng X, Chaudhari R, Wu C, Mehbod AA, Erkan S, Transfeldt EE. Biomechanical evaluation of an expandable meshed bag augmented with pedicle or facet screws for percutaneous lumbar interbody fusion. Spine J. 2010;10:987–93.

Expandable Cages for Thoracic Spinal Deformity

19

Paul E. Kaloostian and Daniel M. Sciubba

19.1 Introduction

Correction of kyphotic deformity of the spine is quite complex, especially in the thoracic spine. A variety of techniques exist for correction of thoracic kyphotic deformity; however, the controversy continues regarding the most efficacious approaches toward improving adequate sagittal balance, obtaining successful fusion of the construct, and providing an adequate scaffold anteriorly to tolerate the forces placed upon the anterior spine. Additionally, these goals must be accomplished while minimizing patient neurological morbidity. The use of an expandable thoracic cage to reconstruct the anterior and middle columns has proven to be a successful method of correcting thoracic kyphotic deformity, especially since 80 % of the axial vector load placed upon the spine is specifically along these particular columns [1].

19.2 Kyphotic Deformity of the Thoracic Spine

There are many different causes of kyphotic deformity in the thoracic spine including traumatic fractures, infection, tumor (both primary and metastatic), inflammatory diseases, and degenerative disease of the spine [2]. Symptoms of progressively worsening thoracic kyphosis include focal intractable thoracic back pain, thoracic radiculopathy due to foraminal stenosis, and myelopathy from narrowing of the spinal canal [3–5]. Neurological findings may include worsening weakness and numbness of lower extremities, hyperreflexia, and bowel/bladder dysfunction [5, 6]. Diagnostic modalities include plain radiographs of the thoracic spine, computerized tomography, and magnetic resonance imaging to determine the degree of kyphosis, bony destruction, extent of infection or tumor growth, as well as spinal cord or nerve root impingement [2, 5] (Figs. 19.1 and 19.2).

19.3 Conservative Management and Treatment of Thoracic Kyphotic Deformity

Patients without significant vertebral body collapse who are asymptomatic or with minimal pain can be managed conservatively. Conservative management generally involves supervised physical and occupational therapy, bracing with thoracolumbar orthoses for comfort, and anti-inflammatory or narcotic medications that are supervised by a pain management specialist. Additionally, close follow-up of these patients is indicated with upright x-rays assessing progression of thoracic kyphotic deformity that may necessitate movement away from conservative management and toward a surgical path [7, 8].

P.E. Kaloostian, M.D. (✉) • D.M. Sciubba, M.D.
The Johns Hopkins Hospital,
Meyer Bldg 5109 600 North Wolfe Street,
Baltimore, MD 21287, USA
e-mail: paulkaloostian@hotmail.com

M.Y. Wang et al. (eds.), *Minimally Invasive Spinal Deformity Surgery*,
DOI 10.1007/978-3-7091-1407-0_19, © Springer-Verlag Wien 2014

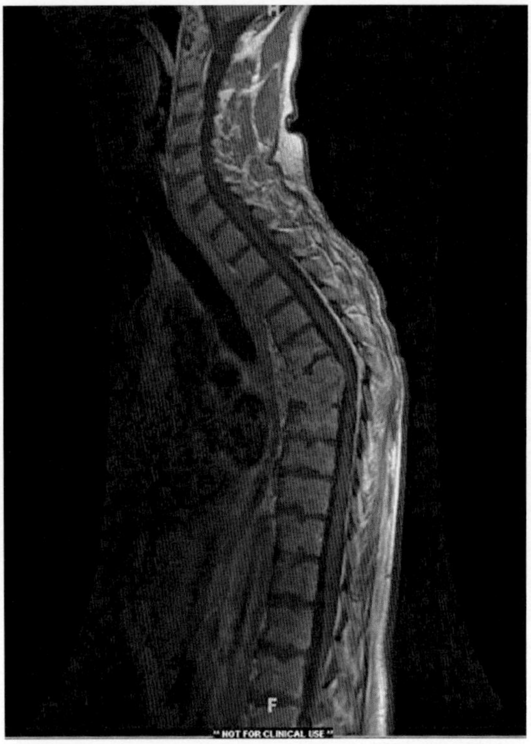

Fig. 19.1 Sagittal T1 MRI thoracic spine with contrast demonstrating severe kyphotic deformity at T6/7 due to infection. The kyphosis, along with epidural enhancing tissue, is encroaching upon the spinal cord

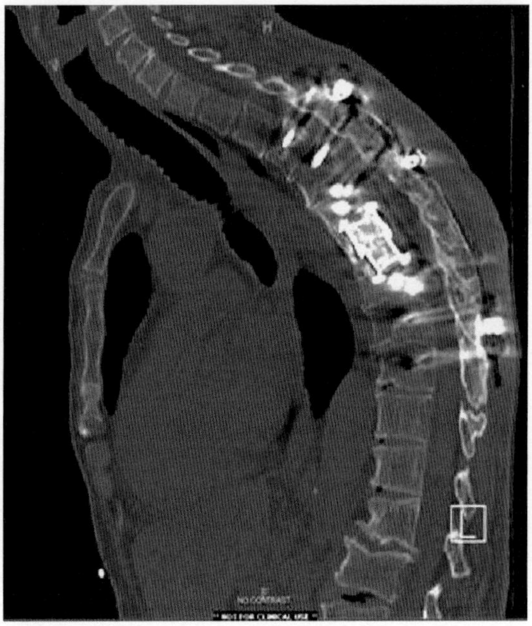

Fig. 19.2 CT scan of the thoracic spine postoperatively demonstrating reconstruction of anterior and middle column via an expandable thoracic cage from a lateral position with elimination of thoracic kyphotic deformity. Second stage of surgery involved posterior instrumentation and fusion

19.4 Indications and Goals for Surgical Correction of Thoracic Kyphotic Deformity

Indications for surgical correction of spinal deformity include instability, deformity, intractable pain, and current or impending neurological compromise [3].

19.5 Surgical Approaches to Treating Thoracic Kyphotic Deformity

A variety of surgical approaches have been studied for correction of thoracic kyphotic deformity with placement of expandable cages. These include open approaches as well as the more recent minimally invasive techniques utilizing percutaneous instrumentation and endoscopic assistance. The goals of kyphotic deformity correction center around altering the main vector of forces drawing the thoracic spine into the kyphotic position. This is mainly done via reconstructing the anterior and middle columns from a variety of different approaches through the use of expandable thoracic cages.

19.5.1 Posterior

19.5.1.1 Laminectomy/Posterolateral Instrumentation/Osteotomy/Fusion

Posterior techniques for ventral thoracic and thoracolumbar pathology have evolved over the years. Laminectomy with Smith-Petersen osteotomies, along with pedicle subtraction osteotomies, has been shown to improve lordosis approximately 6–10° and 15–20°, respectively, via shortening of the posterior elements [9]. However, these techniques are associated with decreased vertebral height and buckling of the posterior spinal ligaments and dura with the possibility of associated cord compression [10]. Additionally, these techniques are associated with significant blood loss and pulmonary complications [11, 12].

The use of long-segment Harrington rod instrumentation may be used to restore thoracic curvature. However, this technique is fraught with morbidity and complications due to the long-segment fusion, possibility of instrumentation failure requiring reoperation, inability to restore the rotational deformity, and possibility of further worsening the preexisting kyphosis upon failure [13]. Additionally, purely posterior pedicle screw instrumentation with fusion may not be able to withstand the physiologic stress from an anterior vector, resulting in hardware failure and progression of the underlying kyphosis [3, 14]. McLain et al. noted progressively worsening deformity during the first 6 months postoperatively after stand-alone posterior kyphotic reduction maneuvers [14]. Multiple studies have demonstrated a failure rate of 20–50 % with solely posterior pedicular fixation and fusion in patients without anterior support [15–17].

19.5.1.2 Laminectomy/Costotransversectomy with Expandable Cage and Posterolateral Instrumentation/Fusion

Laminectomy with costotransversectomy is a technique that has allowed surgeons to access ventral pathology in the thoracic spine. A unilateral approach with laminectomy and removal of the transverse process and portion of the rib head and proximal rib has allowed access down the pedicle and into the affected vertebral body[s] [3]. This allows placement of a thoracic cage anteriorly via a posterior approach between the exiting nerve roots (usually sacrificed in the thoracic spine allowing ample room) to reconstruct the anterior and middle column. Reconstruction of the anterior and middle columns from this approach is typically reinforced by a short-segment pedicle screw instrumentation and posterolateral fusion [18].

Sciubba et al. describe a novel technique of a purely posterior approach with circumferential costotransversectomy and corpectomy toward treating anterior thoracic pathology [3]. They described performing standard bilateral costotransversectomies with transpedicular corpectomy and placement of expandable thoracic cage. They documented seven cases of circumferential costotransversectomies with placement of expandable thoracic cage and noted a kyphosis improvement of 53 % [3]. They calculated a mean kyphotic angle preoperatively of 28.6° and postoperatively of 12.1° [3]. This effect is in accordance with the so-called boundary effect allowing for a greater surface area of anterior axial loading [19].

Snell et al. have also described a similar approach in 15 patients toward treating thoracic kyphotic deformity [20]. They utilized both expandable and non-expandable thoracic cages for reconstruction and noted adequate neurological stabilization and kyphosis reduction in their cohort with two patients improving at least one Frankel grade [20]. The use of expandable cages allows for appropriate distraction of the thoracic spine and provides an adequate surface area along the superior and inferior end plates to facilitate solid fusion [3]. The use of expandable cages, as opposed to fibular and iliac grafts, decreases complications such as end plate penetration due to the large footprint of the expandable cages [12].

Abumi et al. and Oda et al. described the precise benefit of expandable cages as compared to non-expandable cages during spinal reconstruction [21, 22]. They noted the former have a greater in-line distraction capability of the spinal ligaments, which may improve fusion rates [21]. Additionally, the ability to manually distract while noting expansion both visually and radiographically of vertebral height is quite user-friendly in assuring restoration of lordosis and minimizing kyphotic tendency around the normal internal axis of rotation of the thoracic and thoracolumbar spine [3]. Finally, non-expandable cages require one additional step of posterior compression of instrumentation, whereas use of expandable cages may avoid this process [23].

In fact, Knop et al. studied 12 cadaveric spines and biomechanically found more stabilization using an expandable cage compared to the non-expandable cage and noted a decreased need for posterior compression when the expandable cage was used [23]. An additional prospective study using expandable cages by Lange et al. showed successful stabilization of anterior column with no failures in 126 patients with infection, tumor, and traumatic pathology [24]. This led to the development of a larger-size forceps spreader to increase the height of this expandable cage one more level [24]. Keshavarzi et al. retrospectively studied 35 patients from two large centers with thoracic kyphotic deformity due to infection, trauma, and tumor who underwent corpectomy and placement of expandable thoracic cages. They noted early postoperative correction in kyphosis in all, restoration of sagittal alignment at 12 months, and reduction in visual analog pain scale over the 31-month follow-up period [25].

Overall, this technique avoids the morbidity of a large thoracoabdominal and/or transthoracic exposure while completely decompressing neural structures, stabilizing the anterior and middle columns, and restoring adequate sagittal balance. The autograft obtained from the initial decompression can be utilized within the cage itself, allowing for successful fusion via osteoconductive and osteoinductive properties of stem cells. Lastly, supplementing posterior instrumentation with an anterior expandable cage allows for minimizing hardware failure and potentially decreasing the rate of pseudoarthrosis [26].

19.5.2 Anterolateral

Anterior and anterolateral techniques for thoracolumbar kyphotic treatment include the transthoracic-transpleural thoracotomy, thoracoscopy using endoscopic approaches, and a more standard thoracoabdominal/retropleural approach [5]. These techniques have all been well described and utilized in treating this pathology. Compared to the posterior techniques described above, many claimed that patients with respiratory dysfunction and significant comorbidities often are not candidates for this anterior-anterolateral approach in accessing the anterior thoracic spine [3, 5]. Complications noted via these approaches include persistent pleural effusions, hemothorax, chylothorax, and dural-pleural fistulae [27, 28]. Additionally, these procedures typically will obviate the need for a second stage surgery for posterior pedicle instrumentation and fusion at some point, which increases operative time for the patient as well as morbidity and blood loss [5].

Ventrolateral transthoracic minimally invasive techniques, including the mini-open and endoscopic approaches, have become more popular given the morbidity documented with conventional open transthoracic and thoracoabdominal approaches to the thoracic spine [29, 30]. Scheuffler et al. retrospectively studied 38 patients with thoracic and thoracolumbar spondylosis, trauma, or metastasis who underwent minimally invasive vertebral body replacement with cages using an anterolateral retropleural (ALRA) or a combined lateral extrapleural/extraperitoneal thoracolumbar approach (CLETA). They noted successful completion of each surgery without conversion to conventional open approach, 19.3° of average kyphotic correction, and results that are similar to those of standard open and endoscopic techniques [2, 31, 32]. The authors noted the reduction of sagittal deformity exclusively by anterior distraction using expandable cages with no subsidence or loss of correction over an 18-month follow-up period [2]. In three severely osteopenic patients in this series, cement augmentation was done at the adjacent vertebrae [2]. In a select group of patients with preexistent pulmonary disease, the ALRA and CLETA minimally invasive approaches have been shown in small studies to reduce the perioperative risks commonly encountered with the conventional endoscopic and anterolateral transthoracic approaches [2]. Additionally, diminished operative time, decreased intraoperative blood loss, absence of post-thoracotomy pain, and successful sagittal/coronal deformity correction are all favorable factors with these minimally invasive approaches [33].

Conclusion

As detailed in this chapter, the treatment of thoracic kyphotic deformity is quite diverse. Treatment options include conservative management for asymptomatic or minimally symptomatic patients and surgical management for patients with worsening kyphotic deformity, intractable pain, radiculopathy, and myelopathy. Surgical techniques include posterior costotransversectomy (unilateral or circumferential) with corpectomy and posterolateral instrumentation and fusion, open lateral thoracoabdominal or anterolateral transthoracic corpectomy with cage placement and lateral plating, and minimally invasive anterolateral retropleural or combined extraperitoneal thoracoabdominal approaches. In all cases, goals of surgery should be clearly documented and include decompression of neural structures, treatment of spinal instability, pain control, and correction of spinal deformity [5]. Through the approaches mentioned above and utilization of expandable thoracic cages, these goals may be accomplished. Despite the various pros and cons presented above, a randomized controlled and blinded study comparing the use of expandable and non-expandable cages along with a study comparing the utility of the various approaches described has yet to be done.

References

1. Magerl F, Aebi M, Getzbein SD, et al. A comprehensive classification of thoracic and lumbar injuries. Eur Spine J. 1994;3:184–201.
2. Scheuffler K. Technique and clinical results of minimally invasive reconstruction and stabilization of the thoracic and thoracolumbar spine with expandable cages and ventrolateral plate fixation. Neurosurgery. 2007;61:798–809.
3. Sciubba DM, Gallia G, McGirt M, et al. Thoracic kyphotic deformity reduction with a distractible titanium cage via an entirely posterior approach. Neurosurgery. 2007;60 Suppl 2:223–31.
4. Denis F. The three column spine and its significance in the classification of acute thoracolumbar spinal injuries. Spine. 1983;8:817–31.
5. Yoo C, Ry S, Park J. Fracture-related thoracic kyphotic deformity correction by single-stage posterolateral vertebrectomy with circumferential reconstruction and stabilization. J Spinal Disord Tech. 2009;22(7):492–501.
6. Bradford DS, McBride GC. Surgical management of thoracolumbar spine fractures with incomplete neurologic deficits. Clin Orthop Relat Res. 1987;218:201–16.
7. Fidler MW. Remodeling of the spinal canal after burst fractures. J Bone Joint Surg Br. 1988;70:730–2.
8. Ha KI, Hand SH, Chung M, et al. A clinical study of the natural remodeling of burst fractures of the lumbar spine. Clin Othop. 1996;323:210–4.
9. Goel MK. Vertebral osteotomy for correction of fixed flexion deformity of the spine. J Bone Joint Surg Am. 1968;50:287–94.
10. Micheli LJ, Hall JE. Complications in the treatment of adult spinal deformities. In: Epps Jr CH, editor. Complications in orthopedic surgery. Philadelphia: Lippincott, Williams & Wilkins; 1994.
11. Baba H, Maezawa Y, Kamitani K, et al. Osteoporotic vertebral collapse with late neurological complications. Paraplegia. 1995;33:281–9.
12. Knop C, Lange U, Bastian L, et al. Biomechanical compression tests with a new implant for thoracolumbar vertebral body replacement. Eur Spine J. 2001; 10:30–7.
13. Benzel EC. Biomechanics of spine stabilization. New York: Thieme Medical; 2001.
14. McLain RF, Sparling E, Benson DR. Early failure of short-segment pedicle instrumentation for thoracolumbar fractures. A preliminary report. J Bone Joint Surg Am. 1993;75:162–7.
15. Carl AL, Tromanhauser SG, Roger DJ. Pedicle-screw instrumentation for thoracolumbar burst fractures and fracture-dislocations. Spine. 1992;17(Suppl 8J): S317–24.
16. Kuklo TR, Polly TW, Owens BD, et al. Measurement of thoracic and lumbar fracture kyphosis: evaluation of intraobserver, interobserver, and technique variability. Spine. 2001;26:61–6.
17. Louis CA, Gauthier VY, Louis RP. Posterior approach with Louis plates for fractures of the thoracolumbar and lumbar spine with and without neurological deficits. Spine. 1998;23:2030–40.
18. Benson DR, Burkus JK, Montesano PX, et al. Unstable thoracolumbar and lumbar burst fractures treated with the AO fixateur interne. J Spinal Disord. 1992;5:335–43.
19. Yerby SA, Bay BK, Toh E, et al. The effect of boundary conditions on experimentally measured trabecular strain in the thoracic spine. J Biomech. 1998;31:192–5.
20. Snell BE, Nasr FF, Wolfla CA. Single-stage thoracolumbar vertebrectomy with circumferential reconstruction and arthrodesis: surgical technique and results in 15 patients. Neurosurgery. 2006;58 Suppl 2:S263–9.
21. Abumi K, Panjabi MM, Duranceau J. Biomechanical evaluation of spinal fixation devices. Part III. Stability provided by six spinal fixation devises and interbody bone grafts. Spine. 1989;14:1249–55.

22. Oda I, Cunningham BW, Abumi K, et al. The stability of reconstruction methods after thoracolumbar total spondylectomy: an in vitro investigation. Spine. 1999;24:1634–8.
23. Knop C, Lange U, Bastian L, et al. Three-dimensional motion analysis with Synex. Comparative biomechanical test series with a new vertebral body replacement for the thoracolumbar spine. Eur Spine J. 2000;9:472–85.
24. Lange U, Knop C, Bastian L, et al. Prospective multicenter study with a new implant for thoracolumbar vertebral body replacement. Arch Orthop Trauma Surg. 2003;123:203–8.
25. Keshavarzi S, Newman CB, Ciacci JD, et al. Expandable titanium cages for thoracolumbar vertebral body replacement: initial clinical experience and review of the literature. Am J Orthop. 2011;40(3):E35–9.
26. Kaneda K, Taneichi HJ, Abumi K, et al. Anterior decompression and stabilization with the Kaneda device for thoracolumbar burst fractures associated with neurological deficits. J Bone Joint Surg Am. 1997;79:69–83.
27. Cybulski GR, Stone JL, Opesanmi O. Spinal cord decompression via a modified costotransversectomy approach combined with posterior thoracic instrumentation for management of metastatic neoplasms of the thoracic spine. Surg Neurol. 1991;35:280–5.
28. Findlay GF. Adverse effects of the management of malignant spinal cord compression. J Neurol Neurosurg Psychiatry. 1984;47:761–8.
29. Bohlman HH, Zdeblick TA. Anterior excision of herniated thoracic discs. J Bone Joint Surg Am. 1988;20:1038–47.
30. Elsaghir H. Endoscopic medial parascapular approach to the thoracic spine. Surg Endosc. 2005;19:389–92.
31. Oskouian RJ, Shaffrey CI, Whitehill R, et al. Anterior stabilization of three column thoracolumbar spinal trauma. J Neurosurg Spine. 2006;5:18–25.
32. Uchida K, Kobayashi S, Nakajima H, et al. Anterior expandable strut cage replacement for osteoporotic thoracolumbar vertebral collapse. J Neurosurg Spine. 2006;4:454–62.
33. Kossmann T, Jacobi D, Trentz O. The use of a retractor system (Synframe) for open, minimally invasive reconstruction of the anterior column of the thoracic and lumbar spine. Eur Spine J. 2001;10:396–402.

Expandable Cages for Lumbar Spinal Deformity

20

Michael Y. Wang

20.1 Introduction

Interbody fusion has particular advantages in the setting of adult spinal deformity (ASD). Compared to an intertransverse posterolateral fusion, interbody fusion (1) has a more robust fusion rate due to the improved local vascularity and load sharing present at the endplates, (2) permits anterior release and height restoration for correction of the deformity in the coronal and sagittal planes, (3) allows for bilateral indirect decompression of the neural foramina by restoring interbody height, and (4) in select cases can assist in vertebral de-rotation in the axial plane. These advantages with interbody fusion have led to a plethora of techniques for approaching the disc space, preparing the graft recipient site, and interbody spacer placement.

However, the various surgical techniques that have been developed for interbody fusion all increase the complexity of a spinal operation. A typical posterolateral fusion involves preparation of the pars interarticularis, facets, and transverse processes by exposing the bony surfaces, decorticating them, and placement of onlay grafting materials. These sites are typically already well exposed during an open spinal deformity operation. Performing an additional interbody fusion necessitates additional steps, including accessing the disc space, removal of the disc and cartilaginous endplate, preparation of the bony endplate for fusion, and placement of both graft materials and a spacer to maintain or restore interbody height. These steps require additional operative time, engender more blood loss, and expose critical neurovascular structures to mechanical injury.

Thus, most traditional spinal deformity surgeons will selectively include an interbody fusion only at the most critical segments. For example, the lumbosacral junction, which is at higher risk of nonunion, will often be supplemented with an interbody fusion to stress shield the sacral screws. Similarly, selective release and interbody fusion at the apex of a curve may result in more complete deformity correction. Only with the advent of MIS deformity surgery has the concept of multilevel lumbar interbody fusion (i.e., relying primarily upon interbody fusion at all or most-treated levels) for spinal deformity reemerged.

20.2 Approaches to the Intervertebral Disc

Numerous approaches are available for approaching an interbody fusion with relative merits and drawbacks:

Anterior – Anterior lumbar interbody fusion (ALIF) is a well-proven technique which typically involves a mini-open retroperitoneal route

M.Y. Wang, M.D., FACS
Departments of Neurological Surgery
and Rehab Medicine, University of Miami Miller
School of Medicine, 1095 NW 14th Terrace,
Lois Pope Life Center, D4-6, Miami, FL 33136, USA
e-mail: mwang2@med.miami.edu

M.Y. Wang et al. (eds.), *Minimally Invasive Spinal Deformity Surgery*,
DOI 10.1007/978-3-7091-1407-0_20, © Springer-Verlag Wien 2014

of access (see Chap. 34). Endoscopic methods have been utilized (primarily transperitoneal) but were largely abandoned due to high rates of complications and sympathectomy effects. ALIF has the advantages of providing complete release of the anterior longitudinal ligament (ALL) to increase segmental lordosis, exposing the maximal endplate area in preparation for fusion, and permits the placement of a graft with the largest footprint possible. Disadvantages include the risks of approach-related complications such as vascular or hollow viscus injury, postoperative ileus, need for an approach surgeon, limitations in approaching the mid-lumbar spine (from retroperitoneal vessels), and limitations from scarring due to previous retroperitoneal surgery. ALIF is thus ideal for achieving segmental lordosis and fusing the lumbosacral junction (L4–S1) as an adjunct to a posterior operation (Fig. 20.1).

Lateral – Open lateral approaches have been used for decades to access the mid-lumbar spine. Originally used for the treatment of Pott's disease, this method later found utility for managing thoracolumbar fractures and releasing the mid-lumbar spine for ASD pathologies. This method has the morbidities associated with the ALIF approach and originally also required an extensive disruption of the soft tissues via the thoracoabdominal approach. Its use has been largely supplanted by less invasive methods such as the extreme lateral interbody fusion (XLIF) and direct lateral interbody fusion (DLIF). These approaches are discussed extensively in Chaps. 24, 25, 26, 27, 28, 29, 30, 31, and 32. Expandable cages also have potential applications in this arena.

Oblique – A new method approaching the spine from an intermediary approach has also been developed (Fig. 20.2). Limited data are available on the safety and efficacy of this approach, particularly for treating spinal deformities, but the oblique lateral interbody fusion (OLIF) has the advantages of accessing the spine posterolaterally without any bone removal. More data is needed on the safety and efficacy of this method for treating spinal deformities.

Trans-sacral – Approaching the lumbosacral junction via a low incision through the presacral

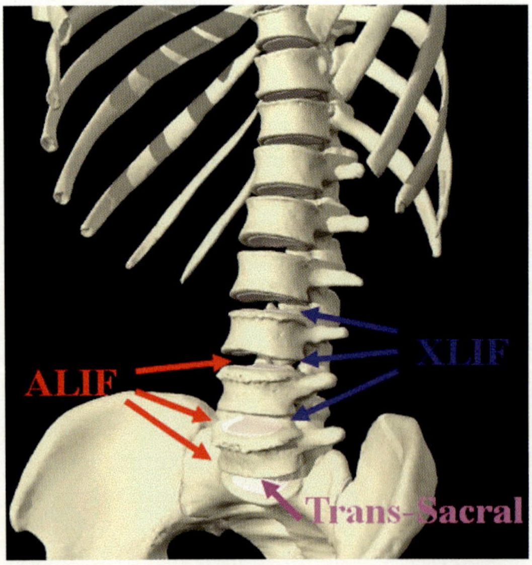

Fig. 20.1 Preferential access routes to the interbody space at varying spinal segments

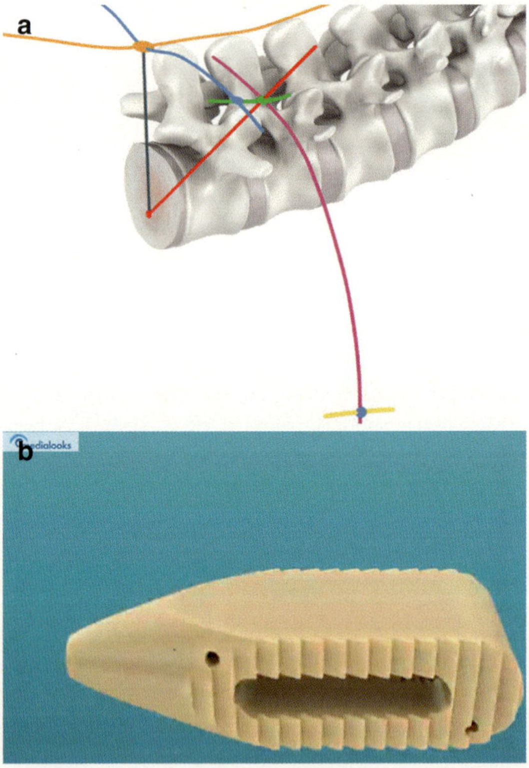

Fig. 20.2 Oblique lateral interbody fusion. (**a**) Access is through Kambin's triangle, and (**b**) a cannulated and bulleted cage is inserted through the inferior neuroforamen

fat pad has also been popular (see Chap. 35). This method, which allows an interbody fusion at L5–S1 and occasionally L4–5, has the advantage of allowing for an anterior interbody spacer to be placed at the lumbosacral junction with the patient in the prone position. This accomplishes the goal of stress shielding the sacral screws while not excessively prolonging the operation with a second position surgical approach.

Posterior – Because the above approaches are covered in other chapters in this textbook, this discussion on expandable cages will focus on the use of these devices in minimally invasive posterior surgeries.

20.3 Problems with Traditional Posterior Interbody Cages

Posterior lumbar interbody fusion (PLIF) has been a widely utilized technique since its introduction by Ralph Cloward a half century ago [2]. This method is robust as it completely treats a spinal segment with decompression, fixation, and fusion. It is effective as a treatment for segmental correction of spinal deformities [5].

While powerful as a technique, rates of new neural symptoms can be seen in as many as 7 % of patients undergoing PLIF. Much of this has been attributed to the neural retraction needed for cage placement. Thus, the technique of transforaminal lumbar interbody fusion (TLIF) was innovated by Harms. This method approaches the disc space more laterally and from only one side, thus reducing the likelihood of nerve root retraction and its attendant clinical problems. Regardless, both methods typically involve some amount of nerve root manipulation, particularly to place an appropriately sized graft.

With the advent of MIS PLIF and TLIF, new problems emerged, much of this was related to interbody graft undersizing. This was due to less complete disc space preparation and a reduced ability to distract upon pedicle screws to allow cage placement. While potentially acceptable in cases of degenerative disease, treatment of ASD requires special attention to spinal alignment and maintenance/restoration of lordosis.

20.4 Kambin's Triangle and the Geometry of Interbody Cages

Placement of an interbody grafts involves adequate disc space clearance and preparation, selection of an ideal height spacer, management of neural tissues, and graft insertion. Creation of a corridor of space requires an understanding of the geometry of these corridors. While selection of the ideal spacer height is a relatively straightforward but arbitrary decision, the confines limiting cage placement are to some degree fixed and real. The relationship of the traversing and exiting nerve roots, lateral removal of the facet joint, scarring and adhesions, and the elasticity of the neural elements all influence the available space for cage placement. Furthermore, the cage shape, route of entry, and the trajectory of approach all affect the space needed.

In a previous report by Barnes et al., it was shown that, in order to achieve a predefined spacer height, placement of a cylindrical cage would have to require more nerve root retraction than a rectangular cage. They investigated this in a cohort of 49 patients. Clinically, this translated to a 13.6 % rate of permanent nerve root injuries in patients with cylindrical cages vs. 0 % in rectangular cages [1]. Currently, nearly all cylindrical cages have been replaced by impacted rectangular implants.

The method of cage application is also critical. Because lateral facet joint removal can allow significant exposure of the disc space in the transverse plane, an "insert and rotate" technique allows for efficient disc space preparation. In almost all cases, a 13 mm spreader or scraper can be placed with minimal nerve root retraction transversely (in the plane of the disc). Once ventral to the neural elements, the spreader or scraper can be rotated 90° in to the longitudinal axis, increasing interbody height. The cages can be placed in a similar manner.

Kambin's triangle is defined as the space between the traversing nerve root/lateral thecal sac, the exiting nerve root, and the vertebral endplate (Fig. 20.3). Reliable entry into the disc space percutaneously has been well established

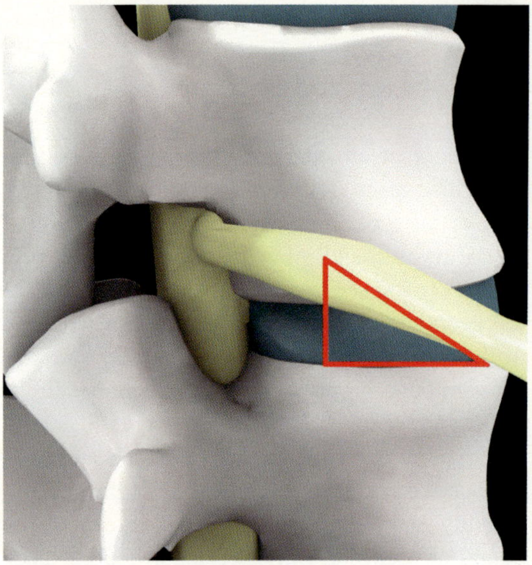

Fig. 20.3 Kambin's triangle

through this route. Because use of this corridor does not require neural retraction (or potentially even visualization), it is an important confine. The typical maximal cylindrical passage through Kambin's triangle is 7 mm. Thus, cages that can be inserted through this space and expanded inside the disc space present the opportunity for truly MIS or percutaneous interbody fusion.

20.5 The Role of Expandable Cages

One of the "Holy Grails" of MIS surgery has been the ability to place a relatively large implant through a smaller soft tissue or bony opening. Proper contact of the endplates is necessary for anterior load sharing and a successful arthrodesis. For ASD, this also affords the opportunity to distract the disc height symmetrically or asymmetrically in order to correct a kyphoscoliosis. In general three types of expandable cages are available:

Micromechanical – These cages are typically of a lower height that can be "jacked up" after placement to elevate the intradiscal space (Fig. 20.4). Because of the mechanical nature of these devices, they can typically place significant force selectively in the rostral-caudal plane and this action can be controlled. Furthermore, these devices can often be reduced in height as well to adjust placement. Disadvantages include a more limited footprint on the endplates and an inability to fuse the contact surface between cage and bone.

In Situ Assembly Modular – These devices are mechanical in nature and are assembled with the body. Modularized components are attached together after placement into the disc space. These devices have the same footprint disadvantages as micromechanical cages but have the potential to be placed from a smaller access route (Fig. 20.5).

In Situ Assembly-Contained Deformables – These devices are assembled in the disc space. However, the components are "flowable" either due to their small size or their liquid nature. Semisolid implants rely on the concept of "granular packing" within a containment bag to achieve a final solid structure (Fig. 20.6) [6]. Liquid implants are still theoretical for ASD and polymerize in situ. These implants are currently limited to the application of annular repair after microdiscectomy, but they hold a promising future for deformity correction.

20.6 Case Illustration

A 53-year-old male presented with severe and intractable back and leg pain. He had failed all conservative measures and was found to have symptoms predominantly due to a spondylolisthesis. After full discussion on the various surgical alternatives for treatment, the patient elected to undergo an L4/5 MIS TLIF (Fig. 20.7).

The surgical technique involved a midline skin incision followed by selective unilateral opening of the soft tissue envelope at the levels of the disc space. A hemilaminotomy was used on the side of the leg pain to expose the exiting L4 and traversing L5 nerve roots. The disc is then removed in a fashion similar to an aggressive microdiscectomy, with care to properly prepare the vertebral endplates for fusion by denuding them of cartilage. Disc space preparation was accomplished using "insert and rotate" shaver dilators, rongeurs, and curettes through a 7 mm

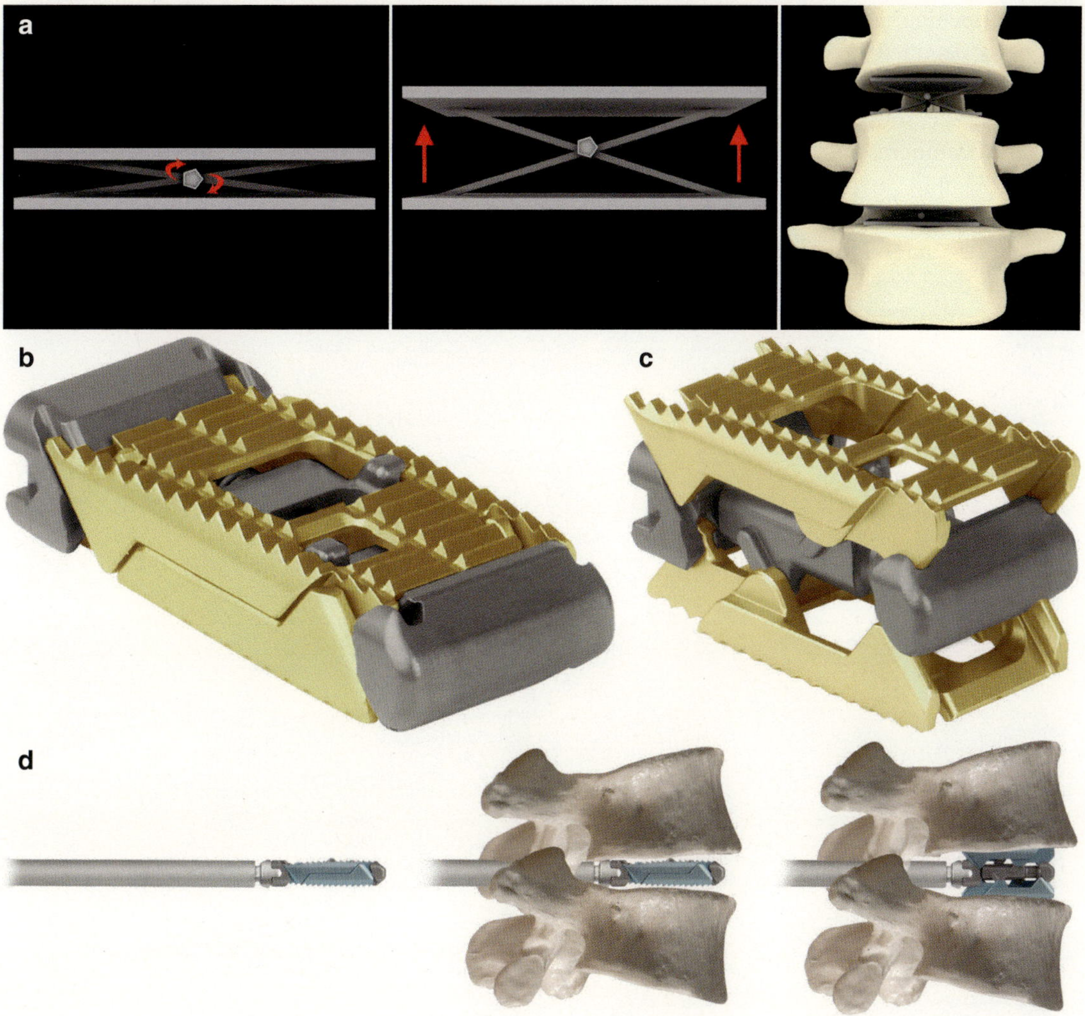

Fig. 20.4 (**a**) Intervertebral height restoration using a micromechanical cage elevates the disc space similar to a car jack. (**b–d**) Example of a micromechanical expandable TLIF cage

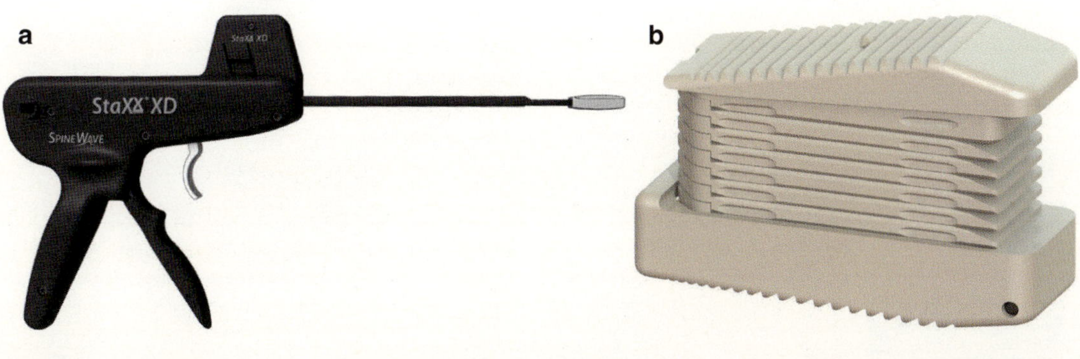

Fig. 20.5 (**a**) Example of an in situ assembly modular cage inserter. (**b**) The implant is composed of PEEK leaflets which stack together to elevate the disc space after insertion

annular opening. After the vertebral endplates had been denuded of cartilage, 1/2 of a small rhBMP-2 kit (2.1 mg) was placed into the anterior disc space, followed by autograft bone saved from the decompression.

A 25 mm expandable interbody cage (Spineology™, Minneapolis, Minnesota) was filled internally with allograft paste (demineralized bone matrix). This elevated the disc space providing for fusion, correcting the spondylolisthesis, and indirect decompression of the nerve roots bilaterally. It should be noted that the use of rhMP-2 and Spineology™ cages in this setting is an off-label use per Food and Drug Administration (FDA) guidelines [3, 4]. After crimping the cage shut to seal it, the area was washed with irrigation to remove any allograft carrier matrix. This is followed by percutaneous screw and rod placement without manipulation of the hardware to correct the spondylolisthesis.

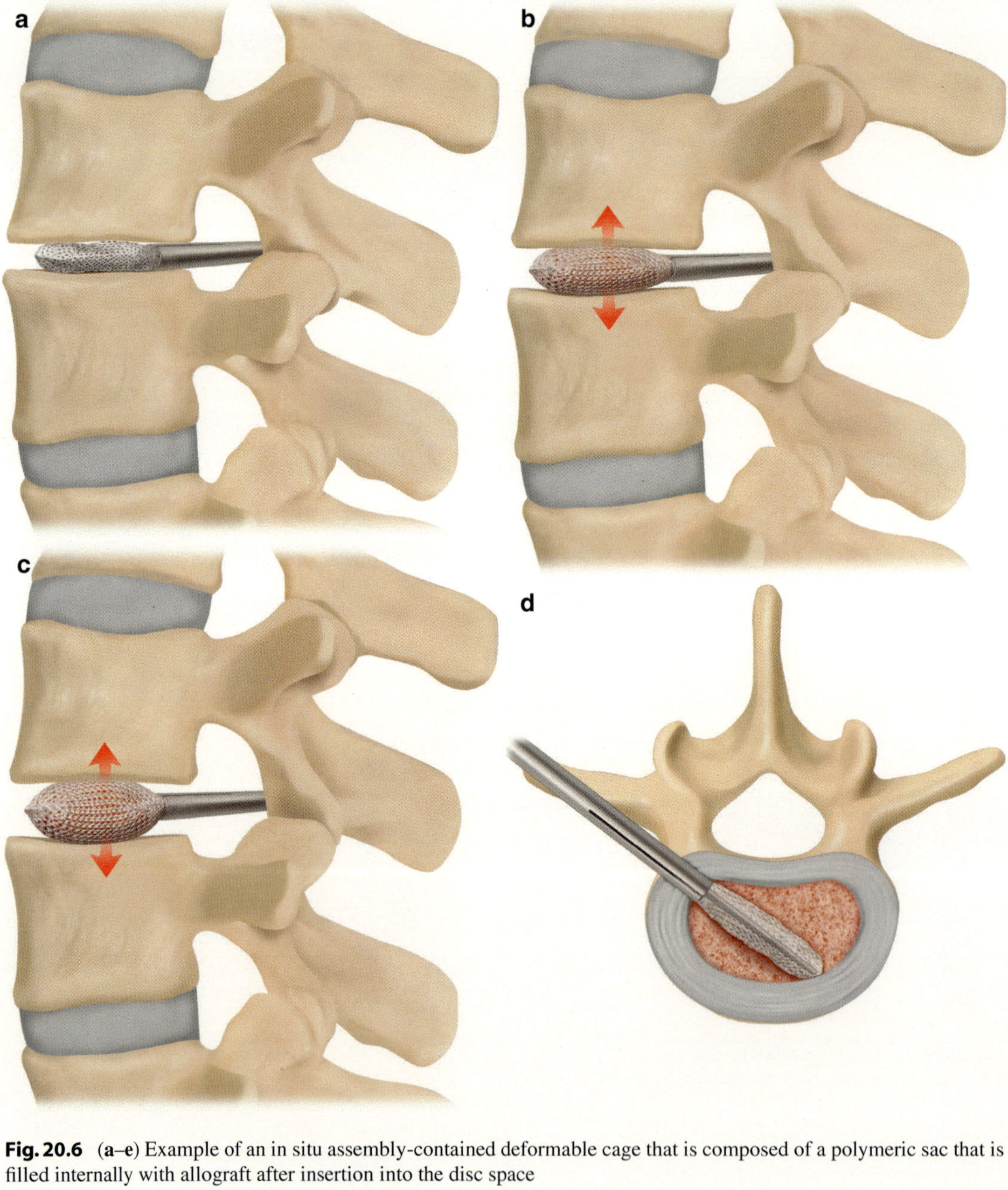

Fig. 20.6 (**a–e**) Example of an in situ assembly-contained deformable cage that is composed of a polymeric sac that is filled internally with allograft after insertion into the disc space

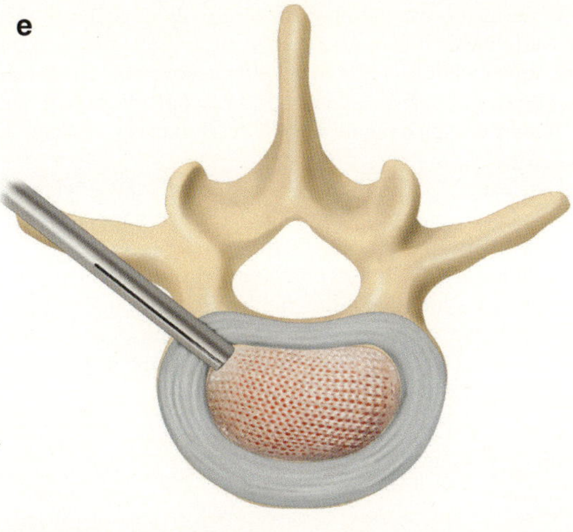

Fig. 20.6 (continued)

Postoperatively the patient had a rapid recovery with improvement of both leg and back pain.

Conclusions

Expandable cages offer the opportunity to significantly reduce the morbidity of MIS ASD surgeries. Powerful anterior corrective forces can potentially be applied through these implants, and several options already exist and are commercially available. In addition, a tall cage can be inserted through a collapsed disc space more easily. The ideal implant has yet to be developed, but regardless of the spacer used, successful arthrodesis is critical to the long-term success of any ASD surgery.

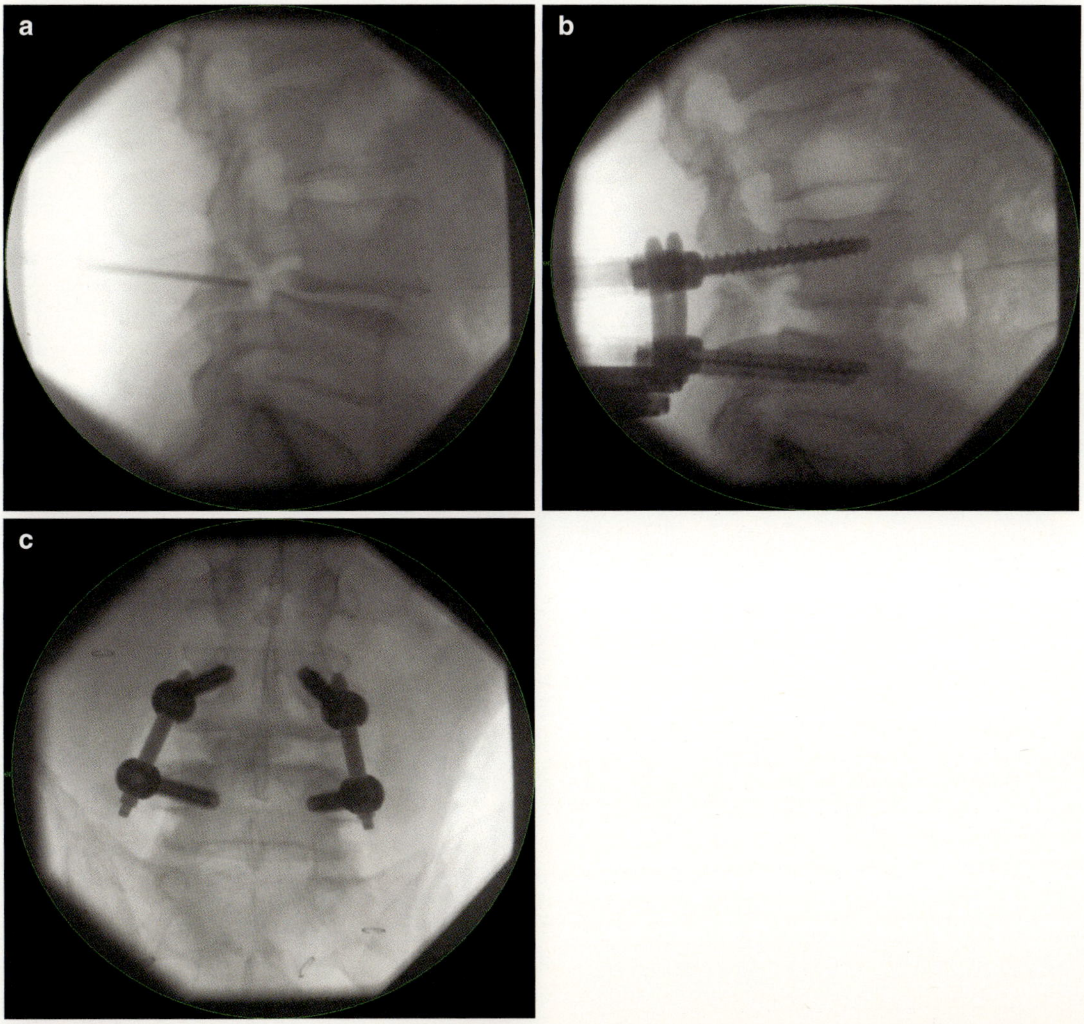

Fig. 20.7 (**a–c**) Treatment of an L4/5 spondylolisthesis using an inflatable cage to restore anterior column height. This method allows easy access through Kambin's triangle into a collapsed disc space without nerve root retraction

References

1. Barnes B, GE R, Haid R, Subach B, McLaughlin M. Allograft implants for posterior lumbar interbody fusion: results comparing cylindrical dowels and impacted wedges. Neurosurgery. 2002;51:1191–8.
2. Brantigan J, Neidre A, Toohey J. The lumbar I/F cage for posterior lumbar interbody fusion with the variable screw placement system: 10-year results of a Food and Drug Administration clinical trial. Spine J. 2004;4:681–8.
3. Burkus JK, Transfeldt EE, Kitchel SH, Watkins RG, Balderston RA. Clinical and radiographic outcomes of anterior lumbar interbody fusion using recombinant human bone morphogenetic protein-2. Spine. 2002; 27:2396–408.
4. Glassman SD, Carreon L, Djurasovic M, Campbell MJ, Puno RM, Johnson JR, Dimar JR. Posterolateral lumbar spine fusion with INFUSE bone graft. Spine J. 2007;7:44–9.
5. Heary R, Karimi R. Correction of lumbar coronal plane deformity using unilateral cage placement. Neurosurg Focus. 2010;28:E10.
6. Wang MY. Improvement of sagittal balance and lumbar lordosis following less invasive adult spinal deformity surgery with expandable cages and percutaneous instrumentation. J Neurosurg Spine. 2013;18:4–12.

21 Lumbar Endoscopic Fusion

Gun Choi, Guilherme Pereira Corrêa Meyer, and Daniel H. Kim

21.1 Introduction

Spinal fusions have been performed for nearly a century for a variety of conditions. Interbody fusion is an effective method and it is associated with high fusion rates [1]. Traditionally, the ability to achieve adequate exposure to perform these procedures required an open surgical approach. However, with the advent of newer techniques and technology, combined with an improved understanding of surgical anatomy, newer minimally invasive techniques have been developed [2, 3].

At the same time, the endoscope is a powerful tool. It allows us a good illumination and visualization of spaces that were only seen through large exposures. For this reason it is used in several different medicine fields. For lumbar spine it is not different. Several advantages are related to minimally invasive approaches like less intraoperative blood loss, less postoperative pain, decreased postoperative narcotic usage, early ambulation, and decreased length of hospital stay [3–6].

Indications for an endoscopic fusion are similar to a conventional fusion surgery. It includes grade I or II spondylolisthesis, recurrent disc herniations, severe discogenic back pain, instability, and pseudarthrosis. There are relatively few contraindications to minimally invasive instrumentation: obesity (body mass index (BMI) >40), advanced spondylolisthesis (grade 3 or 4), three or more levels, and previous surgery if instrumentation removal is needed.

Here we describe four different types of lumbar endoscopic fusions: endoscopically assisted transforaminal lumbar interbody fusion (ETLIF), laparoscopic anterior lumbar interbody fusion (LALIF), endoscopic lateral lumbar interbody fusion (ELLIF), and percutaneous endoscopic lumbar interbody fusion (PELIF) (Fig. 21.1).

G. Choi, MD, PhD
Director of Endoscopic Spine Center,
Hanyang Medical College,
Wooridul Spine Hospital, Seoul, Korea

G.P.C. Meyer, MD
Hospital Albert Einstein,
Av. Jurua, 706, Alphaville Industrial, São Paulo

D.H. Kim, MD, FAANS, FACS (✉)
Department of Neurosurgery,
Reconstructive Peripheral Nerve Surgery,
University of Texas Medical School at Houston,
6400 Fannin, Suite 2800, Houston, TX 77030, USA

Baylor College of Medicine, Houston, TX, USA
e-mail: daniel.h.kim@uth.tmc.edu

21.2 ETLIF

In 1952 Cloward described the posterior lumbar interbody fusion procedure (PLIF) [7], and later Harms and Rolinger introduced the transforaminal lumbar interbody fusion (TLIF) in 1982 for the management of degenerative spinal disorders that necessitate interbody fusions [8]. TLIF has the advantage of less neural retraction in comparison to PLIF during the cage insertion [9]. Moreover there is no need to expose the epidural

M.Y. Wang et al. (eds.), *Minimally Invasive Spinal Deformity Surgery*,
DOI 10.1007/978-3-7091-1407-0_21, © Springer-Verlag Wien 2014

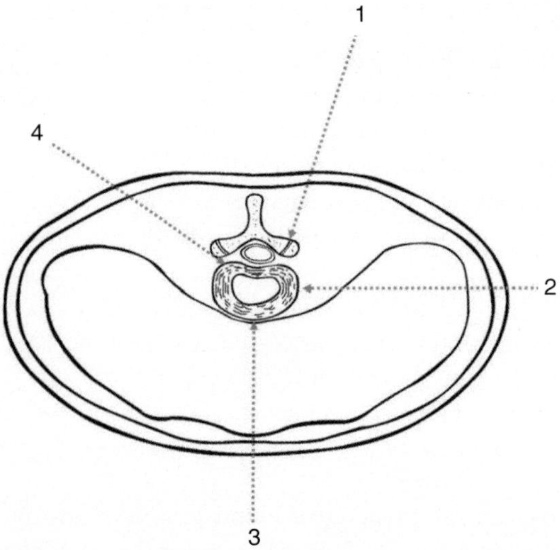

Fig. 21.1 Different endoscopic approaches to the spine: *1*, endoscopically assisted transforaminal lumbar interbody fusion (ETLIF); *2*, endoscopic lateral lumbar interbody fusion (ELLIF); *3*, laparoscopic anterior lumbar interbody fusion (LALIF); *4*, percutaneous endoscopic lumbar interbody fusion (PELIF)

space bilaterally [10]. ETLIF combines the advantages of TLIF with a minimal access exposure. The inherent muscle damage from subperiosteal dissections and retraction that have been demonstrated objectively through several studies is believed to adversely affect clinical outcomes [11–15]. ETLIF decreases muscle damage by splitting the muscles fibers without cutting or significantly retracting them. Tubular retractors with the assistance of an endoscope view can provide a minimally invasive exposure. There is no need for a microscope once it is possible to see clearly the neuro structures and even inside the disc space in order to check the adequate endplate preparation. Moreover, the microscope has a propensity for contamination because of unknown contact with unsterile parts of the surgeon, and it can be a source of infection [16].

21.2.1 Indications: Special Considerations

ETLIF is specially indicated in case of unilateral foraminal stenosis. This allows direct foraminal decompression. If bilateral foraminal decompression is needed, a bilateral approach for adequate decompression should be used [17–19]. It's also a particularly useful approach because there is no need for an access surgeon.

21.2.2 Surgical Technique

After a carefully preoperative planning and evaluation, the patient is brought to the operation room. Somatosensory evoked potential (SSEP) can be used to increase the safety of the procedure in special cases. Patient is prone positioned and care is made to insure adequate padding of all pressure points. The surgeon should stand on the same side of the approach that usually corresponds to the most symptomatic side. In case there is no difference between sides, a right-handed surgeon should stay on the patients left side. Fluoroscopy is used to confirm the level. The 2.5-cm incision is placed 3–4 cm from the midline, and it goes from the superior pedicle to the inferior pedicle centered on the disc space. A Steinmann is placed vertically under lateral fluoroscopy toward the facet complex over the pathological disc space. After confirming the correct positioning, serial soft tissue dilators are introduced (METRx; Medtronic Sofamor Danek, Memphis, TN). For ETLIF a 20-mm or larger working channel is needed.

A monopolar cautery is used to dissect the soft tissue and expose the lamina, isthmus, and facet joint (Fig. 21.2a).

It is safer to begin laterally where bone is apparent. To maximize the working space is essential to remove all the soft tissue overhanging the anatomic structures. If the medial facet, lateral interlaminar window, and lamina are not clearly seen, the working channel should be repositioned.

Next step consists in a generous hemilaminectomy and facetectomy to expose the lateral aspect of the dural sac and the superior and inferior nerve roots (Fig. 21.2b).

The endoscope magnifies the view. Surgeon hands may obstruct the vision when working in small fields like tubular retractors with a microscope. Endoscopic vision eliminates this drawback. High-speed drills, osteotomes, and Kerrison punches are used. The bone removed and spared is

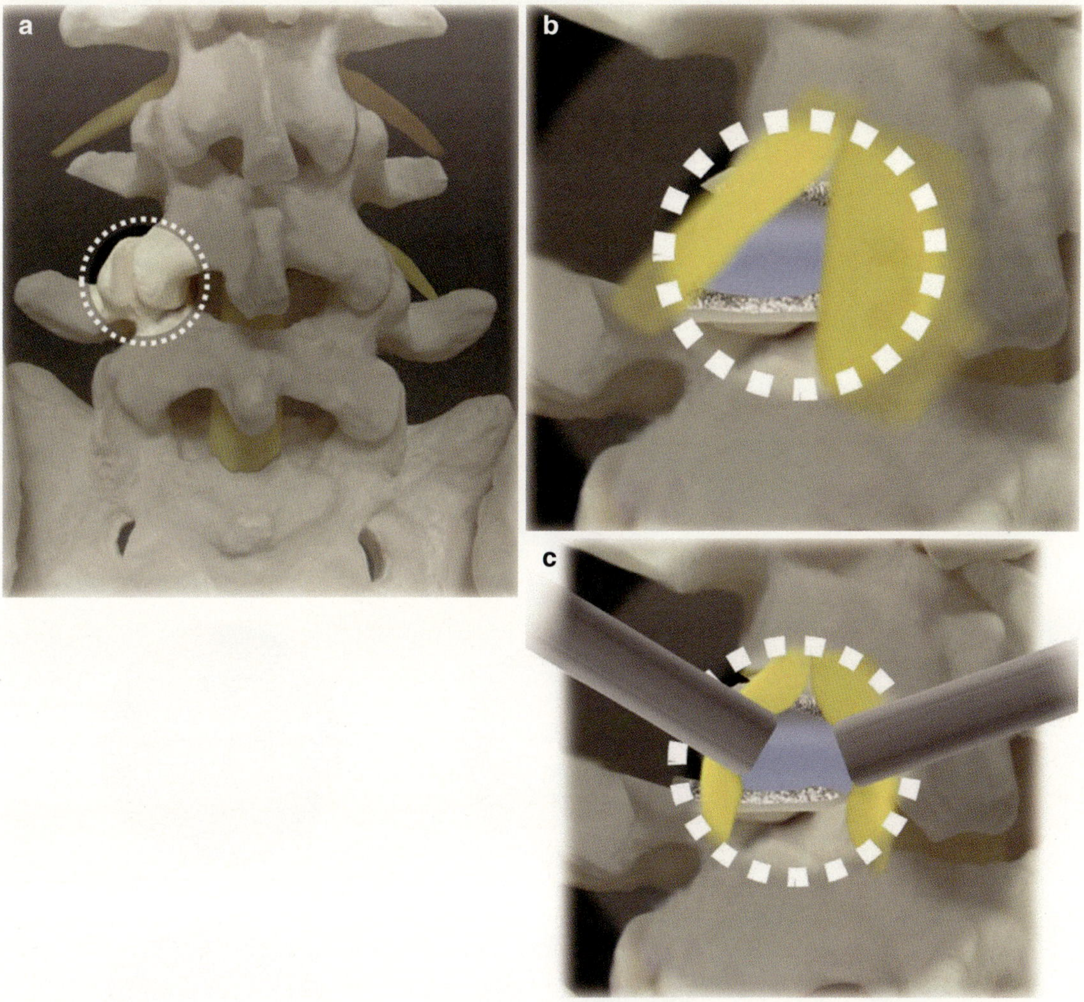

Fig. 21.2 (**a**) The working channel should be centered on the facet joint with the disc space beneath it. It is important to see the medical facet, lateral interlaminar window, and lama. (**b**) After removing the facet joint and some lamina, the disc, exiting and traversing root, is exposed. (**c**) Gently retracting and protecting the neuro structures, we can access the disc and proceed with the discectomy

later used as autograft in the interbody fusion. After visualization of the nerve roots, the exiting nerve root is protected or gently retracted laterally. Dural sac and traversing nerve are gently retracted medially to expose the disc space (Fig. 21.2c).

Epidural veins overlaying the disc space may be cauterized with a bipolar cautery. At this moment discectomy is done with a scalpel no.15. The disc material and endplate preparation is done with curettes, pituitary rongeurs, reamers, and plate scrapers using standard technique. The cage's size is measured in preoperative exams and confirmed using a trial. Disc space is then partially filled with graft. We usually use allograft mixed with autograft collected from the laminotomy site. The cage is also filled up with this mixture of grafts. Chisel is then used to create space for the cage insertion. Endoscopic view allows a better visualization and increases the safety during these steps (Fig. 21.3).

Fluoroscopic view is used in the lateral position to confirm the appropriate cage depth. At this step the working channel should be angled to the opposite side. This allows a better angle for the cage placement (Fig. 21.4).

After the cage insertion, the pedicle screws are inserted percutaneously. Insertion of pedicle screws through a midline approach requires

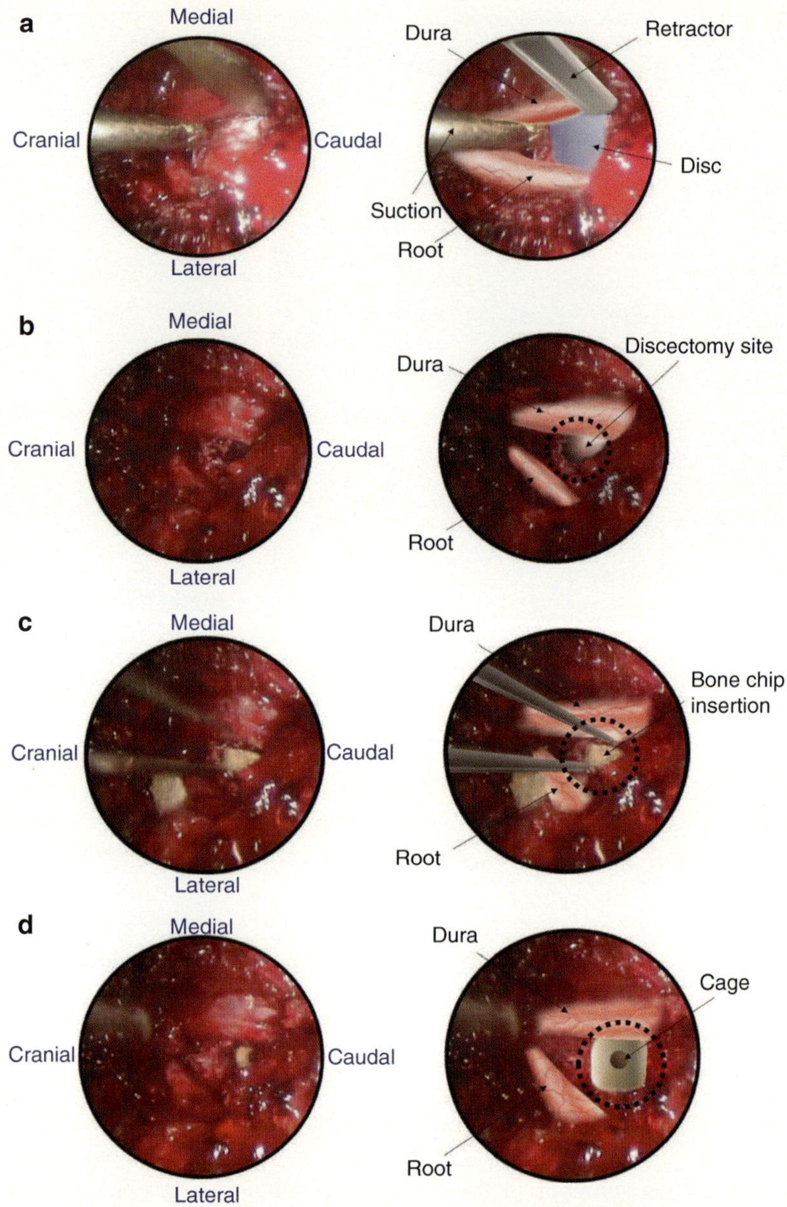

Fig. 21.3 Endoscopic images. (**a**) Exposure. (**b**) Discectomy. (**c**) Bone chip insertion. (**d**) Cage insertion

massive retraction of the multifidus muscle, subjecting the muscle to high retraction pressures and disruption of its osseo-tendinous attachments and neurovascular supply [14]. Percutaneous screws avoid such muscular injuries. The working channel and endoscope are removed and the procedure is done using the C-arm.

The percutaneous pedicle screw technique begins with a Jamshidi-type trocar needle that is placed under fluoroscopic control through the previous incision. In the opposite site, the screws are placed through separate incisions. A true anteroposterior view with the spinous process centered between each pedicle and a flat superior endplate of the corresponding vertebra and a lateral view with the pedicles and endplate parallels are essential. This can avoid inadvertent malpositioning of the screws. Once the needles are correctly positioned inside the pedicle, the stylets are removed and guide wires inserted (Fig. 21.5).

The guide wire is then used to direct cannulated taps and screws into the pedicle. C-arm

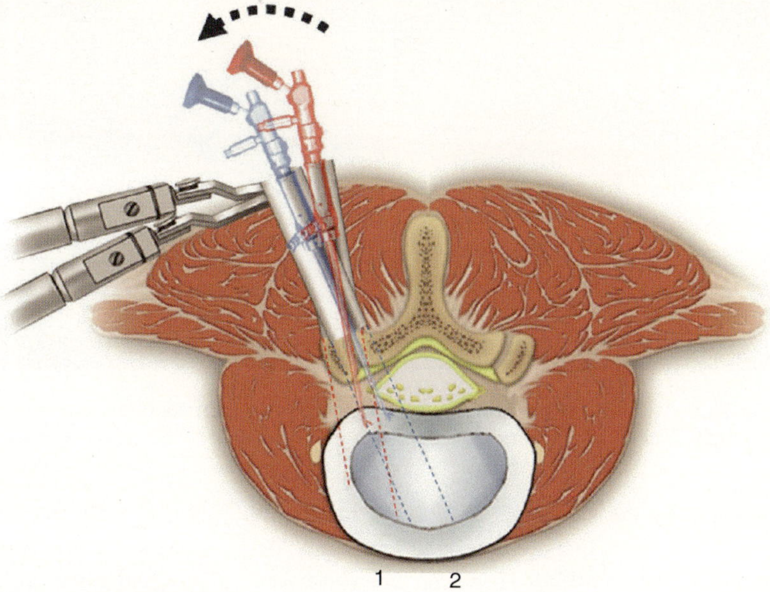

Fig. 21.4 After preparing the endplate, the retractor and endoscope are angled. We should see bleeding endplates without breakage. The endoscope is removed and the cage is inserted

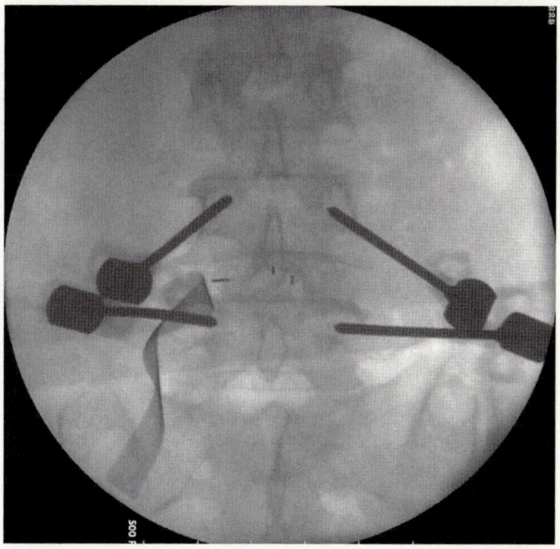

Fig. 21.5 Percutaneous placement of Jamshidi needles through the pedicle. Needle stylets are replaced by guide wires. The needles are removed and taps create the pathway for the screws

lateral view is important to ensure that the K wire is not advancing. Once the pedicle screws are positioned, the rods are placed percutaneously and then connected. We change the patient's position into lordosis to avoid a "flat back" before fixing the rods. C-arm is used in lateral view and then in AP view to confirm the appropriate implants positioning (Fig. 21.6).

The wound is irrigated, hemostasis is confirmed, and the fascia and skin are closed in a layered fashion. A subfascial drain might be placed for 24 h.

21.3 LALIF

Laparoscopic lumbar discectomy was described in 1991 by Obenchain [20]. The technique was then modified to allow anterior fusion and posterior instrumentation. The use of an anterior approach preserves the posterior muscles and avoids related complications. Moreover, the cages can be bigger when compared to posterior and posterolateral approaches. In addition the laparoscopic approach allows good visualization, decreases the blood loss, and has excellent cosmetic results. However anterior approaches have potential injury to large vessels and retrograde ejaculation as their main drawbacks, and LALIF requires long learning curve [21].

Due to the vascular anatomy at the L4–5 disc level where the large abdominal vessels bifurcate and override the disc space, the technical feasibility differs significantly between L4–5 and L5–S1 levels.

For L5–S1 LALIF have good results quite similar to mini-open ALIF. Blood loss and hospital stay are decreased, and the clinical outcome is

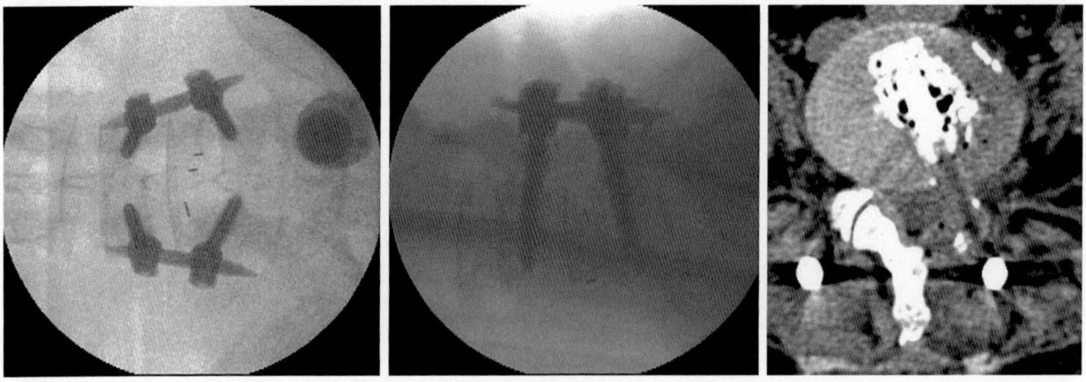

Fig. 21.6 After ETLIF posterior percutaneous screws are inserted. C-arm intraoperatively confirms the good positioning of the implants. Postoperative CT shows good positioning of the cage and bone graft around it

statistically the same [22, 23]. It's a minimally invasive surgery that preserves the important posterior lumbar muscles. However, operative time was higher in the LALIF group [22, 23], and some studies showed a higher retrograde ejaculation rate when compared to ALIF (5.1 % vs. 2.3 %) but without statistical significance [21].

For the L4–5 level, LALIF doesn't show the same good results. Due to anatomic considerations, the rate of complications is higher [21]. The incidence of retrograde ejaculation is over 10 % [21], and some studies report a conversion to an open procedure in 67 % [24].

No conclusion regarding either the superiority or inferiority of LALIF to the open or mini-open ALIF can be drawn, because of the lack of data with a high level of evidence [21]. However, some spine surgeons are abandoning this procedure and switching to the mini-open ALIF. On the other hand, Beutler et al. published a description of LALIF using the da Vinci Robotic Surgical System for anterior lumbar interbody fusion [25]. He considered the visualization inside the disc space and surrounding structures better than current open and laparoscopic techniques. The future role of LALIF still remains to be followed closely.

21.3.1 Indications: Special Considerations

LALIF is indicated as a stand-alone procedure for patients with DDD, low-grade spondylolisthesis, and post-laminectomy syndrome. A stand-alone LALIF fully preserves posterior muscles and decreases postoperative pain related to dissection. If needed, posterior percutaneous screws increase the stability and may be added. Special considerations must be done for male patients, L4–5 level, and previous abdominal surgery. Those are not formal contraindications but may increase the complications.

21.3.2 Surgical Technique

Here we describe the technique for L5–S1 LALIF. The patient is placed supine on a radiolucent table, and straps are placed on the patient's ankles to prevent sliding because a steep Trendelenburg's position is required during the procedure. This allows the abdominal viscera to move cranially out of the pelvis (Fig. 21.7).

Equipment in the room is positioned to allow the surgeon an adequate view of both the C-arm image and the video monitor. Pillows are placed under the patient's hips to accentuate lumbar lordosis at the lumbosacral junction. It's also important to prevent knees hyperextension by placing a pillow under them. The arms are placed at the patient's side, low enough to prevent interference with the fluoroscopic lateral view (Fig. 21.7). A nasogastric tube and Foley catheter are used to decompress the stomach and bladder, respectively. Both catheters are removed at the end of the procedure. Patients are advised that an open laparotomy may be needed in case of uncontrolled bleeding or poor visualization of the lumbar spine, in addition to other potential complications.

The fluoroscopic equipment is then brought into place before the incisions are made to verify the midline. It is important to obtain adequate fluoroscopic views for proper intraoperative visualization of the vertebral bodies and to estimate instruments trajectory. Four incisions are used. The two lower paramedian incisions allow placement of portals for the working forceps (Fig. 21.8).

The incision for the interbody channel and devices is centered over the midline suprapubic region and measures 2–4 cm in length. The viewing camera is placed through the curvilinear umbilical incision.

The patient is placed in a steep Trendelenburg's position to mobilize the abdominal contents out of the pelvic inlet and allow a good visualization of the L5–S1 disc level. The sacral promontory is identified and confirmed by fluoroscopy (Fig. 21.9a).

The peritoneum is then opened and special care must be taken in male patients. Unipolar cautery increases the rate of retrograde ejaculation and should be avoided. It is preferable to use a blunt dissector with a gentle sweeping motion to mobilize the presacral sympathetic plexus. In female patients, monopolar electrocautery can be used to expose the anterior face of the vertebral bodies and disc space.

Lying anterior to the disc space, the middle sacral artery and vein can be recognize (Fig. 21.9b). Preoperative MRI and CT may help to identify the relationship between these vessels and the midline. Artery and vein should be divided and ligated. C-arm is used to establish the correct midline. If the midline cannot be accurately identified, the surgeon should consider an open conversion because higher rates of

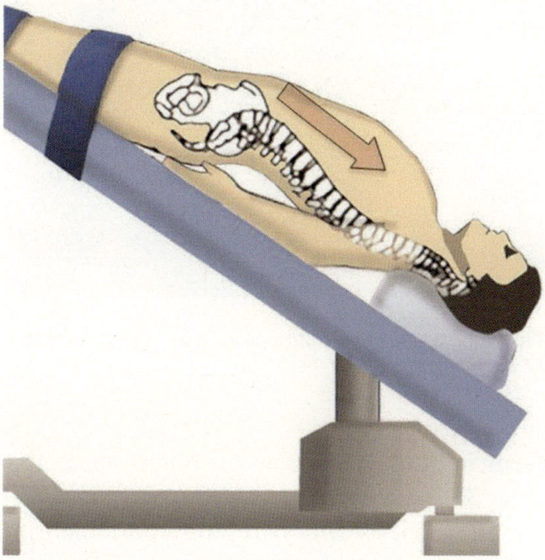

Fig. 21.7 A steep Trendelenburg's position allows the abdominal content to move cranially out of the pelvis. The patient's arms are placed under the lumbosacral spine to allow good visualization of the spine under C-arm. A pillow is placed under the knees to prevent hyperextension

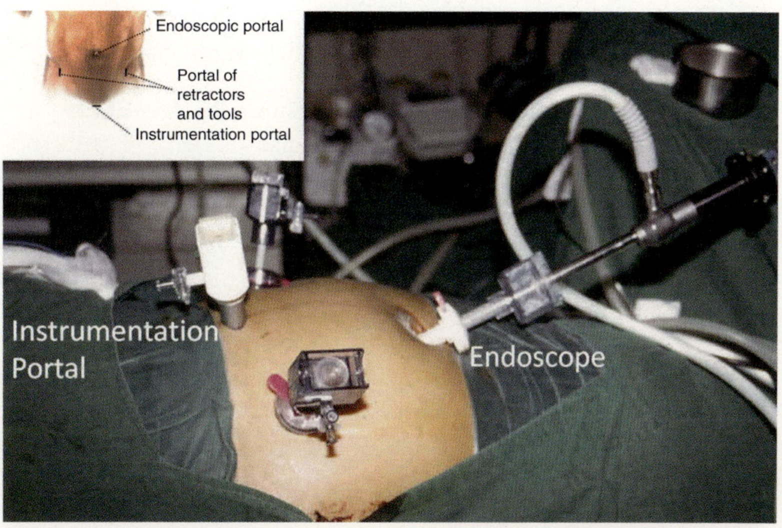

Fig. 21.8 Four routinely incisions. Two paramedian incisions provide conduits for the working forceps. The viewing camera is placed through an umbilical incision. The working channel is placed through a midline suprapubic incision measuring 2–4 cm in length

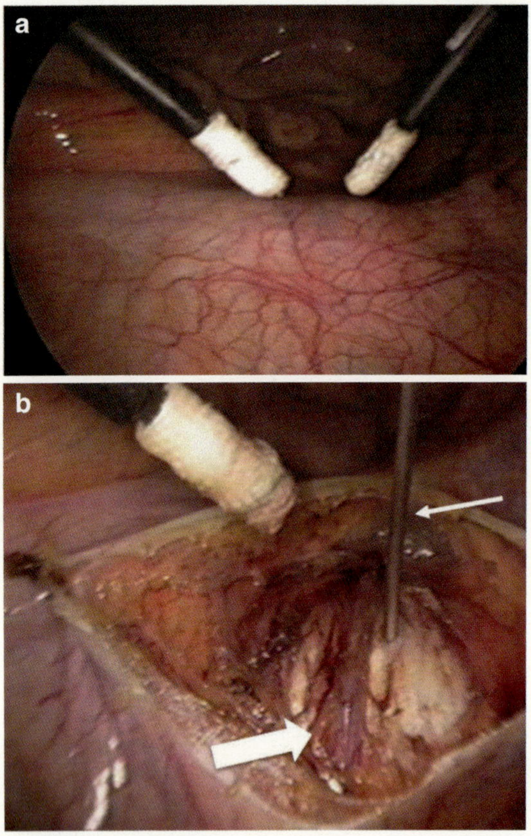

Fig. 21.9 (**a**) The sacral promontory is identified and confirmed by fluoroscopy. (**b**) Posterior peritoneum incised and the middle sacral vessels exposed. Marking needle (*fin arrow*) and middle sacral vessels (*wide arrow*)

complication are more likely [26]. The left iliac vein protrudes more anteriorly and may require more retraction.

Next step consists in removing the disc material with trephines and pituitary rongeurs. It is important to maintain the instruments parallel to the endplates. Progressively larger distractors are then tamped into the disc space to restore the disc height to the appropriate level and to provide tension for the annulus fibrosis. Ideally the collapsed disc space should be distracted to reach its original size. The implant should be filed with graft and must be inserted in adequate alignment (Fig. 21.10a). Once again the restoration of the disc space height should be checked. The empty spaces around the implants should also be filled up with bone graft to increase the fusion rate and

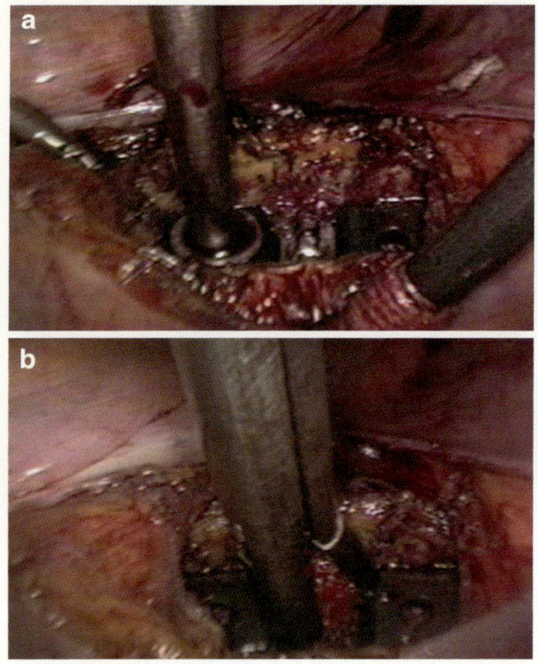

Fig. 21.10 (**a**) Cage insertion. (**b**) Graft insertion between cages

facilitate its recognition in follow-up exams (Fig. 21.10b). At the end of the procedure, AP and lateral views certify the proper positioning of the implants. All the instruments are removed, the pneumoperitoneum is deflated, the peritoneum is closed, and the abdominal incisions are sutured.

Percutaneous pedicle screws may be used, but LALIF can be done as a stand-alone procedure (Fig. 21.11).

21.4 ELLIF

ELLIF is a retroperitoneal approach that has the advantage of not penetrating the abdominal cavity and thus obviates the risk of small bowel obstruction or postoperative intraperitoneal adhesions [27]. Additionally, as the autonomic plexus is not dissected, there is a reduced risk of retrograde ejaculation in comparison with transperitoneal techniques [28]. Moreover, the anterior longitudinal ligament and posterior longitudinal ligament

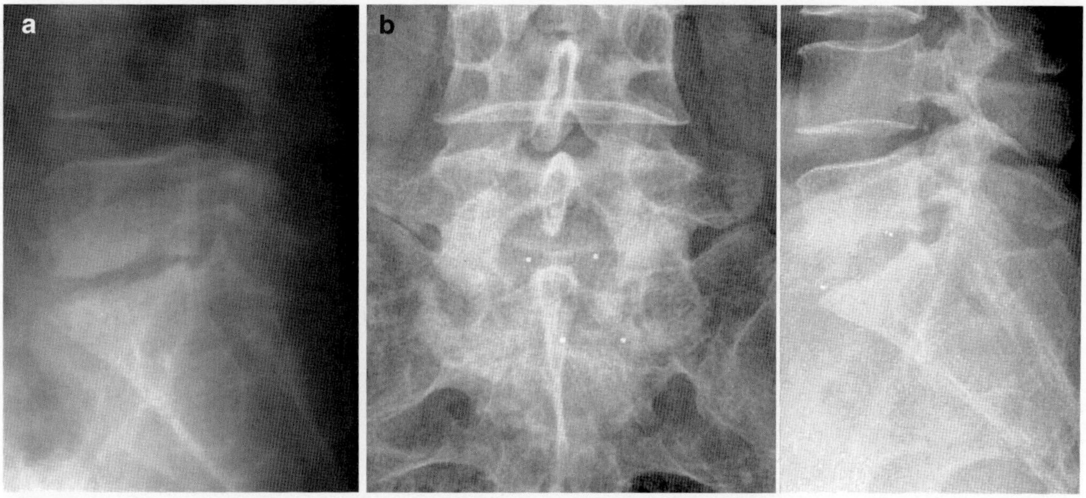

Fig. 21.11 Preoperative (**a**) and postoperative (**b**) images showing restoration of L5–S1 disc height and good implants positioning

are not violated with the lateral retroperitoneal approach. ELLIF allows placement of a wider cage in comparison with ETLIF. This provides good support for the endplates reducing subsidence and provides indirect foraminal decompression [29].

Lower lumbar levels are more prone to degenerative diseases and require fusion more frequently than higher levels [6]. However, the access to the disc space must be orthogonal to the endplates, and the iliac crest may overlap the lumbar lower levels. This can make ELLIF inadequate for L5–S1 and sometimes for L4–5 levels (Fig. 21.12).

In addition, a large mass of psoas muscle containing lumbosacral nerve roots may need to be mobilized causing postoperative leg pain, psoas weakness, or paresthesia [30, 31].

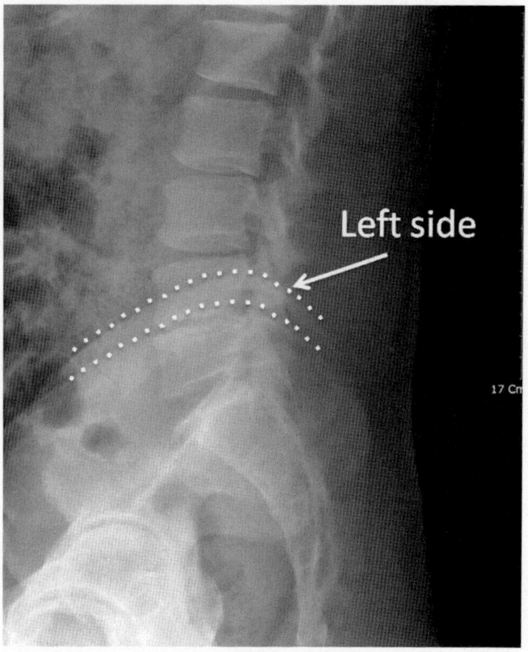

Fig. 21.12 High iliac crest, especially on the left side, making a lateral approach not feasible

21.4.1 Indications: Special Considerations

ELLIF is particularly best suited for higher lumbar levels. There is less lumbosacral nerve roots, and they are located more posteriorly making this technique even safer. It allows placement of a large cage that provides good support for the endplates.

21.4.2 Surgical Technique

The patient lies in lateral decubitus position on a radiolucent table with side rails to accommodate robotic arms. A left-sided approach is preferred to

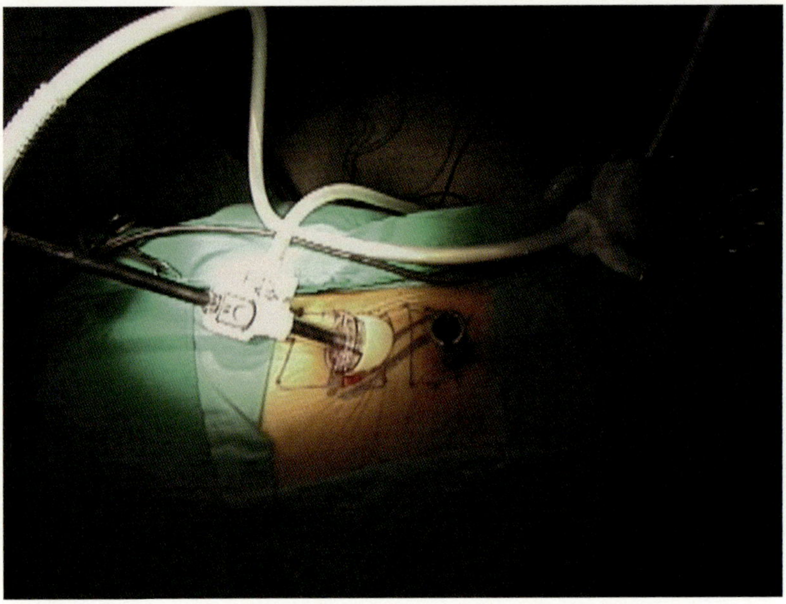

Fig. 21.13 ELLIF provides a retroperitoneal approach to the spine, while the endoscope allows a clear visualization of the operation field. The working portal should lie directly over the desired disc space

a right-sided approach, because it is easier to dissect the aorta. The 1-cm incision is made according to the level that will be addressed. Lateral C-arm fluoroscopic image is used to confirm the level, and patient's midaxillary line is another landmark used. The working portal should lie directly over the desired disc space (Fig. 21.13).

The retroperitoneal space can be dissected with surgeon's finger or balloon insufflation. The peritoneum is not penetrated and lies anteriorly. The retroperitoneal fat and the surface of the psoas muscle are identified. Usually, the genitofemoral nerve is visualized on the surface of the psoas muscle. At this juncture, a dissection balloon, such as that manufactured by Origin (Menlo Park, CA), can be filled with 1 l of normal saline or air to dissect the retroperitoneal layer. This creates a working space to triangulate the endoscope. Usually three portals are used: working portal for pituitary rongeurs, curettes, a high-powered burr, or Kerrison rongeurs. A second portal is used for the 10-mm laparoscope and a third for posterior retraction of the psoas.

The segmental vessels are ligated and divided and the discs space is exposed. If needed, another portal can be used for suction in case of intense bleeding. The psoas muscle is retracted posteriorly, and the retroperitoneal fat and ureter are retracted anteriorly (Fig. 21.14). The disc material is removed and the endplates prepared. It is important to reach the contralateral side of the vertebral endplate. Otherwise this could lead to a cage malpositioning and iatrogenic scoliosis.

The disc space height must be restored to enlarge the foramen and restore the segmental lordosis. The fusion cage is packed with allograft or autogenous iliac graft. It is also recommended to pack additional bone graft around the cage. Posterior percutaneous screws augmentation can be used to improve stability, but the procedure can also be in a stand-alone fashion (Fig. 21.15).

21.5 PELIF

TLIF has proven to be a successful option for interbody access and fusion [32, 33]. The cage increases the disc space height and consequently the foraminal area. However, the facets and part of the lamina have to be removed for implantation of a cage with an adequate size. It is also not a thoroughly percutaneous procedure.

Percutaneous endoscopic lumbar interbody fusion (PELIF) is possible with the use of expandable cages that can be inserted without removing the facets. B-Twin (Disc-O-Tech Medical Technologies Ltd., Herzliya, Israel) is an example of expandable cage that can be used for PELIF

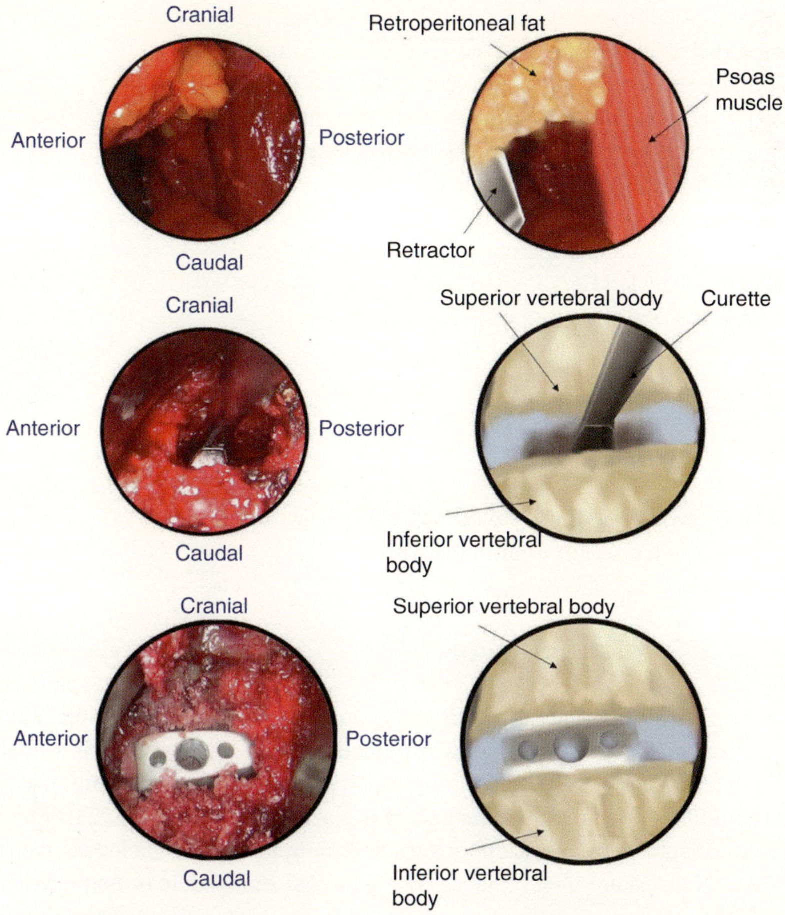

Fig. 21.14 (**a**) Retroperitoneal fat is retracted anteriorly and psoas muscle can be seen clearly. Psoas is then retracted posteriorly. (**b**) The disc material is removed and the endplates prepared. (**c**) After adequate endplate preparation, the cage filled with graft is inserted, while retractors hold psoas muscle posteriorly and retroperitoneal fat anteriorly

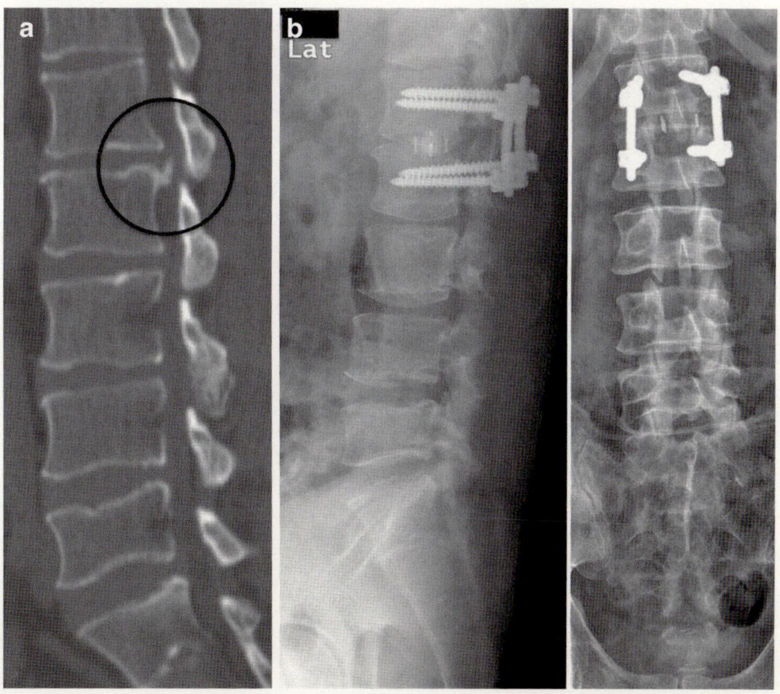

Fig. 21.15 (**a**) Sagittal CT image shows a calcified disc herniation. (**b**) Lateral and AP postoperative X-rays after decompression and fusion using ELLIF technique

(Fig. 21.16). It is made of titanium and when collapsed, five fins are enclosed within a cylinder 5 mm in diameter. Following placement within the disc space by a single-use delivery system, the implant is expanded fin by fin until it is 25-mm long and up to 15 mm in diameter. Upon completion of the process, the device self-locks. The final configuration is trapezoid and there are three available size options: 9.5/11, 11.5/13, and 13.5/15. Preoperative X-rays are useful for proper size selection.

21.5.1 Indications: Special Considerations

This procedure is best suited for patients with discogenic back pain or mild instability.

21.5.2 Surgical Technique

After undergoing general anesthesia, the patient is placed in the prone position on a radiolucent operative table. The skin entry point lies 6–8 cm from the midline [34]. An 18-gauge needle is placed in the disc space through Kambin's triangle in both sides. Needles are then replaced by a guide wire, and conically tipped dilators are slipped over it into the disc space. After that, a 7.5-mm working cannula is slipped into the disc space.

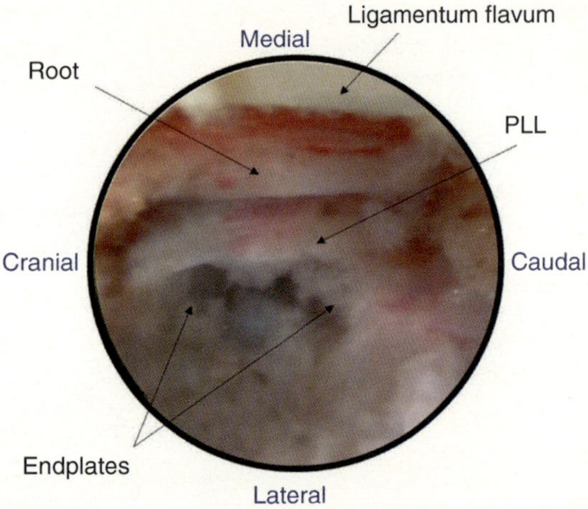

Fig. 21.17 Endoscopic anatomy: ligamentum flavum under the facet joint, traversing nerve root, posterior longitudinal ligament (*PLL*), and cranial and caudal endplates can be seen in this image

Endoscopic visualization of the local anatomy is done before disc removal and endplate preparation (Fig. 21.17).

This adds safety to the procedure. The whole procedure is monitored using fluoroscopy (Fig. 21.18).

Blunt dissection of the annulus avoids expulsion of any bone graft. Removal of the disc material was performed under endoscopic view with the Ho:YAG laser and forceps. Endplate preparation can be done using radiofrequency ablation, specially designed burr, or abrasive cutters [35, 36]. Implant diameter was verified by insertion of the trial implants into the intervertebral space. This confirms what was measured in preoperative exams. Graft is packed in the disc space. Allograft with demineralized bone matrix or autograft can be used. Expandable holders are inserted then (B-Twin). Since the first fin is opened perpendicularly to the endplates, adjustments can be made at this stage by turning the delivery system 90° to reposition. After complete implants placement, more graft is inserted into the disc space.

This procedure can also be done as a standalone modality, or posterior percutaneous pedicle screws may be used to increase stability (Fig. 21.19). Fusion is verified during routine follow-up exams (Fig. 21.20).

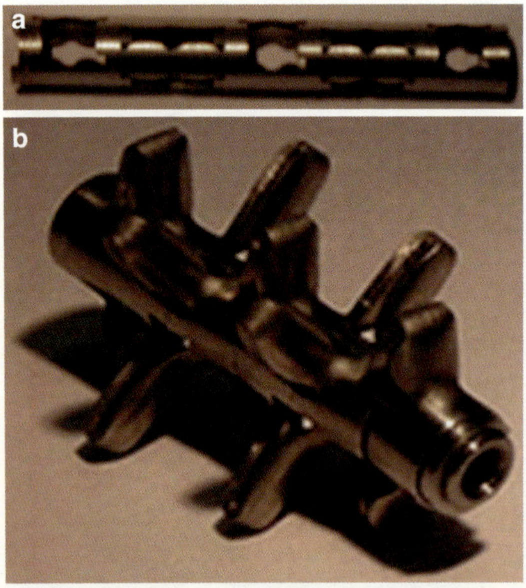

Fig. 21.16 (**a**) The B-Twin ESS in its reduced configuration. The five sets of fins are enclosed within a cylinder 5 mm in diameter. (**b**) Expanded configuration

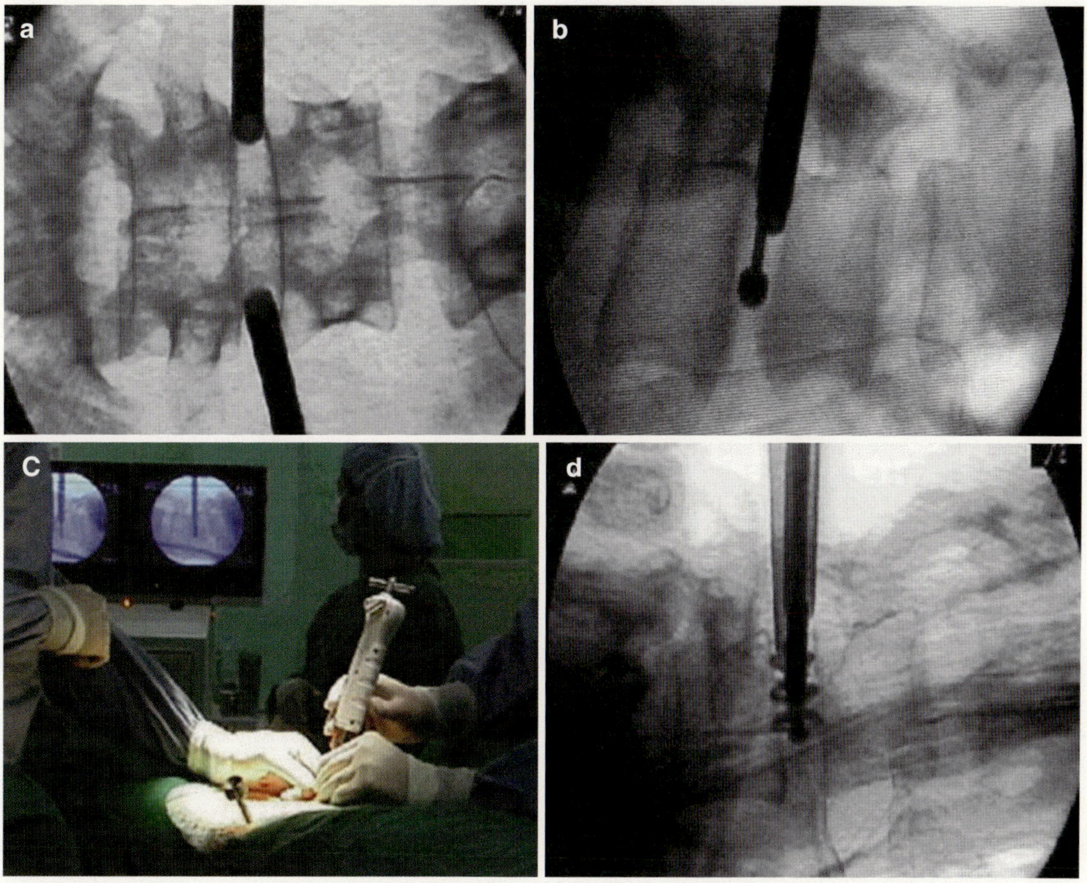

Fig. 21.18 (**a**) PELIF is performed through posterolateral biportal channels that are placed *inside* the disc space trough Kambin's triangle. (**b**) Preparing endplates using specially designed burr. (**c**) On the *bottom right*, inserting a specially designed expandable cage/holder under constant C-arm view. (**d**) The expandable cages stabilize the segment, and bone graft is placed *around* the implants

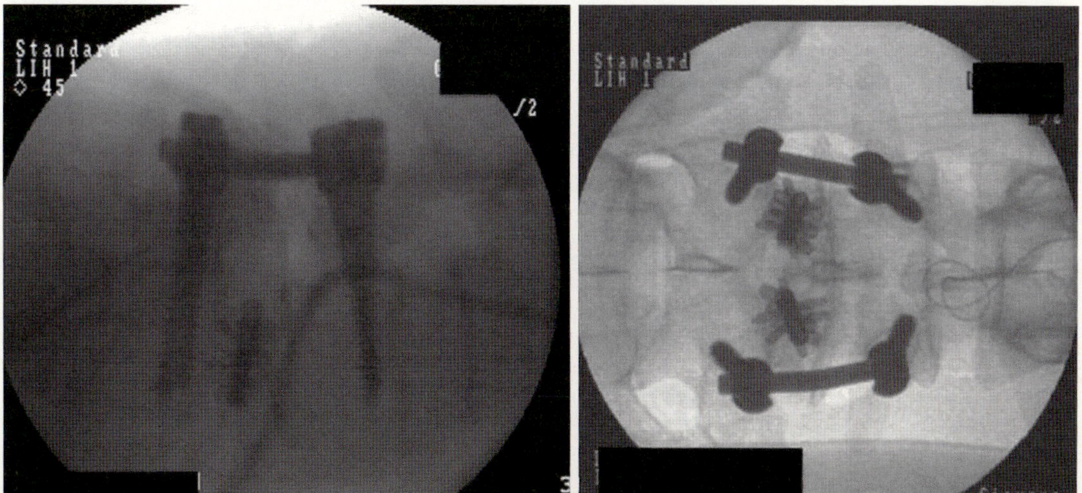

Fig. 21.19 Posterior percutaneous pedicle screws increase the stability after PELIF

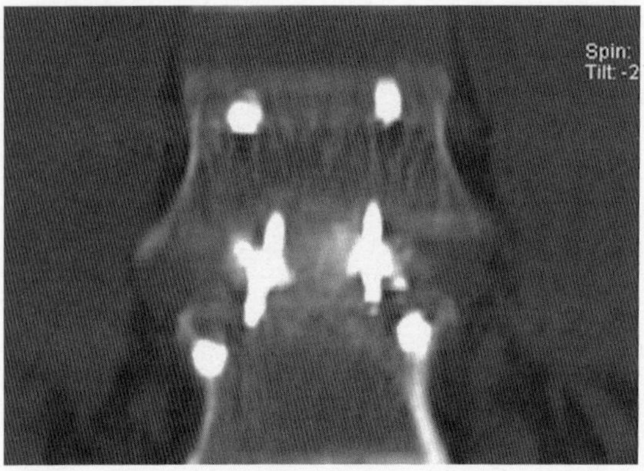

Fig. 21.20 CT scan done after 12 months showing a solid bone bridge in the disc space between the implants

21.6 Final Considerations

Medicine is an evolving science, and newer products with higher technology are constantly offered to spine surgeons and patients every year. Endoscopic fusion techniques are still crawling, and we still don't have comparative prospective trials to identify which technique is the best. Innovation, better equipment, and more studies are still to come. There is no doubt that there is a room for endoscopic fusion techniques. Time and studies will provide adequate information so we can choose the most suitable ones.

References

1. Herkowitz HN, Rothman RH, Simeone FA. Rothman-Simeone, the spine. 5th ed. Philadelphia: Saunders Elsevier; 2006.
2. Shen FH, Samartzis D, Khanna AJ, Anderson DG. Minimally invasive techniques for lumbar interbody fusions. Orthop Clin North Am. 2007;38(3):373–86. abstract vi.
3. Foley KT, Holly LT, Schwender JD. Minimally invasive lumbar fusion. Spine (Phila Pa 1976) 2003;28 Suppl 15:S26–35.
4. Fessler RG. Minimally invasive percutaneous posterior lumbar interbody fusion. Neurosurgery. 2003;52(6): 1512.
5. Isaacs RE, Podichetty VK, Santiago P, Sandhu FA, Spears J, Kelly K, et al. Minimally invasive microendoscopy-assisted transforaminal lumbar interbody fusion with instrumentation. J Neurosurg Spine. 2005;3(2):98–105.
6. Kim DH, Choi G, Lee SH. Endoscopic spine procedures. New York: Thieme; 2011.
7. Cloward RB. The treatment of ruptured lumbar intervertebral disc by vertebral body fusion. III. Method of use of banked bone. Ann Surg. 1952;136(6):987–92.
8. Harms J, Rolinger H. A one-stager procedure in operative treatment of spondylolistheses: dorsal traction-reposition and anterior fusion (author's transl). Z Orthop Ihre Grenzgeb. 1982;120(3):343–7.
9. Ray CD. Threaded titanium cages for lumbar interbody fusions. Spine (Phila Pa 1976). 1997;22(6):667–79; discussion 79–80.
10. Holly LT, Schwender JD, Rouben DP, Foley KT. Minimally invasive transforaminal lumbar interbody fusion: indications, technique, and complications. Neurosurg Focus. 2006;20(3):E6.
11. Kawaguchi Y, Matsui H, Tsuji H. Back muscle injury after posterior lumbar spine surgery. Part 2: Histologic and histochemical analyses in humans. Spine (Phila Pa 1976). 1994;19(22):2598–602.
12. Kawaguchi Y, Matsui H, Tsuji H. Back muscle injury after posterior lumbar spine surgery. Part 1: Histologic and histochemical analyses in rats. Spine (Phila Pa 1976). 1994;19(22):2590–7.
13. Sihvonen T, Herno A, Paljarvi L, Airaksinen O, Partanen J, Tapaninaho A. Local denervation atrophy of paraspinal muscles in postoperative failed back syndrome. Spine (Phila Pa 1976). 1993;18(5):575–81.
14. Datta G, Gnanalingham KK, Peterson D, Mendoza N, O'Neill K, Van Dellen J, et al. Back pain and disability after lumbar laminectomy: is there a relationship to muscle retraction? Neurosurgery. 2004;54(6):-1413–20; discussion 20.
15. Kim DY, Lee SH, Chung SK, Lee HY. Comparison of multifidus muscle atrophy and trunk extension muscle strength: percutaneous versus open pedicle screw fixation. Spine (Phila Pa 1976). 2005;30(1):123–9.
16. Bible JE, O'Neill KR, Crosby CG, Schoenecker JG, McGirt MJ, Devin CJ. Microscope sterility during spine surgery. Spine (Phila Pa 1976). 2012;37(7): 623–7.
17. Karikari IO, Isaacs RE. Minimally invasive transforaminal lumbar interbody fusion: a review of techniques and outcomes. Spine (Phila Pa 1976) 2010;35 Suppl 26:S294–301.
18. Shunwu F, Xing Z, Fengdong Z, Xiangqian F. Minimally invasive transforaminal lumbar interbody fusion for the treatment of degenerative lumbar diseases. Spine (Phila Pa 1976). 2010;35(17): 1615–20.
19. Villavicencio AT, Burneikiene S, Roeca CM, Nelson EL, Mason A. Minimally invasive versus open transforaminal lumbar interbody fusion. Surg Neurol Int. 2010;1:12.
20. Obenchain TG. Laparoscopic lumbar discectomy: case report. J Laparoendosc Surg. 1991;1(3):145–9.
21. Inamasu J, Guiot BH. Laparoscopic anterior lumbar interbody fusion: a review of outcome studies. Minim Invasive Neurosurg. 2005;48(6):340–7.

22. Regan JJ, Yuan H, McAfee PC. Laparoscopic fusion of the lumbar spine: minimally invasive spine surgery. A prospective multicenter study evaluating open and laparoscopic lumbar fusion. Spine (Phila Pa 1976). 1999;24(4):402–11.
23. Chung SK, Lee SH, Lim SR, Kim DY, Jang JS, Nam KS, et al. Comparative study of laparoscopic L5-S1 fusion versus open mini-ALIF, with a minimum 2-year follow-up. Eur Spine J. 2003;12(6):613–7.
24. Cowles RA, Taheri PA, Sweeney JF, Graziano GP. Efficacy of the laparoscopic approach for anterior lumbar spinal fusion. Surgery. 2000;128(4):589–96.
25. Beutler WJ, Peppelman WC, Jr., Dimarco LA. The da Vinci robotic surgical assisted anterior lumbar interbody fusion: technical development and case report. Spine (Phila Pa 1976). 2012;38:356–63.
26. McLaughlin MR, Zhang JY, Subach BR, Haid Jr RW, Rodts Jr GE. Laparoscopic anterior lumbar interbody fusion. Technical note. Neurosurg Focus. 1999; 7(6):e8.
27. Levrant SG, Bieber EJ, Barnes RB. Anterior abdominal wall adhesions after laparotomy or laparoscopy. J Am Assoc Gynecol Laparosc. 1997;4(3):353–6.
28. Than KD, Wang AC, Rahman SU, Wilson TJ, Valdivia JM, Park P, et al. Complication avoidance and management in anterior lumbar interbody fusion. Neurosurg Focus. 2011;31(4):E6.
29. Oliveira L, Marchi L, Coutinho E, Pimenta L. A radiographic assessment of the ability of the extreme lateral interbody fusion procedure to indirectly decompress the neural elements. Spine (Phila Pa 1976) 2010;35 Suppl 26:S331–7.
30. McAfee PC, Regan JJ, Geis WP, Fedder IL. Minimally invasive anterior retroperitoneal approach to the lumbar spine. Emphasis on the lateral BAK. Spine (Phila Pa 1976). 1998;23(13):1476–84.
31. Arnold PM, Anderson KK, McGuire Jr RA. The lateral transpsoas approach to the lumbar and thoracic spine: A review. Surg Neurol Int. 2012;3 Suppl 3: S198–215.
32. Yan DL, Pei FX, Li J, Soo CL. Comparative study of PILF and TLIF treatment in adult degenerative spondylolisthesis. Eur Spine J. 2008;17(10):1311–6.
33. Ames CP, Acosta FL Jr., Chi J, Iyengar J, Muiru W, Acaroglu E, et al. Biomechanical comparison of posterior lumbar interbody fusion and transforaminal lumbar interbody fusion performed at 1 and 2 levels. Spine (Phila Pa 1976). 2005;30(19):E562–6.
34. Wun Chul Choi CWP, Sang Ho Lee. Percutaneous endoscopic lumbar interbody fusion. J Minim Invasive Spinal Tech. 2002;2:6–7.
35. Aryan HE, Ames CP, Szandera B, Nguyen AD, Acosta Jr FL, Taylor WR. Coblation of spinal endplates in preparation for interbody spinal fusion. J Clin Neurosci. 2006;13(3):349–52.
36. Leu HF, Hauser RK. Percutaneous endoscopic lumbar spine fusion. Neurosurg Clin N Am. 1996;7(1): 107–17.

Minimally Invasive Osteotomy Techniques

22

Michael Y. Wang

22.1 Introduction

Unlike adolescent scoliosis, adult spinal deformities are frequently associated with a rigid spine. The last decade has witnessed major advances in the understanding of how to treat these problems, and one of the major developments has been an increasing understanding of the need for various osteotomies to mobilize the spine prior to correction of the deformity. Destabilizing osteotomies, which remove bone in the anterior or posterior spinal columns, allow the spine to become mobile in the sagittal and/or coronal planes. This destabilization prior to reconstruction is particularly important in the setting of osteoporosis where spinal fixation can be poor and screw pullout is a major concern.

Prior to the surgical intervention, the surgeon must plan the radiographic goals of the deformity operation. An increasing body of evidence has indicated that maintenance or restoration of sagittal balance is one of the most critical factors that will determine the clinical outcome for the patient. As such, the surgeon will have to plan for the appropriate type, number, and location of osteotomies to accomplish the desired surgical goal. Through the work of Shaffrey and Schwab, it is now recognized that the major radiographic determinants of a good long-term outcome relate to sagittal balance. In planning, the surgeon's goals should be to match the lumbar lordosis to the pelvic incidence within 10° and achieve a sagittal vertical axis made less than 5 cm (Chap. 6) [1, 2].

22.2 Classification of Osteotomies

A variety of osteotomy techniques have been developed for the treatment of adult spinal deformities. Recently, classification schemes have been developed to improve the surgeon's ability to plan deformity corrections (Table 22.1). This grading scheme recognizes that increasing destabilization of the spine through its various columns also provides for greater corrective power.

22.3 Posterior Column Osteotomies (Grades I and II)

For patients with flexibility of the disc spaces, a series of posterior column osteotomies can achieve significant deformity correction. In the realm of open surgery, these osteotomies are typically described as a Smith Peterson or Ponte osteotomy. The essence of the technique involves removal of sufficient spinous process, lamina, and facet bone to allow compression posteriorly between pedicle screws with the

M.Y. Wang, M.D., FACS
Departments of Neurological Surgery
and Rehab Medicine, University of Miami Miller
School of Medicine, 1095 NW 14th Terrace Lois
Pope Life Center, D4-6, Miami, FL 33136, USA
e-mail: mwang2@med.miami.edu

M.Y. Wang et al. (eds.), *Minimally Invasive Spinal Deformity Surgery*,
DOI 10.1007/978-3-7091-1407-0_22, © Springer-Verlag Wien 2014

Table 22.1 Classification of osteotomy techniques as described by Lenke

	Anatomical Resection	Description	Surgical approach Modifiers
Grade 1	Partial Facet Joint	Resection of the inferior facet and joint capsule at a given spinal level	**A/P** (anterior soft tissue release combined with posterior resection) **P** (posterior approach only)
Grade 2	Complete Facet Joint	Both superior and inferior facets at a given spinal segment are resected with complete ligamentum flavum removal; other posterior elements of the vertebra including the lamina, and the spinous processes may also resected	**A/P** (anterior soft tissue release combined with posterior resection) **P** (posterior approach only)
Grade 3	Pedicle/Partial Body	Partial wedge resection of a segment of the posterior vertebral body and a portion of the posterior vertebral elements with pedicles	**A** (anterior release) **P** (posterior approach only) **A/P** (both)
Grade 4	Pedicle/Partial Body/Disc	Wider wedge resection through the vertebral body; includes a substantial portion of the posterior vertebral body, posterior elements with pedicles and includes rejection of at least a portion of one end plate with the adjacent intervertebral disc	**A** (anterior release) **P** (posterior approach only) **A/P** (both)
Grade 5	Complete Vertebra and Disc	Complete removal of a vertebra and both adjacent discs (rib resection in the thoracic region)	**A** (anterior release) **P** (posterior approach only) **A/P** (both)
Grade 6	Multiple Vertebrae and Disc	Resection of more than one entire vertebra and adjacent discs. Grade 5 resection and additional adjacent vertebral resection	**A** (anterior release) **P** (posterior approach only) A/P (both)

axis of sagittal rotation centered on the posterior vertebral body. This stretches the anterior longitudinal ligament and expands the anterior disc.

A single-level osteotomy will yield between 3° and 5° of lordosis. As such, posterior column osteotomies would typically be performed at three or more consecutive vertebral levels and can be used in the thoracic and/or lumbar spine. Since the adult population typically presents with scoliosis or kyphoscoliosis, these osteotomies would preferentially be compressed on the convexity of a scoliosis. An open surgery allows for bilateral osteotomies in the thoracic and/or lumbar spine. For minimal access surgery, no option yet exists for thoracic posterior column osteotomies. However, in the lumbar spine multilevel MIS TLIF, surgery can achieve unilateral facetectomies. When combined with interbody height restoration, this approach can lead to meaningful deformity correction, even in a rigid spine (Figs. 22.1 and 22.2).

The application of MIS TLIF typically requires some degree of facet removal to access the disc space safely. If a full facetectomy is desired, this can be performed efficiently through a small mini-open approach or a large tubular dilator retractor. An osteotome can be used to remove the lateral facet to access the neuroforamen. The medial facet can then be removed by drilling or use of an osteotome. A typical three-level osteotomy can be accomplished in minutes, so long as an extensive unilateral laminotomy or central decompression is not necessary.

It must be emphasized that use of facet osteotomies requires mobility of the intervertebral disc or the release of the anterior column. In a multilevel TLIF, this can be accomplished with disc removal and application of expandable cages. In addition, if increased lordosis is desired, the surgeon would typically approach along the side of the *concavity* of the scoliosis. Compression of the osteotomies then will increase lordosis as well as straighten the scoliosis.

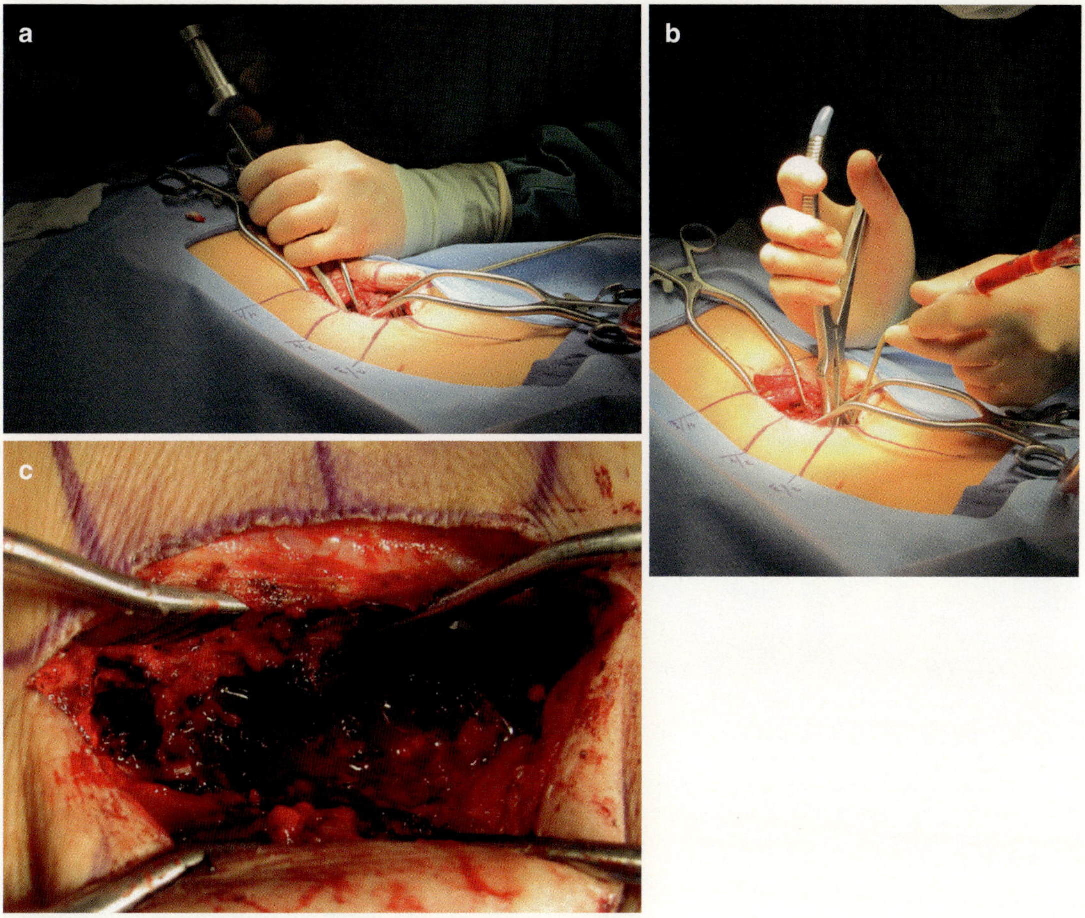

Fig. 22.1 A mini-open unilateral approach allows the surgeon to access multiple facet joints of interest while preserving much of the dorsal musculature and ligamentous attachments. (**a**) An osteotome or (**b**) Leksell rongeur can then be used to remove the facet joint efficiently at (**c**) multiple levels

22.4 Three-Column Osteotomies (Grades III through IV)

Significantly more corrective power can be achieved using a three-column osteotomy. Three-column techniques include the pedicle subtraction osteotomy (PSO) and vertebral column resection, Grades III–IV and Grades V–VI, respectively.

The morbidity of open Grades III–IV osteotomies stems from (1) the deconditioned and debilitated patient population, (2) the need for long-segment fusion and instrumentation, (3) the significant amount of deformity correction achieved at the time of surgery, (4) the prolonged anesthetic times, (5) the blood loss at the osteotomy site, (5) the high prevalence of this being a revision operation, and (6) the risk to surrounding neural elements with osteotomy closure.

To date, no publications have emerged demonstrating a true MIS invasive vertebral column resection in humans, and tubular retractor-based approaches for three-column osteotomy have been limited to cadaveric studies. In the report by Voyadis et al. [3] nine cadavers underwent a bilateral PSO procedure. While the degree of lordosis created was not specified, it appeared to

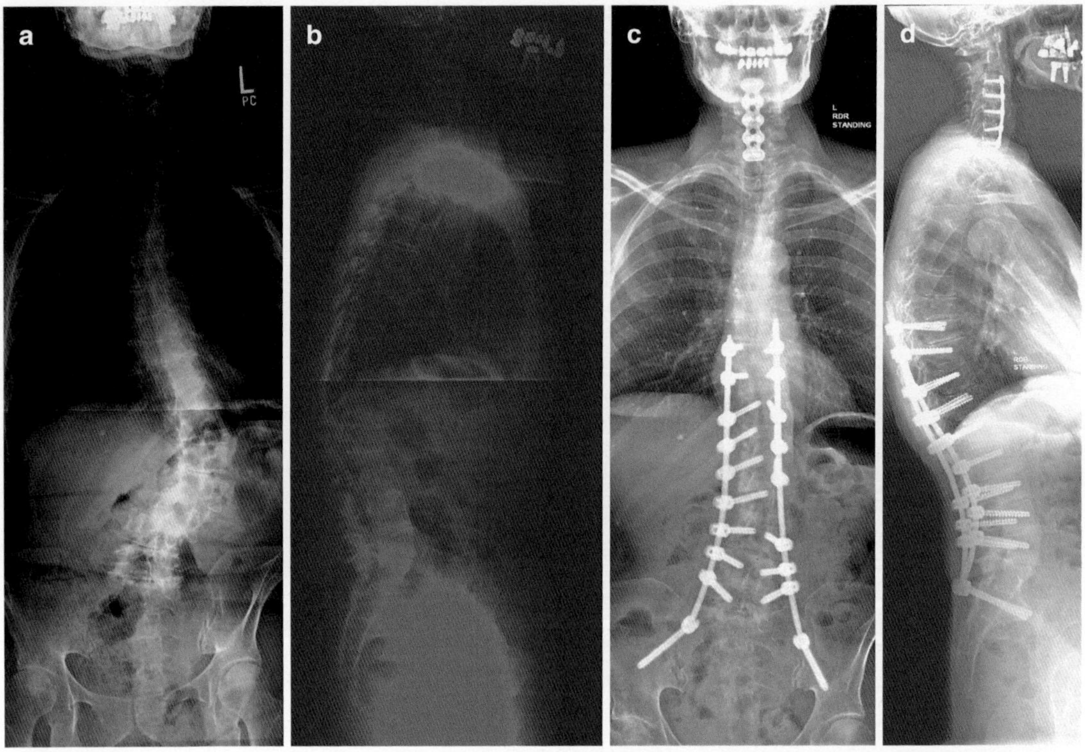

Fig. 22.2 (**a** and **b**) Preoperative and (**c** and **d**) postoperative long cassette X-rays demonstrating the powerful effect of four levels of facet osteotomies (L2-S1) combined with expandable interbody cages in a four-level MIS TLIF procedure to mobilize the spine. The hardware spans from T9 to the pelvis with facet joint fusions at T9-L2

be more "modest" than with open surgery. In the clinical setting, de-cancellation and cortical bone removal are less challenging than controlling and managing the osteotomy closure and protection of the neural elements.

However, advances have recently been made in less invasive PSO methods [4]. This has been driven by the high complication rates associated with these relatively morbid operations. We have recently begun performing the PSO procedure using a mini-open technique. This exposure, similar to a single-level lumbar fusion, allows for direct visualization of neural elements, management of blood loss, and control of wedge closure [4].

22.5 Mini-Open PSO Surgical Technique

The surgical procedure is performed with the patient prone on a Jackson table. A midline skin incision is made from the lower thoracic area to the sacrum allowing for a subcutaneous dissection which exposes the muscle fascia. All subsequent steps are performed through the fascia as opposed to using multiple stab incisions, which are cosmetically less favorable and result in more blood loss.

A bilateral subperiosteal dissection is then taken laterally at the level of the intended PSO (L2 or L3). The extent of the exposure should be so that the transverse processes of the PSO level L3 are exposed. Interbody fusion below the level of the PSO is undertaken with multiple MIS TLIF's.

At the PSO site, the spinous process, lamina, and facets are removed with a rongeur. The nerve roots above and below the pedicle are skeletonized. The PSO pedicles are then removed entirely using rongeurs and the high-speed drill. A bilateral de-cancellation osteotomy is then performed with successively larger curettes to remove two cones of cancellous bone from the vertebral body. The de-cancellation is extended medially and laterally. Sponges are then used to dissect and secure the lateral vertebral wall and its associated vasculature. A Leksell rongeur is then used to remove the lateral vertebral body wall bilaterally in a wedge-shaped pattern to match the de-cancellation.

Control of the spine is then achieved by placing percutaneous pedicle screws at least three levels above and below the PSO site prior to final osteotomy destabilization. Four rods are then bent to the appropriate lordosis and passed through each set of screw heads above and below the PSO. Set screws are then used to loosely attach each of the four rods to its respective set of screws. This prevents any catastrophic vertebral translation during completion of the osteotomy.

Finally, the posterior vertebral body wall and posterior longitudinal ligament are removed by retracting the thecal sac medially on each side successively. The wedge osteotomy is then closed by bringing the cranial and caudal rod holders towards one another. The lumbar region develops lordosis, and the soft tissue and skin is seen to go from taught to slackened. Once the wedge is closed, the neural elements are inspected to be sure there is no cauda equina or nerve root impingement. A rod-to-rod connector is then placed on the end of each rod at the PSO site where the tip is exposed (Figs. 22.3, 22.4, 22.5, 22.6, and 22.7). The set screws are then finally tightened.

22.6 Future Directions

The use of MIS techniques to treat spinal deformity is improving with advances in surgical technique, intraoperative imaging, anesthetic management, and spinal implants. While destabilizing osteotomies remain a cornerstone of open adult deformity surgery, this remains an era in crucial need of advancement for MIS spinal surgery. Future studies on large patient cohorts

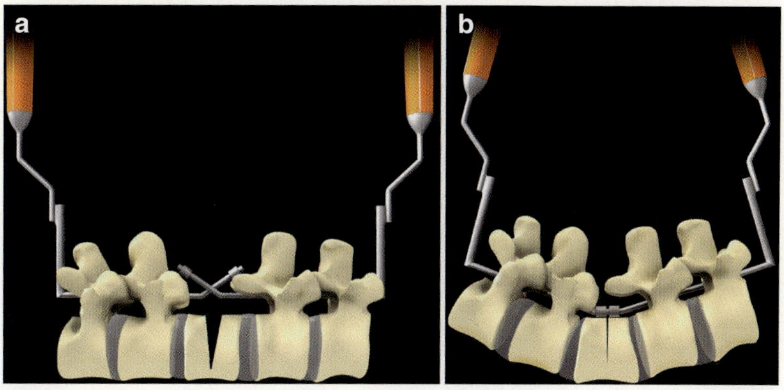

Fig. 22.3 An artist's depiction of a four-rod cantilever technique which can be used to correct kyphoscoliosis across a mini-open pedicle subtraction osteotomy. (**a**) Prior to correction. (**b**) After correction

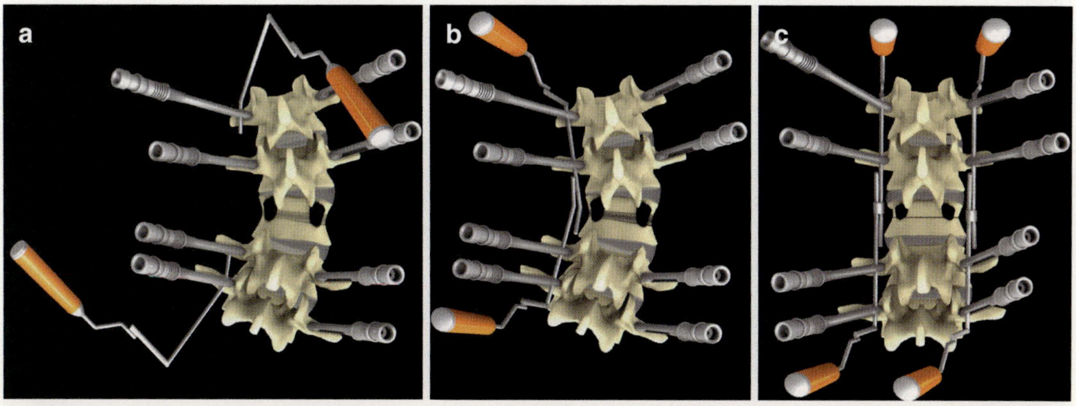

Fig. 22.4 Simultaneous correction in the coronal plane using the four-rod technique. (**a**) Prior to insertion of the rods. (**b**) Prior to correction. (**c**) After correction

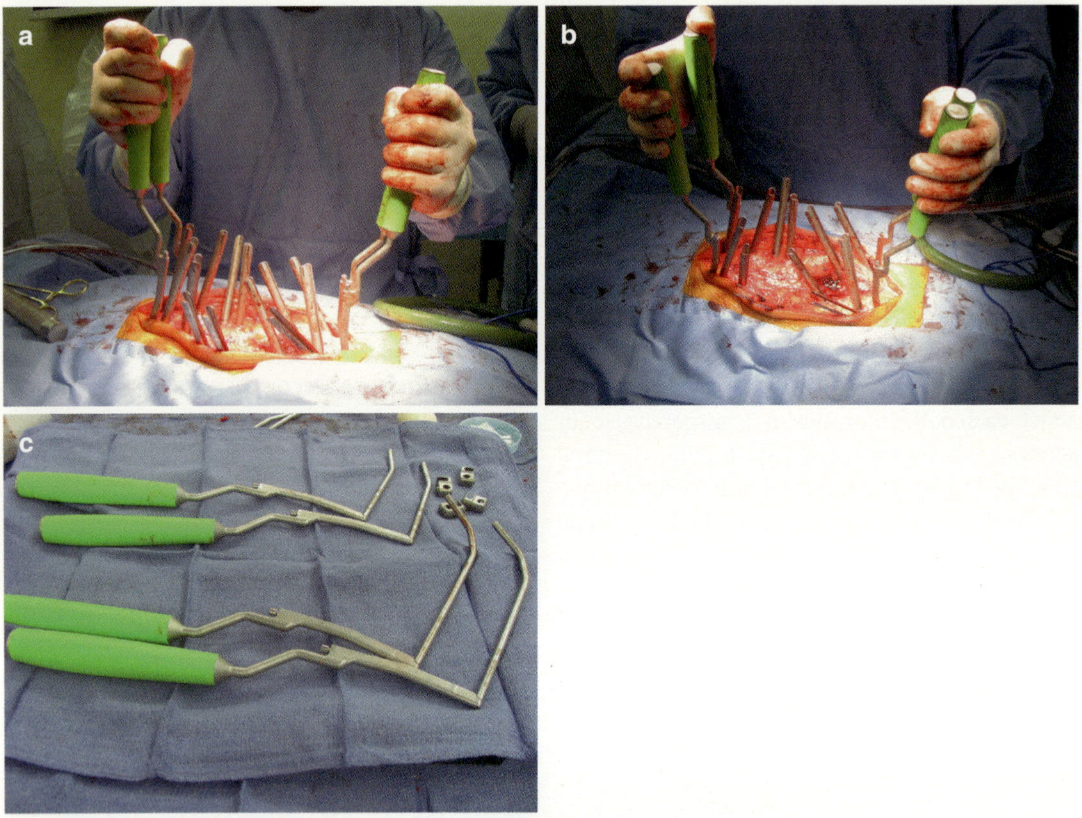

Fig. 22.5 (**a–c**) Intraoperative photos of a four-rod method to correct kyphoscoliosis. Note the use of rod holder extensions to both drive and control the wedge closure. Reduced rod bending also minimizes metal fatigue promoting hardware durability

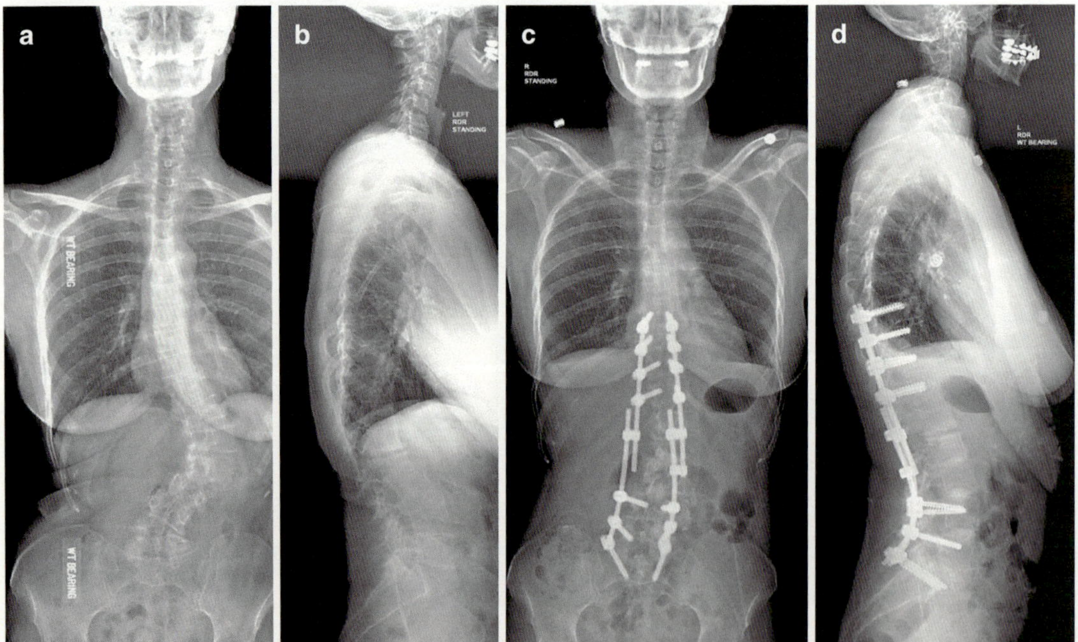

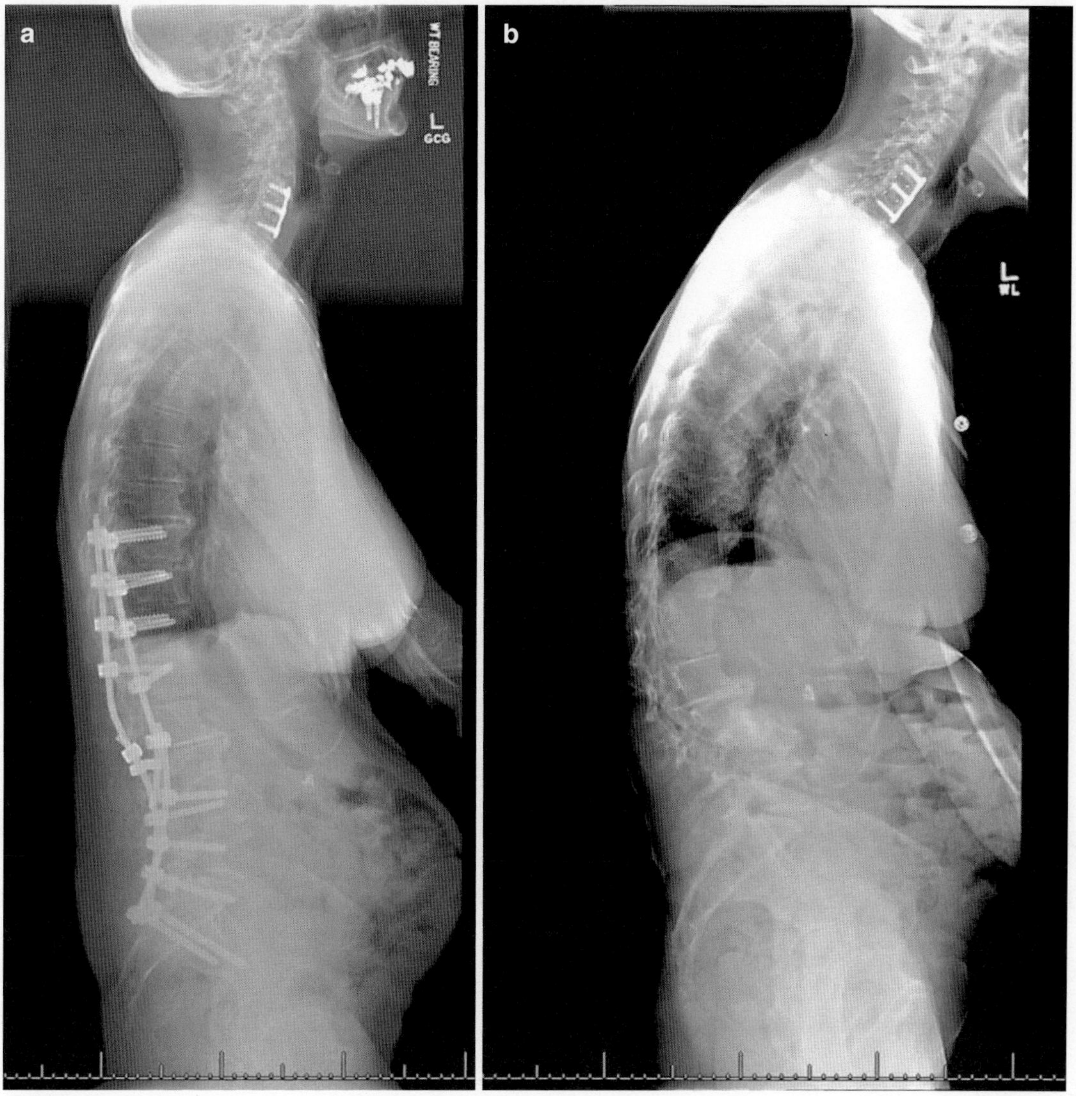

Fig. 22.7 (**a** and **b**) Case example of a more severe case of coronal and sagittal deformity treated with a mini-open PSO and multi-level TLIF

Fig. 22.6 (**a–d**) Case example of a patient with kyphoscoliosis undergoing a mini-PSO at the L2 level with an L3-S1 MIS TLIF. This is supplemented with T9-S1 percutaneous instrumented fusion undergoing less invasive high-grade osteotomies will be needed to validate the effectiveness of the techniques. However, such solutions are needed by an ever growing population of elderly spinal deformity patients.

References

1. Lafage V. Likelihood of reaching Minimal Clinically Important Difference (MCID) in Health Related Quality of Life (HRQOL) measures: prospective analysis of operative and non–operative treatment of Adult Spinal Deformity (ASD), in AANS/CNS Joint Spine Section Meeting. Phoenix; 2013.
2. Lafage V, Smith J, Bess S, Schwab F, Ames C, Klineberg E, Arlet V, Hostin R, Burton D, Shaffrey C, Group. ISS. Sagittal spino-pelvic alignment failures following three column thoracic osteotomy for adult spinal deformity. Eur Spine J. 2012;21:698–704.
3. Voyadis J, Gala V, O'Toole J, Eicholz K, Fessler R. Minimally invasive posterior osteotomies. Neurosurgery. 2008;63:A204–10.
4. Wang M, Madhavan K. Mini-open pedicle subtraction osteotomy: surgical technique. World Neurosurg. Available online 5 October 2012.

Part IV

Lateral Approaches

Thoracoscopic Approaches 23

Jonathan D. Choi and Robert E. Isaacs

The anatomy of the thoracic spine with a narrow thoracic spinal canal, the sensitivity of the spinal cord to minimal retraction, the ribcage, and the proximity to the lungs, heart, great vessels, and the diaphragm make selection of surgical approach to the thoracic spine of utmost importance. Spine surgeons first started treating patients with thoracic herniated discs through a posterior approach by laminectomy with or without discectomy. In 1969, Perot and Munro compiled 91 cases of thoracic herniated disc treated from a dorsal approach. Of the 91 patients, 16 became paraplegic and 6 died [1]. Of the patients with disc herniations in the central portion of the canal, the rate of paraplegia was 26 % and mortality was 9 %. The poor results highlighted the sensitivity of the spinal cord to retraction and the difficulty in treating anterior thoracic spine pathology. To obtain a more direct visualization and minimize retraction of the spinal cord, posterolateral (including transpedicular and transfacet), lateral (including costotransversectomy and extracavitary), and transthoracic approaches were developed.

Lesions in the vertebral body or located in the central anterior spinal canal benefit from a transthoracic approach for direct visualization of the pathology and the ventral dura to avoid retraction on the spinal cord. The transthoracic approach was initially done via open thoracotomy, in most cases requiring a thoracic surgeon to assist with the approach, a chest tube postoperatively, having a high rate of intercostal neuralgia (reported to be as high as 50 %), and having the risk of damage to the lung, heart, and great vessels [2, 3]. The open surgical approaches had significant morbidity related to the approach itself. Fessler and Sturgill reported the transthoracic approach was associated with intercostal neuralgia, pneumonia, atelectasis, hemothorax, and chylothorax [4]. In an effort to reduce the morbidity of the approach while retaining effectiveness and safety, minimally invasive alternatives to open thoracotomy have been developed, namely, thoracoscopic and mini-open transthoracic endoscopic approaches.

Minimally invasive alternatives to open thoracotomy were made possible by adoption of endoscopic and fiberoptic technology. The first endoscopic device for medical use was developed in Germany in 1806 by Philipp Bozzini and first adapted for thoracoscopy in 1910 by Hans Christian Jacobaeus [5, 6]. In the 1970s, fiberoptic and endoscopic video camera technology increased the use of thoracoscopy [7–9]. In 1993, Mack and colleagues and Rosenthal and colleagues were the first to perform spinal surgery with thoracoscopy [10, 11]. Since then, thoracoscopy has been applied to various spinal pathologies and shown to be advantageous over thoracotomy.

Thoracoscopic spinal surgery is performed with the patient in the lateral decubitus position with the ipsilateral arm abducted and placed on an armrest. The patient is intubated with a dual lumen tube for single-lung ventilation and

J.D. Choi, M.D. • R.E. Isaacs, M.D. (✉)
Spine Surgery, Duke University Medical Center, Durham, NC, USA
e-mail: robert.isaacs@dvm.duke.edu

M.Y. Wang et al. (eds.), *Minimally Invasive Spinal Deformity Surgery*,
DOI 10.1007/978-3-7091-1407-0_23, © Springer-Verlag Wien 2014

collapse of the ipsilateral lung. The side of approach is dictated by anatomy and location of the lesion. Above T11, the side of approach is dictated by the location of the lesion and the anatomy of the aorta, vena cava, and azygos vein. At T11 and T12, the liver blocks downward retraction of the diaphragm and requires a left-sided approach unless a right-sided approach is absolutely required [12, 13]. C-arm fluoroscopy is used to localize the target level [2, 3]. Typically three to four ports are inserted through 1.0–1.5 cm skin incisions and blunt dissection over the superior aspect of the rib to avoid injury to the neurovascular bundle running underneath the rib [14]. One port is placed in the posterior axillary line directly lateral to the pathology, and the other ports are placed on the anterior axillary line [14]. The first port is placed blindly and has the greatest risk for injury to the lung. Risk is minimized by single-lung ventilation and collapse of the ipsilateral lung. The subsequent ports are inserted under endoscopic visualization from the first port. The patient is then rolled ventrally by 15–30° to let the lung fall away from the operative site, and a fan retractor can be used to hold the lung out of view. The operator stands on the ventral side of the patient with the first assistant. A second assistant stands opposite the main operator. Pleural adhesions are taken down, and the ribs are counted internally to localize the target level again in addition to use of fluoroscopy. At this point the spinal column is exposed for the operation. The camera can then be fixed to a table mounting system if desired. Subsequent spinal dissection is specific to the pathology addressed such as herniated disc, infection, scoliosis, tumor, or interbody fusion [14–17]. The critical concepts common to these surgeries are that the rib head articulates with superior aspect of the same numbered vertebral body, just below or at the level of the disc space. Dissection and drilling is done for adequate visualization of normal dura above and below the lesion and creation of defect into which pathology can be delivered away from the spinal cord to prevent any retraction on the spinal cord. Once the pathology is addressed, a chest tube is placed and the chest incisions closed. The chest tube is kept until output is less than 100 mL/day [3]. If a dural defect is encountered, the chest tube is kept on water seal only and a lumbar drain is placed.

An example of these key surgical concepts is the procedure for removing a centrally located herniated disc as seen here in preoperative MRI (Fig. 23.1) and CT films (Fig. 23.2) of a patient treated with mini-open transthoracic endoscopic technique. The pleura over the target disc space is incised and the segmental vessels ligated and clipped. The proximal 2 cm of rib is then drilled

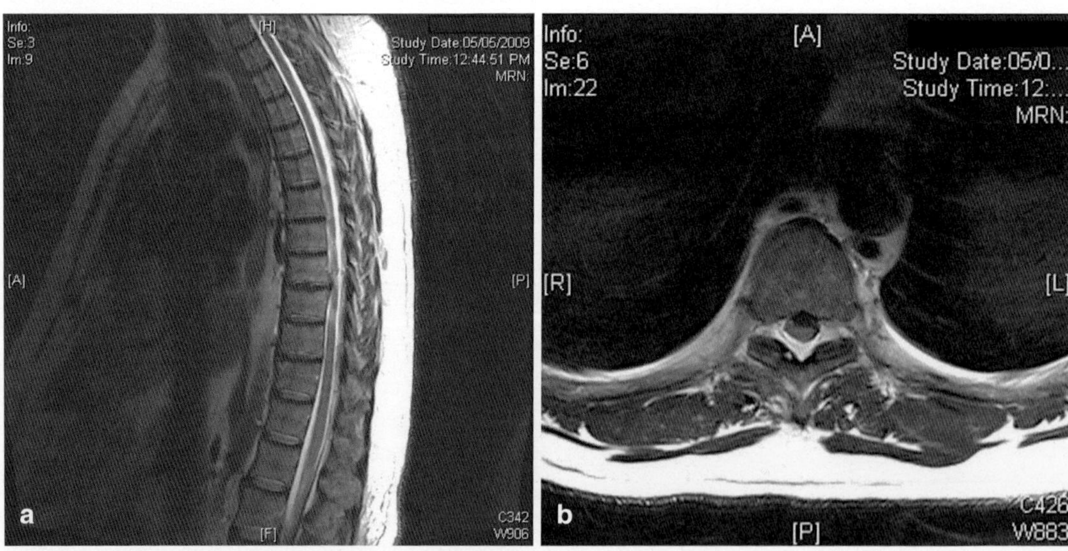

Fig. 23.1 Thoracic herniated disc on MRI. (**a**) A T8-9 herniated disc on sagittal MRI. (**b**) Axial MRI showing a left sided paracentral disc at T8-9 deforming the spinal cord without significant cord signal abnormality

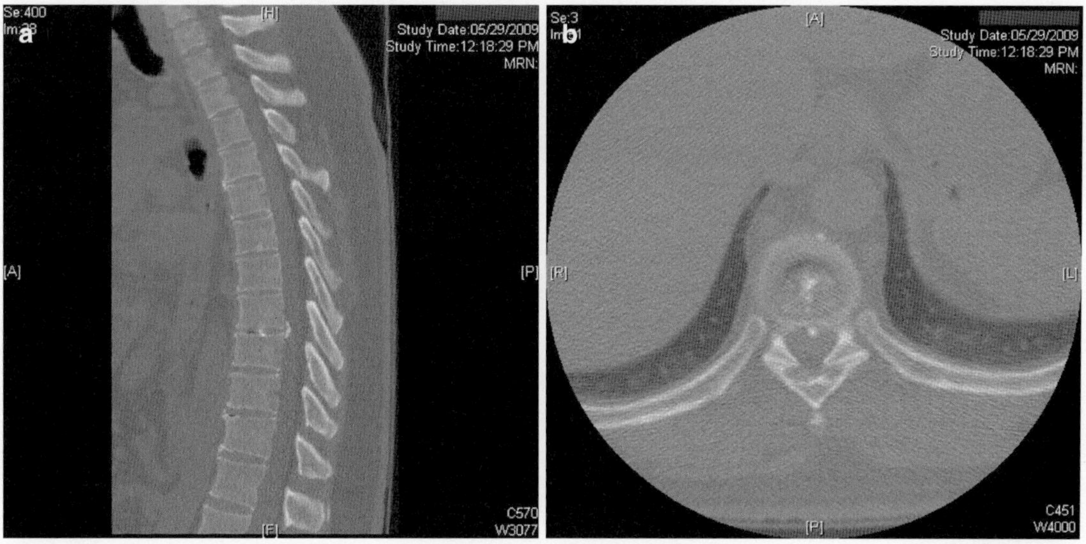

Fig. 23.2 Thoracic herniated disc on CT. (**a**) A T8-9 herniated disc on sagittal CT. (**b**) Axial CT showing calcification in the T8-9 disc herniation

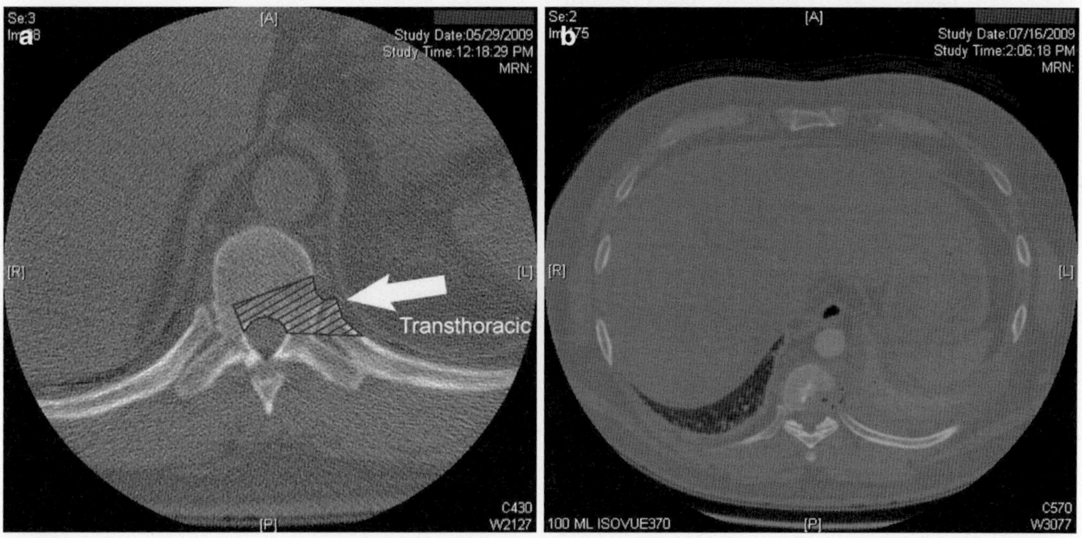

Fig. 23.3 Anterior transthoracic approach for discectomy. (**a**) The disc is removed and a wedge shaped cavity is drilled into the posterior aspect of the vertebral bodies above and below the disc space. This provides a cavity to safely deliver the calcified disc away from the dura, avoiding any manipulation or retraction the spinal cord. (**b**) Postoperative CT scan

and removed, saving the bone for autograft if needed. The superior half of the inferior pedicle is drilled down to define the lateral aspect of the spinal canal. Then the disc is incised and disc material removed, leaving the posterior aspect of the disc to be removed later. A wedge-shaped cavity is then drilled by removing the posterior aspects of the superior and inferior vertebral bodies until normal dura is seen above and below the herniated disc fragment. For a large herniated disc, this may require partial or full vertebrectomies above and below the disc interspace. After the cavity is formed, the herniated disc is carefully delivered into the cavity without manipulating the spinal cord. This bony defect can be seen in the postoperative CT scan in Fig. 23.3. If a dural erosion is found after herniated disc removal, the dura can be primarily repaired or a dural graft with fibrin glue can be placed. Placement of an interbody graft is not necessary for small bony defects, as few patients require reoperation for loss of stability [2, 3]. However, if a large defect is created, a rib graft can be placed. Some authors advocate standard placement of an interbody graft after discectomy to minimize risk of delayed postoperative kyphosis and axial pain [18–21].

A comparison of thoracoscopy and open thoracotomy was performed by Rosenthal and Dickman. They reported on 55 patients that underwent thoracoscopic herniated disc removal and 18 patients that underwent open thoracotomy [3]. They found that mean operative time for thoracoscopic disc removal was 3 h and 25 min, 1 h less operative time than thoracotomy. In addition, when compared to thoracotomy, thoracoscopy resulted in one-half the blood loss (327 vs. 683 mL), one-half the duration of chest tube drainage, and less than one-half of the length of hospital stay (6.5 vs. 16.2 days). Complications included hemothorax from intercostal vessel and segmental vessel bleeding, transient intercostal neuralgia, and two patients with retained fragments of disc material. Only 16 % of patients experienced intercostal neuralgia as opposed to 50 % of the patients who had a thoracotomy due to decreased intercostal retraction. Contraindications to thoracoscopy include patients unable to undergo single-lung ventilation or patients with significant pleural adhesions. The development of thoracoscopy alleviates much of the morbidity of the open thoracotomy approach while maintaining effectiveness in treating the pathology.

Despite showing clear benefits in reducing approach-related morbidity, thoracoscopy has been slow to be adopted by spine surgeons for a number of reasons: lack of 3D visualization, minimal tactile feedback, steep learning curve requiring specialized training in the lab prior to clinical use, and expensive equipment and instrumentation [22–25]. The mini-open transthoracic endoscopic approach was first described by Isaacs and colleagues to accomplish the same goals of reducing approach-related morbidity, but with tools and techniques more familiar to and readily adaptable by the minimally invasive spine surgeon [26]. Our study showed the feasibility and safety of using instrumentation developed for the eXtreme Lateral Interbody Fusion (XLIF) approach to treat a variety of pathologies including thoracic disc herniation, pathologic fractures from tumor, degenerative scoliosis, discitis, and adjacent level disease from prior fusions. The patient is positioned in the same way as for the thoracoscopic approach. The patient is then intubated with a single-lumen tube as the ipsilateral lung does not need to be collapsed for the procedure, allowing for both lungs to be ventilated throughout the procedure. A single 4 cm incision is made directly lateral to the level of interest, and the spine can be approached via either an extrapleural approach or transpleural approach. In the transpleural approach, the lung is deflated digitally and a dilator is slid down the posterior ribcage until it is safely docked on the spine. Sequential dilators are placed until a three-blade MaXcess XLIF-T system is inserted and docked on the spine with the help of fluoroscopy. An intraoperative photo of the mini-open transthoracic endoscopic setup is seen in Fig. 23.4. The view through the endoscope in the same setup is seen in Fig. 23.5. Limitations occur with tube technology as one proceeds more cephalad in the thoracic spine. Floating ribs do not provide a significant obstacle to distraction, but only limited intercostal distraction is possible as one moves higher into the thoracic spine. Some authors suggest using thoracoscopy to take down adhesions and directly visualize placement of the tubular retractor to avoid injury to the lungs [27]. Once the system is docked, a microscope can be used with bayonetted instruments to provide three-dimensional visualization of the anatomy, or a 30° endoscope can be inserted for visualization. A chest tube is inserted if the approach is transpleural. If the approach is extrapleural, a chest tube is not needed. If a chest tube is placed, it can be removed in the postoperative recovery room if a portable film shows no residual pneumothorax.

In a study by Uribe et al. examining the experience with mini-open transthoracic approach for disc herniation in 60 patients, the

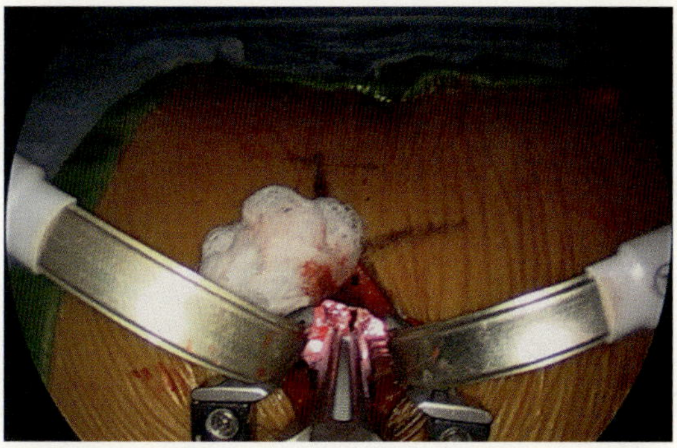

Fig. 23.4 Mini-open transthoracic endoscopic equipment setup. The surgeon stands on the ventral side of the patient. At the top of the photograph is the patient's back. There are three blades with fiber-optic lighting attached to two blades. The discectomy can be seen in the bottom of the surgical site

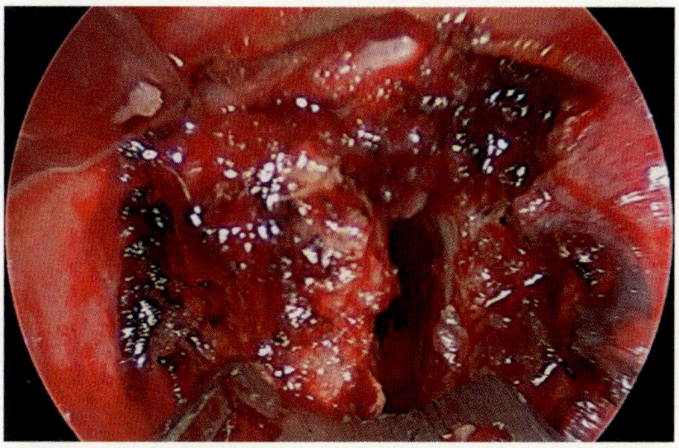

Fig. 23.5 Endoscopic view of the discectomy using a mini-open transthoracic endoscopic approach as seen with the same orientation and setup as in the photograph from Figure 23.4. The rib head overlying the disc space has been removed and the discectomy has been started

complication rate was 15 % compared to 28.4 % in previously reported minimally invasive approaches and 36.7 % in open approaches [28]. No patient in the study experienced intercostal neuralgia. Outcomes were consistent with previous reports in the minimally invasive literature with 80 % with excellent or good outcomes, 15 % unchanged, and 5 % with poor outcomes. This exceeds the reported outcomes for open approaches of 64.4 % with excellent or good outcome. The mini-open transthoracic approach avoids the approach morbidity of open thoracotomy while using techniques familiar to the minimally invasive spine surgeons, offering direct visualization of the ventral dura and achieving improved patient outcomes. Advantages of mini-open transthoracic endoscopic surgery over thoracoscopy are summarized in Fig. 23.6 and include surgeon familiarity with instrumentation, dual-lung ventilation, option of extrapleural dissection obviating the need for chest tube placement, and the freedom to choose endoscopic visualization or the use of the operative microscope with three-dimensional visualization. The disadvantages include inability to directly visualize retractor system placement and inability to take down pleural adhesions safely.

Both thoracoscopic and mini-open transthoracic endoscopic approaches have been applied to the treatment of idiopathic and degenerative thoracic spine deformity. Thoracoscopic anterior release has been used to treat large (>70° Cobb measurements) stiff curves, hyperkyphosis, or lordosis traditionally treated with open thoracotomy [29]. Sucato et al. described a technique of performing the thoracoscopic anterior release with the patient in the prone position, allowing for dual-lung ventilation and obviating the need to change patient position for the posterior instrumentation and fusion [30, 31]. The advantages of thoracoscopy over open thoracotomy for anterior release and fusion are decreased anterior operative time, decreased blood loss and chest tube drainage, and more complete disc excision with comparable correction of deformity and similar complication rates [32]. For an in-depth discussion of the indications and outcomes for treating idiopathic scoliosis with video-assisted thoracoscopic surgery (VATS), please refer to Al-Sayyad et al. retrospective Cincinnati series on 100 consecutive patients treated with VATS [33]. Degenerative, spondylitis, traumatic, and metastatic thoracic deformity have also been treated successfully with both thoracoscopic and mini-open transthoracic endoscopic techniques [26, 34, 35]. Kai-Michael Scheufler reported a series of patients treated with retropleural mini-open transthoracic endoscopic vertebral body replacement cages and ventrolateral plate fixation with equivalent correction of deformity, reduced perioperative morbidity and pain, expedited ambulation, no need

	Thoracoscopy	Mini-open transthoracic
Positives	Four 1–1.5 cm skin incisions Minimal retraction on the neurovascular bundle Direct visualization of intrathoracic approch and ability to take down pleural adhesions Internal counting of ribs for additional intra-op localization	One 4 cm skin incision Minimal retraction on the neurovascular bundle Tools are easily adapted by the spine surgeon familiar with the XLIF approach Flexibility of 2-D endoscope or 3-D operating microscope use Approach can be extrapleural, preventing need for a chest tube Dual lung ventilation during the case without need for lung collapse
Negatives	Step learning curve with instruments unfamiliar to the spine surgeon 2-D visualization Requires dual lumen ET tube intubation with lung collapse Thoracic spine cases are a minority making it difficult to maintain technical proficiency	Blind intrathoracic approach with risk of pleural injury there are adhesions Slightly more retraction of the ribspace is required as compared to thoracoscopy Narrower field of view of the intrathoracic anatomy

Fig. 23.6 Minimally invasive anterior thoracic approaches. Thoracoscopy and mini-open transthoracic endoscopic techniques have unique advantages and disadvantages but both offer decreased approached related morbidity as compared to conventional open thoracotomy

for chest tube placement, and earlier hospital discharge as compared to conventional open surgery [35]. These recent reports highlighted the ability to treat thoracic spinal deformity with minimally invasive techniques that achieve comparable deformity correction as compared to open thoracotomy with significant reduction in approach-related morbidity.

The surgical treatment of thoracic spinal pathology has evolved rapidly over the last 20 years. Thoracoscopic and mini-open transthoracic endoscopic approaches were developed from advances in optical and lighting technology to improve the safety and efficacy of thoracic spine surgery. Both techniques require appropriate training, practice, and continued use to maintain the operative skills learned. By adopting the thoracoscopic and/or mini-open transthoracic endoscopic whether with or without endoscopy techniques, today's minimally invasive spine surgeon can safely and effectively address anterior thoracic spine pathology and minimize the approach-related morbidity associated with open thoracotomy.

References

1. Perot Jr PL, Munro DD. Transthoracic removal of midline thoracic disc protrusions causing spinal cord compression. J Neurosurg. 1969;31(4):452–8. Epub 1969/10/01.
2. Burke TG, Caputy AJ. Treatment of thoracic disc herniation: evolution toward the minimally invasive thoracoscopic technique. Neurosurg Focus. 2000;9(4):e9. Epub 2006/07/13.
3. Rosenthal D, Dickman CA. Thoracoscopic microsurgical excision of herniated thoracic discs. J Neurosurg. 1998;89(2):224–35. Epub 1998/08/04.
4. Fessler RG, Sturgill M. Review: complications of surgery for thoracic disc disease. Surg Neurol. 1998;49(6):609–18. Epub 1998/06/24.
5. Bush RB, Leonhardt H, Bush IV, Landes RR. Dr. Bozzini's Lichtleiter. A translation of his original article (1806). Urology. 1974;3(1):119–23. Epub 1974/01/01.
6. Hc J. Possibility of the use of the cystoscope for investigation of serous cavities. Munchen Med Wochenschr. 1910;57:2090–2.
7. Miller JI, Hatcher Jr CR. Thoracoscopy: a useful tool in the diagnosis of thoracic disease. Ann Thorac Surg. 1978;26(1):68–72. Epub 1978/07/01.
8. Newhouse MT. Thoracoscopy: diagnostic and therapeutic indications. Pneumologie. 1989;43(2):48–52. Epub 1989/02/01.

9. Das K, Rothberg M. Thoracoscopic surgery: historical perspectives. Neurosurg Focus. 2000;9(4):e10. Epub 2006/07/13.
10. Mack MJ, Regan JJ, Bobechko WP, Acuff TE. Application of thoracoscopy for diseases of the spine. Ann Thorac Surg. 1993;56(3):736–8. Epub 1993/09/01.
11. Rosenthal D, Rosenthal R, de Simone A. Removal of a protruded thoracic disc using microsurgical endoscopy. A new technique. Spine. 1994;19(9):1087–91. Epub 1994/05/01.
12. Bohlman HH, Zdeblick TA. Anterior excision of herniated thoracic discs. J Bone Joint Surg Am. 1988;70(7):1038–47. Epub 1988/08/01.
13. Dickman CA, Rosenthal D, Karahalios DG, Paramore CG, Mican CA, Apostolides PJ, et al. Thoracic vertebrectomy and reconstruction using a microsurgical thoracoscopic approach. Neurosurgery. 1996;38(2):279–93. Epub 1996/02/01.
14. Oskouian Jr RJ, Johnson JP, Regan JJ. Thoracoscopic microdiscectomy. Neurosurgery. 2002;50(1):103–9. Epub 2002/02/15.
15. Lall RR, Smith ZA, Wong AP, Miller D, Fessler RG. Minimally invasive thoracic corpectomy: surgical strategies for malignancy, trauma, and complex spinal pathologies. Minim Invasive Surg. 2012;2012:213791. Epub 2012/08/14.
16. Visocchi M, Masferrer R, Sonntag VK, Dickman CA. Thoracoscopic approaches to the thoracic spine. Acta Neurochir (Wien). 1998;140(8):737–43; discussion 43–4. Epub 1998/11/12.
17. Rosenthal D, Marquardt G, Lorenz R, Nichtweiss M. Anterior decompression and stabilization using a microsurgical endoscopic technique for metastatic tumors of the thoracic spine. J Neurosurg. 1996;84(4):565–72. Epub 1996/04/01.
18. Khoo LT, Smith ZA, Asgarzadie F, Barlas Y, Armin SS, Tashjian V, et al. Minimally invasive extracavitary approach for thoracic discectomy and interbody fusion: 1-year clinical and radiographic outcomes in 13 patients compared with a cohort of traditional anterior transthoracic approaches. J Neurosurg Spine. 2011;14(2):250–60. Epub 2011/01/11.
19. Currier BL, Eismont FJ, Green BA. Transthoracic disc excision and fusion for herniated thoracic discs. Spine. 1994;19(3):323–8. Epub 1994/02/01.
20. Korovessis PG, Stamatakis MV, Baikousis A, Vasiliou D. Transthoracic disc excision with interbody fusion. 12 patients with symptomatic disc herniation followed for 2–8 years. Acta Orthop Scand Suppl. 1997;275:12–6. Epub 1997/12/31.
21. Otani K, Yoshida M, Fujii E, Nakai S, Shibasaki K. Thoracic disc herniation. Surgical treatment in 23 patients. Spine. 1988;13(11):1262–7. Epub 1988/11/01.
22. Ringel F, Stoffel M, Stuer C, Totzek S, Meyer B. Endoscopy-assisted approaches for anterior column reconstruction after pedicle screw fixation of acute traumatic thoracic and lumbar fractures. Neurosurgery 2008;62(5 Suppl 2):ONS445–52; discussion ONS52–3. Epub 2008/07/18.
23. McAfee PC, Regan JR, Fedder IL, Mack MJ, Geis WP. Anterior thoracic corpectomy for spinal cord decompression performed endoscopically. Surg Laparosc Endosc. 1995;5(5):339–48. Epub 1995/10/01.
24. McAfee PC, Regan JR, Zdeblick T, Zuckerman J, Picetti 3rd GD, Heim S, et al. The incidence of complications in endoscopic anterior thoracolumbar spinal reconstructive surgery. A prospective multicenter study comprising the first 100 consecutive cases. Spine. 1995;20(14):1624–32. Epub 1995/07/15.
25. Khoo LT, Beisse R, Potulski M. Thoracoscopic-assisted treatment of thoracic and lumbar fractures: a series of 371 consecutive cases. Neurosurgery. 2002;51 Suppl 5:S104–17. Epub 2002/09/18.
26. Karikari IO, Nimjee SM, Hardin CA, Hughes BD, Hodges TR, Mehta AI, et al. Extreme lateral interbody fusion approach for isolated thoracic and thoracolumbar spine diseases: initial clinical experience and early outcomes. J Spinal Disord Tech. 2011;24(6):368–75. Epub 2010/12/15.
27. Yanni DS, Connery C, Perin NI. Video-assisted thoracoscopic surgery combined with a tubular retractor system for minimally invasive thoracic discectomy. Neurosurgery 2011;68 (1 Suppl Operative):138–43; discussion 43. Epub 2011/01/06.
28. Uribe JS, Smith WD, Pimenta L, Hartl R, Dakwar E, Modhia UM, et al. Minimally invasive lateral approach for symptomatic thoracic disc herniation: initial multicenter clinical experience. J Neurosurg Spine. 2012;16(3):264–79. Epub 2011/12/20.
29. Newton PO, Wenger DR, Mubarak SJ, Meyer RS. Anterior release and fusion in pediatric spinal deformity. A comparison of early outcome and cost of thoracoscopic and open thoracotomy approaches. Spine. 1997;22(12):1398–406. Epub 1997/06/15.
30. Sucato DJ, Elerson E. A comparison between the prone and lateral position for performing a thoracoscopic anterior release and fusion for pediatric spinal deformity. Spine. 2003;28(18):2176–80. Epub 2003/09/23.
31. Sucato DJ, Erken YH, Davis S, Gist T, McClung A, Rathjen KE. Prone thoracoscopic release does not adversely affect pulmonary function when added to a posterior spinal fusion for severe spine deformity. Spine. 2009;34(8):771–8. Epub 2009/04/15.
32. Son-Hing JP, Blakemore LC, Poe-Kochert C, Thompson GH. Video-assisted thoracoscopic surgery in idiopathic scoliosis: evaluation of the learning curve. Spine. 2007;32(6):703–7. Epub 2007/04/07.
33. Al-Sayyad MJ, Crawford AH, Wolf RK. Video-assisted thoracoscopic surgery: the Cincinnati experience. Clin Orthop Relat Res. 2005;434:61–70. Epub 2005/05/03.
34. Krasna MJ, Jiao X, Eslami A, Rutter CM, Levine AM. Thoracoscopic approach for spine deformities. J Am Coll Surg. 2003;197(5):777–9. Epub 2003/10/31.
35. Scheufler KM. Technique and clinical results of minimally invasive reconstruction and stabilization of the thoracic and thoracolumbar spine with expandable cages and ventrolateral plate fixation. Neurosurgery 2007;61(4):798–808; discussion -9. Epub 2007/11/08.

Role of Neuromonitoring in Minimally Invasive Lateral Approaches to the Spine

24

Khoi D. Than, Anthony C. Wang, Brian Bush, Paul Park, and Frank La Marca

24.1 Introduction

Minimally invasive approaches allow surgeons to achieve clinical outcomes similar to traditional open approaches but with decreased blood loss, postoperative pain, and length of hospital stay. In 1998, a minimally invasive retroperitoneal transpsoas approach to the lumbar spine was described that provided surgeon access to the anterior lumbar spine with less morbidity than that associated with the traditional retroperitoneal approach [1] while providing equivalent biomechanics [2]. In this procedure, the patient is typically placed in the right lateral decubitus position (so as to avoid the liver). Incisions are planned with the aid of fluoroscopy over the appropriate disc space(s) and the retroperitoneum is entered. The disc spaces are then sequentially accessed through the psoas muscle using a guidewire, dilators, and tubular retractor. Discectomy can then be performed, followed by placement of an interbody spacer. This procedure can be "stand alone" or supplemented with posterior instrumentation.

In this chapter, we review the relevant anatomy that must be considered during the lateral transpsoas approach, as well as the different types of neuromonitoring techniques that are used to maintain neural integrity. Subsequently, we review the literature on the topic of neuromonitoring in minimally invasive lateral approaches to the spine, followed by a summary of recommendations for those surgeons who utilize this versatile surgical technique.

K.D. Than (✉) • A.C. Wang • B. Bush • P. Park
Department of Neurosurgery, University of Michigan, Ann Arbor, MI, USA
e-mail: khoi@med.umich.edu

F. La Marca
University of Michigan, Ann Arbor, MI, USA

24.2 Anatomy

The primary structure at risk during a lateral approach to the lumbar spine is the lumbar plexus (Fig. 24.1). The lumbar plexus has contributions from the subcostal nerve of T12 and the ventral divisions of the L1–L5 nerve roots. The lumbar plexus has seven major branches: (1) obturator nerve (L2–L4), which supplies the adductor muscles of the leg; (2) femoral nerve (L2–L4), which supplies hip flexors and knee extensors; (3) iliohypogastric nerve (L1), which supplies sensation to the buttock and hypogastric regions; (4) ilioinguinal nerve (L1), which supplies sensation to the groin and external genitalia; (5) genitofemoral nerve (L1–L2), which supplies sensation to the genitalia and central portion of the inguinal ligament; (6) lateral femoral cutaneous nerve (L2–L3), which supplies sensation to the anterolateral thigh; and (7) lumbosacral trunk (L4–L5), which descends to join the sacral plexus. Femoral nerve injury is extremely debilitating and often results in the inability to ambulate.

A number of cadaveric studies have detailed the anatomy of the lumbar plexus in relation to the psoas major muscle and the lumbar vertebral

M.Y. Wang et al. (eds.), *Minimally Invasive Spinal Deformity Surgery*,
DOI 10.1007/978-3-7091-1407-0_24, © Springer-Verlag Wien 2014

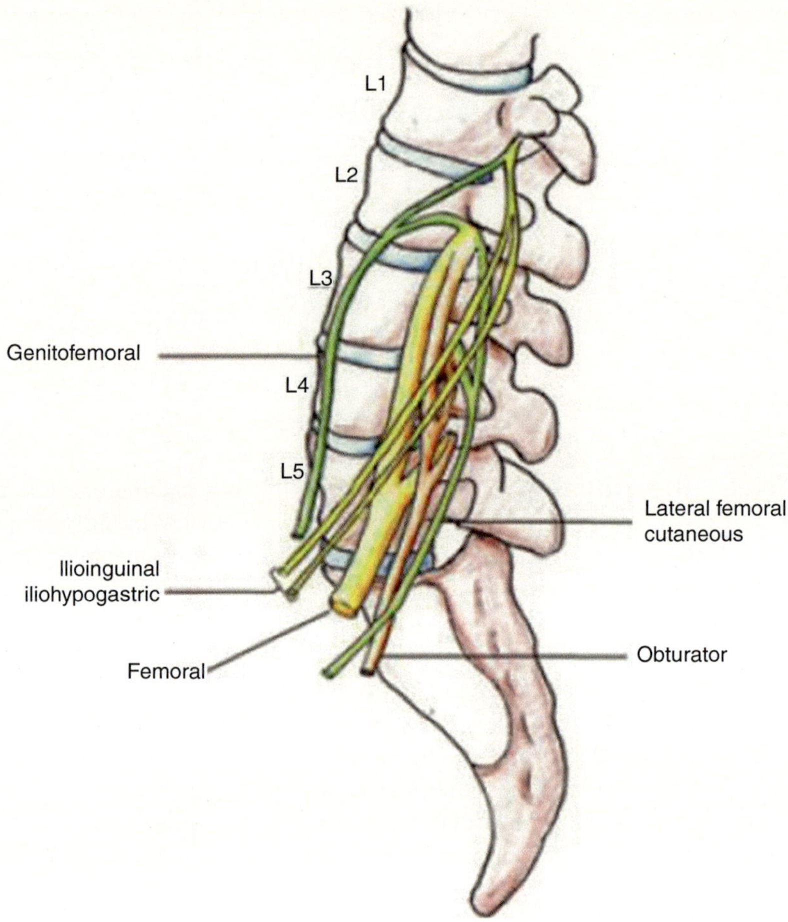

Fig. 24.1 Schematic drawing of the lumbar plexus from the lateral view (Courtesy of Dr. Juan S. Uribe)

bodies. These studies have generally divided the vertebral bodies into "safe working zones," defined by the absence of a crossing lumbar plexus branch. Four zones comprise the vertebral bodies: Zone 1 is the most ventral quarter of the vertebral body, Zone II is the middle anterior quarter, Zone III is the middle posterior quarter, and Zone IV is the most dorsal quarter (Fig. 24.2). One of the first of these cadaveric studies was conducted by Benglis et al. [3] in 2009 using three cadavers. These authors found that the lumbosacral plexus lies on the dorsal surface of the psoas muscle, within a cleft formed between the junction of the transverse process and vertebral body. The plexus was most dorsally positioned at L1–L2 (at the posterior endplate, i.e., Zone IV, at this level) and was found to migrate ventrally then caudally down the lumbar spine. The safe zones identified by this study were Zones I–III at L1–L2, L2–L3, and L3–L4 and Zones I–II at L4–L5. The authors thus suggested positioning the dilators and tubular retractors at the anterior half of the disc spaces.

In a more comprehensive analysis of 20 cadavers, Uribe et al. [4] found that all parts of the lumbar plexus, including the nerve roots, were contained within the substance of the psoas muscle dorsal to Zone IV. An important exception to this was the genitofemoral nerve, which originates at L1–L2, courses obliquely along Zone II at L2–L3, emerges superficially and anterior from the medial border of the psoas muscle at L3–L4, and courses along Zone I at L4–L5. Thus, the authors refined the safe zones of Benglis et al. to be Zone III at L1–L2, L2–L3, and L3–L4 and the midpoint of the vertebral body (Zone II/III demarcation) at L4–L5.

Two other cadaveric studies have further modified the safe working zones at each lumbar disc space. In a study of eight cadavers, Guerin

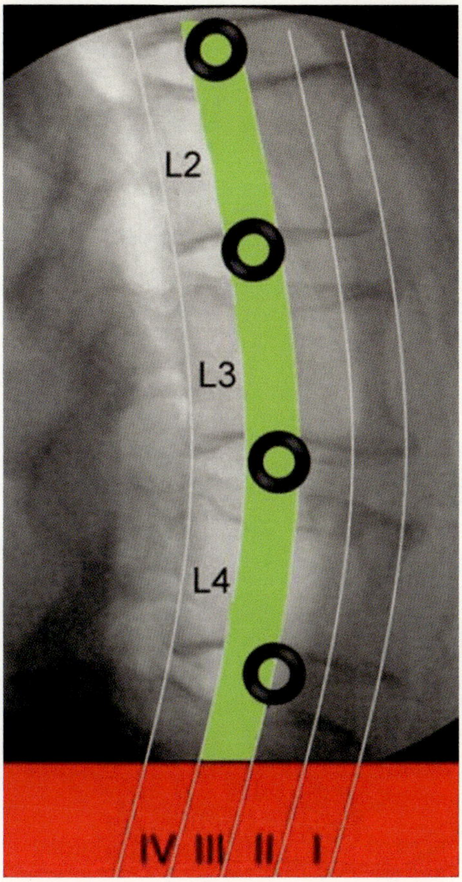

Fig. 24.2 Lateral radiograph of the lumbar spine demonstrating division of the vertebral bodies into four zones (*Zones I–IV*) from anterior to posterior. The relative "safe zone" (*Zone III*) is depicted in *green*. The recommended safe working zones to prevent direct nerve injury are indicated with *black circles* at each level (Courtesy of Dr. Juan S. Uribe)

et al. [5] found the safe zones to be Zones II–III at L1–L2, Zone III at L2–L3 and L3–L4, and Zone II at L4–L5. An early study of 30 cadavers by Moro et al. [6] found the safe zones to be Zones I–III at L1–L2 and L2–L3; these authors were concerned about injury to the genitofemoral nerve anywhere near the L3–L4 and L4–L5 disc spaces.

Analyzing the aforementioned data, the strictest safe working zones are as follows:

- L1–L2: Zone III, as advocated by Uribe et al. [4]
- L2–L3: Zone III, as advocated by Uribe et al. [4] and Guerin et al. [5]
- L3–L4: Zone III, as advocated by Uribe et al. [4] and Guerin et al. [5]
- L4–L5: Zone II, as advocated by Guerin et al. [5]

It deserves noting that Guerin et al. expressed significant concern regarding the sheer quantity of neurovascular structures at L4–L5 and advocated that other routes of access (transforaminal lumbar interbody, posterior lumbar interbody, or anterior lumbar interbody) be considered at that level.

In an important study, Dakwar et al. [7] dissected six cadavers in order to detail the anatomy of the lumbar plexus branches outside of the psoas muscle, i.e., in the retroperitoneum and abdominal wall musculature. The authors identified four nerves particularly at risk during retroperitoneal dissection: the subcostal, iliohypogastric, ilioinguinal, and lateral femoral cutaneous nerves. These nerves are also at risk for retraction injury. In order to minimize the risk of injury, the authors advocated "sequential and gentle muscle dilation with blunt instruments (hemostat forceps) until the vertebral column is identified." They also emphasized "early identification of the posterior wall of the retroperitoneum (quadratus lumborum muscle) and gentle dissection of the space from posterior to anterior and superior to inferior until the transverse process and the psoas muscle are identified at the target level, to avoid injury to the main nerves that run freely in the retroperitoneal cavity."

Injury to the nerves that supply the abdominal wall can result in abdominal flank bulge; thus, understanding this relevant anatomy is also essential. The abdominal wall consists of four major muscle groups: the rectus abdominis, transverse abdominis, and external and internal oblique muscles. The T11 and T12 intercostal nerves provide most of the innervation to the abdominal wall musculature [8], specifically via the subcostal nerve, which travels underneath the transversus abdominis muscle to innervate the rectus abdominis and external oblique muscles (Fig. 24.3) [7]. The iliohypogastric and ilioinguinal nerves also provide innervation, specifically to the internal oblique and transverse abdominis muscles. Special care must be taken to avoid severing, cauterizing, suturing, or otherwise injuring these nerves during exposure and closure.

Anatomical positioning for the minimally invasive lateral retroperitoneal transpsoas approach is worth mentioning (Fig. 24.4). Patients are placed

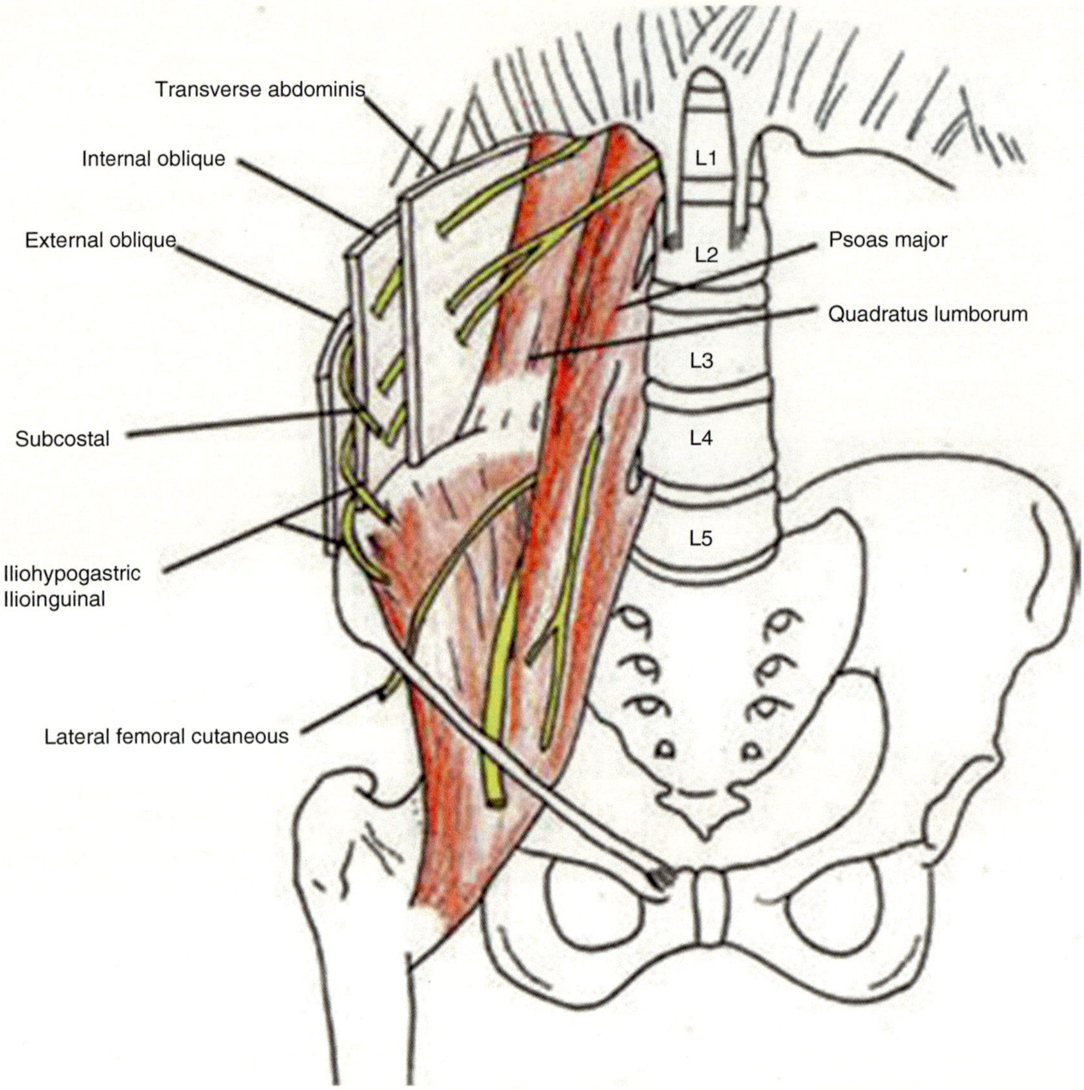

Fig. 24.3 Illustration demonstrating the trajectory of the four main nerves traveling outside the psoas muscle in the retroperitoneum along the posterior abdominal wall and within the abdominal muscles

in the lateral decubitus position with right-side down, and an axillary roll protects the axilla. The dependent (right) arm is supinated and outstretched on an arm rest with the elbow padded. The nondependent (left) arm is pronated and raised, also with the elbow padded. In a series of 1,000 consecutive spine surgeries with patients in five different positions, Kamel et al. [9] found that the lateral decubitus position was associated with the highest incidence (7.5 %) of position-related upper extremity somatosensory-evoked potential (SSEP) changes. This was thought attributable to vertical forces that compress the brachial plexus and the first rib. Thus, adequate padding and keeping the patient's limbs in unstressed positions is paramount to minimizing iatrogenic nerve injury.

24.3 Types of Monitoring

The three standard intraoperative neuromonitoring modalities used during spinal surgery are SSEPs, motor-evoked potentials (MEPs), and

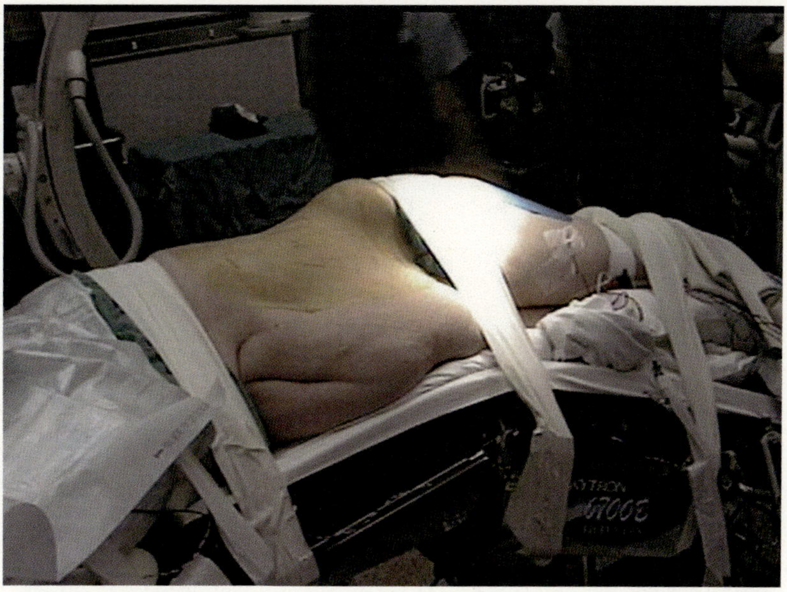

Fig. 24.4 Patient in the lateral decubitus position with the table broken

electromyography (EMG). Each of these modalities has been proposed to play an important role at specific stages of surgery. During spinal surgery, it has been suggested that neurophysiological testing helps to avoid unforeseen neuronal or vascular injury, reduces the risk of a permanent postoperative deficit, and provides localization of specific nerve roots. SSEPs comprise signals recorded from multiple positions along the afferent pathway of primarily proprioceptive tracts. These are transmitted via the dorsal columns of the spinal cord. As mentioned above, when patients are positioned laterally, SSEPs can be particularly useful in possibly identifying and reversing impending damage to peripheral nerves within both upper and lower extremities (by repositioning the extremity of concern) [9]. A peripheral disturbance in neuronal transmission may be resultant of stretch or compression in any of the extremities in this lateral position. As an example, the peripheral nerve(s) in the top arm, primarily at the site of the brachial plexus, can be stretched if proper padding techniques are not administered. The bottom arm can also experience similar strain as nerve(s) can be compressed if the head is not positioned properly in a neutral fashion and/or an axillary roll is inappropriately placed. Furthermore, compression of the ulnar nerve can occur in either of the arms if they are not adequately padded. The break in the surgical table can cause the bottom leg to be compressed or the top leg to be stretched past its functional threshold. It is of utmost importance for the neuromonitoring team to have reliable peripheral SSEP responses (recorded from Erb's point in the upper extremities and the popliteal fossa in the lower extremities) to distinguish between changes caused by positioning, surgical manipulation, pharmacological events, or underlying physiological issues.

MEPs are elicited by transcranial activation of the motor cortex and are transmitted through the lateral corticospinal tracts of the cord, exiting at each nerve root level, continuing transmission of the signal to the motor axons that innervate each of the designated muscles. MEPs have been proposed to be a very sensitive test for assessment of motor function and may allow for more rapid identification of potential damage to neural structures. Although further study is needed, some practitioners feel that effective MEP methods and techniques can give additional prognostic information for the assessment of patient outcomes.

From a technical perspective, EMG electrodes are placed in the muscles that supply the nerve(s) that may be at risk during a given procedure. For the lateral approach, these muscles include the iliopsoas, vastus lateralis, biceps femoris,

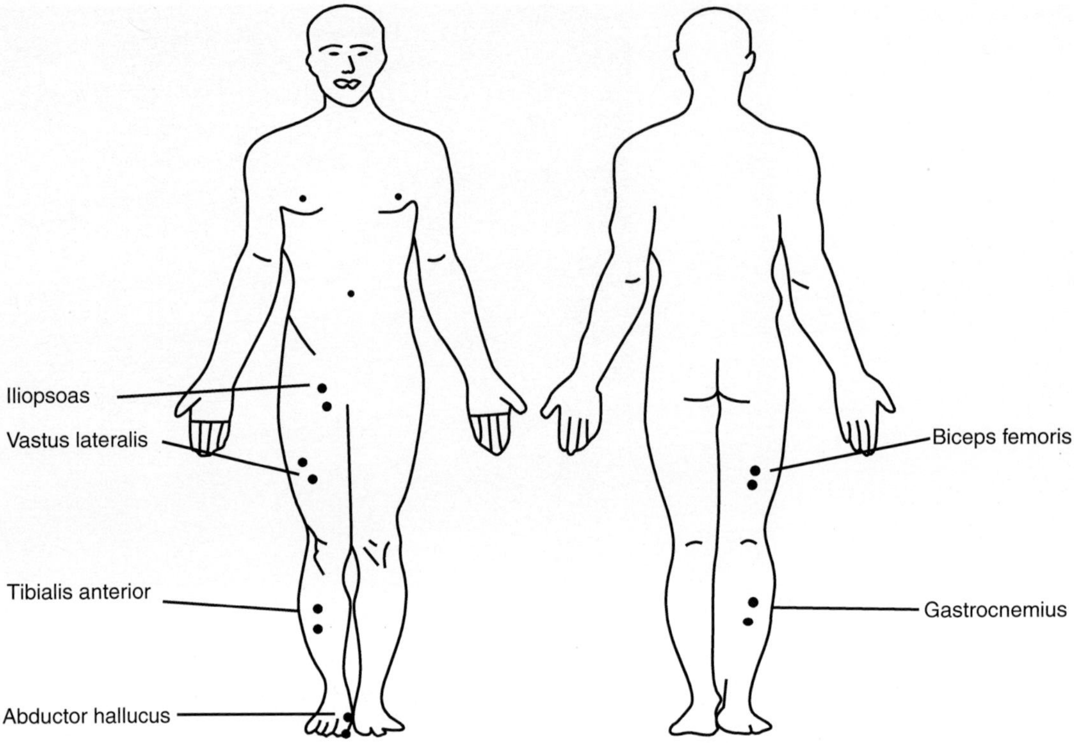

Fig. 24.5 Diagram for placement of EMG leads for lateral approaches to the spine

tibialis anterior, gastrocnemius, and abductor hallucis muscles (Fig. 24.5). Depending upon the neuromonitoring group's protocol, the electrodes used to monitor MEP responses may be sufficient to also monitor the EMG. However, in general, more extensive coverage of muscles is applied to EMG monitoring than is to MEP monitoring. It should be noted that any electrodes used to monitor EMG can theoretically be used to record MEP responses as well; two additional cortical stimulating electrodes are placed to add MEPs as a modality when requested. Both SSEP and EMG monitoring are limited in the information each can give the surgical and neuromonitoring teams (such as an ischemic event at an individual root level). Thus, MEPs may provide the surgeon with more data that can assist with surgical decision-making.

For the minimally invasive lateral transpsoas approach, the most common and beneficial neuromonitoring technique is EMG. EMG can provide real-time feedback, allow for surgical correspondence with specific nerve roots, and safely guide retractors. There are two forms of EMG: (1) free-running, which assesses continuously for evidence of nerve root manipulation, and (2) triggered, where nerves are intentionally stimulated to elicit a response (Figs. 24.6 and 24.7). EMG has high sensitivity but low specificity in predicting postoperative neurologic deficits and thus is frequently used in combination with other forms of neuromonitoring [10, 11].

The use of EMG is essential during the minimally invasive lateral transpsoas approach. In a literature review, Uribe et al. [12] concluded that the use of EMG during lateral approaches has decreased the incidence of neurologic deficit from 30 % to less than 1 % [13–16]. In this review, the authors describe a method by which the femoral nerve can be reliably positioned posterior to the retractor, thus minimizing the risk of injury by retraction. By rotating the directional EMG probe, ideal positioning relative to the femoral nerve can be confirmed by observing high stimulation thresholds anteriorly and low stimulation thresholds posteriorly. (Stimulation thresholds refer to the amount of current required to activate a nerve. Low thresholds indicate close proximity to nerve, whereas high thresholds indicate further distance from it.)

In a prospective, multicenter, industry-sponsored trial, Tohmeh et al. [17] enrolled 102 patients undergoing extreme lateral interbody fusion (XLIF) at L3–L4 and/or L4–L5 to

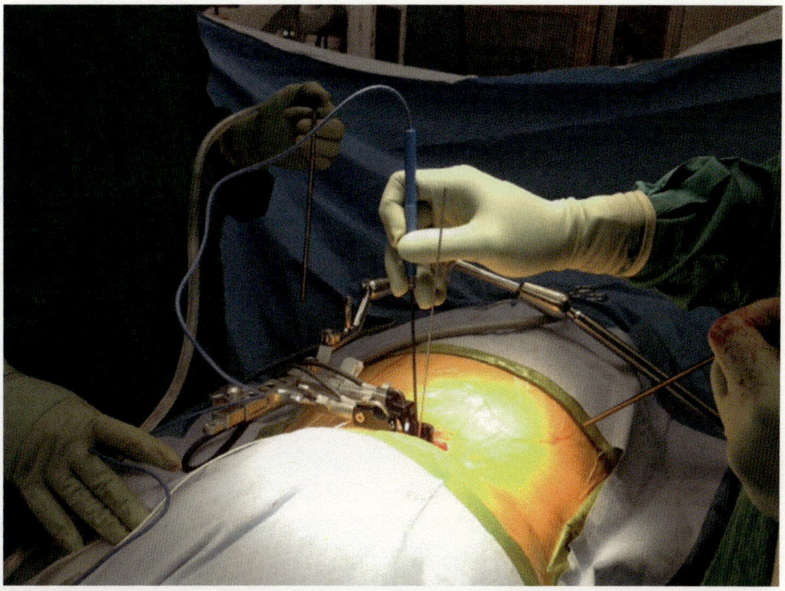

Fig. 24.6 Nerve stimulators are used to assess for nearby nerves prior to expansion of the tubular retractor

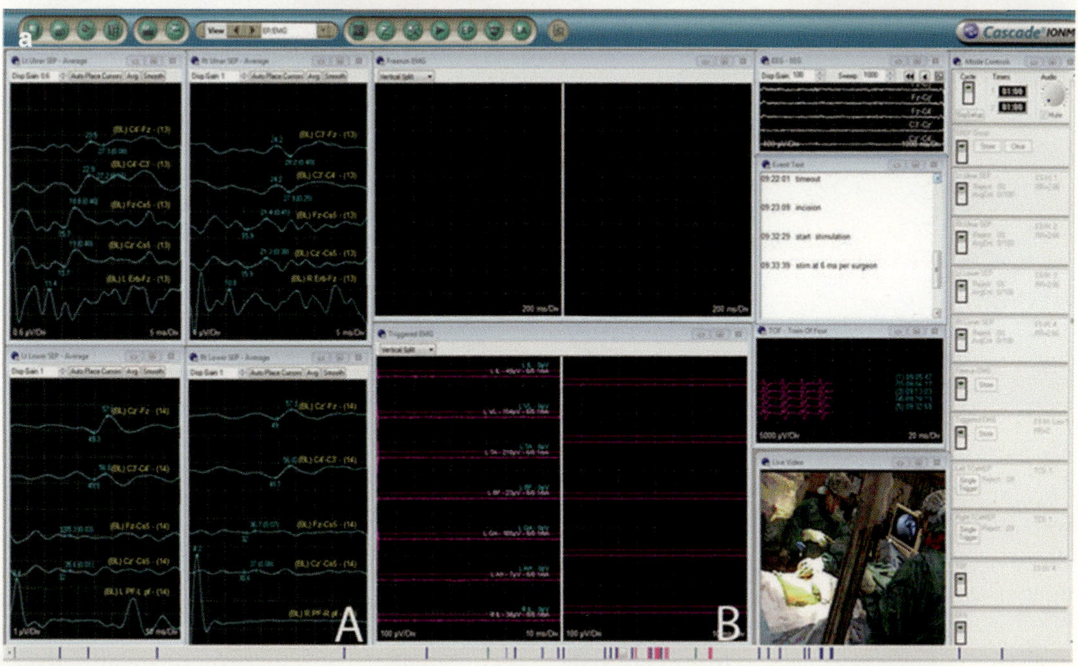

Fig. 24.7 (**a**) Panel A shows baseline SSEP recordings during a lateral transpsoas interbody fusion. Panel B shows baseline EMG. (**b**) Panel A shows stable SSEP recordings. Panel B shows a triggered EMG of the *left* iliopsoas, vastus lateralis, and biceps femoris at 2 mA. (**c**) Enlarged picture of triggered EMG

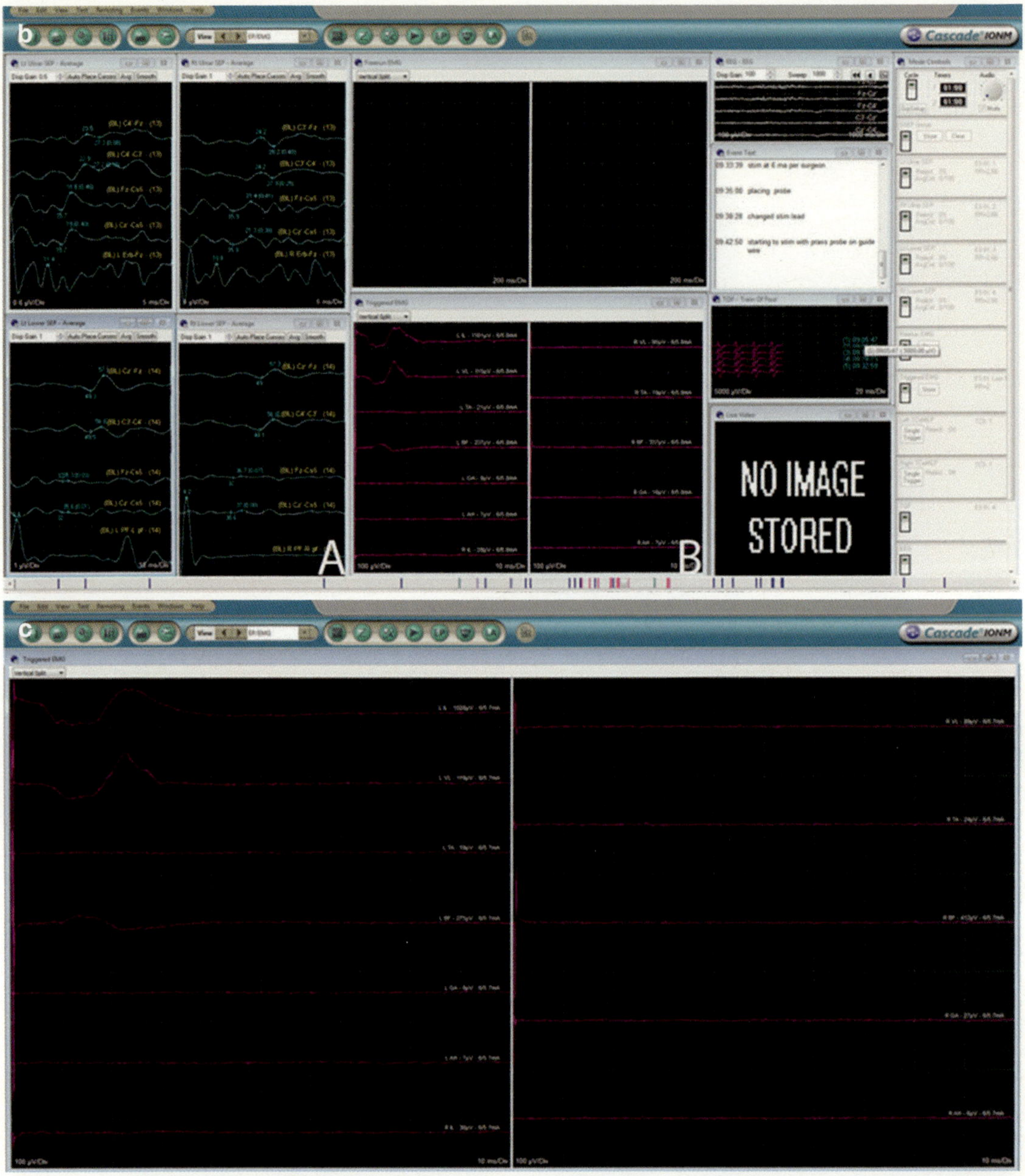

Fig. 24.7 (continued)

receive intraoperative real-time EMG recordings. Recordings were taken using three successive dilators at three points: surface of the psoas muscle, middle of the psoas muscle, and on the spine itself. Recordings were made at four points (posterior, superior, anterior, and inferior) in a 360° rotational field. Zones III and IV were targeted in the vast majority (90 %) of cases. The authors found that lumbar plexus nerves were encountered in 55.7 % of all cases and, more commonly, posteriorly 63 %. The feedback provided by EMG allowed the authors to adjust their surgical trajectory. Postoperatively, transient hip flexion weakness occurred in 27.5 % of patients, and transient upper medial thigh sensory loss occurred in 17.6 %. Three other motor deficits (two patients with knee extension weakness and one patient with ankle dorsiflexion weakness) were encountered, but all had resolved by 6 months postoperatively. Given the variable location of the nerves and the good long-term outcomes of the patients, this authors' study supported the use of real-time EMG during the minimally invasive lateral transpsoas approach.

One emerging neuromonitoring modality that has recently entered the field for use in this and other spine surgeries is mechanomyography (MMG). One potential drawback of EMG is its susceptibility to electrical interference, which can result in a poor signal-to-noise ratio and, hence, the aforementioned low specificity. Using MMG, electrically stimulated probes induce nerve root depolarization. Special sensors (accelerometers that are not susceptible to electrical interference) are placed on correlating muscle groups and detect the mechanical activity (movement) of muscle contraction after nerve stimulation. This feedback is delivered in real time to the surgeon in a fashion similar to EMG activity. Application of this modality to spine surgery is still under development and, to date, no published studies exist that examine its practicality or efficacy. Preliminary results, however, suggest that MMG has faster detection and higher sensitivity than EMG [18].

24.4 Outcomes in Lateral Spine Surgery

The most worrisome complication after any spine surgery is postoperative motor deficits. In a prospective, non-randomized, multicenter, industry-sponsored trial, Isaacs et al. [19] performed XLIF on 107 patients (322 levels) with degenerative scoliosis. Thirty-six patients (33.6 %) had some evidence of postoperative weakness, with 80.6 % of such patients suffering from hip flexion weakness. This was transient in the vast majority of cases (86.2 %). Seven patients (6.5 %) were considered to have a "major" motor deficit, defined as a postoperative decrease in motor grade by more than two grades at any point and/or having no evidence for improvement by 6 months. Only one patient was considered to have an injury of lumbar plexus origin, although further detail was not provided by the authors. The authors did conclude that the risk of experiencing any complication was lower in patients who received stand-alone XLIF compared to supplemental posterior instrumentation; in those who did receive posterior instrumentation, the complication rate was lower in those who had percutaneous screw placement compared to open screw placement. According to this study, "(the) strongest independent predictor of complications was the total number of levels operated per patient." Of note, several important long-term outcome measures were not included in this study, including postoperative sagittal vertical axis measurements and fusion and pseudarthrosis rates.

Cahill et al. [20] retrospectively reviewed 118 patients who had undergone minimally invasive lateral transpsoas interbody fusion at 201 levels, all with continuous EMG monitoring. Ipsilateral nerve injury (specifically of the femoral nerve) occurred in two patients, both at the L4 and L5 levels. This equated to a 4.8 % risk of injury at L4–L5 compared to no neurologic complications at any other level. Echoing the aforementioned conclusions of Guerin et al. [5], these authors also recommended "judicious" use of this surgical procedure at L4–L5. In another study [21], two out of 58 patients suffered iatrogenic femoral nerve injury, although the specific vertebral levels instrumented were not specified. Rarely, contralateral femoral nerve injury can occur. Two such cases have been reported secondary to interbody placement: one due to an osteophyte fracture compressing the contralateral nerve root and another due to a far lateral disc herniation with the same result [22]. Both patients recovered after reoperation for decompression of the injured nerve root.

In the aforementioned Cahill et al. study [20], five patients (4.2 %) suffered from postoperative abdominal paresis/flank bulge, presumably secondary to injury to the T11 and T12 motor nerves during exposure and closure of the abdominal wall. All five cases occurred at the L3–L4 level or higher. A larger multi-institutional study of 568 patients found 10 who developed this complication (1.8 %) [23]. Eight of these patients had resolution of their abdominal wall paresis within 6 months, whereas the other two were lost to follow-up. Conservative treatment of this complication consists of wearing an abdominal corset. To avoid the complication, the authors suggested sequential and gentle muscle dilation with blunt instruments, dissection, and mobilization of any encountered nerves and, in the retroperitoneal space, blunt dissection in a posterior to anterior and superior to inferior trajectory so as to "run with" the trajectory of the nerves.

While motor deficits impact a patient's functionality, sensory changes can also be very bothersome. In a retrospective review of 59 patients who underwent the minimally invasive lateral transpsoas approach, Cummock et al. [24] found that approximately 60 % of patients suffered from postoperative thigh pain, numbness, and/or paresthesias. Half of the patients had resolution of these symptoms at 3 months postoperatively, while 90 % had resolution by 1 year.

The lack of signal changes during intraoperative neuromonitoring does not guarantee that a patient will have normal neurologic function postoperatively. Houten et al. [25] reported two cases of postoperative neurologic deficit (one patient with profound quadriceps weakness and another with antigravity hip flexor and quadriceps weakness) despite normal intraoperative monitoring.

24.5 Recommendations

In summary, while the minimally invasive lateral transpsoas approach is being used increasingly in spine surgery, it can be fraught with complications (specifically, injury to the lumbar plexus). There are a few strategies to employ when utilizing this surgical approach. First, the surgeon must have a good understanding of the safe working zones at each lumbar level. This is simple enough, as the safest zone is Zone III at L1–L2, L2–L3, and L3–L4. At L4–L5, Zone II is the safest, but there should be a low threshold to abort the procedure at this level due to the relatively high risk of neurologic complication. Second, neuromonitoring with EMG should always be used, and trajectories should be adjusted if there is any evidence for firing on EMG. The role of MEP and SSEP monitoring is less clear, although SSEP monitoring may be of benefit to minimize positioning-related brachial plexus injuries.

References

1. McAfee PC, et al. Minimally invasive anterior retroperitoneal approach to the lumbar spine. Emphasis on the lateral BAK. Spine (Phila Pa 1976). 1998;23(13): 1476–84.
2. Laws CJ, et al. Direct lateral approach to lumbar fusion is a biomechanically equivalent alternative to the anterior approach: an in vitro study. Spine (Phila Pa 1976). 2012; 37(10):819–25.
3. Benglis DM, Vanni S, Levi AD. An anatomical study of the lumbosacral plexus as related to the minimally invasive transpsoas approach to the lumbar spine. J Neurosurg Spine. 2009;10(2):139–44.
4. Uribe JS, et al. Defining the safe working zones using the minimally invasive lateral retroperitoneal transpsoas approach: an anatomical study. J Neurosurg Spine. 2010;13(2):260–6.
5. Guerin P, et al. The lumbosacral plexus: anatomic considerations for minimally invasive retroperitoneal transpsoas approach. Surg Radiol Anat. 2012;34(2): 151–7.
6. Moro T, et al. An anatomic study of the lumbar plexus with respect to retroperitoneal endoscopic surgery. Spine (Phila Pa 1976). 2003;28(5):423–8; discussion 427–8.
7. Dakwar E, Vale FL, Uribe JS. Trajectory of the main sensory and motor branches of the lumbar plexus outside the psoas muscle related to the lateral retroperitoneal transpsoas approach. J Neurosurg Spine. 2011; 14(2):290–5.
8. Fahim DK, et al. Avoiding abdominal flank bulge after anterolateral approaches to the thoracolumbar spine: cadaveric study and electrophysiological investigation. J Neurosurg Spine. 2011;15(5):532–40.
9. Kamel IR, et al. The use of somatosensory evoked potentials to determine the relationship between patient positioning and impending upper extremity nerve injury during spine surgery: a retrospective analysis. Anesth Analg. 2006;102(5):1538–42.
10. Paradiso G, et al. Multi-modality neurophysiological monitoring during surgery for adult tethered cord syndrome. J Clin Neurosci. 2005;12(8):934–6.
11. Paradiso G, et al. Multimodality intraoperative neurophysiologic monitoring findings during surgery for

adult tethered cord syndrome: analysis of a series of 44 patients with long-term follow-up. Spine (Phila Pa 1976). 2006;31(18):2095–102.
12. Uribe JS, Vale FL, Dakwar E. Electromyographic monitoring and its anatomical implications in minimally invasive spine surgery. Spine (Phila Pa 1976). 2010;35(Suppl 26):S368–74.
13. Rodgers WB, Gerber EJ, Patterson J. Intraoperative and early postoperative complications in extreme lateral interbody fusion: an analysis of 600 cases. Spine (Phila Pa 1976). 2011;36(1):26–32.
14. Wang MY, Mummaneni PV. Minimally invasive surgery for thoracolumbar spinal deformity: initial clinical experience with clinical and radiographic outcomes. Neurosurg Focus. 2010;28(3):E9.
15. Tormenti MJ, et al. Complications and radiographic correction in adult scoliosis following combined transpsoas extreme lateral interbody fusion and posterior pedicle screw instrumentation. Neurosurg Focus. 2010;28(3):E7.
16. Bergey DL, et al. Endoscopic lateral transpsoas approach to the lumbar spine. Spine (Phila Pa 1976). 2004;29(15):1681–8.
17. Tohmeh AG, Rodgers WB, Peterson MD. Dynamically evoked, discrete-threshold electromyography in the extreme lateral interbody fusion approach. J Neurosurg Spine. 2011;14(1):31–7.
18. Jogani J, Wybo C, Bartol S. Innovation in spine surgery: miracles of MMG. International society for the advancement of spine surgery. 2011. SAS11.
19. Isaacs RE, et al. A prospective, nonrandomized, multicenter evaluation of extreme lateral interbody fusion for the treatment of adult degenerative scoliosis: perioperative outcomes and complications. Spine (Phila Pa 1976). 2010;35(Suppl 26):S322–30.
20. Cahill KS, et al. Motor nerve injuries following the minimally invasive lateral transpsoas approach. J Neurosurg Spine. 2012;17:227–31.
21. Knight RQ, et al. Direct lateral lumbar interbody fusion for degenerative conditions: early complication profile. J Spinal Disord Tech. 2009;22(1):34–7.
22. Papanastassiou ID, Eleraky M, Vrionis FD. Contralateral femoral nerve compression: an unrecognized complication after extreme lateral interbody fusion (XLIF). J Clin Neurosci. 2011;18(1):149–51.
23. Dakwar E, et al. Abdominal wall paresis as a complication of minimally invasive lateral transpsoas interbody fusion. Neurosurg Focus. 2011;31(4):E18.
24. Cummock MD, et al. An analysis of postoperative thigh symptoms after minimally invasive transpsoas lumbar interbody fusion. J Neurosurg Spine. 2011;15(1):11–8.
25. Houten JK, et al. Nerve injury during the transpsoas approach for lumbar fusion. J Neurosurg Spine. 2011; 15(3):280–4.

Lateral Interbody Decompression and Fusion: Which Side to Approach From?

25

Andrew A. Sama

25.1 Background

Bertagnoli et al. initially described lateral lumbar interbody surgery in 2003 when they described the approach to implant prosthetic nuclear devices into the lumbar spine [1]. Ozgur and Pimenta described the extreme lateral transpsoas approach for interbody fusion in 2006 [2]. Over the last 7 years, the popularity and applications for minimally invasive lateral retroperitoneal approaches to the lumbar spine have grown. As the indications and applications have broadened, so have the dilemmas regarding which side to approach. In cases of a one-level fusion for degenerative disc disease, the point may be moot, and the approach should be based on which side appears easier to access on x-ray with respect to the ribs or iliac crest or whether the patient had prior retroperitoneal surgery on one side or the other. In more complex cases with coronal and sagittal deformities, the side of the approach becomes more poignant.

25.2 Anterior Interbody Versus Posterior Interbody

The first thing to decide is whether an anterior or posterior interbody approach is warranted and advisable. It has been demonstrated that both traditional posterior and anterior approaches to the spine are associated with a variety of potential benefits and complications [3–5]. Once the decision to approach anteriorly has been made, then consideration for anterior retroperitoneal transpsoas or anterior-to-the-psoas approaches can be considered. Approaching from the anterior lateral aspect of the spine allows powerful correction of the spine in both the coronal and sagittal planes [6]. It also allows placement of a large interbody spacer with large graft chambers to facilitate fusion. By restoring collapsed disc space height, indirect decompression of the neuroforamina and subarticular lateral recesses can be achieved [7]. Careful evaluation of the facet joints at the proposed fusion sites on preoperative CT scan or MRI is imperative to estimate how much distraction and elevation of the disc space will be possible from the lateral approach. If the facets are ankylosed, it is not likely that the surgeon will be able to correct the collapsed disc space or the deformity anteriorly alone. In these cases, a posterior approach for release of the facets and correction of the deformity is advisable prior to any interbody work. If the facets are not ankylosed and an anterior, lateral, or transpsoas approach is contemplated, the surgeon must decide on whether to perform a traditional anterior approach, a direct transpsoas approach, or an anterior-to-the-psoas lateral approach. In cases with severe loss of lumbar lordosis, or in the presence of lumbar kyphosis, release of the anterior longitudinal ligament may be necessary for optimal correction. Release of the anterior

A.A. Sama, M.D.
Department of Orthopaedic Surgery,
Weill Cornell Medical College, 523 East 72 Street,
New York, NY 10021, USA
e-mail: samaa@hss.edu

M.Y. Wang et al. (eds.), *Minimally Invasive Spinal Deformity Surgery*,
DOI 10.1007/978-3-7091-1407-0_25, © Springer-Verlag Wien 2014

longitudinal ligament from the transpsoas approach is possible [8, 9] but typically ill advised because of the potential increased risk of injury to the great vessels and difficulty in controlling a bleed if an injury were to occur. The lateral interbody approach also temporarily depends on the integrity of the anterior and posterior longitudinal ligaments to help keep the spacer in place. If the anterior longitudinal ligament is released or ruptured, provisional fixation of the interbody spacer should be considered. Mobilization of the vessels via a traditional anterior approach or even from an anterior-to-the-psoas lateral approach allows for safer access to release the anterior longitudinal ligament and correct the severe sagittal deformity than posterior or transforaminal interbody approaches.

25.3 Approaching from the Concave or Convex Side of the Spine

Several factors should come into consideration when determining the side of the lateral approach, especially in deformity cases. Things to consider include the approach that would allow the best access to the greatest number of levels in order to achieve correction of the deformity. A general rule of thumb is to allow the alignment and approachability of the L4–5 disc to be the guide if it is to be included in the fusion. A good set of lumbar or scoliosis x-rays in the anterior-posterior and lateral planes are usually adequate to begin planning the approach (Fig. 25.1). The films should be analyzed to determine if the patient has scoliosis or spondylolisthesis in the anterior-posterior or lateral planes. Depending on the presence of one or more of these deformities, the approach that gives access to the L4–5 disc is usually preferred. Once the analysis of the scoliosis or lumbar x-rays has been completed and the surgeon has decided on the provisional approach, careful evaluation of the preoperative MRI (Fig. 25.2) should be undertaken to assess the position of the psoas muscle, the lumbar plexus, and the great vessels with respect to the fusion levels under consideration [10–13].

25.4 Concave Approach

Fortunately, approaching from the side that allows access to the L4–5 disc obliquity is usually approaching from the concavity of a lumbar scoliosis (Fig. 25.3). When approaching from the concavity, the surgeon is able to access multiple levels from one well-placed incision as depicted in Fig. 25.3. Once the decision to approach from the concavity has been made, the surgeon should consider addressing the cephalad or most caudal levels first rather than addressing the apical levels first which will correct the deformity and likely make access to the higher or lower levels more difficult because they will be further displaced upward under the ribs or lower into the pelvis, respectively. Angled instrumentation to access and prepare the disc spaces is now available from most manufacturers. These angled cob elevators, pituitary rongeurs, and curettes allow the surgeon to access, prepare, and release the disc while preserving the end plates.

By addressing the curvature from the concavity, a significant amount of correction can be achieved in the coronal and sagittal plane deformities. Releasing the annulus of each disc and distracting the more collapsed side of the disc allow for the most significant correction. Approaching from the concavity also allows approach to the upper lumbar levels with less likelihood of entering the chest (Fig. 25.4). The operating table can be used to help correct the deformity when approaching from the concave side of the curve by flexing the break in the table (Fig. 25.5).

Care must be taken when approaching from the concave side to avoid excessive bony destruction. This is especially true in patients with large bridging osteophytes on the concavity of the curve. Using an osteotome to enter the disc space under fluoroscopic guidance in the anterior-posterior view from the concavity of the curve can help minimize bony destruction (Fig. 25.8). The position of the segmental vessels must also be considered with a concave-sided approach [14, 15]. The segmental arteries can be bunched together and may be prone to injury when removing concave osteophytes. Again, using the fluoroscopic guidance to be sure the trajectory of the

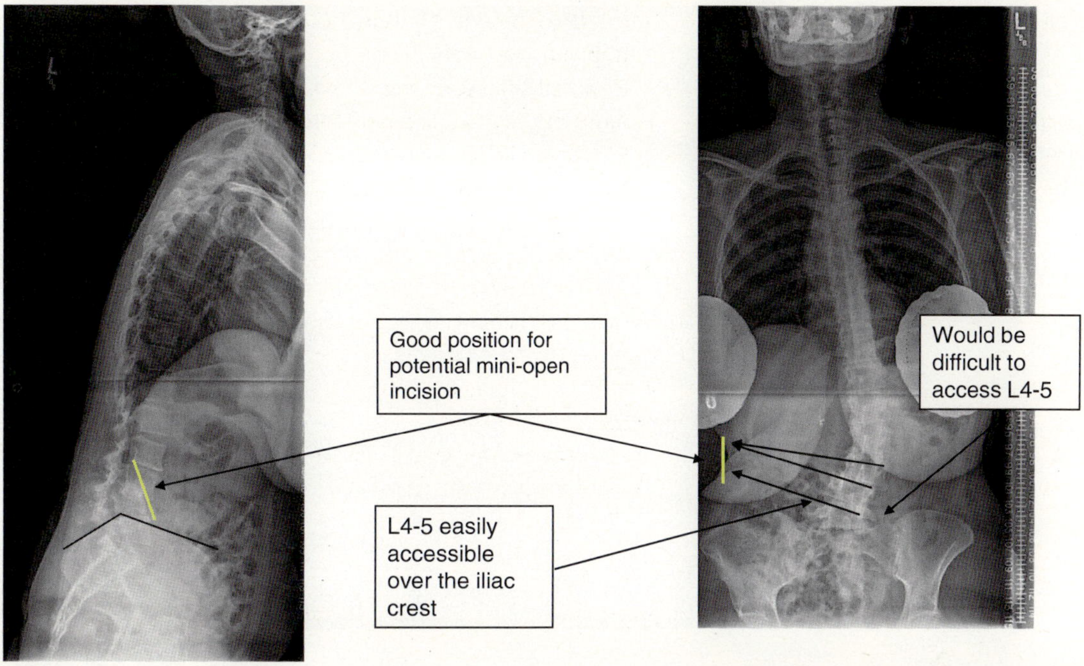

Fig. 25.1 Standing Anteriorposterior and Lateral Scoliosis x-rays showing coronal and sagittal decompensation

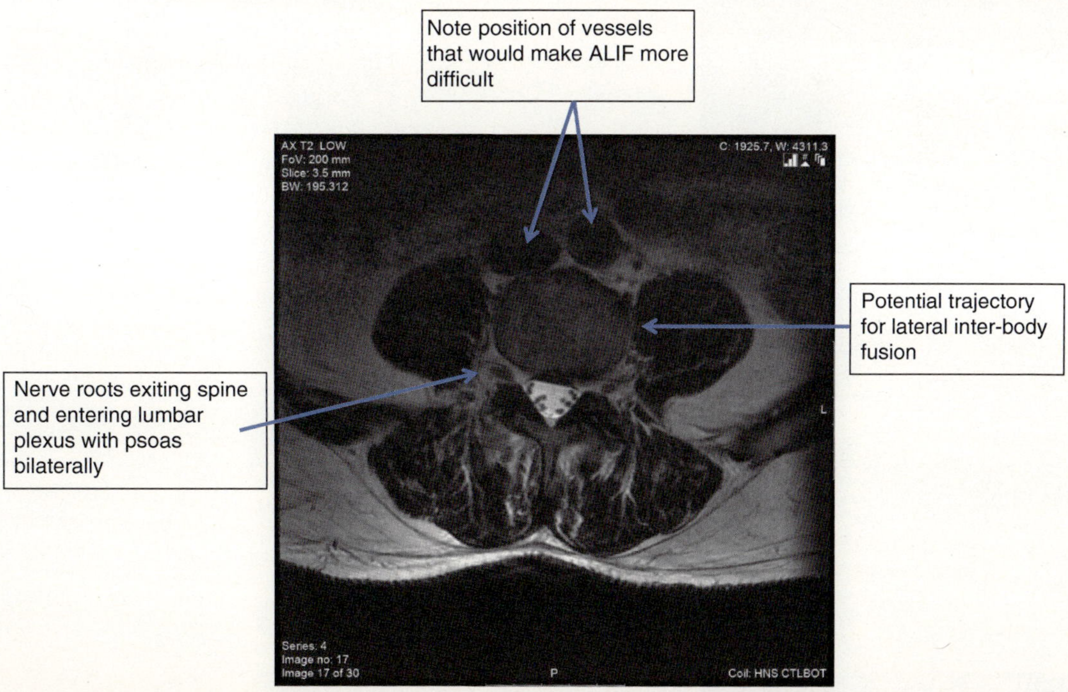

Fig. 25.2 Axial T2 Weighted slice through lumbar segment to illustrate position of the psoas

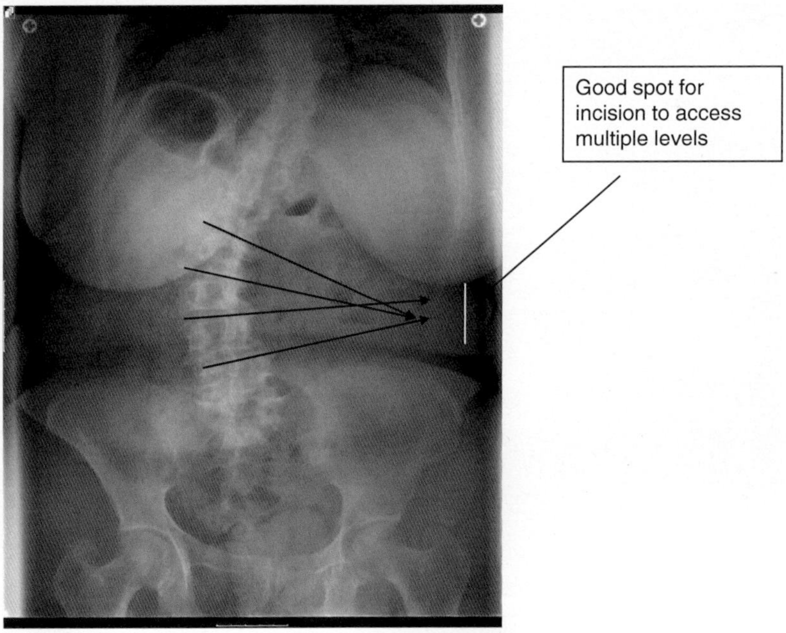

Fig. 25.3 Posterioranterior x-ray of the lumbar spine with lines drawn along endplates of each vertebrae demonstrating how to localize incision site

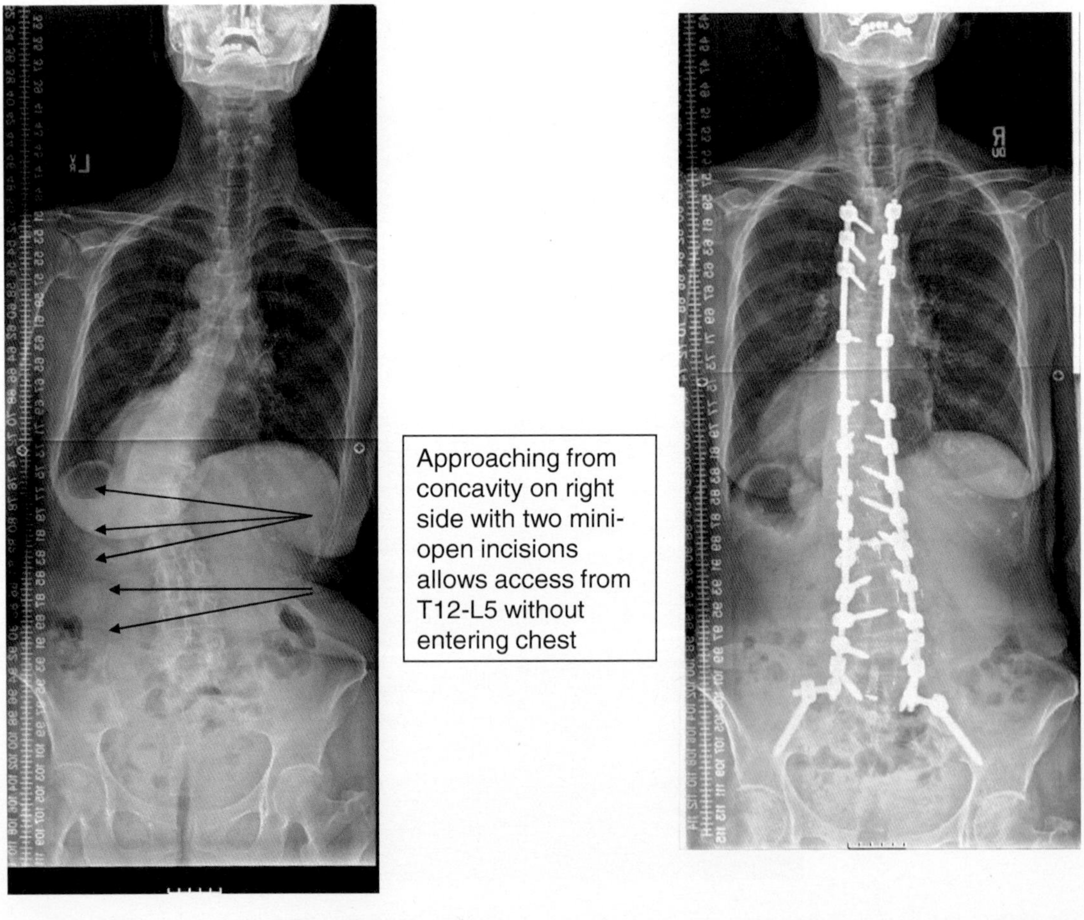

Fig. 25.4 Preoperative and postoperative posterioranterior standing scoliosis x-rays showing the correction achieved

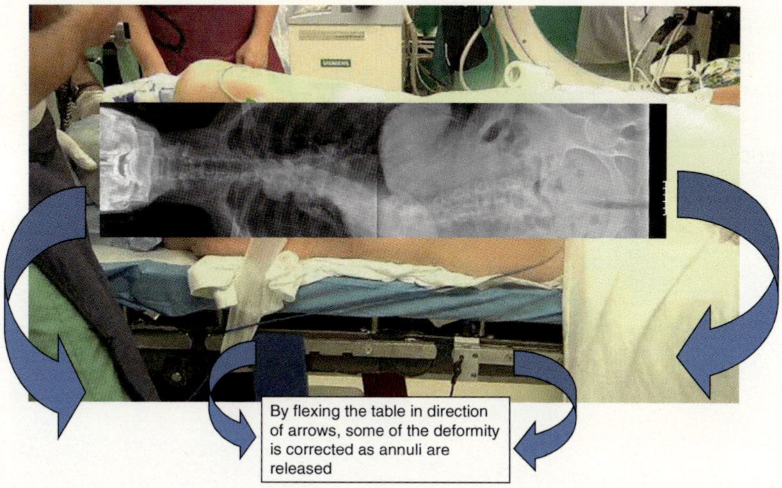

Fig. 25.5 Clinical photograph of patient on operating table in left lateral decubitus postion with superimposed posterioranterior scoliosis x-ray demonstrating approach from concave side and how flexing the operating table would facilitate access to the spine

osteotome remains in the plane of the disc will minimize the likelihood of injury to the segmental vessels.

In 30 cases of adult degenerative scoliosis, improvement of Oswestry Disability Index, Short Form-12, and Visual Analog scores for back pain improved by approach from the concave side at 130 levels without any increase in perioperative complications [16].

25.5 Convex Approach

In cases of a large lumbar scoliosis with extreme coronal decompensation, approach from the concavity may not be possible except to access the lower lumbar levels. Due to the extreme degree of coronal deformity and lumbar curvature in these cases, the upper lumbar disc spaces may actually be vertical and directed perpendicular to the floor when the patient stands, making approach from the concavity difficult if not impossible (Fig. 25.6). These upper discs may be brought into a more approachable position in patients with flexible curves, but in patients with rigid curves, the levels may not be approachable with a lateral technique without entering into the thoracic cavity usually from the convex side. In cases where approach to the lower levels can be facilitated by approach from either the concave or convex sides of the curve, partial correction can be achieved. This partial correction may make the upper lumbar levels more approachable through a second incision in a more orthogonal plane to the upper lumbar disc spaces usually from the concavity through a second incision to facilitate fusion if necessary (Fig. 25.7).

In cases where multiple incisions may be needed, especially when approaching a curve from the convexity, the lower lumbar incision is made where it will afford the best approach to the L4–5 level. It is usually possible to have access to L3–4 and L4–5 with this incision. Where the second, more cephalad incision will allow access to the L1–2 and L2–3 levels. Working in the disc space to release the annulus is somewhat easier coming from the convexity (Fig. 25.8).

25.6 Other Considerations

In patients with unilateral radicular pain associated with foraminal stenosis or secondary to scoliosis, approach on the ipsilateral side as the radiculopathy may serve a dual purpose. First, it provides the best opportunity to release and correct the deformity thereby opening the ipsilateral foramen and providing thorough indirect decompression. Second, it mitigates the likelihood of having a neuropraxia related to the approach on the side contralateral to the presenting symptoms. [7, 17–23]

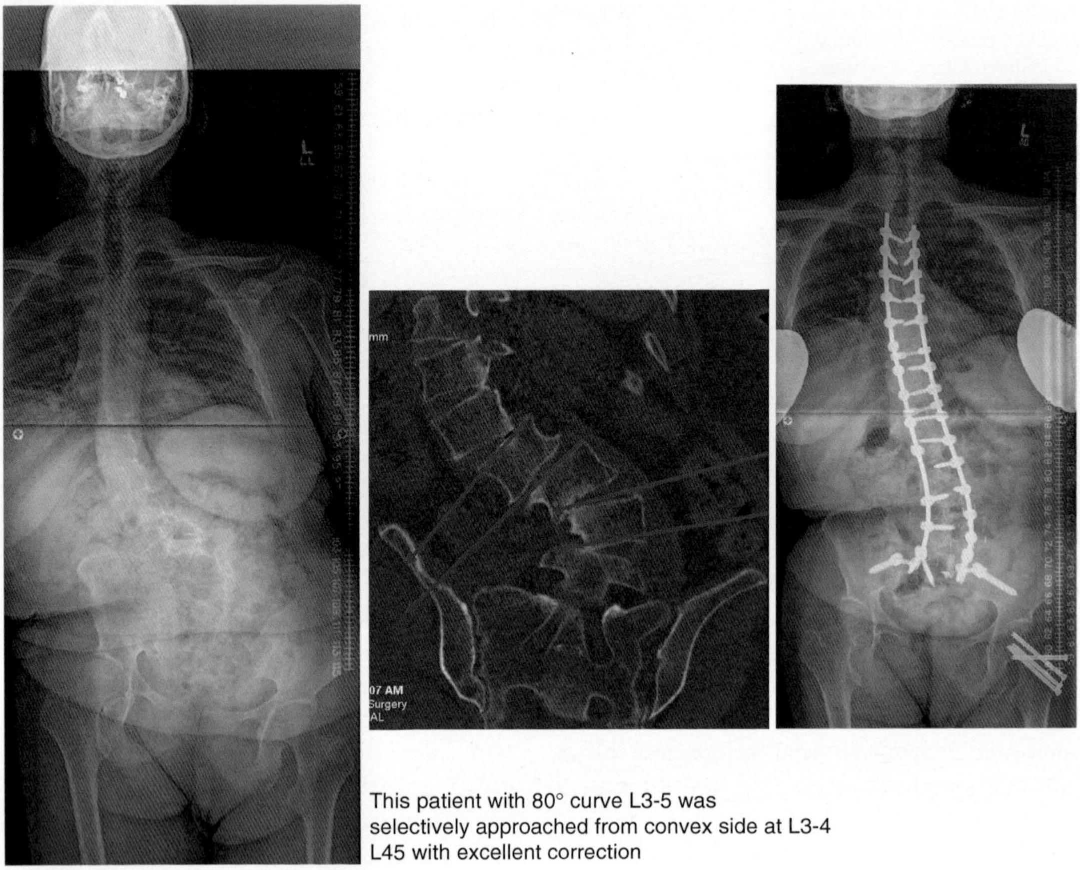

Fig. 25.6 Standing Anteriorposterior scoliosis x-ray and coronal CT scan image showing the difficulty that would be encountered with an attempt at access from the concave side in this patient. Anteriorposterior standing scoliosis x-ray showing final correction after approach from the convex side and posterior realignment

Regardless of the side of the approach, a good practice is to advise patients undergoing anterior or lateral transpsoas surgery that they are likely to have thigh pain, numbness, or mild weakness secondary to local irritation associated with the dissection and retraction around the psoas and the lumbar plexus. The majority of these postoperative symptoms should resolve within 6 weeks postoperatively. [7, 17–23]

In patients who have previously had retroperitoneal surgery, it is prudent to avoid the side of the prior retroperitoneal approach if possible. If lateral surgery is contemplated from the side of the prior retroperitoneal approach, consultation with a general or vascular surgeon may be warranted. Patients who have had prior radiation treatment to the lumbar or abdominal area may also require special consideration in planning for the lateral approach (Fig. 25.9).

For cases that require access to the upper lumbar or lower thoracic levels, approaching from the patient's right side may aid in avoiding

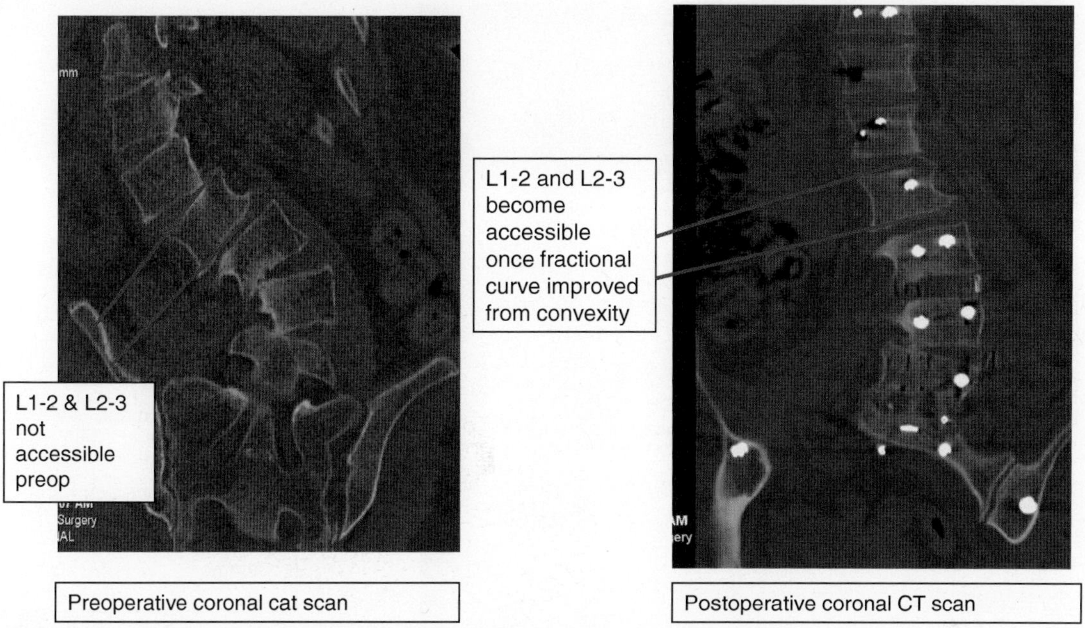

Fig. 25.7 Preoperative and postoperative coronal CT scan images showing lumbar spine

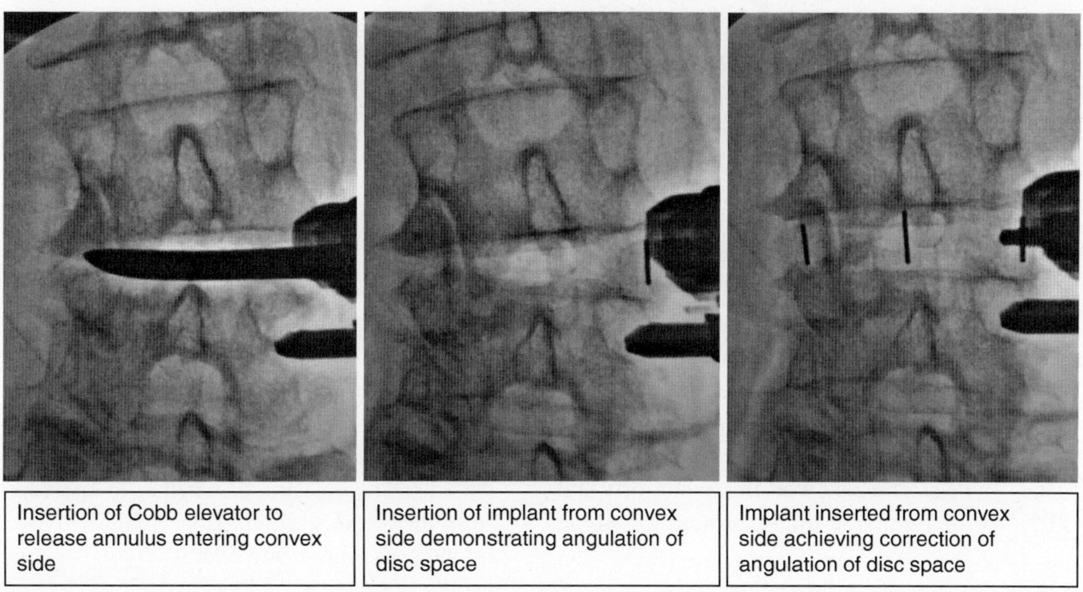

Fig. 25.8 Intraoperative floroscopic Anteriorposterior images showing release of the disc space and insertion of the interbody cage correcting the coronal segmental deformity and restoring disc space height

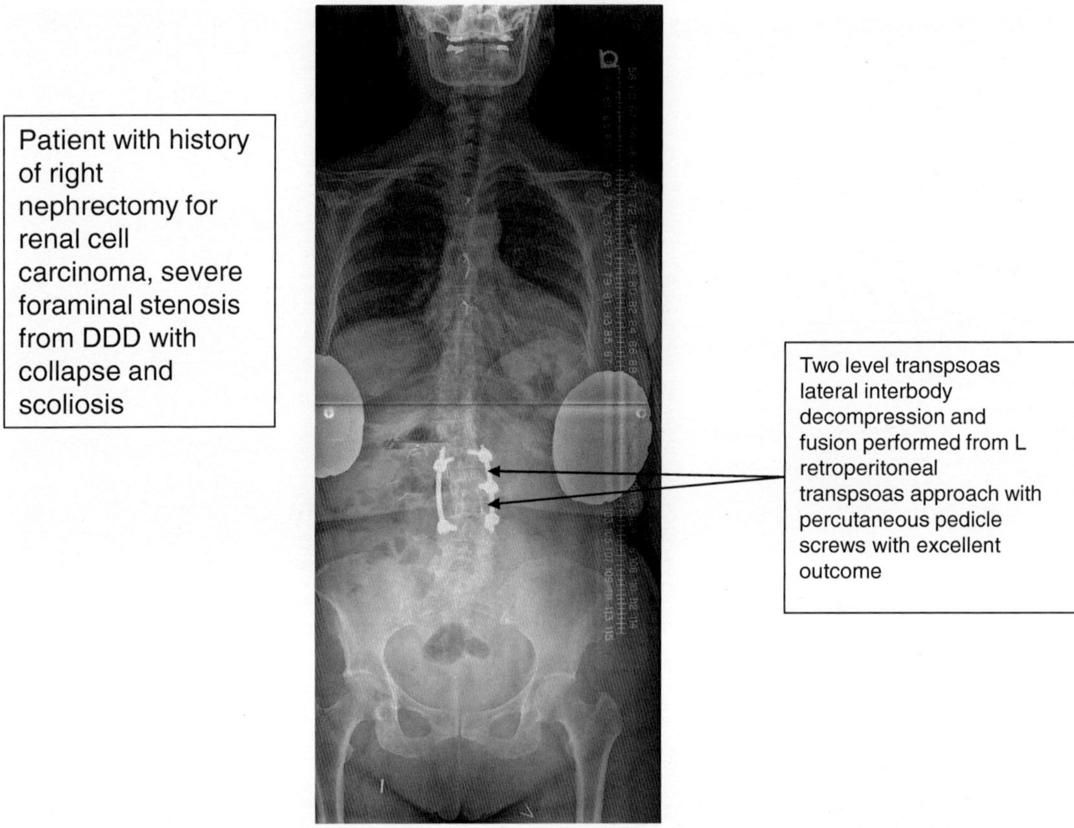

Fig. 25.9 Standing Anteriorposterior scoliosis x-ray showing correction with selective apical fusion throught the lateral approach and with posterior percutaneous pedicle screws in a patient with prior retroperitoneal surgery

entry into the chest given that the right hemidiaphragm is usually higher than the left. Oftentimes, dissection onto one of the lower ribs and subperiosteal dissection above that rib allows for a safe approach. If necessary the rib can be removed for bone graft or to allow access. Once the rib has been removed, a retropleural plane can be established working posteriorly and inferiorly to reach the upper lumbar vertebrae and discs.

The position of the psoas and lumbar plexus should be evaluated on the MRI. If there is a difference from right to left in the position of the psoas, the approach is safest on the side where the psoas is located more posteriorly and closest to the vertebral body [10, 12].

Conclusion

In summary, the anterior lateral approach to the spine is a powerful tool in the treatment of lumbar conditions that require fusion. Studies have shown that it can be applied safely and effectively. There are issues unique to the approach that must be considered and discussed with patients. The decision of whether to approach from the left or the right side should be based on the pathology being addressed and the surgeon's preference. Guidelines to consider are outlined above. Whichever the side selected, it should be the side that affords the safest approach to the desired levels to be addressed in order to achieve the best correction of the condition for which the surgery was indicated.

References

1. Bertagnoli R, Vazquez RJ. The Anterolateral TransPsoatic Approach (ALPA): a new technique for implanting prosthetic disc-nucleus devices. J Spinal Disord Tech. 2003;16:398–404.
2. Ozgur BM, Aryan HE, Pimenta L, et al. Extreme Lateral Interbody Fusion (XLIF): a novel surgical technique for anterior lumbar interbody fusion. Spine J. 2006;6:435–43.
3. Fantini GA, Pappou IP, Girardi FP, et al. Major vascular injury during anterior lumbar spinal surgery: incidence, risk factors, and management. Spine (Phila Pa 1976). 2007;32:2751–8.
4. Rajaraman V, Vingan R, Roth P, et al. Visceral and vascular complications resulting from anterior lumbar interbody fusion. J Neurosurg. 1999;91:60–4.
5. Lin PM. Posterior lumbar interbody fusion technique: complications and pitfalls. Clin Orthop Relat Res, 1983:180:154; http://www.springer.com.
6. Acosta FL, Liu J, Slimack N, et al. Changes in coronal and sagittal plane alignment following minimally invasive direct lateral interbody fusion for the treatment of degenerative lumbar disease in adults: a radiographic study. J Neurosurg Spine. 2011;15:92–6.
7. Sharma AK, Kepler CK, Girardi FP, et al. Lateral lumbar interbody fusion: clinical and radiographic outcomes at 1 year: a preliminary report. J Spinal Disord Tech. 2011;24:242–50.
8. Deukmedjian AR, Le TV, Baaj AA, et al. Anterior longitudinal ligament release using the minimally invasive lateral retroperitoneal transpsoas approach: a cadaveric feasibility study and report of 4 clinical cases. J Neurosurg Spine. 2012;17:530–9.
9. Uribe JS, Smith DA, Dakwar E, et al. Lordosis restoration after anterior longitudinal ligament release and placement of lateral hyperlordotic interbody cages during the minimally invasive lateral transpsoas approach: a radiographic study in cadavers. J Neurosurg Spine. 2012;17:476–85.
10. Kepler CK, Bogner EA, Herzog RJ, et al. Anatomy of the psoas muscle and lumbar plexus with respect to the surgical approach for lateral transpsoas interbody fusion. Eur Spine J. 2011;20:550–6.
11. Hu WK, He SS, Zhang SC, et al. An MRI study of psoas major and abdominal large vessels with respect to the X/DLIF approach. Eur Spine J. 2011;20:557–62.
12. Kirchmair L, Lirk P, Colvin J, et al. Lumbar plexus and psoas major muscle: not always as expected. Reg Anesth Pain Med. 2008;33:109–14.
13. Uribe JS, Arredondo N, Dakwar E, et al. Defining the safe working zones using the minimally invasive lateral retroperitoneal transpsoas approach: an anatomical study. J Neurosurg Spine. 2010;13:260–6.
14. Shimizu S, Tanaka R, Kan S, et al. Origins of the segmental arteries in the aorta: an anatomic study for selective catheterization with spinal arteriography. AJNR Am J Neuroradiol. 2005;26:922–8.
15. Kawahara N, Tomita K, Baba H, et al. Cadaveric vascular anatomy for total en bloc spondylectomy in malignant vertebral tumors. Spine (Phila Pa 1976). 1996;21:1401–7.
16. Caputo AM, Michael KW, Chapman Jr TM, et al. Clinical outcomes of extreme lateral interbody fusion in the treatment of adult degenerative scoliosis. ScientificWorldJournal. 2012;2012:680643.
17. Isaacs RE, Hyde J, Goodrich JA, et al. A prospective, nonrandomized, multicenter evaluation of extreme lateral interbody fusion for the treatment of adult degenerative scoliosis: perioperative outcomes and complications. Spine (Phila Pa 1976). 2010;35:S322–30.
18. Pumberger M, Hughes AP, Huang RR, et al. Neurologic deficit following lateral lumbar interbody fusion. Eur Spine J. 2012;21:1192–9.
19. Rodgers WB, Gerber EJ, Patterson J. Intraoperative and early postoperative complications in extreme lateral interbody fusion: an analysis of 600 cases. Spine (Phila Pa 1976). 2011;36:26–32.
20. Banagan K, Gelb D, Poelstra K, et al. Anatomic mapping of lumbar nerve roots during a direct lateral transpsoas approach to the spine: a cadaveric study. Spine (Phila Pa 1976). 2011;36:E687–91.
21. Tormenti MJ, Maserati MB, Bonfield CM, et al. Complications and radiographic correction in adult scoliosis following combined transpsoas extreme lateral interbody fusion and posterior pedicle screw instrumentation. Neurosurg Focus. 2010;28(3):E1–7.
22. Le TV, Burkett CJ, Deukmedjian AR, et al. Postoperative lumbar plexus injury following lumbar retroperitoneal transpsoas minimally invasive lateral interbody fusion. Spine (Phila Pa 1976). 2012.
23. Arnold PM, Anderson KK, McGuire Jr RA. The lateral transpsoas approach to the lumbar and thoracic spine: a review. Surg Neurol Int. 2012;3:S198–215.

Stand-Alone Lateral Surgery for Spinal Deformity

26

Amir Ahmadian and Juan S. Uribe

26.1 Introduction

Spinal deformity is term used to define many different types of pathologies in either adult or pediatric patients; hence, it can include both congenital and degenerative defects. Pediatric or adolescent scoliosis/deformity and its treatment are beyond the scope of this chapter. Furthermore, a stand-alone lateral construct in pediatric spine deformity is not well established in the current literature, and hence posterior or combined techniques are mainly used. Adult spinal deformity is characterized by spinal curvature >10° with associated derangement of spinopelvic alignment [1, 2]. Adult scoliosis consists of primary degeneration that developed over time after skeletal maturity most likely secondary to asymmetric degeneration of discs, osteoporosis, and vertebral body compression fractures or progressive idiopathy that developed prior to skeletal maturity. Presenting symptoms of this condition primarily include radiculopathy, chronic low back pain and neurogenic claudication caused by concurrent spinal stenosis.

Classification of type and progression of adult deformity both radiographically and clinically is critical to the treatment paradigm [3]. Timing of surgical intervention, surgical approach, and length of constructs for operative stabilization or correction have been controversial. Minimally invasive spine surgery (MIS) was initially developed to address morbidity associated with traditional, open spinal surgery. As the field has continued to advance, MIS techniques have been implemented in the treatment of adult spinal deformity (ASD). One such technique is the minimally invasive lateral retroperitoneal transpsoas interbody fusion (MIS-LIF), which was first described by Pimenta in 2001 [4, 5]. This approach has been used to deliver stand-alone interbody cages. Indications for operative intervention remain the same across any surgical approach and include progression of deformity, pain, and neurological deficits. Stand-alone MIS lateral constructs are relatively new to the previously established surgical paradigms. Patient selection is key in any surgical intervention but particularly in the decision for a lateral MIS stand-alone construct.

A. Ahmadian, M.D • J.S. Uribe, M.D (✉)
Department of Neurological Surgery,
University of South Florida, Tampa, FL, USA
e-mail: juansuribe@gmail.com

26.2 Patient Selection

Once the decision to proceed with surgical intervention is made, selecting the most appropriate and patient specific approach can be challenging. There are no "one size fits all" constructs for spinal deformity. Stand-alone lateral constructs should be reserved for patient who at unacceptably high operative risk for alterative conventional or MIS combined approaches. Patients with unrelievable pain, progressive degenerative scoliosis with advanced age, significant co-mobility,

M.Y. Wang et al. (eds.), *Minimally Invasive Spinal Deformity Surgery*,
DOI 10.1007/978-3-7091-1407-0_26, © Springer-Verlag Wien 2014

and significant anesthetic risk should be considered for less invasive interventions. Additionally, to consider a lateral stand-alone construct, the radiographic evaluation should exhibit reasonable coronal/sagittal balance. Finally, all patients being considered for stand-alone constructs should be evaluated for degree of osteopenia or osteoporosis. The vertebral body end-plate strength is greatly dependent on the bone density [6]. Patient with osteoporosis or advanced osteopenia should not be considered for stand-alone lateral fusion but rather a nonoperative treatment options or a limited decompression. However, this can lead to a deformity progression and worsening of symptoms.

26.3 Advantages and Disadvantages

As previously stated, the decision for surgical intervention and approach, particularly lateral, is multifactorial. Morbidity of surgical approach required postoperative care, operative/anesthetic risk, and a patient's preoperative medical comorbidities are of particular importance in proceeding with a lateral stand-alone construct. The risk profile of anterior, posterior, lateral, and combined approaches is different and must be considered [7–10]. Minimally invasive techniques (MIS) have potentially less surgical and postoperative morbidity [11, 12]. There are certain advantages to MIS lateral approach that make stand-alone feasible. It is not a destabilizing technique as compared to the posterior approaches in which important stabilizing structures have to be violated to gain access to the intervertebral disc space. In addition, it is associated with shorter operative time and decreased blood loss [5, 13]. The MIS lateral approach also allows for generous discectomy and end-plate preparation allowing placement of larger interbody implant placement from one diaphysis to the other, with less likely device subsidance [14, 15]. On the other hand, the MIS lateral approach allows access to more levels with less vascular risk and preservation of anterior longitudinal ligament (ALL) as compared to the traditional anterior interbody fusion (ALIF). The risk of lumbar plexus injury is greater for lateral techniques particularly in the lower lumbar levels with a relative preservation of sympathetic plexus which is a particular concern associated with a direct anterior approach. Furthermore, compared to posterior approaches, there is increase risk to retroperitoneal organs and vessels.

26.4 Biomechanics

Biomechanical comparisons between the stand-alone lateral and stand-alone ALIF have demonstrated its increased rigidity to promote arthrodesis [16]. Stand-alone lateral is more rigid in lateral bending and flexion-extension when compared to stand-alone ALIF [16]. Though the biomechanical advantage of a lateral stand-alone construct is its favorable rigidity in all six basic movements, it falls short to the addition of unilateral and bilateral pedicle screws, which are much more rigid overall. Stand-alone construct should be reserved for patients free of any significant gross instability. Patients with instability would best be treated with additional spinal instrumentation. For similar reasons, stand-alone constructs may not be optimal for gross deformity correction, though it does have a very limited application in this patient population. In addition, a unified bilateral pedicle screw and rod construct provides stability across multiple segments as compared to a lateral stand-alone construct, which stabilizes one segment at a time and protects subsidence. Phillips et al. presented radiographic evaluation of a cohort of patient with lumbar stand-alone constructs and who exhibited no loss of Cobb angle, with minimal improvement in lumbar lordosis of 9.8 % and 18.7°, respectively [17]. As expected spinopelvic parameters significantly improve with addition of posterior instrumentation, which emphasizes the importance of patient selection of stand-alone constructs.

26.5 Anatomical Considerations

Retroperitoneal transpsoas approach involved traversing the nerves of the lumbar plexus both within and outside of psoas muscle. There are four major nerves traveling outside of the psoas muscle and include subcostals (T12), iliohypogastric (L1), ilioinguinal (L1), and lateral femoral cutaneous (L2–L3) nerves. They originate from the posterior border of the psoas muscle and descend obliquely through the retroperitoneal space. These free nerves are most vulnerable at the initial stages of the approach during abdominal muscle and retroperitoneal dissection superficial to the psoas and hence necessitate delicate blunt dissection [18]. The genitofemoral (L1–L2) nerve initially travels within the psoas muscle, across the L2/L3 disc space, for a short distance before emerging and continuing on the anterior surface of the muscle.

The L2, L3, and L4 roots merge to form the femoral nerve which courses deep within the psoas muscle to pass under the inguinal ligament prior to giving off cutaneous (medial/intermediate femoral cutaneous/infrapatellar branch/saphenous nerve) and muscular branches. Variation in proximal trajectory of the femoral nerve has been described as it transverses the psoas muscle [19, 20]. Though anatomical variations to the lumbar plexus have been described in the literature, large population studies to establish a more accurate measure of the prevalence of the surgically relevant variability are lacking [21, 22]. Variations in trajectory of the femoral nerve should be strongly considered when establishing an operative corridor with utilization of directional EMG monitoring to prevent nerve injury. Finally, the obturator nerve (L2–L4) courses through psoas muscle posterior to the femoral nerve. It emerges from the medial aspect of the psoas muscle and travels just lateral to the sacrum prior to exiting the pelvis though the obturator foramen. Finally, the sympathetic plexus runs on the anterior surface of the vertebral body and is at risk especially with lateral corpectomies or anterior longitudinal ligament (ALL) releases.

The fibers of the sympathetic plexus/ganglion are found along the lateral edge of the ALL and have communicating branched with lumbar plexus nerves. The communicating branches consist of the white (presynaptic) and gray (postsynaptic) rami communicans. Moreover, these fibers generally reside at the inferior aspect of the vertebral body.

The intended trajectory of the lateral retroperitoneal dissection is mid-vertebral body in the A-P plane for placement of intervertebral cage. The approach is anterior to the neural foramen and hence vulnerable to lumbar nerves injury rather than specific root injury. Lumbar nerves have contributor from multiple roots, therefore a much more clinically significant outcome if injured. All nerves of the lumbar plexus have a dermal sensory representation, except for the intrinsic motor branches supplying the psoas muscle. Clinical diagnosis of specific lumbar plexus nerve injuries can sometime depend on overlapping sensory deficits, which can make diagnostic evaluation more difficult.

26.6 Operative Considerations

Intraoperative consideration of a lateral approach to any type of spinal deformity is uniform and includes understanding of regional anatomy, avoidance of lumbar plexus injury, preservation of the ALL, adequate end-plate preparation, and restoration of disc height. However, with stand-alone constructs a great emphasis is made on utilization of vertebral ring apophysis and hence on implant width or "footprint" to increase fusion bed area and more importantly to protect the implants from subsidence. Available width cages include 18, 22, and 26 mm width and lordotic up to 30° (Coroent, Nuvasive CA). Large-diameter implants are less likely to subside compared to small-diameter cages, possibly related to a more efficient transfer of force to the end plate [23–25]. Utilization of dense bone of the vertebral ring apophysis for load bearing is a key concept for stand-alone lateral fusion as to minimize the subsidence risk.

The preoperative planning is critical to ensure that the patient is a good surgical candidate. Preoperative imaging should include a magnetic resonance imaging (MRI) to ensure that abdominal blood vessels will not hinder access to the desired disc space and an A-P X-ray to determine which side will provide the best access, especially at L4/5, in relation to the iliac crest. The patient is then placed in the lateral position with the optimal side facing up. Placing the concave side of a scoliotic deformity facing up can facilitate correction by improving access to the L4/5 disc space, allowing access to multiple levels through fewer incisions and release of soft tissue on the contracted side hence permitting placement of asymmetric cages. The legs are flexed maximally at the knee and hip to relax tension on the psoas muscle and lumbar plexus nerves. A roll is placed beneath the axilla to prevent brachial plexus injury, and a roll is placed under the iliac crest to facilitate deformity correction and promote flexion at the iliac crest for improved access to the L4/5 level. Intraoperative fluoroscopy is then used to position the patient in such a manner that a symmetric A-P image with the pedicles equidistant from the spinous processes is achieved. It is essential that these images be as accurate and symmetric as possible to prevent inadvertently dissecting too far anteriorly or posteriorly. In multilevel procedures, the position should be reevaluated at every level to address rotational deformity and changes related to implant placement.

Once properly positioned, the patient is taped and secured to the table. If needed, the table is flexed at the level of the iliac crest just enough to give access to the disc space. Excessive flexion of the table can put tension on the lumbar plexus and potentially promote nerve injury. The incision is fluoroscopically guided and marked at the middle of the disc space based on the anatomic safe zones [26]. If multiple disc spaces are being approached, separate fascial incisions are made for each disc space to help stabilize the retractor and to minimize abdominal muscles dissection. Once the fascial incision over the area of interest is completed, the external oblique, internal oblique, and transversus abdominis muscles are identified and bluntly dissected until the transversalis fascia and retroperitoneal space are encountered. The psoas muscle is palpated. Sequential dilators are then used to dilate the psoas muscle and stimulated using triggered EMG (t-EMG). The position of the femoral nerve can be estimated by the location of the sharp decreases in the t-EMG threshold. Ideally, the sharp decreases will be present when stimulating with the dilator posteriorly and increased thresholds present anteriorly; thus, the femoral nerve can be estimated to be posterior to the dilators. This orientation will allow placement and opening of the retractor with minimal risk of nerve injury. Once the t-EMG stimulation with the final dilator verifies decreased threshold responses posteriorly and increased threshold responses anteriorly, the retractor is then placed. Once it is confirmed that disc space is visualized and no nerves are present in the surgical field, lateral X-ray is obtained to check the position of the retractor in relation to the disc space. The shim blade is advanced into the disc space firmly with image guidance using A-P fluoroscopy.

Once the retractor is in final position, the rest of the procedure must be performed as efficiently and quickly as possible to reduce the duration of retraction of the lumbar plexus. With careful attention to keeping instruments in a vertical orientation, a combination of box cutter disc shaver, pituitary rongeur, rasp, and curettes are utilized to prepare the disc space. Depending on the preoperative X-ray, a straight or lordotic polyetheretherketone (PEEK) interbody cage, filled with a variety of biologics, is then placed (Fig. 26.1).

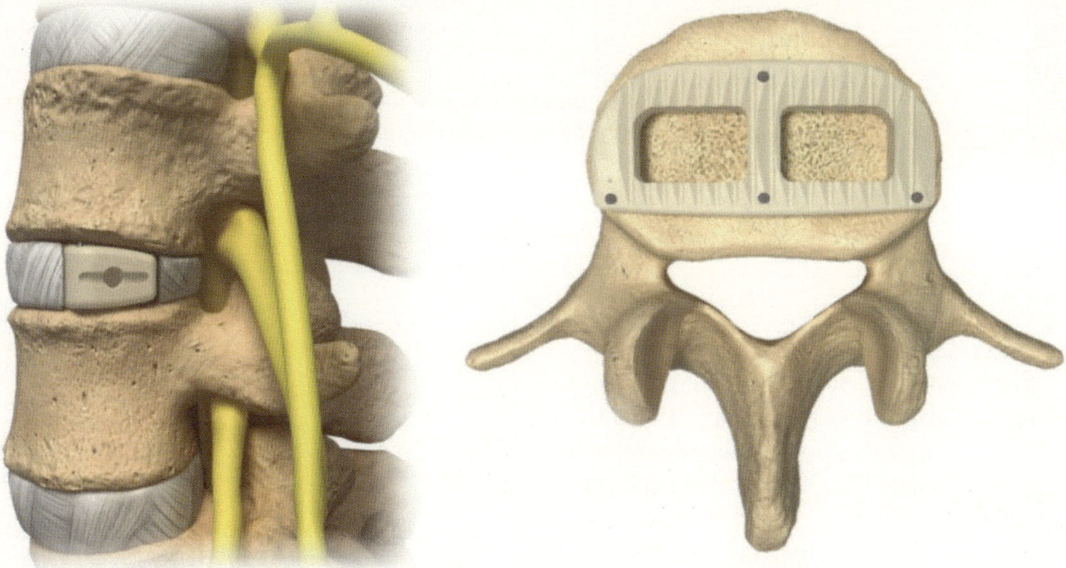

Fig. 26.1 Lordotic cage placed in the intervertebral disc space. Note that it spans the lateral endplate on both the right and left sides of the apophyseal ring, which is the region with the strongest endplate bone

26.7 Case Illustration

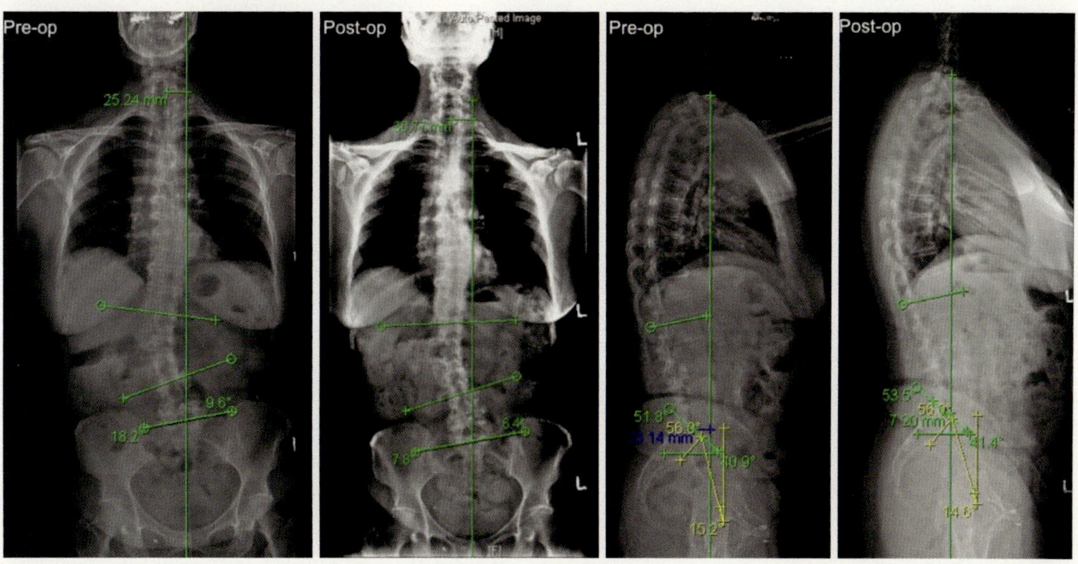

The patient is a 73-year-old female present with complaint of progressive chronic back pain over 10 years. She has failed conservative therapy that included physical therapy and pain management. She underwent left MIS lateral interbody fusion as stand-alone construct. Standing scoliosis films show:

	Preop	Postop
Coronal Cobb angle	18.2	7.8
SVA	2.3 cm	0.7 cm
CSVL	2.5 cm	3.0 cm
Sacral slope	40.9°	41.4°
Pelvic incidence	56°	56°
Pelvic tilt	15.2°	14.6°
Lumbar lordosis	51.8°	53.5°
Fractional curve	9.6°	6.4°

Conclusions

The importance of understanding the differing risk characteristics of an aging population with spinal deformity cannot be overstated. Lateral stand-alone surgery for adult spinal deformity is a viable option in very selective patient population. Combined approaches for correction of spinal deformity provide the best chance for correction of spinopelvic alignment and neural decompression. However, certain patients may have unacceptable risk with combined or more invasive procedures. A patient's comorbid medical condition can affect postoperative outcomes [27, 28]. In this select few of patients who have failed conservative therapies, spine practitioners may consider a stand-alone construct. The advantages of the MIS-LIF include minimization of muscle dissection/trauma, shorter operative time, relatively decreased blood loss, preservation of anterior/posterior longitudinal ligaments, maximization of interbody cage size, indirect foraminal decompression, and relatively earlier postoperative mobilization. MIS-LIF is a safe feasible alternative to traditional surgical approaches in a selected group of patients with adult spinal deformity.

References

1. Birknes JK, White AP, Albert TJ, Shaffrey CI, Harrop JS. Adult degenerative scoliosis: a review. Neurosurgery. 2008;63 Suppl 3:94–103.
2. Aebi M. The adult scoliosis. Eur Spine J. 2005;14(10):925–48.
3. Smith JS, Shaffrey CI, Kuntz C, Mummaneni PV. Classification systems for adolescent and adult scoliosis. Neurosurgery. 2008;63 Suppl 3:16–24.
4. Pimenta L. Lateral endoscopic transpsoas retroperitoneal approach for lumbar spine surgery. VIII Brazilian spine meeting, Belo Horizonte, Minas Gerais, Brazil; 2001.
5. Ozgur BM, Aryan HE, Pimenta L, Taylor WR. Extreme Lateral Interbody Fusion (XLIF): a novel surgical technique for anterior lumbar interbody fusion. Spine J. 2006;6(4):435–43.
6. Oxland TR, Lund T. Biomechanics of stand-alone cages and cages in combination with posterior fixation: a literature review. Eur Spine J. 2000;9 Suppl 1:S95–101.
7. Than KD, Wang AC, Rahman SU, et al. Complication avoidance and management in anterior lumbar interbody fusion. Neurosurg Focus. 2011;31(4):E6.
8. Asha MJ, Choksey MS, Shad A, Roberts P, Imray C. The role of the vascular surgeon in anterior lumbar spine surgery. Br J Neurosurg. 2012;26:499–503.
9. Lee P, Fessler RG. Perioperative and postoperative complications of single-level minimally invasive transforaminal lumbar interbody fusion in elderly adults. J Clin Neurosci. 2012;19(1):111–4.
10. Mehta VA, McGirt MJ, Garces Ambrossi GL, et al. Trans-foraminal versus posterior lumbar interbody fusion: comparison of surgical morbidity. Neurol Res. 2011;33(1):38–42.
11. Pelton MA, Phillips FM, Singh K. A comparison of perioperative costs and outcomes in patients with and without workers' compensation claims treated with minimally invasive or open transforaminal lumbar interbody fusion. Spine (Phila Pa 1976). 2012 Oct 15;37(22):1914-9. doi: 10.1097/BRS.0b013e318257d490. PMID:22487713.
12. Adogwa O, Parker SL, Bydon A, Cheng J, McGirt MJ. Comparative effectiveness of minimally invasive versus open transforaminal lumbar interbody fusion: 2-year assessment of narcotic use, return to work, disability, and quality of life. J Spinal Disord Tech. 2011;24(8):479–84.
13. Rodgers WB, Gerber EJ, Rodgers JA. Lumbar fusion in octogenarians: the promise of minimally invasive surgery. Spine (Phila Pa 1976). 2010;35(Suppl 26):S355–360.
14. Eck JC, Hodges S, Humphreys SC. Minimally invasive lumbar spinal fusion. J Am Acad Orthop Surg. 2007;15(6):321–9.
15. Benglis DM, Elhammady MS, Levi AD, Vanni S. Minimally invasive anterolateral approaches for the treatment of back pain and adult degenerative deformity. Neurosurgery. 2008;63 Suppl 3:191–6.
16. Cappuccino A, Cornwall GB, Turner AW, et al. Biomechanical analysis and review of lateral lumbar fusion constructs. Spine (Phila Pa 1976). 2010;35(Suppl 26):S361–367.
17. Phillips FM, Khan S. Early radiographic outcomes of XLIF in minimally invasive treatment of adult scoliosis: results from a prospective multicenter nonrandomized study of 107 patients. Paper presented at: 27th annual: disorders of the spine and peripheral nerves, Phoenix; 2011.

18. Dakwar E, Vale FL, Uribe JS. Trajectory of the main sensory and motor branches of the lumbar plexus outside the psoas muscle related to the lateral retroperitoneal transpsoas approach. J Neurosurg Spine. 2011;14(2):290–5.
19. Davis TT, Bae HW, Mok MJ, Rasouli A, Delamarter RB. Lumbar plexus anatomy within the psoas muscle: implications for the transpsoas lateral approach to the L4-L5 disc. J Bone Joint Surg Am. 2011;93(16):1482–7.
20. Anloague PA, Huijbregts P. Anatomical variations of the lumbar plexus: a descriptive anatomy study with proposed clinical implications. J Man Manip Ther. 2009;17(4):e107–14.
21. Matejcik V. Anatomical variations of lumbosacral plexus. Surg Radiol Anat. 2010;32(4):409–14.
22. Moro T, Kikuchi S, Konno S, Yaginuma H. An anatomic study of the lumbar plexus with respect to retroperitoneal endoscopic surgery. Spine (Phila Pa 1976). 2003;28(5):423–8; discussion 427–8.
23. Pearcy MJ, Evans JH, O'Brien JP. The load bearing capacity of vertebral cancellous bone in interbody fusion of the lumbar spine. Eng Med. 1983;12(4):183–4.
24. Closkey RF, Parsons JR, Lee CK, Blacksin MF, Zimmerman MC. Mechanics of interbody spinal fusion. Analysis of critical bone graft area. Spine (Phila Pa 1976). 1993;18(8):1011–5.
25. Lowe TG, Hashim S, Wilson LA, et al. A biomechanical study of regional endplate strength and cage morphology as it relates to structural interbody support. Spine (Phila Pa 1976). 2004;29(21):2389–94.
26. Uribe JS, Arredondo N, Dakwar E, Vale FL. Defining the safe working zones using the minimally invasive lateral retroperitoneal transpsoas approach: an anatomical study. J Neurosurg Spine. 2010;13(2):260–6.
27. Baron EM, Albert TJ. Medical complications of surgical treatment of adult spinal deformity and how to avoid them. Spine (Phila Pa 1976). 2006;31(Suppl 19):S106–18.
28. Akbarnia BA, Ogilvie JW, Hammerberg KW. Debate: degenerative scoliosis: to operate or not to operate. Spine (Phila Pa 1976). 2006;31(Suppl 19):S195–201.

Complications of the Lateral Lumbar Transpsoas Approach

27

Adam S. Kanter and Matthew B. Maserati

The lateral transpsoas approach to the spine, popularized by Pimenta and colleagues in their 2006 landmark technical report [12], has gained increasingly widespread use by spine surgeons seeking to perform lumbar interbody fusion in a minimally disruptive fashion. Essentially an adaptation of the retroperitoneal approach to the spine, the technique may be viewed as a paradigm shift in interbody fusion, offering a unique and innovative solution to the problem of achieving robust reconstruction of the anterior column while avoiding injury to critical stabilizing structures of the spine. The lateral approach offers advantages over PLIF/TLIF in that retraction of the intraspinal neural elements is entirely avoided, along with the attendant complications of cerebrospinal fluid (CSF) leak, trauma to the exiting and traversing nerve roots, epidural fibrosis, and arachnoiditis. As experience with the lateral approach grows, however, it has become clear that the technique is associated with its own unique set of approach-related complications. An understanding of these complications and their potential causes is clearly critical for any surgeon attempting the technique.

Some complications of the lateral approach – such as those related to transgression of the psoas muscle and retraction of the lumbar plexus that travels through it – are unique to this particular approach; other complications are similar to those encountered in the traditional approaches to lumbar interbody fusion, including end-plate violation, graft migration, and nonunion, but which may occur under slightly different circumstances during the lateral approach.

With the goal of establishing a systematic, stepwise approach to complications and their avoidance in lateral approach surgery, we have grouped complications according to the stage of the procedure during which they are encountered: (1) positioning injuries, (2) complications encountered during exposure and traverse of the psoas muscle, (3) complications associated with the performance of discectomy and graft placement, and (4) delayed complications. In the following sections, we review each group of complications and offer strategies—culled from the available literature and formulated from the authors experience – to avoid them.

27.1 Complications of Positioning

Complications associated with positioning for the lateral approach are generally neurologic or soft tissue related. Neurologic complications of positioning are typically transient and include painful thigh dysesthesias and/or proximal leg weakness due to traction neurapraxia of the ipsilateral lumbar plexus, ipsilateral hip flexor weakness from psoas stretching, and traction or compression peripheral neuropathy (such as contralateral

A.S. Kanter, M.D. (✉) • M.B. Maserati, M.D.
Department of Neurological Surgery,
University of Pittsburgh Medical Center,
Pittsburgh, PA, USA
e-mail: kanteras@upmc.edu

M.Y. Wang et al. (eds.), *Minimally Invasive Spinal Deformity Surgery*,
DOI 10.1007/978-3-7091-1407-0_27, © Springer-Verlag Wien 2014

axillary or ulnar neuropathy from insufficient padding of the contralateral upper extremity in the lateral decubitus position). Soft tissue complications consist predominantly of pressure ulcers over the sites of bony prominences of the dependent hip and shoulder and may be successfully treated with topical antibiotic emollients.

Careful attention to several nuances of positioning is critical if such injuries are to be avoided, particularly given the nonanatomic position in which the patient is placed and tightly secured to the operating table. Complication avoidance should begin as in any operation with careful padding of bony prominences such as the contralateral hip, elbow, shoulder, knee, and ankle. An axillary roll should be used, and hyperextension of the arm should be avoided. These measures serve to limit compression or traction on the ulnar, axillary, peroneal, and posterior tibial nerves and protect against the development of pressure ulcers.

Some stretching of the ipsilateral psoas and lumbar plexus is unavoidable when "breaking" the bed at the level of the hip to enlarge the costopelvic angle. While not necessary in every patient, this maneuver is generally required for access to the L4–L5 level and when operating within the concavity of a scoliotic deformity and should be performed judiciously. Placement of a roll under the contralateral hip may in some cases decrease or eliminate the need to "break" the operating table and may result in less stretching of the ipsilateral psoas and lumbar plexus.

27.2 Complications Associated with Exposure and Psoas Traverse

Whereas traditional approaches to the lumbar spine rarely require entry into the retroperitoneum, the lateral approach takes advantage of this corridor to gain access to the ventral aspect of the spinal column without disrupting the posterior musculo-osseoligamentous stabilizing structures. With navigation of this often-unfamiliar anatomy comes the potential for complications, many of them unique to the lateral approach. While the risk of injury to the spinal nerves is likely less than with traditional posterior or posterolateral approaches, the potential for neurologic complications during the lateral approach is significant, due in large part to the need for transgression of the psoas muscle through which the lumbar plexus travels.

Assiduous use of active neuromonitoring (EMG) minimizes the risk of direct injury to the spinal nerves and motor branches of the lumbar plexus but does not herald impending injury to the sensory branches, including the genitofemoral, ilioinguinal, and iliohypogastric nerves (Fig. 27.1). Injury to the genitofemoral nerve, which emerges from the ventral aspect of the psoas muscle around the L3–L4 level and is therefore most frequently at risk during the transpsoas approach, is thought to be responsible for postoperative painful dysesthesias of the ipsilateral groin and anteromedial thigh. It is difficult to distinguish this injury from thigh pain resulting from a general lumbar plexus traction neurapraxia and/or direct psoas trauma; regardless postoperative thigh pain of some form has been reported in most series as an early, typically transient, complication [15, 18, 19]. Indeed, in their review of the largest series published to date, Rodgers et al. report that transient thigh pain and hip flexor weakness – which they attribute to direct psoas trauma – is a nearly universal finding [16]. Cummock et al., in a recent publication, have provided some initial data on the duration of these symptoms, which in their experience resolve by 3 months in 50 % of patients and by 1 year in greater than 90 % of patients [3]. In our experience, some patients also complain of dysesthetic pain extending ventrally from the flank incision(s), which may be due to injury to cutaneous nerves and responds in most cases to neuromodulatory medications such as gabapentin and pregabalin.

Although rare, the motor nerve injuries could happen during the minimally invasive lateral interbody fusion procedures. Cahill et al. reported a single-center experience of 118 consecutive patients who underwent lateral interbody fusions at 201 lumbar intervertebral disc levels. The authors noted 4.8 % injury risk of femoral nerve

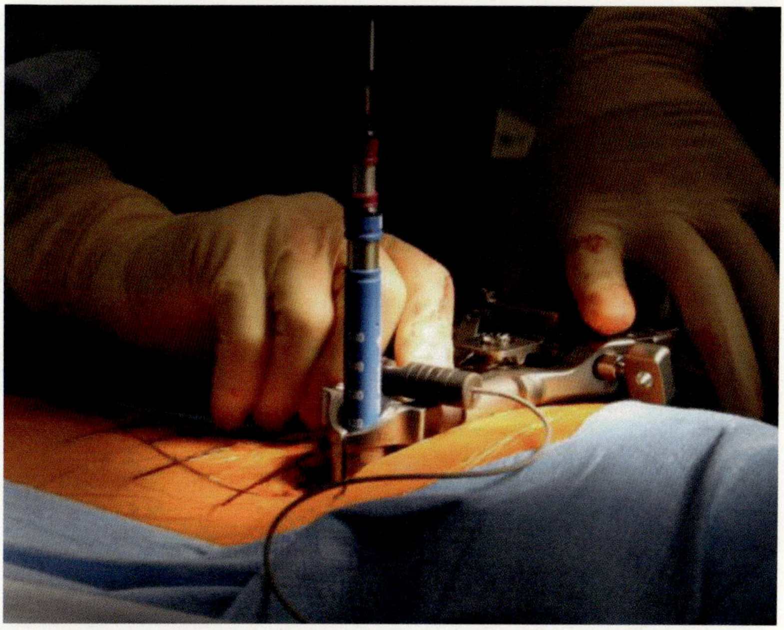

Fig. 27.1 Serial dilators and the retractor itself are each inserted utilizing EMG neuromonitoring to detect nerve proximity and location thus minimizing the risk of neural injury during psoas transgression

at the L4–L5 level and 0 % injury risk at other lumbar spine levels [2]. At the L4–L5 disc space, the lumbosacral plexus is more anterior compared to other disc levels. The femoral nerve can be located as far anteriorly as the midpoint of the disc space at L4–L5 [20], explaining the higher risk of femoral nerve injury at L4–L5 levels during minimally invasive lateral approaches.

In the same article, Cahill et al. also documented a 4.2 % incidence of postoperative abdominal flank bulge [2]. Similarly, Dakwar et al. reported a 1.8 % incidence of abdominal wall paresis after minimally invasive lateral transpsoas interbody fusion [5]. Most of the patients with abdominal wall paresis resolved at the 6-month follow-up visit. Fahim et al. performed a detailed anatomical analysis to study the etiology of abdominal flank bulge after anterolateral approaches to the thoracolumbar spine [7]. They found that T11 and T12 intercostal nerves are the major contributions to the anterolateral abdominal wall innervation. The occurrence of postoperative abdominal flank bulge is most likely due to muscle denervation caused by T11 and T12 intercostal nerves injury. The authors speculated that the nerves could be injured during the rib dissection to gain access to the upper level of the lumbar interbody space, from the crush or stretch injury when retractor is used to expand the intercostal space or during dissection of the three layers of the abdominal musculature, especially when Bovie electrocautery is used for the dissection through the muscle layers.

While the spine surgeon is acutely aware of the potential for neurologic injury during surgery, perhaps the most devastating complications of the lateral transpsoas interbody fusion procedure are injuries to the vascular and visceral contents of the retroperitoneum. Regardless of the side of approach, the colon and great vessels lie in close proximity to the ventral spinal column – the ascending colon and inferior vena cava (IVC) on the right and the descending colon and aorta on the left. Anterior mobilization of the peritoneal contents through the posterolateral incision is the first and most critical step upon entry into the retroperitoneum, and – particularly in very thin patients and in the setting of significant rotational deformity – these viscera are frequently seen and/or felt along the surgical corridor.

Bowel injury is most likely to occur as a result of sharp division of the transversalis fascia, excessively vigorous blunt dissection of the peritoneum, or pincer action of the retractor blades. Even when recognized intraoperatively, injury to the colon is a potentially disastrous complication,

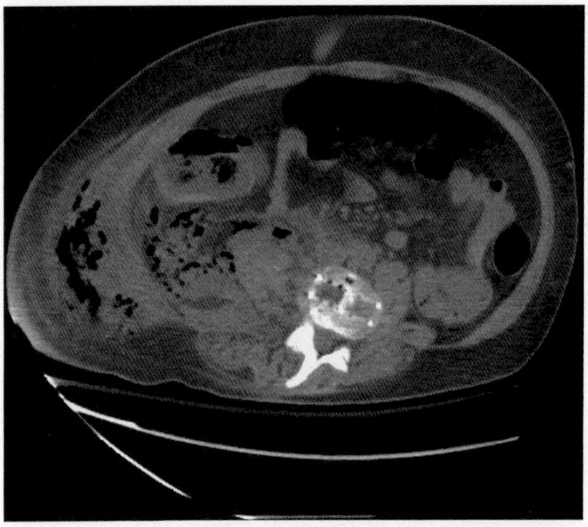

Fig. 27.2 An unappreciated descending colon injury with fecal extravasation into the retroperitoneal space led to catastrophic sepsis. An acute abdomen did not present due to the containment of the contents within the retroperitoneal cavity; thus, bowel injury can remain relatively silent for days following injury

frequently necessitating the performance of a diverting colostomy and close observation for development of a retroperitoneal abscess. The consequences of occult bowel injury may be catastrophic [19] (Fig. 27.2). The kidneys are also at risk during exposure and transit of the retroperitoneal space and may be injured as a result of sharp entry into the retroperitoneum at the more rostral levels of the lumbar spine or excessive retractor opening [9]. Finally, the ureters travel on the ventral surface of the psoas muscle and, particularly in the setting of rotational deformity, may be encountered during retractor placement.

Similarly, injury to the great vessels during the lateral approach has been reported and carries with it the potential for massive intraoperative blood loss, postoperative retroperitoneal hematoma with or without hemodynamic instability, and delayed pseudoaneurysm formation [17, 19]. The great vessels are at risk particularly in the setting of severe rotational deformity, in which the vessels are often displaced from their typical locations anterior to the spine. Injury may result from aggressive dissection along the ALL or from pincer action of the retractor against the spine. Also at risk – particularly with excessive opening of the rostral and caudal blades of the retractor – are the segmental spinal arteries. Although injury to the segmental arteries is much less likely to be hemodynamically significant, and rarely has any consequences for spinal cord perfusion (except perhaps at L1), it remains a potential source of intraoperative bleeding and, if not controlled, of postoperative retroperitoneal hematoma [11, 18].

At the thoracolumbar junction, the thoracic cavity replaces the retroperitoneum in the approach to the ventral spine. Violation of the parietal pleura is common during the dissection and typically does not require specific management. The visceral pleura is, however, occasionally breached and if the defect is significant should be treated with placement of a small chest tube. Even in the absence of a large recognized defect, a pleural effusion or hemopneumothorax may develop postoperatively and, when significant, requires placement of a draining catheter [9, 19].

Avoidance of approach-related complications begins prior to incision, ensuring that the patient is positioned so that a true lateral image and an anteroposterior image are projected with the fluoroscope at right angles to the floor. This decreases the likelihood of bringing the abdominal viscera further into the operative corridor. When planning the incision(s), it may be advantageous to consider the local pattern of Langer's lines as the risk of transection of cutaneous nerves – and of the postoperative flank and anterior abdominal wall dysesthetic pain syndromes thought to result therefrom – may be less when the incision(s) are made parallel to these lines. Next, confirmation of proper entry into the retroperitoneum is critical, facilitated by careful preoperative review of magnetic resonance or computed tomography imaging. The authors utilize the posterolateral incision in most lateral approach cases (and in *all* cases involving rotational deformity) and emphasize the importance of blunt finger dissection at a 45° angle to the plane of the spine, so as not to lose one's orientation and risk entrapment of peritoneum. Passage through the transversalis fascia and into the retroperitoneum is typically achievable without the need for sharp dissection, avoidance of which may limit the risk of injury to the retroperitoneal viscera. Thorough, gentle mobilization of the peritoneal viscera anteriorly, away from the operative corridor, is critical.

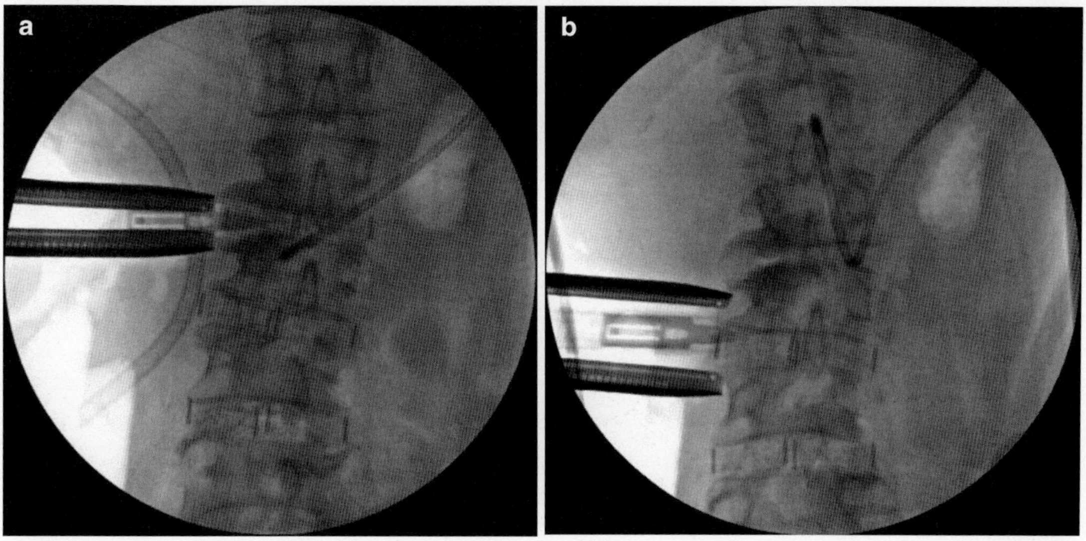

Fig. 27.3 It is important to (**a**) limit the rostral-caudal retractor blade opening to only what is necessary to successfully complete the discectomy and implant the cage; (**b**) excessive blade retraction can lead to injury to the psoas muscle, lumbar plexus, segmental arteries, and other vital structures that lie within and adjacent to the lateral spine

As an additional protection against the development of infectious complications in the event of a bowel injury, a preoperative bowel preparation may be considered. Given the extremely low incidence of bowel injury reported thus far [9, 15, 16, 19], this is probably only necessary for complex cases, such as in the setting of significant deformity.

After the flank incision is made, careful blunt dissection to connect the two corridors will permit safe descent of the dilators onto the psoas muscle. Some surgeons advocate direct inspection of the psoas in the depths of the corridor by temporary insertion of the retractor, prior to dilation of the psoas. This additional step may allow the surgeon to better plan his initial entry into the psoas muscle so as to avoid the genitofemoral nerve. During dilation of the psoas muscle, real-time, directional EMG monitoring should be used to safely position the retractor away from the nerve roots. An in-depth understanding of the position of the lumbar contributions to the lumbar plexus within the psoas muscle is critical if injury to the plexus is to be avoided during retractor placement. Elegant cadaveric and radiographic studies have demonstrated that these contributions become progressively more ventral as one proceeds caudally down the lumbar spine and have defined safe working zones at each level [1, 8, 20]. Even with avoidance of direct trauma to the neural elements, however, the roots and proximal portions of the lumbar plexus are at risk of stretch injury from excessive retractor opening. For this reason, it is advisable to open the retractor blades only enough to permit the discectomy and graft insertion, which also helps to avoid injury to the segmental arteries and psoas muscle (Fig. 27.3). Once the retractor is docked on the lateral annulus, proper orientation should again be confirmed with an anteroposterior fluoroscopic image. Any soft tissue remaining in the depths of the field should be carefully dissected away, using an EMG-equipped ball-tipped probe to ensure that no neural elements have crept into the field during retractor manipulation and placement.

27.3 Complications Encountered During Discectomy and Graft Placement

The main concern during discectomy and graft insertion is for violation of the bony vertebral end plate(s) and disruption of the ALL with the

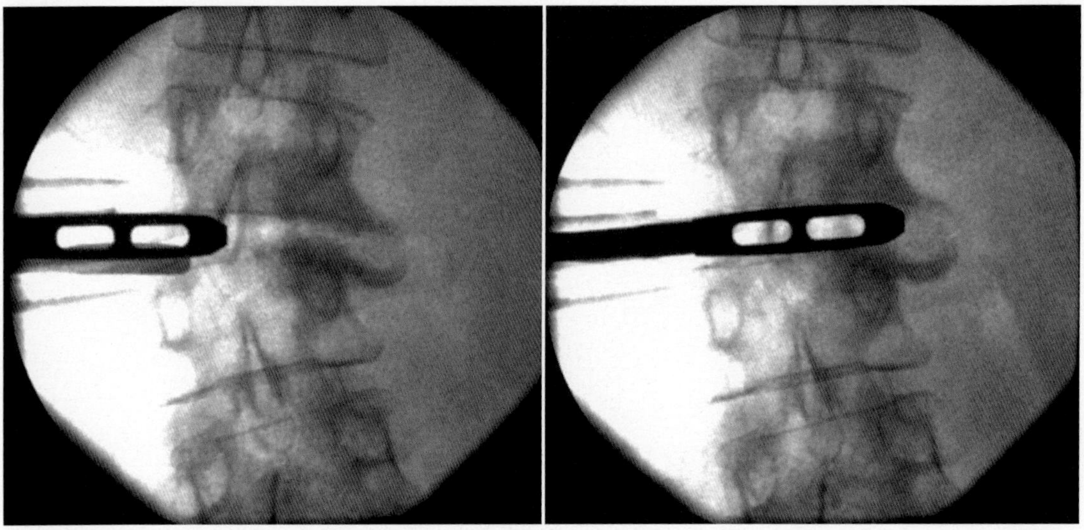

Fig. 27.4 Distraction of the disc space with steel trials sequentially increasing in size enables safe final graft placement while limiting end-plate trauma and the risk of PEEK cage fracture due to excessive impact forces

attendant risks of graft malposition, subsidence, and migration. Also worthy of mention, however, is the potential for many of the injuries – previously discussed in the context of the exposure and retractor placement – to occur on the *contralateral* side as a result of maneuvers during the discectomy and graft insertion steps of the procedure. It is essential, using fluoroscopic imaging if necessary, to remain aware at all times of the depth of insertion of the instruments used during the discectomy. This is particularly true when using the Cobb elevator to open the contralateral portion of the annulus fibrosus and break any bridging anterolateral osteophytes (Fig. 27.4), which risks injury to the contralateral nerve root and psoas muscle and may lead to the development of a contralateral retroperitoneal hematoma [13]. All of the visceral structures discussed in the preceding section – including the ureter, kidney, pleura, lung parenchyma, and great vessels – might theoretically be injured on the side opposite the approach, particularly in the setting of rotational deformity.

Although not yet reported to have occurred as a complication of the lateral approach, a dural tear is a theoretical possibility, particularly if the retractor is docked dorsally and the posterior longitudinal ligament (PLL) is inadvertently breached during the annulotomy or discectomy portion of the procedure. If PLL disruption does occur intraoperatively, dorsal extrusion of the cage can occur either acutely or at a delayed point in recovery, potentially leading to neural compression and injury (Fig. 27.4).

The anterior longitudinal ligament (ALL) is a powerful stabilizing structure and must be protected throughout the procedure, particularly if no posterior fixation is planned. Disruption of the ALL introduces the potential for the development of ventral cage misplacement or migration as well as segmental hyperlordosis with resultant foraminal narrowing. This may be avoided by early identification of the ALL immediately following retractor placement and by placement of an instrument (such as a modified Scoville retractor) directly anterior to the ALL, which serves as a visual marker of the location of the ventral border of the spine throughout the procedure. In the event of ALL disruption, the surgeon may elect to use one of the newer generation grafts, which permits screw fixation of the graft to the vertebral body.

With regard to preparation of the end plates for arthrodesis, it is essential to avoid violation of the bony end plate, which can lead to graft subsidence and to vertebral body fracture [6, 10, 11,

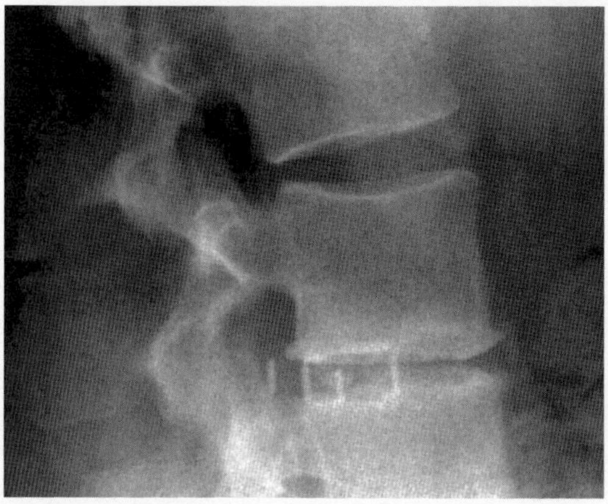

Fig. 27.5 Note the dorsal protrusion of the intervertebral cage that occurred 3 weeks postoperatively, presumably due to intraoperative disruption of the PLL and a lack of posterior compression and supplemental stabilization

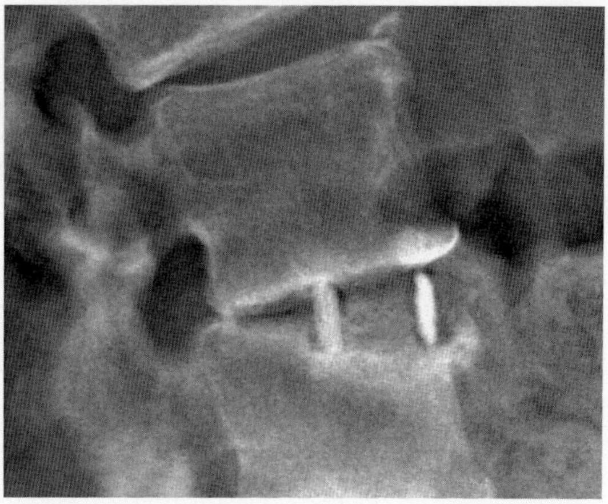

Fig. 27.6 Graft subsidence can occur due to a variety of surgical factors, although most commonly due to overly aggressive end-plate preparation. Additionally, placement of oversized grafts in the rostral-caudal plane has been found to induce subside at a greater rate and in a delayed fashion more so than appropriately sized interbody grafts

15, 16, 18, 20, 21] (Fig. 27.5). The nucleus pulposus and cartilaginous end plate should be removed with care, and distraction of the disc space should be executed judiciously and only after the contralateral annulus fibrosus and bridging osteophytes have been disrupted (Fig. 27.6). Following the discectomy, an appropriately sized graft should be chosen. Size is important as too tall a graft risks injury to the end plates and too wide a graft risks overhang [14]. The graft should then be inserted under fluoroscopic visualization, taking care to maintain a trajectory that is parallel to the end plates (Fig. 27.7). Safe graft insertion into the intervertebral space is rarely complicated when a complete and meticulous discectomy is followed by serial distraction with appropriately sized trails.

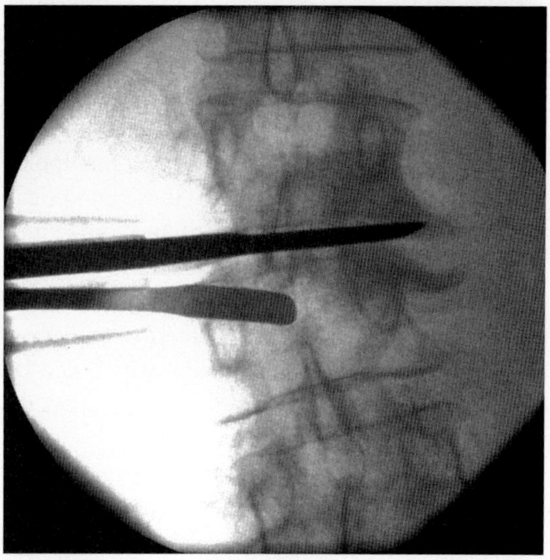

Fig. 27.7 The surgeon must be careful when tamping through the contralateral annulus fibrosus and fracturing bridging osteophytes to enable planar intervertebral distraction and not to injure the adjacent neural and visceral structures on the contralateral side

27.4 Complications Encountered in the Postoperative Period

Postoperative complications of the lateral transpsoas interbody fusion procedure include graft-related, soft tissue, and gastrointestinal problems. Nonunion has only rarely been reported – perhaps due to frequent off-label use of bone morphogenetic protein (BMP) – and in one study occurred equally in instrumented and non-instrumented constructs [18]. The large graft footprint and ease of accomplishing a thorough discectomy and end-plate preparation are powerful catalysts to arthrodesis and probably underlie the high fusion rates reported thus far. Delayed subsidence or migration has been reported and is theoretically more likely to occur in the absence of posterior fixation [4, 10, 11, 15, 16, 18]; however, delayed subsidence is less likely to occur in the absence of intraoperative end-plate violation.

Wound infection has been reported but remains a rare occurrence, as for most minimally invasive procedures, likely due to small incision size and minimal tissue trauma [9, 10, 18, 19]. Routine antisepsis measures, including preoperative administration of intravenous antibiotics and copious antibiotic irrigation prior to closure, remain the principal defense against infectious complications. Another wound complication that has been reported is that of incisional hernia [15, 16]. This complication may be avoided in most cases by ensuring reapproximation of the fascia and lateral abdominal wall prior to skin closure.

Finally, paralytic ileus [9, 15, 16, 19] and gastric volvulus [15, 16] have been reported following the lateral approach, with the latter requiring surgical repair. These complications are likely the result of intolerance of the abdominal contents to manipulation associated with their anterior mobilization prior to retractor insertion. Care should thus be taken to minimize such manipulation, although it is not likely that these complications can be entirely avoided with a procedure such as the lateral transpsoas interbody fusion. This is particularly true when one considers the consequences of insufficient anterior mobilization of the bowel and peritoneum, which can be potentially catastrophic.

Conclusions

The lateral approach to the lumbar spine is a powerful new tool that provides direct access to the anterior spinal column without many of the limitations of traditional anterior and posterior approaches, affording unparalleled access to the intervertebral space without the need for transgression of the neural elements or abdominal viscera. It is ligament sparing and muscle sparing, offering advantages over PLIF and TLIF procedures, and does not require the assistance of an access surgeon such as with the ALIF procedure. Furthermore, complications such as durotomy, arachnoiditis, and epidural fibrosis – problems with which spine surgeons have become all too familiar – are not of significant concern with the lateral approach.

Still, the lateral approach is itself associated with a host of potential approach-related complications. Neurologic complications are a significant concern with the lateral approach and are primarily the result of blunt or traction injury to the lumbar plexus or one of its branches such as the genitofemoral nerve. Direct trauma to the psoas muscle, even when minimal, typically produces transient anterior thigh pain and hip flexor weakness in many patients. Of great concern is the potential for catastrophic injuries to the retroperitoneal viscera, principally the colon and great vessels. Finally, the potential for graft-related complications, including end-plate violation and subsidence, is significant particularly if discectomy and end-plate preparation are too aggressive and if too large a graft is chosen.

Avoidance of these complications, as for any surgery, begins with selection of an appropriate candidate for the lateral transpsoas interbody fusion procedure. In particular, attention should be paid to any history of abdominal surgery, to the presence of rotational deformity, and to the relative contribution of posterior spondylotic changes to the stenosis being treated. Careful examination of preoperative imaging and constant awareness of the proximity of the retroperitoneal contents are critical to avoiding visceral injury. Positioning should be accomplished while minimizing traction on the lumbar plexus. Continuous EMG monitoring should be used throughout the approach and psoas traverse to prevent injury to the motor components of the plexus. Limiting retractor opening to the minimum required for discectomy and graft insertion decreases the potential for injury to the psoas muscle and the lumbar plexus.

Using these strategies, it is possible to safely and effectively perform the lateral approach even in the setting of severe rotational deformity. The lateral approach procedure is a uniquely powerful tool in the contemporary spine surgeon's armamentarium.

References

1. Benglis DM, Vanni S, Levi AD. An anatomical study of the lumbosacral plexus as related to the minimally invasive transpsoas approach to the lumbar spine. J Neurosurg Spine. 2009;10:139–44.
2. Cahill KS, Martinez JL, Wang MY, Vanni S, Levi AD. Motor nerve injuries following the minimally invasive lateral transpsoas approach. J Neurosurg Spine. 2012;17:227–31.
3. Cummock MD, Vanni S, Levi AD, Yu Y, Wang MY. An analysis of postoperative thigh symptoms after minimally invasive transpsoas lumbar interbody fusion. J Neurosurg Spine. 2011;15:11–8.
4. Daffner SD, Wang JC. Migrated XLIF cage: case report and discussion of surgical technique. Orthopedics. 2010;33:518.
5. Dakwar E, Le TV, Baaj AA, Le AX, Smith WD, Akbarnia BA, et al. Abdominal wall paresis as a complication of minimally invasive lateral transpsoas interbody fusion. Neurosurg Focus. 2011;31:E18.
6. Dua K, Kepler CK, Huang RC, Marchenko A. Vertebral body fracture after anterolateral instrumentation and interbody fusion in two osteoporotic patients. Spine J. 2010;10:e11–15.
7. Fahim DK, Kim SD, Cho D, Lee S, Kim DH. Avoiding abdominal flank bulge after anterolateral approaches to the thoracolumbar spine: cadaveric study and electrophysiological investigation. J Neurosurg Spine. 2011;15:532–40.
8. Guerin P, Obeid I, Gille O, Bourghli A, Luc S, Pointillart V, et al. Safe working zones using the minimally invasive lateral retroperitoneal transpsoas approach: a morphometric study. Surg Radiol Anat. 2011;33:665–71.
9. Isaacs RE, Hyde J, Goodrich JA, Rodgers WB, Phillips FM. A prospective, nonrandomized, multicenter evaluation of extreme lateral interbody fusion for the treatment of adult degenerative scoliosis: perioperative outcomes and complications. Spine (Phila Pa 1976). 2010;35:S322–30.
10. Karikari IO, Grossi PM, Nimjee SM, Hardin C, Hodges TR, Hughes BD, et al. Minimally invasive lumbar interbody fusion in patients over seventy years of age: analysis of peri- and post-operative complications. Neurosurgery. 2011;68:897–902.
11. Oliveira L, Marchi L, Coutinho E, Pimenta L. A radiographic assessment of the ability of the extreme lateral interbody fusion procedure to indirectly decompress the neural elements. Spine (Phila Pa 1976). 2010;35:S331–7.
12. Ozgur BM, Aryan HE, Pimenta L, Taylor WR. Extreme Lateral Interbody Fusion (XLIF): a novel surgical technique for anterior lumbar interbody fusion. Spine J. 2006;6:435–43.
13. Papanastassiou ID, Eleraky M, Vrionis FD. Contralateral femoral nerve compression: an unrecognized complication after extreme lateral interbody fusion (XLIF). J Clin Neurosci. 2011;18:149–51.
14. Regev GJ, Haloman S, Chen L, Dhawan M, Lee YP, Garfin SR, et al. Incidence and prevention of intervertebral cage overhang with minimally invasive lateral approach fusions. Spine (Phila Pa 1976). 2010;35:1406–11.
15. Rodgers WB, Cox CS, Gerber EJ. Early complications of extreme lateral interbody fusion in the obese. J Spinal Disord Tech. 2010;23:393–7.
16. Rodgers WB, Gerber EJ, Patterson J. Intraoperative and early postoperative complications in extreme lateral interbody fusion: an analysis of 600 cases. Spine (Phila Pa 1976). 2011;36:26–32.
17. Santillan A, Patsalides A, Gobin YP. Endovascular embolization of iatrogenic lumbar artery pseudoaneurysm following extreme lateral interbody fusion (XLIF). Vasc Endovascular Surg. 2010;44:601–3.
18. Sharma AK, Kepler CK, Girardi FP, Cammisa FP, Huang RC, Sama AA. Lateral lumbar interbody fusion: clinical and radiographic outcomes at 1 year: a preliminary report. J Spinal Disord Tech. 2011;24:242–50.
19. Tormenti MJ, Maserati MB, Bonfield CM, Okonkwo DO, Kanter AS. Complications and radiographic correction in adult scoliosis following combined transpsoas extreme lateral interbody fusion and posterior pedicle screw instrumentation. Neurosurg Focus. 2010;28:E7.
20. Uribe JS, Arredondo N, Dakwar E, Vale FL. Defining the safe working zones using the minimally invasive lateral retroperitoneal transpsoas approach: an anatomical study. J Neurosurg Spine. 2010;13:260–6.
21. Youssef JA, McAfee PC, Patty CA, Raley E, DeBauche S, Shucosky E, et al. Minimally invasive surgery: lateral approach interbody fusion: results and review. Spine (Phila Pa 1976). 2010;35:S302–11.

Minimally Invasive Anterior Column Reconstruction for Sagittal Plane Deformities

28

Armen Deukmedjian and Juan S. Uribe

28.1 Introduction

Many factors are involved in the surgical management of adult spinal deformity, including maintenance of coronal and sagittal balance as well as spinopelvic harmony [1–5]. Adult spinal deformity (ASD) is believed to develop because of asymmetrical degeneration of discs, osteoporosis, and vertebral body compression fractures [6]. Presenting symptoms of this condition primarily include radiculopathy, chronic low back pain, and neurogenic claudication caused by concurrent spinal stenosis [7, 8].

Studies by Schwab et al. [9, 10], Glassman et al. [11, 12], and others [13] have demonstrated that in the treatment of congenital and acquired deformity, correction of sagittal alignment to an SVA (sagittal vertical axis) < 5 cm leads to improved HRQOL outcomes. With a positive sagittal alignment, there is increased stress on the axial musculature, which in turn leads to abnormal degenerative changes in the disc spaces, resulting in further imbalance and serving a self-perpetuating cycle. A high postoperative SVA also increases the risk for pseudarthrosis, adjacent segment disease, and proximal functional kyphosis [14–16]. Although currently no practice guidelines exist regarding MIS sagittal deformity correction, in addition to the SVA, here are a few key questions that should be addressed during the treatment decision-making process:

1. Is the thoracic kyphosis within the normal range of 20°–40°? [17]
2. Is the lumbar lordosis within 9° of the pelvic incidence? [1, 4, 18]
3. Is the pelvic tilt < 25°?
4. How many degrees of sagittal correction is the goal?
5. Are MIS techniques feasible or would traditional open procedures be indicated?

Despite the many benefits of minimally invasive surgery (MIS), one of the limitations of MIS techniques is that up until now they have been unable to improve sagittal balance significantly [19]. Sagittal imbalance is traditionally managed with posterior shortening osteotomies, anterior lengthening maneuvers, or both. Classically, closing wedge osteotomies include a Smith-Petersen osteotomy (SPO), a pedicle subtraction osteotomy (PSO), or a vertebral column resection (VCR), which have been reported to have a 41 % complication rate in ASD [20, 21]. Major complications in revision adult deformity surgery were reported by Cho et al. to be 34 % in a retrospective review of 141 patients [22].

For these reasons, alternative minimally invasive techniques with reduced morbidity are being proposed for improving sagittal balance in ASD. A few examples of this cutting-edge

Figures 28.1, 28.2, 28.3, 28.4, 28.5, and 28.6 and some text reproduced with permission from the Journal of Neurosurgery: Spine.

A. Deukmedjian, M.D. (✉) • J.S. Uribe, M.D.
University South Florida, Tampa, FL, USA
e-mail: juansuribe@gmail.com

M.Y. Wang et al. (eds.), *Minimally Invasive Spinal Deformity Surgery*,
DOI 10.1007/978-3-7091-1407-0_28, © Springer-Verlag Wien 2014

technology that will be explored in this chapter include:

1. Sectioning the anterior longitudinal ligament (ALL) with placement of a hyperlordotic cage [23, 24] (anterior column release-ACR)
2. Lateral transpsoas hybrid PSO/VCR

Also, less invasive facetectomy in conjunction with the prior techniques can potentially provide additional lordosis when compression is applied to the construct having the interbody implant as a pivot. In addition, a recent report demonstrates that significant sagittal correction can be achieved using multilevel MIS transforaminal lumbar interbody fusions (TLIF) in conjunction with percutaneous pedicle screw fixation, which in itself is a hybrid open-MIS technique that will need to be explored further [25]. Up to this point, literature on these techniques has been scarce, and most reports are scattered with no homogeneity or agreement on techniques. We will attempt here to systematically describe several MIS options in the treatment of sagittal imbalance, as well as the anatomy encountered from the lateral approach.

28.2 Patient Selection

In addition to technological advancements in spine instrumentation that allow us to treat different pathologies more efficiently, our understanding of the optimal relationship between the spine and pelvis has evolved. We now understand that if certain spinopelvic parameters are realized during surgical management, patient satisfaction and overall outcomes are improved, as well as a potential reduction in adjacent segment disease. The goals often cited are:

1. Sagittal vertical axis < 5 cm
2. Pelvic incidence within 9° of lumbar lordosis
3. Pelvic tilt < 25°

In the not-so-distant past, it was adequate to work up a patient with intractable low back pain with a lumbar x-ray only. However, given what we now know about spinopelvic harmony, it almost seems an injustice to our patients to not obtain standing spine x-rays with a 36″ cassette. Although at this point the majority of spine surgeons are not analyzing sagittal balance and pelvic parameters, it seems that national spine organizations for both neurosurgery and orthopedic surgery are encouraging their members to embrace these new philosophies. Hopefully in the near future, 3′ standing x-rays of the entire spine will be available to all spine surgeons and performed on all patients evaluated for surgery. It must be realized that it can be dangerous to treat all patients the same and that each patient must be treated on an individual basis. However, much like with minimally invasive surgery, each patient should be viewed with a "new eye," with the goal of safely attaining spinopelvic harmony in the most minimalistic manner possible.

28.3 Advantages and Disadvantages

As discussed previously, open surgical techniques for the correction of sagittal imbalance include posterior shortening osteotomies/VCR and anterior release. With anterior release, historically there has been significant approach-related morbidity, limiting its utility [26]. Posterior osteotomies are also limited by long operative times, heavy blood loss, significant postoperative pain, and possible neurologic compromise related to the manipulation of neural elements. However, even given the significant morbidity associated with a PSO, it is currently the most effective means of improving sagittal balance, assuming a 30° correction per level of PSO. It also enables the surgeon to provide direct neural decompression. Though less evidence exists regarding MIS ALL release, recent literature suggests that through the lateral transpsoas approach, we are able to achieve 10–15° of sagittal correction per level of ALL released, with much shorter operative times and reduced morbidity [23, 27, 28]. However, we must be aware that further study is necessary to be able to reliably reproduce MIS techniques for the correction of sagittal imbalance.

28.4 Anterior Longitudinal Ligament Section via the Lateral Transpsoas Approach

Recent advances in minimally invasive spine surgery allow for options in the treatment of spinal deformity, as many new techniques may offer similar or even improved clinical and radiographic outcomes with less morbidity than conventional approaches [29]. In particular, the lateral retroperitoneal or retropleural approach allows access to the spine with minimal tissue disruption along a relatively bloodless plane and has been shown to preserve coronal and sagittal balance [30, 31]. However, in cases of fixed sagittal imbalance, ALL release (anterior column release-ACR) may be useful to restore proper alignment, as it can potentially provide sagittal correction similar to an SPO based on emerging data [23, 27, 32]. This requires further investigation as the technique becomes more utilized.

As with any operation, meticulous preoperative planning and identification of appropriate candidates for ACR is essential. We realize that this is an evolving technique still with much left to discover; however, we hope that in describing our method of performing an ACR, surgeons may be encouraged to attempt or modify this procedure with a goal of continuous improvement.

Releasing the ALL is technically demanding and requires a thorough understanding of the regional anatomy of the lateral retroperitoneal or retropleural approach to the spine. Though it reduces some complications associated with posterior approaches, it is associated with its own unique set of risks in addition to those related to the standard MIS lateral access. As with other MIS techniques, there is a significant learning curve and this will likely foster initial skepticism given the potential complications associated with an ACR. However, the potential benefit to patients is significant and thus should be explored further.

As with preoperative evaluation for any planned lateral retroperitoneal approach, it is essential to evaluate the patient's MRI to determine the course of the great vessels and where the bifurcation occurs [33, 34]. In addition, care must be taken not to injure the ilioinguinal, iliohypogastric, or lateral femoral cutaneous nerves when accessing the retroperitoneum [34–36].

However, given its posterior to anterior course along the iliopsoas muscle at the most frequently accessed levels (L2/3 and L3/4), the genitofemoral nerve is particularly at risk. Depending on its course, opening the retractor may cause a neuropraxia that is likely dependent on both the timing and amount of stretch of the nerve. Risk of injury to this nerve may also occur when performing anterior interspace dissection to reach the ALL [37]. Although the use of directional electrophysiologic monitoring can help minimize nerve injury during the lateral approach, the genitofemoral nerve is mainly sensory and unable to be monitored without scrotal or labial electrodes [38].

Another pitfall comes with dissecting the sympathetic plexus and great vessels off the ALL using the curved custom retractor, which carries the risk of a potentially catastrophic aortic or IVC injury. The target of the retractor blade is the plane of dissection dorsal to the sympathetic plexus/great vessels and ventral to the ALL. However, a unique problem associated with this procedure is dissection in the plane ventral to the sympathetic plexus and dorsal to the great vessels. If this occurs unbeknownst to the surgeon, inadvertent damage may be done to the sympathetic plexus unilaterally. At this point ramifications of such an injury have been unexamined and require further study. It is likely that injuries occur during these dissections to the gray and white rami communicantes, which connect the sympathetic plexus to the spinal nerve roots and generally run on the lateral aspect of the inferior third of the vertebral bodies. However, given the many overlapping connections existing between these structures, it is unlikely that injury at one or two levels will produce any significant clinical consequence.

After reaching the contralateral interspace with the retractor, a fresh 11-blade rather than monopolar electrocautery should be used to incise the ALL in order to prevent thermal injury to the sympathetic plexus and nearby vascular structures. Opening the intradiscal distractor should then produce a "fish-mouth" deformity at the disc space. If this does not occur, it is likely that the ALL is not fully cut. The variety of hyperlordotic cages (10°–30°) enables the surgeon to fit each disc space appropriately. It should be placed between the anterior and middle third of the disc space, which is anterior to the suggested position of a lumbar interbody cage placed from the lateral decubitus position [37, 39]. The purpose of this is to provide ligamentotaxis of the posterior longitudinal ligament (PLL) and indirect foraminal decompression at that level. One or two transversely oriented screws are used for the sole purpose of securing the cage and preventing ventral migration into the peritoneal cavity. The mechanical stability provided by these screws is likely negligible.

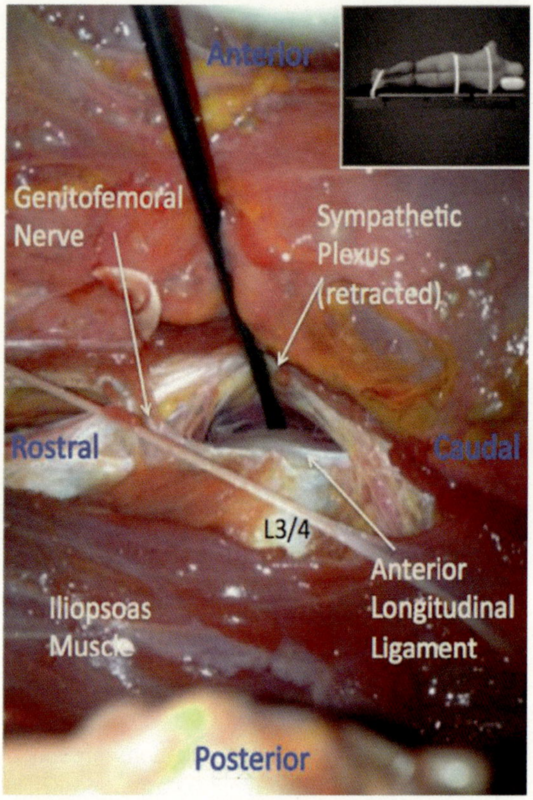

Fig. 28.1 Sympathetic plexus. Photograph during cadaveric dissection demonstrating the sympathetic plexus retracted off the anterior longitudinal ligament at the L3/4 disc space. Note the genitofemoral nerve crossing the disc space moving posterior to anterior. Inset demonstrates the position of the cadaver during dissection

28.5 Anatomic Consideration

28.5.1 Anterior Longitudinal Ligament

The ALL is a strong band of fibers extending along the anterior aspect of the vertebrae. It widens as you move caudad along the spine and is thicker in the thoracic than the cervical or lumbar region [40–42]. In the lumbar spine, the ALL traverses the anterior aspect of all VB and disc spaces and is composed of three layers: superficial, intermediate, and deep. The superficial layer traverses four or five vertebral bodies, while the intermediate layer covers two or three vertebral bodies. The deep layer of the ALL covers only the individual vertebral bodies and attaches from one VB to the next. The ALL is thinner and wider at the level of the disc but thicker and narrower at the vertebral bodies. Also, it is more strongly adherent to the intervertebral disc than the middle of the vertebral body, making mobilization at the disc space difficult. There are oval apertures at the lateral aspect of the ligament to allow passage of vessels (Fig. 28.1) [40–42].

28.5.2 Lumbar/Sympathetic Plexus

Neural structures at risk during this procedure are similar to those in the standard lateral approach [37, 39, 43]. However, because it courses dorsal to ventral in the psoas major, of all the lumbar plexus nerves, the genitofemoral nerve (L1, 2) is especially at risk as it crosses the L2/3 and L3/4 disc spaces. At the caudal end of the L4 VB, it has moved anterior to run along with the sympathetic plexus.

The sympathetic plexus is a paired bundle of nerves running along the anterolateral border of the vertebral bodies in the lumbar spine that functions as part of the autonomic nervous system via fibers to the inferior mesenteric ganglion [40, 41]. It lies along the lateral border of

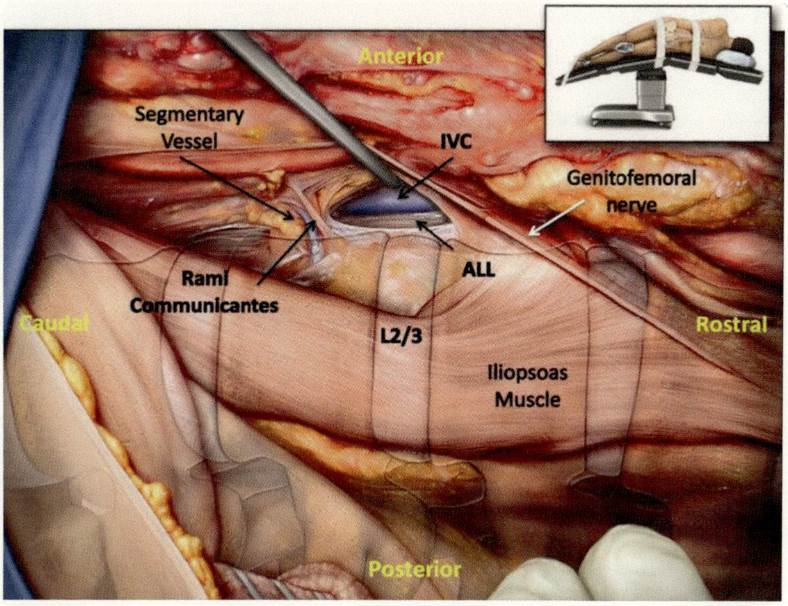

Fig. 28.2 Anterior longitudinal ligament and sympathetic plexus. Illustrated photograph during cadaveric dissection demonstrating the relationship between the anterior longitudinal ligament and the sympathetic plexus. Note the complex network of communicating nerves in connection with the sympathetic plexus. Inset demonstrates the position of the cadaver during dissection

the ALL, where it meets the psoas major, and may be encountered during an ACR (Fig. 28.2). It is in communication with the lumbar plexus, with information arriving at the paravertebral ganglia through the white rami communicantes and leaving via the gray rami communicantes. These communicating fibers run along the inferolateral aspect of the VB and generally are not encountered at the disc space where an ACR is performed.

28.5.3 Great Vessels

The aorta and the IVC lie along the left and right anterior lumbar VB border, respectively. Even when intimately associated with the ALL, there is an adipose-lined anatomic plane allowing dissection dorsal to the great vessels. There are generally four paired lumbar (segmental) arteries, which arise from the aorta and course laterally around the vertebral body, thus avoiding the disc space [41, 43–45]. [44, 45] The aorta bifurcates into the right and left common iliac arteries 18 mm rostral to the L4/5 disc space, while the right and left common iliac veins converge to form the IVC within 2 mm of the L4/5 disc space (Fig. 28.3) [33].

Retroperitoneal transpsoas approach involves traversing the nerves of the lumbar plexus both within and outside of the psoas muscle. There are four major nerves traveling outside of the psoas muscle, namely, subcostal (T12), iliohypogastric (L1), ilioinguinal (L1), and lateral femoral cutaneous (L2–L3) nerves. They originate from the posterior border of the psoas muscle and descend obliquely through the retroperitoneal space. These free nerves are most vulnerable at the initial stages of the approach during abdominal muscle and retroperitoneal dissection superficial to the psoas muscle and hence necessitate delicate blunt dissection [35]. The genitofemoral (L1–L2) nerve initially travels within the psoas muscle, across the L2/3 disc space, for a short distance before emerging and continuing on the anterior surface of the muscle.

The L2, L3, and L4 roots merge to form the femoral nerve which courses deep within the psoas muscle to pass under the inguinal ligament prior to giving off the cutaneous (medial/intermediate femoral cutaneous/infrapatellar branch/saphenous nerve) and muscular branches. Variation in proximal trajectory of the femoral nerve has been described as it traverses the psoas muscle [46, 47]. Though anatomical variations of the lumbar plexus have been described in the

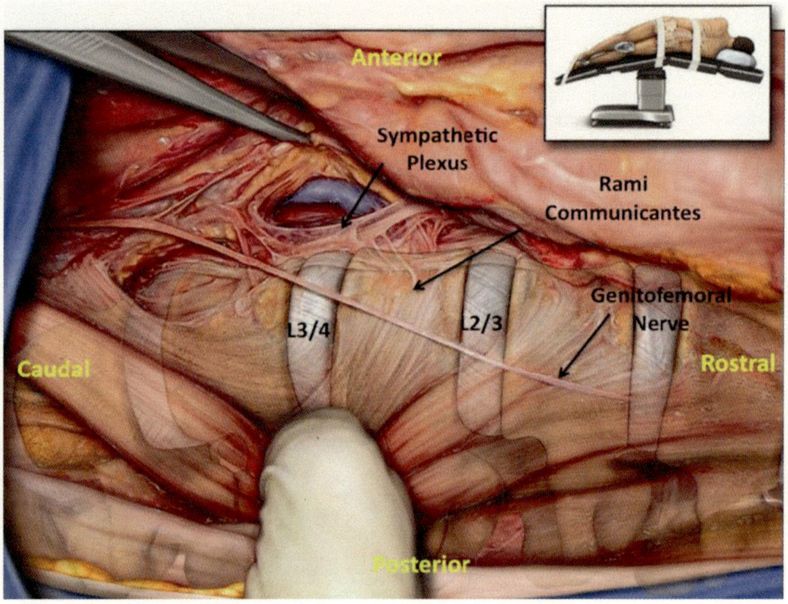

Fig. 28.3 Great vessels. Illustrated photograph during cadaveric dissection in the right lateral decubitus position (*inset*). Note the inferior vena cava ventral to the anterior longitudinal ligament on the contralateral side. The aorta here is being retracted. Notice also the lumbar segmental artery arising from the aorta. The sympathetic plexus is being retracted with the aorta

literature, large population studies to establish a more accurate measure of the prevalence of the surgically relevant variability are lacking [48, 49]. Variations in the trajectory of the femoral nerve should be strongly considered when establishing an operative corridor with utilization of directional EMG monitoring to prevent nerve injury. The obturator nerve (L2–L4) courses through the psoas muscle posterior to the femoral nerve. It emerges from the medial aspect of the psoas muscle and travels just lateral to the sacrum prior to exiting the pelvis though the obturator foramen. Finally, the sympathetic plexus runs on the anterior surface of the vertebral body and is at risk especially with lateral corpectomies or anterior longitudinal ligament (ALL) releases.

The fibers of the sympathetic plexus/ganglion are found along the lateral edge of the ALL and have communicating branches with lumbar plexus nerves. The communicating branches consist of the white (presynaptic) and gray (postsynaptic) rami communicantes. Moreover, these fibers generally reside at the inferior aspect of the vertebral body.

The intended trajectory of the lateral retroperitoneal dissection is mid-vertebral body in the A-P plane for the placement of intervertebral cage. The approach is anterior to the neural foramen and hence vulnerable to lumbar nerve injury rather than specific root injury. Lumbar nerves have contributor from multiple roots, therefore a much more clinically significant outcome if injured. All nerves of the lumbar plexus have a dermal sensory representation, except for the intrinsic motor branches supplying the psoas muscle. The clinical diagnosis of specific lumbar plexus nerve injuries can sometimes depend on overlapping sensory deficits, which can make diagnostic evaluation more difficult.

28.6 Operative Considerations

After the induction of general anesthesia and positioning in the lateral decubitus position, fluoroscopy is utilized to ensure proper orthogonal visualization of the target segment on anterior-posterior and lateral views. The skin is marked using fluoroscopic guidance and then incised. The retroperitoneal space is entered after gentle splitting of the abdominal wall muscles and the transversalis fascia. For multiple levels we use a

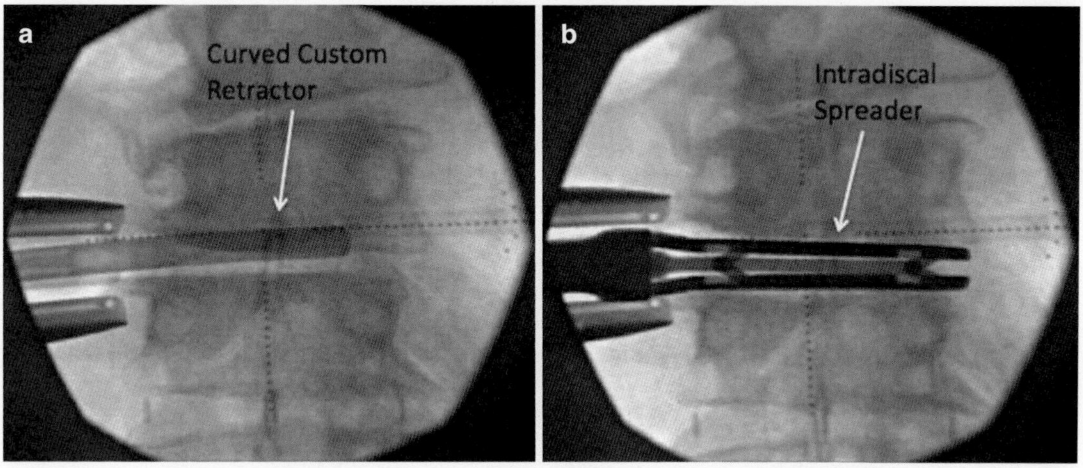

Fig. 28.4 Intraoperative A-P fluoroscopy. (**a**) The curved retractor can be visualized reaching almost entirely across to the contralateral side (**b**) The intradiscal spreader is seen in the process of opening the disc space

single longitudinal skin incision with individual transverse fascial incisions for each level accessed. Serial dilators traverse the psoas muscle and are positioned over the junction of the middle and posterior third of the disc space, using directional electrophysiologic monitoring (NV5®, NuVasive, Inc., San Diego, CA) to guide dilator placement and minimize the risk of lumbar plexus motor nerve injury [37, 38]. A retractor is placed (MaXcess®, NuVasive, Inc., San Diego, CA) and secured by a table-mounted flexible arm while a shim blade anchors the retractor into the disc space [39, 50].

An annulotomy and extensive discectomy are then performed paying careful attention to endplate preparation and preservation. A curved custom retractor is then gently passed along the anterior edge of the ALL and positioned between the large vessels/sympathetic plexus and the ventral aspect of the disc (Fig. 28.4). The great vessels are not visualized at this point, as that amount of dissection would likely place the patient at more risk than simply placing a 1–2 mm retractor. Using a custom disc blade and intradiscal distractor, the ALL is sectioned in a sequential fashion, easing the curved retractor across to the contralateral side of the disc space. Complete ALL release is confirmed when the adjacent VB end plates are mobilized with minimal resistance and there is an obvious "fish-mouth" opening of the ventral disc space.

Once the end plates are prepared, an appropriate-sized PEEK cage is selected (CoRoent® XL-Hyperlordotic, NuVasive, Inc., San Diego, CA). These cages range from 8 to 18 mm in height × 22 mm in width × 50–60 mm in length × 10°–30° lordosis and are packed with allograft of the surgeon's preference. The cages are anchored to the adjacent VB with one or two screws to prevent ventral migration into the peritoneal cavity and loss of indirect decompression (Fig. 28.5).

28.7 Case Illustration

A 66-year-old male presented with severe back pain radiating to the right leg with limited ability to ambulate, with VAS and ODI scores of 22 and 54, respectively. Preoperative imaging showed a thoracolumbar coronal Cobb angle of 54°, SVA of 10 cm, LL of 23°, PI of 67°, PT of 34°, SS of 18°, and SL at L2–4 of 5°.

During stage 1, he underwent MIS lateral interbody fusion from T12–L5 with ALR at T12/L1, L2/3, and L3/4 with placement of hyperlordotic PEEK cages, along with an L5/S1 anterior lumbar interbody fusion (ALIF). Stage

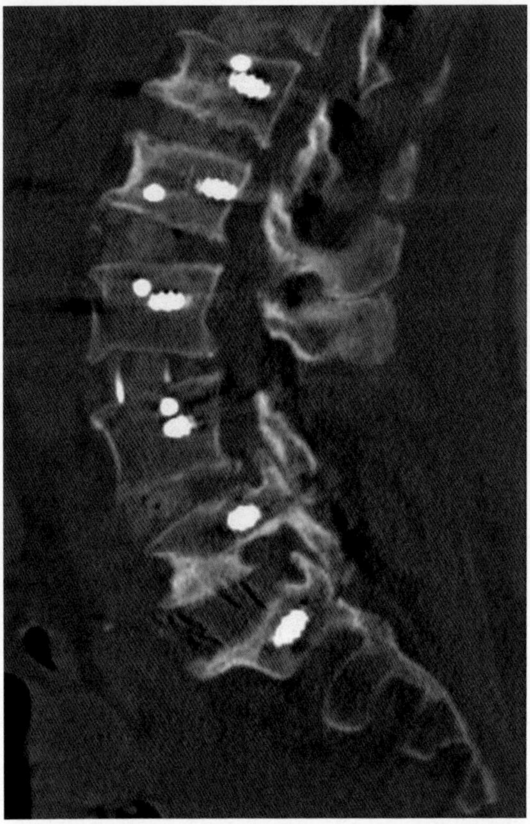

Fig. 28.5 Sagittal CT scan with implanted hyperlordotic cage. Image of the lumbar spine demonstrating a hyperlordotic cage at the L2/3 disc space, with transverse screws traversing the vertebral body

2 consisted of T10–S1 posterior percutaneous pedicle screw fixation. Both procedures were tolerated well and without complication, with a total EBL of <100 cc. His VAS and ODI scores improved to 16 and 30, respectively, and imaging revealed a thoracolumbar coronal Cobb angle of 15°, SVA of 3 cm, LL of 50°, PI of 67°, PT of 25°, SS of 40°, and SL at L2–4 of 25° (Fig. 28.6).

	Preop	Postop
Coronal Cobb angle	54 deg	15 deg
SVA	10 cm	3 cm
Sacral slope	18°	40°
Pelvic incidence	67°	67°
Pelvic tilt	34°	25°
Lumbar lordosis	23°	50°
Segmental lordosis	5°	25°

28.8 Osteotomy via the Lateral Transpsoas Approach: "Hybrid PSO/VCR"

28.8.1 Introduction

For all the reasons stated previously, including morbidity of the posterior osteotomy as well as technical challenges, there has been a drive for a safer and less invasive way to do the osteotomy. Although this subject is in its infancy, we propose a hybrid technique, approaching from both lateral and posterior when performing an osteotomy. This is especially important at the more rostral levels (T12–L2) due to the relative inflexibility in mobilizing the neural structures. Another difficulty with a posterior-only osteotomy is the increased chance of pseudarthrosis at the osteotomy site and subsequent hardware failure. With a hybrid PSO, manipulation of the neural elements is minimized when resecting the PLL (posterior longitudinal ligament) and making the wedge osteotomy. The surgeon is also able to provide interbody fusion at the corresponding rostral/caudal levels, reducing the risk of pseudarthrosis and hardware failure.

28.8.2 Anatomic/Operative Considerations

From the standpoint of the lateral approach, the anatomy and technique is similar to that described previously. The bony resection is that of a lateral corpectomy, also described elsewhere in this volume. However, in our limited experience, we have discovered thus far two different variations in performing the lateral osteotomy:

1. If the patient is fused above and below (e.g., Harrington rods, previous interbody fusions like TLIF/XLIF/DLIF), then the retractor is placed at the level of the vertebral body (VB) and the wedge osteotomy is made with resection of the ipsilateral pedicle and PLL.
2. If the patient is not fused above or below, the retractor is placed at those disc spaces and

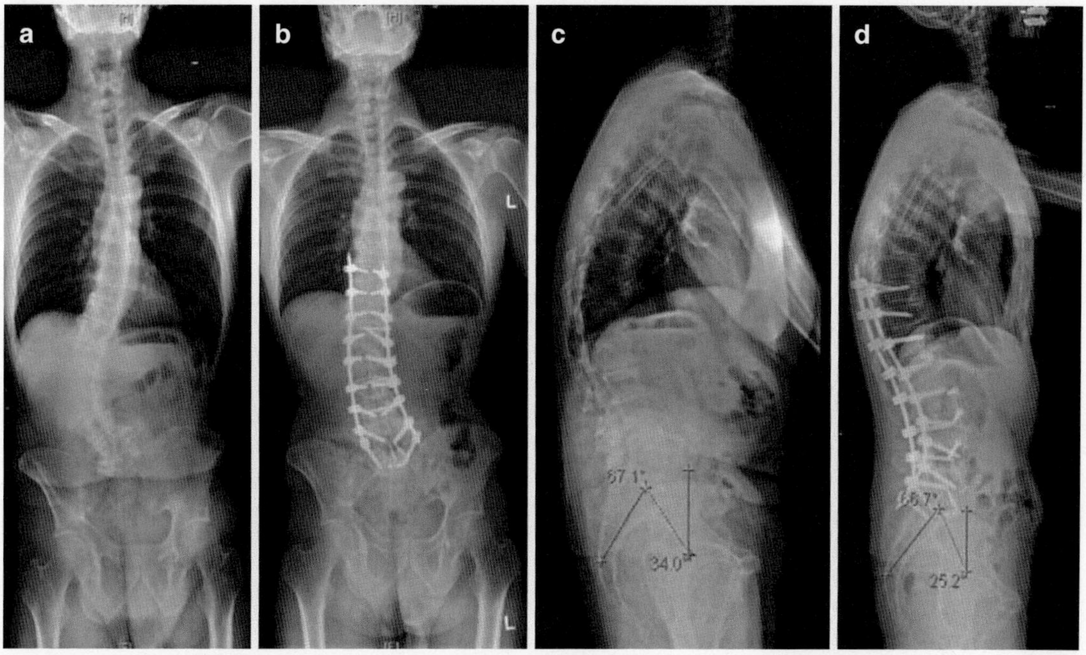

Fig. 28.6 (**a**) Preoperative standing A-P radiograph demonstrating coronal imbalance (Cobb angle = 54°) (**b**) Postoperative standing A-P radiograph demonstrating improved coronal balance (Cobb angle = 15°) (**c**) Preoperative standing lateral radiograph demonstrating a PI of 67.1° and PT of 34° (**d**) Postoperative standing lateral radiograph after T12–S1 interbody fusions and ALR at L2/3 and L3/4, with percutaneous pedicle screw fixation from T10–S1, demonstrating a PI of 66.7° and PT 25.2°

discectomies are performed followed by cage/graft placement. After that is done, the retractor is placed at the level of the VB and the wedge osteotomy/PLL resection is done. This necessitates placement of the retractor three times to avoid unnecessary retraction of the psoas muscle and lumbar plexus.

Above the L1 level the approach will be retropleural and involve releasing the diaphragmatic attachments from the VB and posterior spinal elements. Below L1 the approach should involve a retroperitoneal operation. During the placement of the retractor at the VB and dissection for the osteotomy, one of the main difficulties is manipulation/coagulation of the segmentary vessels, which run along the inferolateral border of the VB, from anterior to posterior. After coagulation, the osteotomy is performed using a drill, osteotome, rongeur, etc. In order to avoid buckling of the dura when closing the osteotomy from the back, it is necessary to fully resect the PLL and expose the dura. This also includes the removal of the ipsilateral pedicle.

The second stage, which we recommend doing shortly after the first stage, should involve laminectomy, bilateral facetectomy, and removal of the contralateral pedicle. This is followed by closure of the osteotomy in standard fashion as described elsewhere. The hybrid osteotomy, nascent in its description, has advantages and disadvantages similar to all other surgical techniques:

Potential advantages:

1. Less blood loss
2. Minimal manipulation of neural elements
3. Direct visualization of vascular structures and anterior thecal sac
4. Ability to do interbody fusion at the index level

Disadvantages:

1. Two surgical procedures
2. Learning curve with MIS techniques

28.9 Case Illustration

The patient is a 69-year-old male status post L2–S1 fusion in 2000. He developed proximal junctional kyphosis and had the fusion extended to T10 in 2009 with no correction of positive sagittal balance at that time. His current complaints include low back pain with radiation into bilateral gluteal region.

In the lateral position, he underwent posterior removal of his L1 pedicle screws and the rod connecting T12–L2. A small oblique incision was then made in the standard fashion of a thoracolumbar corpectomy (please see prior descriptions of the technique). Dissection was taken down to the lateral aspect of the L1 VB in the retropleural plane, and a retractor was placed. Using an osteotome, a portion of the VB was then resected in a wedge shape through to the contralateral side, and autologous bone kept for subsequent arthrodesis. Finally, using a combination of rongeuring and high-speed drilling, the ipsilateral pedicle was resected (Figs. 28.7a, b, c and 28.8a, b).

In the next phase of the reconstruction, the patient was placed in the prone position, and the posterior bony elements were resected (spinous process, laminae, facets, transverse processes). The pedicle on the contralateral side from the side of the approach was also resected, and rods were placed connecting the rostral and caudal ends of the construct. Using a compression device, the osteotomy was closed under direct vision (Figs. 28.8c and 28.9a, b). Pre- and postoperative lateral x-rays are displayed in Fig. 28.10.

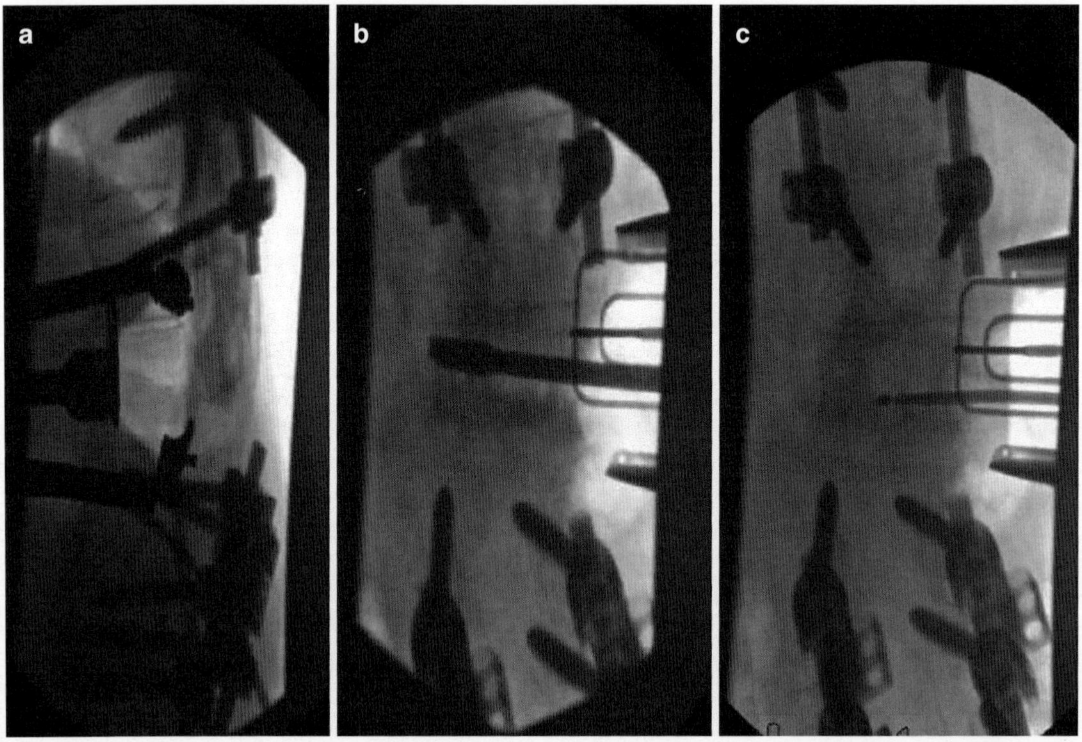

Fig. 28.7 Intraoperative fluoroscopy during various stages of the osteotomy in the lateral position. (**a**) Lateral fluoroscopy showing retractor placement at the lateral aspect of the L1 VB. As is seen on this x-ray, there is adequate exposure of the ventral portion of the ipsilateral pedicle to perform a resection. **b/c** A-P x-ray demonstrating osteotome (**b**) and drill (**c**) use

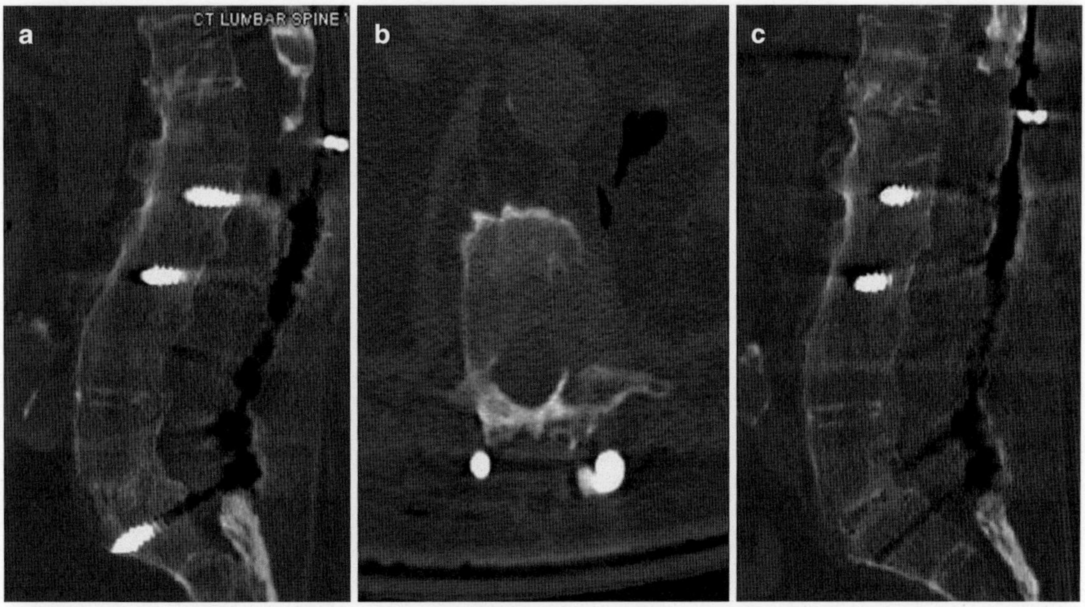

Fig. 28.8 CT images. **a/b**. Sagittal (**a**) and axial (**b**) slices taken with intraoperative CT scan between the two stages, after the lateral osteotomy but before the closure from posterior. Notice the wedge-shaped bony resection in the L1 VB and the absence of the left pedicle. (**b**) Postoperative CT scan after closure of the osteotomy, showing a much improved segmental lordosis at the L1 level

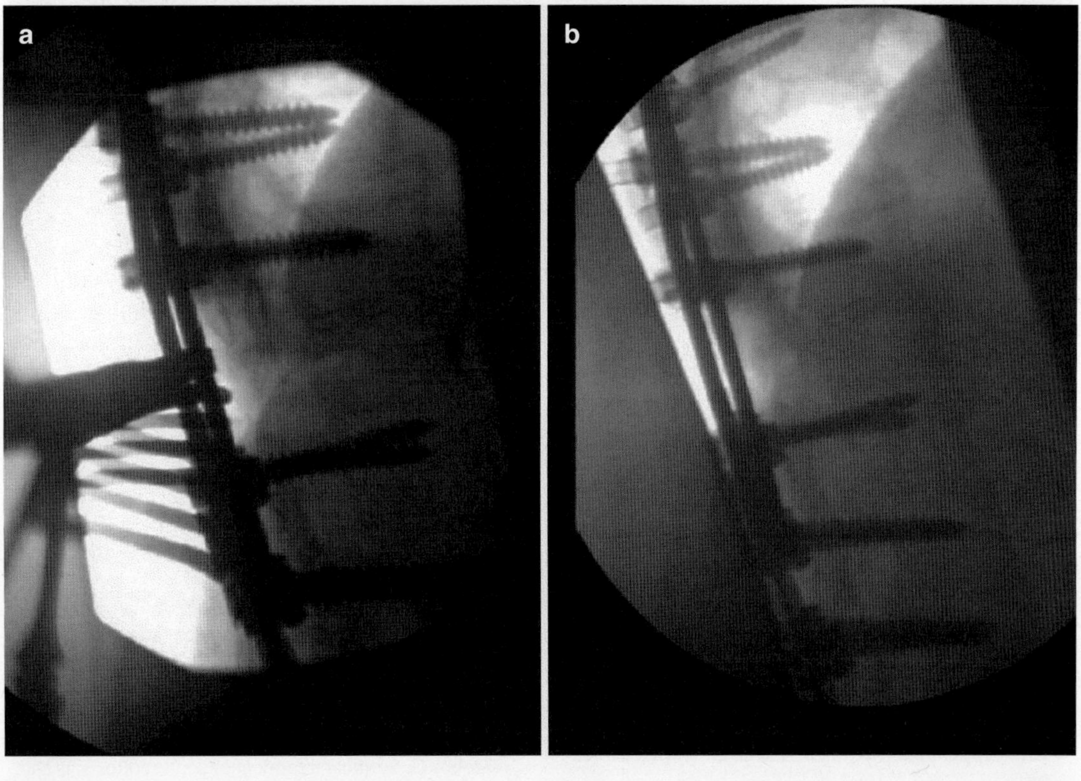

Fig. 28.9 Intraoperative fluoroscopy. (**a**) Demonstrates the placement of the compression device on the rods. (**b**) After closure of the osteotomy

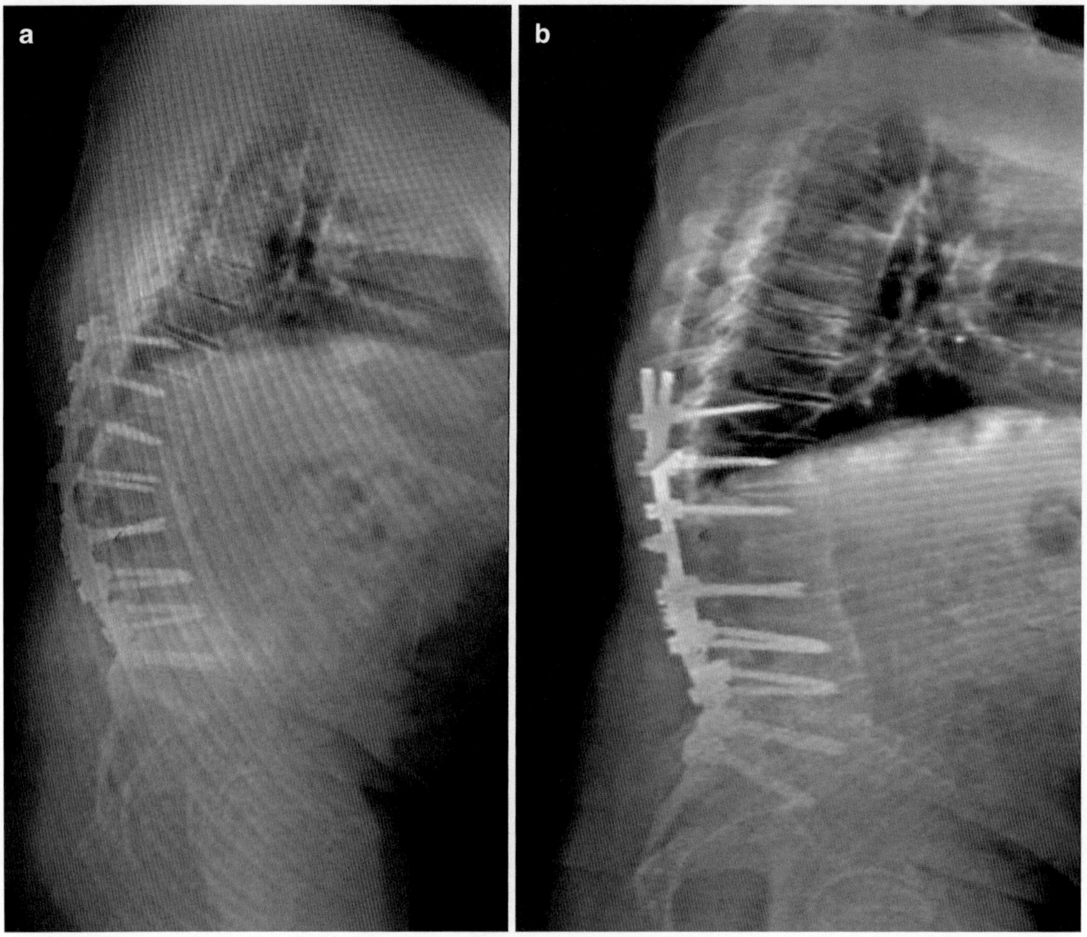

Fig. 28.10 Pre- (**a**) and post-osteotomy (**b**) lateral x-rays demonstrating improvement in overall sagittal balance

Conclusions

Sagittal imbalance is a causative factor of clinical impairment and is of great concern to spine surgeons. It can be managed through anterior lengthening procedures and posterior shortening techniques. Both are historically associated with significant morbidity. Releasing the ALL using the MIS lateral retroperitoneal transpsoas approach **may** provide an alternative to both ALIF and posterior osteotomies for the restoration of segmental lordosis. The specific utility of ALL resection and MIS lateral deformity correction will be better understood as more experience is gained with this approach through clinical applications. The use of the lateral approach to augment a vertebral column resection or pedicle subtraction osteotomy is still being explored, and will require further anatomic and clinical study, but may be on the horizon as a useful adjunct.

Figures 28.1, 28.2, 28.3, 28.4, 28.5, and 28.6 and some text reproduced with permission from the Journal of Neurosurgery: Spine.

References

1. Ames CP, Smith JS, Scheer JK, et al. Impact of spinopelvic alignment on decision making in deformity surgery in adults: A review. J Neurosurg Spine. 2012;16(6):547–64. http://www.ncbi.nlm.nih.gov/pubmed/22443546
2. Kim YB, Lenke LG, Kim YJ, Kim YW, Bridwell KH, Stobbs G. Surgical treatment of adult scoliosis: is anterior apical release and fusion necessary for the lumbar curve? Spine (Phila Pa 1976). 2008;33(10):1125–32.

3. Michael MA, Loughenbury MP, Rao MA, Dunsmuir MR, Millner MP. A survey of current controversies in scoliosis surgery in the United Kingdom. Spine (Phila Pa 1976). 2012;37:1573–8.
4. Schwab F, Patel A, Ungar B, Farcy JP, Lafage V. Adult spinal deformity-postoperative standing imbalance: how much can you tolerate? An overview of key parameters in assessing alignment and planning corrective surgery. Spine (Phila Pa 1976). 2010;35(25):2224–31.
5. Wollowick AL, Glassman SD, Perra JH, Schwab FJ. Patient evaluation and clinical assessment of adult spinal deformity. Instr Course Lect. 2012;61:469–79.
6. Herkowitz HN, Kurz LT. Degenerative lumbar spondylolisthesis with spinal stenosis. A prospective study comparing decompression with decompression and intertransverse process arthrodesis. J Bone Joint Surg Am. 1991;73(6):802–8.
7. Kostuik JP, Israel J, Hall JE. Scoliosis surgery in adults. Clin Orthop Relat Res. 1973;93:225–34.
8. Winter RB, Lonstein JE, Denis F. Pain patterns in adult scoliosis. Orthop Clin North Am. 1988;19(2):339–45.
9. Schwab F, Lafage V, Patel A, Farcy JP. Sagittal plane considerations and the pelvis in the adult patient. Spine (Phila Pa 1976). 2009;34(17):1828–33.
10. Schwab F, Patel A, Ungar B, Farcy JP, Lafage V. Adult spinal deformity-postoperative standing imbalance: how much can you tolerate? An overview of key parameters in assessing alignment and planning corrective surgery. Spine. 2010;35(25):2224–31.
11. Glassman SD, Bridwell K, Dimar JR, Horton W, Berven S, Schwab F. The impact of positive sagittal balance in adult spinal deformity. Spine (Phila Pa 1976). 2005;30(18):2024–29.
12. Glassman SD, Dimar JR, Carreon LY, Campbell MJ, Puno RM, Johnson JR. Initial fusion rates with recombinant human bone morphogenetic protein-2/compression resistant matrix and a hydroxyapatite and tricalcium phosphate/collagen carrier in posterolateral spinal fusion. Spine. 2005;30(15):1694–8.
13. Blondel B, Schwab F, Ungar B, et al. Impact of magnitude and percentage of global sagittal plane correction on health-related quality of life at 2-years follow-up. Neurosurgery. 2012;71(2):341–8; discussion 348.
14. Kim YJ, Bridwell KH, Lenke LG, Rhim S, Cheh G. Pseudarthrosis in long adult spinal deformity instrumentation and fusion to the sacrum: prevalence and risk factor analysis of 144 cases. Spine (Phila Pa 1976). 2006;31(20):2329–36.
15. Schwab FJ, Patel A, Shaffrey CI, et al. Sagittal realignment failures following pedicle subtraction osteotomy surgery: are we doing enough? clinical article. J Neurosurg Spine. 2012;16(6):539–46. http://www.ncbi.nlm.nih.gov/pubmed/22462571. doi: 10.3171/2012.2.SPINE11120. Epub 2012 Mar 30.
16. Jackson RP, Hales C. Congruent spinopelvic alignment on standing lateral radiographs of adult volunteers. Spine (Phila Pa 1976). 2000;25(21):2808–15.
17. Fon GT, Pitt MJ, Thies Jr AC. Thoracic kyphosis: range in normal subjects. AJR Am J Roentgenol. 1980;134(5):979–83.
18. Lafage V, Schwab F, Vira S, Patel A, Ungar B, Farcy JP. Spino-pelvic parameters after surgery can be predicted: a preliminary formula and validation of standing alignment. Spine (Phila Pa 1976). 2011;36(13):1037–45.
19. Hsieh PC, Koski TR, O'Shaughnessy BA, et al. Anterior lumbar interbody fusion in comparison with transforaminal lumbar interbody fusion: implications for the restoration of foraminal height, local disc angle, lumbar lordosis, and sagittal balance. J Neurosurg Spine. 2007;7(4):379–86.
20. Glassman SD, Hamill CL, Bridwell KH, Schwab FJ, Dimar JR, Lowe TG. The impact of perioperative complications on clinical outcome in adult deformity surgery. Spine (Phila Pa 1976). 2007;32(24):2764–70.
21. Yadla S, Maltenfort MG, Ratliff JK, Harrop JS. Adult scoliosis surgery outcomes: a systematic review. Neurosurg Focus. 2010;28(3):E3.
22. Cho SK, Bridwell KH, Lenke LG, et al. Major complications in revision adult deformity surgery: risk factors and clinical outcomes with 2- to 7-year follow-up. Spine (Phila Pa 1976). 2012;37(6):489–500.
23. Deukmedjian AR, Dakwar E, Ahmadian A, Smith DA, Uribe JS. Early outcomes of minimally invasive anterior longitudinal ligament release for correction of sagittal imbalance in patients with adult spinal deformity. Scientific World Journal. 2012;2012:789698.
24. Deukmedjian AR, Le TV, Baaj AA, Dakwar E, Smith DA, Uribe JS. Anterior longitudinal ligament release using the minimally invasive lateral retroperitoneal transpsoas approach: a cadaveric feasibility study and report of 4 clinical cases. J Neurosurg Spine. 2012;17(6):530–9.
25. Wang MY. Improvement of sagittal balance and lumbar lordosis following less invasive adult spinal deformity surgery with expandable cages and percutaneous instrumentation. J Neurosurg Spine. 2013;18(1):4–12.
26. Kim YB, Lenke LG, Kim YJ, et al. The morbidity of an anterior thoracolumbar approach: adult spinal deformity patients with greater than five-year follow-up. Spine. 2009;34(8):822–6.
27. Deukmedjian AR, Le TV, Baaj AA, Dakwar E, Smith DA, Uribe JS. Anterior longitudinal ligament release using the minimally invasive lateral retroperitoneal transpsoas approach: a cadaveric feasibility study and report of 4 clinical cases. J Neurosurg Spine. 2012;17:530–9.
28. Uribe JS, Smith DA, Dakwar E, et al. Lordosis restoration after anterior longitudinal ligament release and placement of lateral hyperlordotic interbody cages during the minimally invasive lateral transpsoas approach: a radiographic study in cadavers. J Neurosurg Spine. 2012;17(5):476–85.
29. Anand N, Baron EM, Thaiyananthan G, Khalsa K, Goldstein TB. Minimally invasive multilevel percutaneous correction and fusion for adult lumbar degenerative scoliosis: a technique and feasibility study. J Spinal Disord Tech. 2008;21(7):459–67.
30. Benglis DM, Elhammady MS, Levi AD, Vanni S. Minimally invasive anterolateral approaches for

the treatment of back pain and adult degenerative deformity. Neurosurgery. 2008;63 Suppl 3:191–6.

31. Dakwar E, Cardona RF, Smith DA, Uribe JS. Early outcomes and safety of the minimally invasive, lateral retroperitoneal transpsoas approach for adult degenerative scoliosis. Neurosurg Focus. 2010;28(3):E8.
32. Uribe JS SD, Dakwar E, Baaj AA, Mundis GM, Turner AW, Cornwall GB, Akbarnia BA. Lordosis restoration after anterior longitudinal ligament release and placement of lateral hyperlordotic interbody cages during the MIS lateral transpsoas approach: a radiographic study in cadavers. Society of Lateral Access Surgeons. San Diego.,2012.
33. Deukmedjian AR, Le TV, Dakwar E, Martinez CR, Uribe JS. Movement of abdominal structures on magnetic resonance imaging during positioning changes related to lateral lumbar spine surgery: a morphometric study: clinical article. J Neurosurg Spine. 2012;16(6):615–23. A review. J Neurosurg Spine. 2012;16(6):547–64. http://www.ncbi.nlm.nih.gov/pubmed/22462569. doi: 10.3171/2012.3.SPINE1210. Epub 2012 Mar 30.
34. Dakwar E, Le TV, Baaj AA, et al. Abdominal wall paresis as a complication of minimally invasive lateral transpsoas interbody fusion. Neurosurg Focus. 2011;31(4):E18.
35. Dakwar E, Vale FL, Uribe JS. Trajectory of the main sensory and motor branches of the lumbar plexus outside the psoas muscle related to the lateral retroperitoneal transpsoas approach. J Neurosurg Spine. 2011;14(2):290–5.
36. Ahmadian A, Deukmedjian AR, Abel N, Dakwar E, Uribe JS. Analysis of lumbar plexopathies and nerve injury after lateral retroperitoneal transpsoas approach: diagnostic standardization. J Neurosurg Spine. 2012;18:289–97.
37. Uribe JS, Arredondo N, Dakwar E, Vale FL. Defining the safe working zones using the minimally invasive lateral retroperitoneal transpsoas approach: an anatomical study. J Neurosurg Spine. 2010;13(2): 260–6.
38. Uribe JS, Vale FL, Dakwar E. Electromyographic monitoring and its anatomical implications in minimally invasive spine surgery. Spine (Phila Pa 1976). 2010;35(Suppl 26):S368–74.
39. Ozgur BM, Aryan HE, Pimenta L, Taylor WR. Extreme Lateral Interbody Fusion (XLIF): a novel surgical technique for anterior lumbar interbody fusion. Spine J. 2006;6(4):435–43.
40. DA Agur AM. Grant's atlas of anatomy. 12th ed. Baltimore: Lippincott Williams & Wilkins/Wolters Kluwer; 2009.
41. Netter F. Atlas of human anatomy. 2nd ed. Teterboro: ICON Learning Systems; 1997.
42. Vidic B. Photographic atlas of the human body. 1st ed. St Louis: The C.V. Mosby Company; 1984.
43. Stulik J, Vyskocil T, Bodlak P, et al. Injury to major blood vessels in anterior thoracic and lumbar spinal surgery. Acta Chir Orthop Traumatol Cech. 2006;73(2):92–8.
44. Arslan M, Comert A, Acar HI, et al. Surgical view of the lumbar arteries and their branches: an anatomical study. Neurosurgery. 2011;68(1 Suppl Operative):16–22; discussion 22.
45. Lolis E, Panagouli E, Venieratos D. Study of the ascending lumbar and iliolumbar veins: surgical anatomy, clinical implications and review of the literature. Ann Anat. 2011;193(6):516–29.
46. Davis TT, Bae HW, Mok MJ, Rasouli A, Delamarter RB. Lumbar plexus anatomy within the psoas muscle: implications for the transpsoas lateral approach to the L4-L5 disc. J Bone Joint Surg Am. 2011;93(16):1482–7.
47. Anloague PA, Huijbregts P. Anatomical variations of the lumbar plexus: a descriptive anatomy study with proposed clinical implications. J Man Manip Ther. 2009;17(4):e107–14.
48. Matejcik V. Anatomical variations of lumbosacral plexus. Surg Radiol Anat. 2010;32(4):409–14.
49. Moro T, Kikuchi S, Konno S, Yaginuma H. An anatomic study of the lumbar plexus with respect to retroperitoneal endoscopic surgery. Spine (Phila Pa 1976). 2003;28(5):423–8; discussion 427–8.
50. Le TV, Uribe JS. The minimally invasive lateral retroperitoneal transpsoas approach. 1st ed. Rijeka: InTech; 2012.

29 MIS Thoracic Interbody Surgery

Kai-Michael Scheufler

29.1 Evolution of MIS Thoracic Interbody Techniques

Surgical techniques for reconstruction of the thoracic and thoracolumbar spine have evolved dramatically within the past 15 years [1, 2, 4, 5, 7, 9, 12, 14, 15, 18, 21, 24, 26–29, 34–36, 38–40, 42, 44–49, 51, 53–55, 57]. Traumatic structural damage to the anterior load-bearing spinal column, disc herniation, spinal neoplasm, spondylitis/spondylodiscitis, and posttraumatic deformity represent the most frequent indications for thoracic interbody surgery [1, 2, 7, 9, 10, 12–14, 23–27, 31, 33, 40, 43, 45, 47, 48, 53, 55, 57]. Anterior column reconstruction to treat spinal trauma, metastasis, and inflammatory lesions has gained increasing importance due to the unfavorable results obtained with exclusively posterior approaches [7, 14, 15, 20, 25, 40, 43, 50, 55].

In addition, comprehensive 3-dimensional correction procedures (columnotomy, wedge osteotomies) for complex thoracolumbar deformity warrant primary-stable reconstruction of the anterior column to prevent instrumentation failure, pseudarthrosis, and subsequent loss of correction. However, standard thoracotomies entail significant muscle dissection (e.g., shoulder girdle during approaches to the upper thoracic spine), as well as lung and rib retraction, potentially resulting in postoperative pulmonary dysfunction (pulmonary contusion, atelectasis, hemothorax, chylothorax, pleural effusion, and adhesion) [9, 12, 13, 19, 20, 36–38, 49, 56]. The major complication rate of a formal open thoracotomy ranges around 11 % [18, 20]. To reduce this approach-related morbidity, a variety of less-invasive techniques has been developed.

Surgical approaches to the thoracic and thoracolumbar can be divided into posterior (laminectomy, pediculofacettectomy [41, 50]), posterolateral (costotransversectomy [39], transverse arthropediculectomy [10], posterolateral extracavitary approach [8, 12, 21, 27, 29, 31, 33, 46, 47]), and anterolateral (open transthoracic transpleural [7, 9, 13, 40, 51] or retropleural thoracotomy [3, 17, 25, 26, 36–38, 45, 48, 54, 55] and video-assisted thoracoscopy [14, 16, 34, 42, 43, 47]). While some of the abovementioned approaches are useful mainly for spinal decompression, only those techniques affording an anterolateral working trajectory to the thoracic spine allow for both comprehensive decompression of the spinal canal and extensive vertebral column manipulation. The latter is an integral part in treating complex thoracic deformity. Correction of severe thoracic hyperkyphosis may require division of the anterior longitudinal ligament (ALL) and therefore mandate surgical control of the prevertebral vessels.

Video-assisted thoracoscopic surgery (VATS) has been demonstrated to be a viable option in the treatment of thoracic disc herniations, traumatic

K.-M. Scheufler, M.D.
Department of Neurosurgery,
Medical University Innsbruck, Innsbruck, Austria
e-mail: kai-michael.scheufler@uki.at

M.Y. Wang et al. (eds.), *Minimally Invasive Spinal Deformity Surgery*,
DOI 10.1007/978-3-7091-1407-0_29, © Springer-Verlag Wien 2014

spinal fractures, and idiopathic scoliosis [1, 2, 14, 16, 34, 42, 43, 47]. Compared to conventional open thoracotomy, VATS has been associated with decreased postoperative pain and overall perioperative morbidity [18, 34, 35, 43, 47]. However, the utility of VATS may be significantly reduced in the treatment of neoplastic and infectious lesions of the thoracic and thoracolumbar spine. Single lung ventilation is frequently not well tolerated by patients in reduced medical condition (due to pulmonary or cardiovascular comorbidity). Iatrogenic dissemination of tumor cells or infectious microorganisms into the thoracic cavity is difficult to avoid in VATS. Moreover, perioperative assessment of pulmonary function in patients undergoing either open or thoracoscopic instrumentation to correct spinal deformity has revealed significant decreases of vital capacity by up to 30 % [19, 56]. Dissection within the spinal canal, handling of large prevertebral vessels, and columnotomy with vertebral body replacement (VBR) are technically challenging features of VATS and require a significant learning curve and specialized training with instructional and laboratory teaching [1, 2, 5, 14, 34, 42, 43, 57]. These factors have prevented wide dissemination of VATS in spinal deformity surgery.

29.2 Anterior Techniques

The lateral transthoracic retropleural [3, 26, 36, 45, 48, 54] and combined retropleural/retroperitoneal approaches [17, 25, 37, 38, 45, 48, 55] provide direct lateral working trajectories to the thoracic and thoracolumbar spine without disruption of pleura and peritoneum, therefore causing minimal postoperative discomfort and pulmonary complications. As the MIS variants represent technical modifications of standard open thoracotomy, the learning curve is less steep than for VATS, and standard spinal instrumentation may be used [45, 54, 55]. Conversion to a standard approach is straightforward and can be performed expeditiously. Double-lumen intubation with deflation and direct retraction of the ipsilateral lung as well as postoperative closed chest drainage is not required. Extrapleural (and retroperitoneal) dissection reduces the risk of injury to the aorta, vena cava, and sympathetic plexus and decreases the likelihood of duropleural cerebrospinal fluid fistulae [7, 17, 19, 34, 36, 45, 54].

The 90° lateral trajectory to the thoracolumbar spine allows the surgeon to identify the thecal sac early during exposure while sparing the nerve roots and intraforaminal radiculomedullary artery [3, 17, 21, 22, 32, 37, 45, 48]. This differentiates the direct lateral approach from the traditional oblique anterolateral access route (which requires at least a partial corpectomy to visualize the thecal sac) as well as the posterolateral extracavitary approach (which entails sacrifice of at least one nerve root during VBR). Table-fixed frame-retractor systems [30, 45, 48, 54] facilitate less-invasive exposure and create sufficient working space for the surgeon to perform discectomy, spondylectomy, spinal canal decompression, VBR, comprehensive correction maneuvers, and ventrolateral screw-plate or screw-rod instrumentation from T3 to L4 [3, 4, 6, 17, 24–26, 40, 44–46, 48, 54, 55]. To facilitate the surgeon's anatomical orientation throughout approaching, canal decompression and spinal instrumentation, the patient is usually placed in a 90° lateral decubitus position. While it is feasible to insert pedicle screws in the lateral decubitus position (especially with spinal image guidance), most surgeons prefer to reposition the patient prone on a bolster frame before commencing with (percutaneous) posterior pedicle-based fixation.

29.3 Posterior Techniques

The posterolateral extracavitary approach [8, 12, 16, 21, 27, 29, 31, 33, 46, 47] has been used for removal of median thoracic disc herniations and oligosegmental vertebral column replacement (VBR) without the need for comprehensive anterior column manipulation. Standard prone positioning allows for simultaneous pedicle screw fixation, resulting in time-efficient workflow. Whereas the originally described techniques involved extensive tissue dissection, recent MIS variants have greatly reduced the invasiveness of the posterolateral extracavitary approach [8, 12, 21, 27, 29, 33, 46]. Contemporary MIS variants of the posterolateral extracavitary approach involve a limited oblique paramedian skin incision (lateral to the erector trunci muscle belly) along a rib at the level of the pathology. In contrast to the anterolateral approaches, only an oblique view of the spinal canal can be obtained, one or more nerve roots need to be sacrificed to perform a VBR [47], and comprehensive manipulation (e.g., correction of hyperkyphosis) is not feasible due to inadequate visualization and control of the prevertebral vessels. Moreover, conversion to a standard size approach entails significant, time-consuming additional tissue dissection, blood loss, and muscle damage [21, 31, 46, 47, 51].

29.4 Indications for MIS Thoracic Interbody Surgery

In the context of spinal deformity surgery, the indications for thoracic columnotomy, interbody instrumentation, and VBR encompass:

- Correction of idiopathic or degenerative thoracic kyphosis and/or kyphoscoliosis
- Part of comprehensive thoracolumbar kyphoscoliosis correction
- Kyphosis due to (osteoporotic) vertebral body collapse
- Bechterew's disease
- Posttraumatic deformity of the thoracic spine
- Postlaminectomy kyphosis
- Anderson's lesion in Bechterew's disease

General indications include:

- Vertebral body replacement for tumor, spondylitis, and spondylodiscitis
- Anterior column reconstruction in spinal trauma
- Pseudarthrosis following posterior thoracic fusion surgery

29.5 Contraindications for MIS Thoracic Interbody Surgery

The following conditions or circumstances may render MIS techniques unsafe, unpractical, or useless:

- Previous ipsilateral thoracotomy (or previous ipsilateral retroperitoneal approach, if a combined thoracolumbar approach is considered)
- Demonstration of neoplastic or inflammatory pleural infiltration on preoperative imaging
- Excessive anticipated depth of operative corridor (based on patient size/preoperative imaging), precluding the safe and efficient use of available tools and instrumentation

Generally, any new MIS technique or technology is associated with a learning curve. Adequate surgeon training, skills, and experience are prerequisite for safe and efficient application of MIS in clinical practice. The choice of technique used in any individual case should be based on the surgical goal and patient safety and should incorporate a bailout option in case the MIS approach needs to be abandoned. This includes availability of a vascular surgeon to manage a potential vascular accident.

29.6 MIS Thoracic Interbody Surgery via Lateral Retropleural Approach

Patients are positioned in a 90° lateral decubitus position with supportive pad spaced at the shoulders, sternum, sacrum, and symphysis (Fig. 29.1). Biplanar fluoroscopy is used to assure exact positioning. A chest pad may be positioned to avoid undue pressure at the dependent shoulder. The operating table may be flexed at the joint underlying the patient's pelvis to improve exposure of the thoracolumbar junction but must be reversed to a neutral position before instrumentation to avoid iatrogenic scoliosis. The approach side is selected according to both local anatomy and pathology. Usually, upper and mid-thoracic lesions (Th4–Th9) are approached from the right side (to avoid the aortic arch overlying the left upper thoracic spine), whereas access from the left is used for thoracolumbar (Th10–L2) lesions (to avoid retraction of the liver) [22, 32, 45, 52, 54]. The arms are secured on padded boards or suspended (Fig. 29.1). To release tension from the iliopsoas muscle on the approach side in thoracolumbar approaches, the hip is flexed.

The rib directly overlying the lesion and the outlines of the affected and adjacent vertebral bodies are marked on the skin under fluoroscopy – schematic line drawing). The length of the

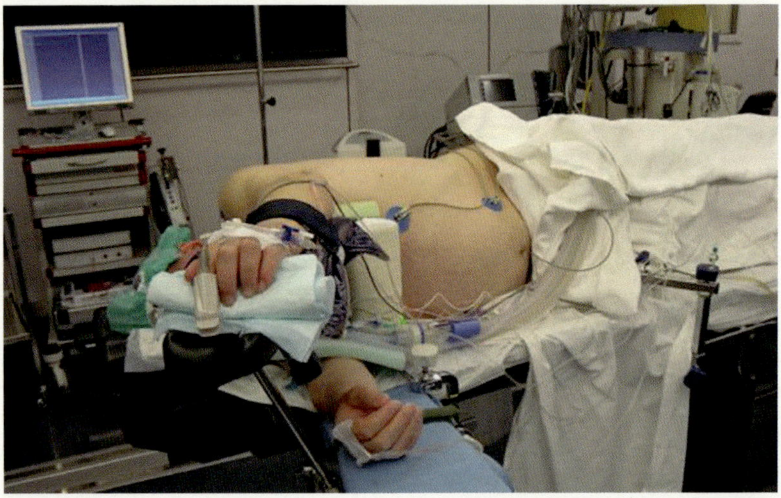

Fig. 29.1 Patient positioning for left lateral MIS approach to the thoracolumbar spine. Arms are abducted, and torso is fixed by supportive pads at the shoulders, sternum, sacrum, and symphysis to assure adequate anatomical orientation by maintaining exact lateral position. Access to the thoracolumbar spine must be kept clear circumferentially, especially if simultaneous posterior instrumentation is intended. The iliac crest is commonly used as fixation point for the image-guidance dynamic reference frame and should therefore also be draped and be accessible during surgery

skin incision depends on the intended procedure. For monosegmental spondylectomy and VBR, a 5–6 cm incision is adequate. Incisional length is extended to 8 cm for bilevel pathology or 10–12 cm for multiple segments – schematic line drawing). Sufficient mobilization of the skin and subcutaneous areolar tissue from the outer chest cage is important to permit soft tissue retraction craniocaudally and ventrodorsally during dissection and instrumentation. This will also allow for lateral instrumentation to be placed through additional thoracoports inserted one or two intercostal spaces above/below the rib resection site – schematic line drawing). An 8 cm rib segment is dissected subperiosteally and removed. The intercostal neurovascular bundle is mobilized off the costal sulcus, covered with a moist sponge and deflected into the chest cavity to avoid retraction-related intercostal neuralgia. Introducing the frame-retractor blades, the parietal pleural is then mobilized from the chest wall using blunt finger dissection or a peanut sponge – schematic line drawing). Mobilization of the parietal pleura is initialized around the rib removal site (i.e., ventrally and near the supra- and infrajacent ribs) before redirecting the retropleural dissection towards the spine. This will minimize the likelihood of pleural tears. The valves of a table-fixed frame retractor [30] are frequently adjusted during this process, facilitating retropleural dissection by keeping the interface between parietal pleura and chest wall under constant tension. The sympathetic chain, segmental vessels, thoracic duct (left-sided approach), and the azygous/hemiazygous veins are contained against the vertebral bodies within this areolar tissue layer [22, 32, 52] – schematic line drawing). Once the rib heads are visualized, an attempt can be made to mobilize the sympathetic chain off the spinal surface along with the pleura. Unlike the thoracic duct and veins, the sympathetic chain may be difficult to preserve and can be divided at the approach level without sequelae. Segmental vessels are isolated, ligated, and divided as dictated by pathology and surgical goal. If the ALL needs to be released during kyphosis correction, the dissection is carried between anterior vertebral surface and vessels to the contralateral side – schematic line drawing). Once the vessels are protected by a wide spatula, the ALL can be divided. Removal of the pedicles at the level of pathology allows for early identification of the spinal canal – schematic line drawing). To address lesions at the thoracolumbar junction, the retropleural and retroperitoneal spaces may need to be connected to gain full access to the spine/spinal canal and to place the instrumentation. The retroperitoneal space is entered by dividing the costal cartilage of the 11th or 12th ribs [22, 32, 37, 52] and the psoas muscle is bluntly split en route to the spine [4, 6, 17, 24, 45, 48, 54]. The extent of associated rib removal depends on both individual anatomy and required surgical access dimensions. In contradistinction to the original descriptions of thoracolumbophrenic access [37, 38], extensive division of the diaphragm itself is not required. Only the most proximal diaphragmatic insertions on the thoracolumbar spine (L1, L2) are dissected off the lateral spinal surface to connect the retropleural and retroperitoneal spaces [11, 17, 45, 55] – schematic line drawing). Overlying skin, soft tissues, pleura, diaphragm, and peritoneal sac are retracted by multiple valves of a table-fixed retractor to allow for simultaneous visualization of supra- and infradiaphragmatic extensions of the combined approach. Closed chest tube drainage usually is not required. If a visceral pleural leak (i.e., air fistula) or a parietal pleural tear should occur that cannot be addressed by direct suture or application of a sealant (e.g., a fibrin-coated collagen sponge), a small chest tube is placed directly through from the approach site. Otherwise, a single large vacuum drain (12Ch) is left in the retropleural space to promote reattachment of the parietal pleura to the chest wall for 3–4 days. Mid-thoracic (true) ribs are approximated and secured with nonabsorbable sutures. The wound is closed anatomically in layers, with the skin either sutured or sealed with cyanoacrylate. Postoperative chest X-rays to exclude clinically relevant pneumo-/hemothorax are obligatory before discharge of the patient from the ICU.

29.7 Extracoelomic Approach to the Thoracolumbar Junction

The thoracolumbar junction may be accessed either via a primarily transthoracic retropleural route [1, 2, 13, 14, 30, 34, 42, 43, 57] (working downward with transdiaphragmatic extension into the retroperitoneal space at L1 or L2) or via a retroperitoneal approach working upward through the insertion of the medial diaphragm arcade [11] with subsequent retropleural dissection along the lateral spine surface [3, 17, 45, 54]. The choice of the most suitable approach is dictated by individual chest cage anatomy (position, angulation, and length of the 10th to 12th ribs), the intended instrumentation, and surgeon preference.

29.8 MIS Thoracic Interbody Surgery via Posterolateral Extracavitary Approach

Our preferred MIS variant of the posterolateral extracavitary approach (PECA) involves partial removal of the proximal 8–10 cm of the rib at the level of the pathology with the patient in regular prone position (Fig. 29.2). The approach side needs to be ipsilateral to the location or major extension of pathology, respectively, since the PECA does not offer a lateral working trajectory tangential to the spinal canal – schematic line drawing). This feature of PECA precludes the treatment of lesions that require radical VBR, comprehensive anterior column manipulation, division of the ALL, or full pedicle-to-pedicle visualization of the spinal canal. However, posterior pedicle screw fixation can easily be performed without repositioning the patient. Therefore, in our hands this approach is a preferred option in the treatment of spinal metastasis, rather than deformity. Like in retropleural thoracotomy, blunt dissection of the parietal pleura commences at the site of rib removal. This retropleural plane is progressively developed to expose the rib head(s) and then the lateral vertebral body wall, up to its anterior border – schematic line drawing). For VBR, at least one spinal nerve root needs to be divided to gain enough space for insertion of the distraction cage. In contradistinction to the lateral retropleural approach, the trajectory during VBR cage insertion is invariably oblique. For lordotic anterior column reconstruction, instrumentation systems allowing for insertion of lordotic

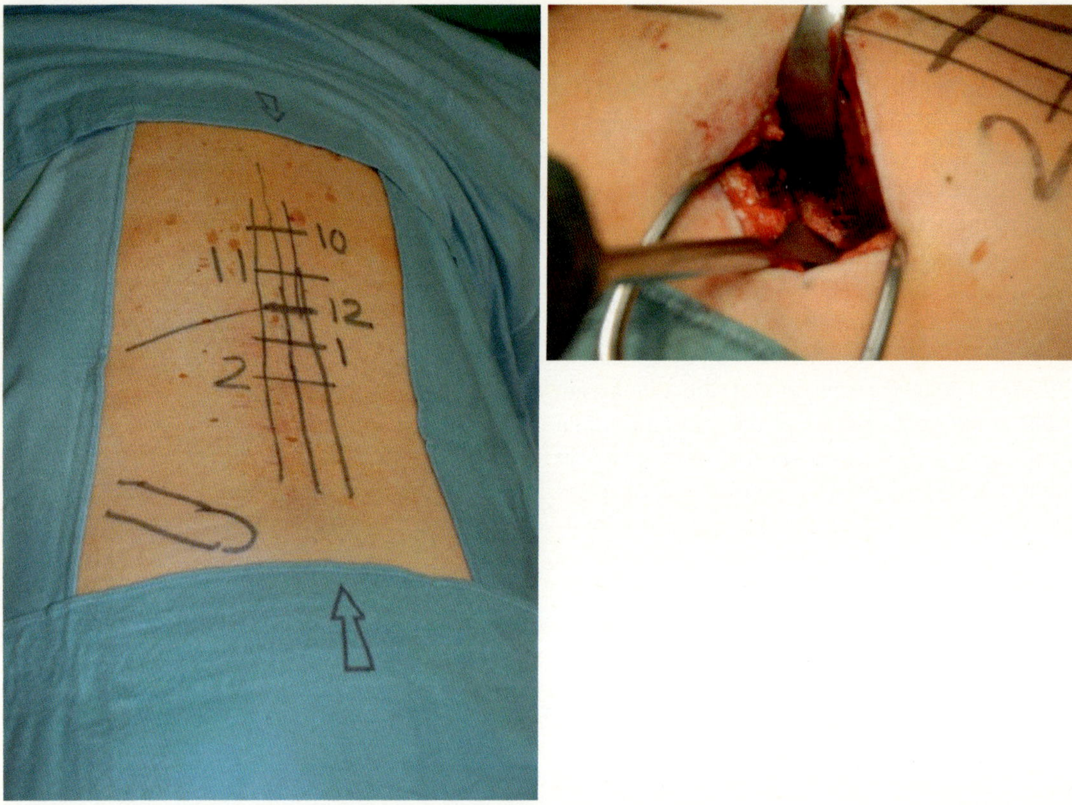

Fig. 29.2 MIS lateral extracavitary approach to Th12. *Left image* – overview showing skin markings of midline, pedicle rows, and positions of Th10–L2 pedicles. *Lower left mark* indicates posterior iliac crest. *Right image* – operative situs following resection of proximal left 12th rib and retropleural dissection to the costovertebral joint. Cobb elevator is placed below rib head. The dissection remains entirely lateral to and therefore spares the erector trunci muscle

VBR devices from variable oblique angles (e.g., Obelisk®, Ulrich Medical, Ulm, Germany) [45, 54] are recommended.

29.9 MIS Corpectomy and Vertebral Body Replacement

Removal of adjacent discs greatly facilitates anatomical orientation during subsequent corpectomy. Discectomy and/or corpectomy is performed using long-handled instruments (chisels, elevators, rongeurs, curettes, or a power burr). If spinal canal decompression is required, the posterior vertebral wall is initially left intact during corpectomy, then progressively thinned down, and finally displaced ventrally into the corpectomy defect with a long slim Cobb dissector, directing it away from the thecal sac – schematic line drawing). Adequacy of decompression may be assessed by either passing a blunt nerve hook along the posterior vertebral surface and below the thecal sac to the contralateral side, epidural contrast medium instillation with subsequent fluoroscopy (intraoperative epidurography), or intraoperative 3D imaging (isocentric C-arm or intraoperative CT technology).

A variety of interbody devices may be used for anterior column reconstruction [1, 15, 29, 33, 40, 45, 47, 53, 54]. Implants of specific interest for deformity surgery are (a) hyperlordotic intervertebral cages (lordosis angle 16°–25°) and distractable VBR cages with variable angle end plates. The individual choice of implant depends on correction requirements, the size of gap that needs to be closed, the number of segments addressed, and availability of instrumentation

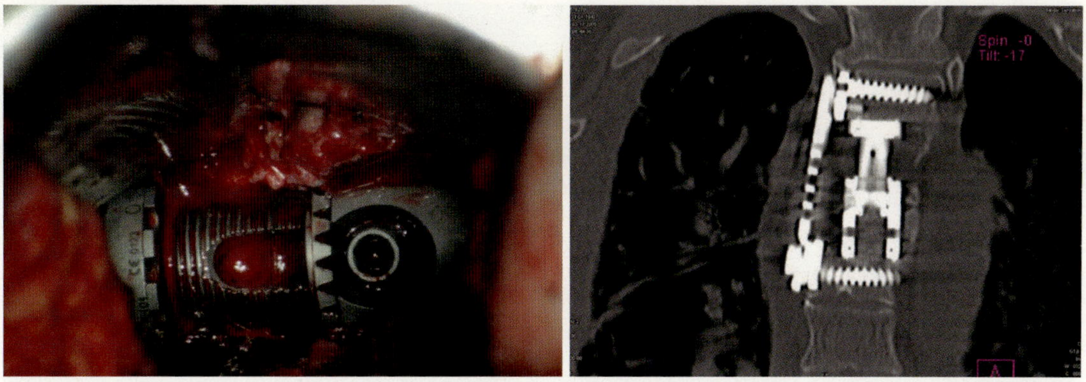

Fig. 29.3 MIS bisegmental (Th4 and Th5) vertebral body replacement (VBR) via right-sided retropleural approach. The aortic arch is overlying the left lateral vertebral surface in the upper thoracic spine. *Left image* – the parietal pleura is held below two retractor blades (*upper image border*); the spinal canal is oriented parallel to *lower image border*. VBR device is fully expanded, and the locking nut is engaged. *Right image* – corresponding postoperative coronal CT reconstruction, demonstrating VBR device and lateral plate

suitable for MIS. We use individually trimmed titanium mesh cylinders as hyperlordotic intervertebral cage to close PSO gaps. For VBR, our preferred implant is a hollow cylindrical titanium distractable device equipped with variable angle end plates (Fig. 29.3) that is manufactured in various sizes to bridge corpectomy voids of up to three segments (Obelisk®, Ulrich Medical, Ulm, Germany) [45, 54]. In the elderly and in patients with questionable or proven poor bone quality, we routinely reinforce the vertebral bodies flanking distractable VBR devices with PMMA (i.e., intraoperative vertebroplasty) to prevent subsidence and vertebral stress fracture (Fig. 29.4).

29.10 MIS Deformity Correction

MIS correction of thoracic hyperkyphosis or scoliosis by interbody techniques involves either multiple thoracic discectomies (Fig. 29.4) or columnotomy (oligosegmental corpectomy) with subsequent (hyper)lordotic intervertebral cage or VBR device insertion (Fig. 29.5). The thoracic and combined thoracoabdominal retropleural/retroperitoneal approaches provide suitable access for such procedures, specifically by granting visualization and control of prevertebral vessels and thecal sac during release and subsequent instrumentation. Spinal deformity correction maneuvers as well as VBR implant size and shape may be planned individually with the aid of specifically designed software, allowing for assessment of correction results and required hardware ahead of the actual intervention. The importance of meticulous surgical planning for successful completion of a complex MIS deformity procedure cannot be overstated. Comprehensive spinal fixation and deformity reduction usually involve either posterior pedicle-based fixation or anterolateral screw-rod fixation (Fig. 29.4). Posterior instrumentation may either be placed prior to or during the anterior procedure [25, 54]. Surgical options include insertion of provisional rods, which are replaced by definitive rods during anterior correction, and image-guided single-step circumferential instrumentation in the lateral decubitus position. Various surgical sequence strategies are currently evolving, as are specific implants, correction tools, as well as integration of surgical image-guidance and planning software.

29.11 Complications Avoidance and Management

The complication profile of MIS deformity procedures generally resembles that of conventional open procedures. Complications specifically related to MIS may arise from inability of the

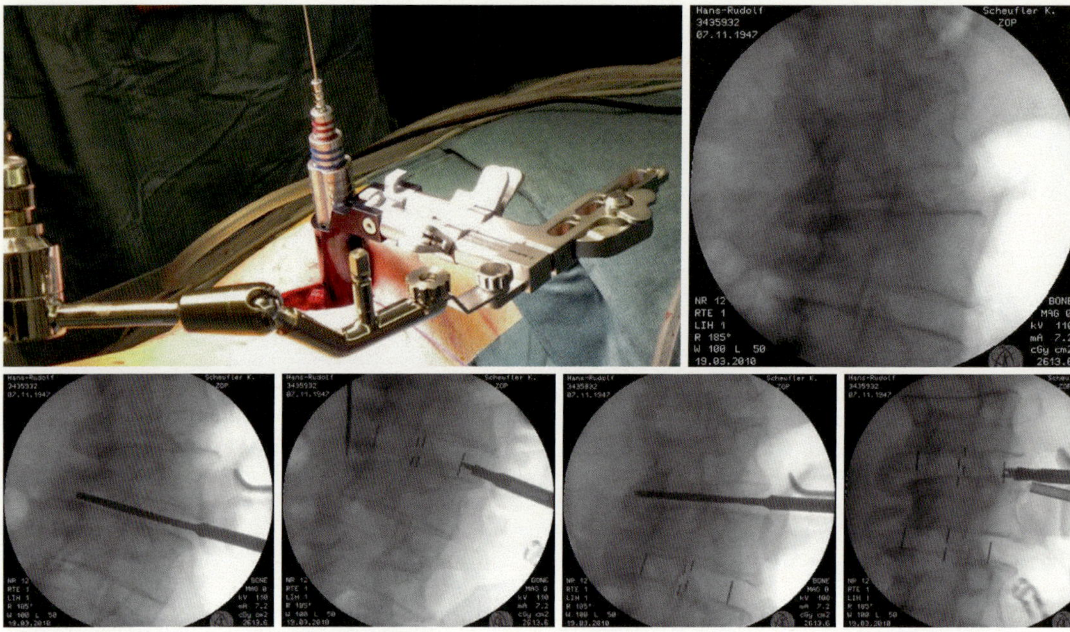

Fig. 29.4 MIS correction of thoracolumbar scoliosis (degenerative adult scoliosis) in a 62-year-old male via left-sided DLIF. *Upper left image* – intraoperative situs after insertion of the tubular retractor. *Upper right image* – initial intraoperative A-P radiograph before correction. Note solid lateral syndesmophytes on concave *right side*, requiring aggressive intersomatic release during correction. *Lower row* – intraoperative radiographs during sequential intersomatic release and insertion of intervertebral cages. Note the frontal correction release following release of syndesmophytes on final image

surgeon to accomplish the surgical goal(s) within the confines of an MIS exposure. In our experience, true MIS-related problems are rare and mostly due to inadequate surgical planning or experience. Few events may warrant conversion to a "standard" size approach:

- Uncontrollable bleeding from laceration of a large vessel in the depth of the operative field
- Inability to safely dissect the soft tissues anterior to the spine in severe rotational scoliosis
- Inability to safely perform anterior instrumentation due to inadequate trajectory in severe rotational scoliosis

Pleural tears or dural lacerations with CSF egress do not warrant access extension. Pleural tears are not uncommon and easy to deal with (direct suture and/or application of fibrin-soaked gelatin sponge) and do not per se warrant insertion of a chest tube. The anesthesia team is asked to increase the PEEP of mechanical ventilation to expand the lung. If there is contact between visceral and parietal pleura, a chest drain is not required. However, if the pleural gap does not close or in case of a visceral pleural tear (air fistula), placement of a chest tube is mandatory. Dural lacerations are best treated by application of fibrin glue and fibrin-soaked gelatin sponge in several layers. In this event, the retropleural drain should be placed more anteriorly and the retropleural space adjacent to the spine obliterated with Floseal (Baxter).

29.12 Clinical Results

The recent steep increase in lateral lumbar fusion procedures may be attributed to the ease and efficacy of the direct lateral approach [4, 6, 17, 21, 24, 45]. Various MIS deformity procedures utilize the unique features offered by the lateral trajectory to the thoracolumbar spine. Both VATS and mini-open lateral trans-/retropleural approach share the lateral route that allows for direct visualization of the vertebral body and anterior spinal

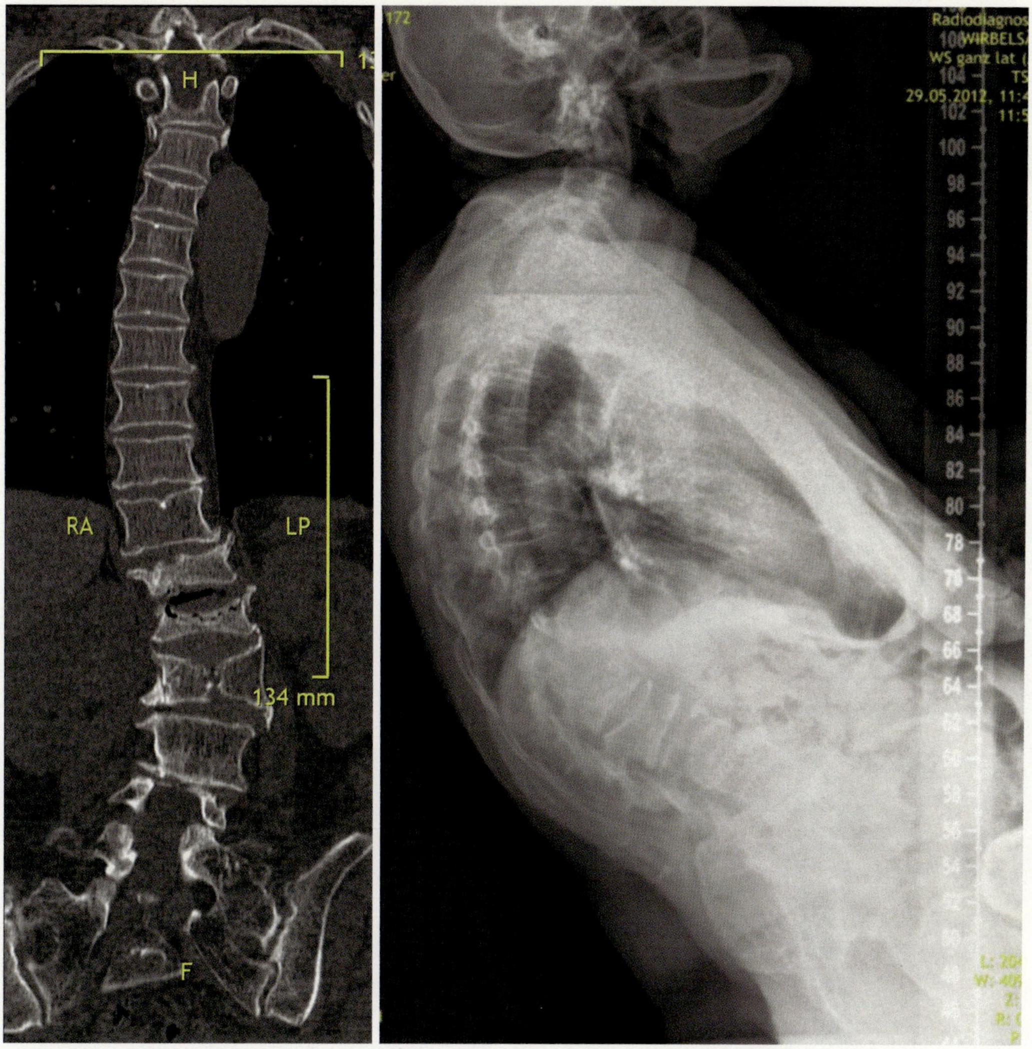

Fig. 29.5 MIS correction of thoracolumbar kyphoscoliosis (degenerative adult scoliosis) in a 67-year-old female via left-sided mini-open combined thoracolumbar extracoelomic approach. *Upper left image* – coronal CT reconstruction demonstrating fracture and lateral rotational displacement of the Th12, L1, and L2 vertebrae. *Upper right image* – full spine standing X-ray showing severe thoracolumbar kyphosis with marked compensatory pelvic retroversion. The patient was unable to walk for pain and sagittal imbalance. *Lower left image* – postoperative coronal CT reconstruction after deformity correction by trisegmental corpectomy/ VBR (Th12–L2), DLIF L3/L4, and L4/L5 and complementary posterior fixation from T8 to sacropelvis. Note PMMA reinforcement of vertebra flanking the VBR device and placement of morcellized rib autograft lateral to the VBR device to promote fusion. *Lower right image* – postoperative sagittal CT reconstruction showing correction of sagittal profile, decompression of the spinal canal

canal, comprehensive anterior correction maneuvers, and high fusion rates [1–4, 12–14, 25, 45, 48, 54]. Both of these features are advantageous for the treatment of fixed thoracic hyperkyphosis and kyphoscoliosis. MIS anterior thoracic interbody surgery has been applied for a variety of indications, including trauma, tumor, infection, and deformity with promising results [1, 3, 14, 17, 25, 43–45, 48, 54]. Readily connecting to the retroperitoneal space, the MIS lateral retropleural approach is specifically suited for complex thoracolumbar interventions requiring anterior release and anterior column support. The complication spectrum of MIS generally resembles that of

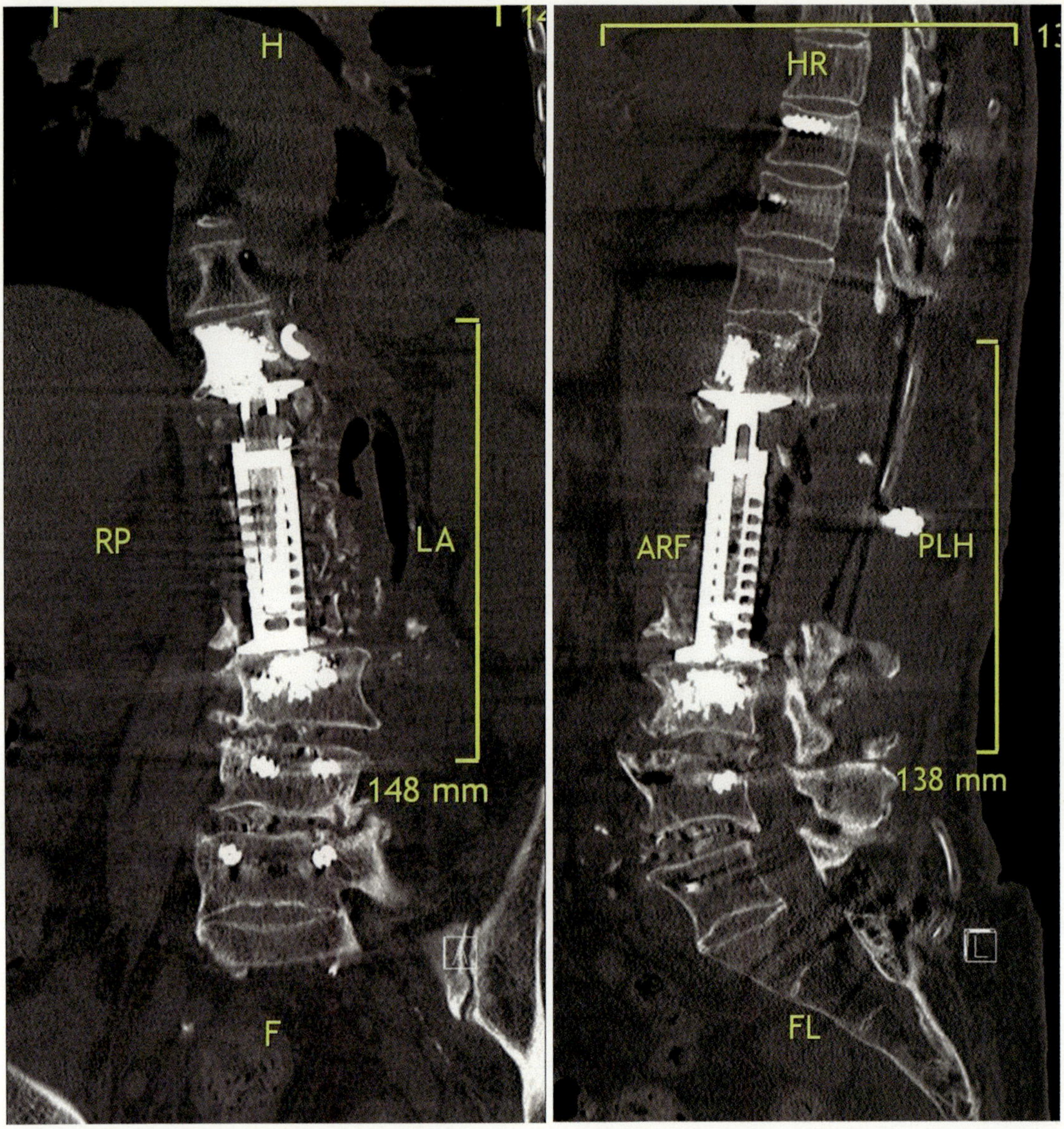

Fig. 29.5 (continued)

conventional "open" surgery, while significant complications such as duropleural fistula may be effectively prevented by using the MIS retropleural approach. Both VATS and mini-open approaches reduce postoperative pain and pulmonary dysfunction and promote early mobilization. In comparison to "standard" open technique [18–20, 27, 35, 45], no study has yet demonstrated significant shortcomings or inferior clinical results of MIS thoracic procedures conducted under the proviso of sound surgical indication making. Moreover, favorable results regarding operative time, intraoperative blood loss, and neurological outcomes have been reported [1–3, 12–14, 25–27, 29, 45, 48, 54, 55]. While MIS thoracic interbody surgery has only recently been introduced to the treatment of spinal deformity, preliminary experience indicates its potential as a powerful adjunct to the surgical armamentarium.

References

1. Amini A, Beisse R, Schmidt MH. Thoracoscopic spine surgery for decompression and stabilization of the anterolateral thoracolumbar spine. Neurosurg Focus. 2005;19:E4.
2. Anand N, Regan JJ. Video-assisted thoracoscopic surgery for thoracic disc disease: classification and outcome study of 100 consecutive cases with a 2-year minimum follow-up period. Spine. 2002;27: 871–9.
3. Barone GW, Eidt JF, Webb JW, Hudec WA, Pait TG. The anterior extrapleural approach to the thoracolumbar junction revisited. Am Surg. 1998;64: 372–5.
4. Benglis DM, Elhammady MS, Levi AD, Vanni S. Minimally invasive anterolateral approaches for the treatment of back pain and adult degenerative deformity. Neurosurgery. 2008;63:191–6.
5. Bergey DL, Villavicencio AT, Goldstein T, Regan JJ. Endoscopic lateral transpsoas approach to the lumbar spine. Spine. 2004;29:1681–8.
6. Bertagnoli R, Vazquez RJ. The Anterolateral TransPsoatic Approach (ALPA): a new technique for implanting prosthetic disc-nucleus devices. J Spinal Disord Tech. 2003;16:398–404.
7. Bohlman HH, Zdeblick TA. Anterior excision of herniated thoracic discs. J Bone Joint Surg Am. 1988; 20:1038–47.
8. Capener N. The evolution of lateral rhachotomy. J Bone Joint Surg Br. 1954;36-B:173–9.
9. Chen LH, Chen WJ, Niu CC, Shih CH. Anterior reconstructive spinal surgery with Zielke instrumentation for metastatic malignancies of the spine. Arch Orthop Trauma Surg. 2000;120:27–31.
10. Chi JH, Dhall SS, Kanter AS, et al. The Mini-Open transpedicular thoracic discectomy: surgical technique and assessment. Neurosurg Focus. 2008;25: 1–5.
11. Dakwar E, Ahmadian A, Uribe JS. The anatomical relationship of the diaphragm to the thoracolumbar junction during the minimally invasive lateral extracoelomic (retropleural/retroperitoneal) approach. J Neurosurg Spine. 2012;16:359–64.
12. Delfini R, Di Lorenzo N, Ciappretta P, et al. Surgical treatment of thoracic disc herniation: a reappraisal of Larson's lateral extracavitary approach. Surg Neurol. 1996;45:517–23.
13. Deviren V, Kuelling FA, Poulter G, Pekmezci M. Minimal invasive anterolateral transthoracic transpleural approach: a novel technique for thoracic disc herniation. A review of the literature, description of a new surgical technique and experience with first 12 consecutive patients. J Spinal Disord Tech. 2011;24:E40–8.
14. Dickman CA, Rosenthal D, Karahalios DG, et al. Thoracic vertebrectomy and reconstruction using a microsurgical thoracoscopic approach. Neurosurgery. 1996;38:279–93.
15. Dvorak MF, Kwon BK, Fisher CG, Eiserloh 3rd HL, Boyd M, Wing PC. Effectiveness of titanium mesh cylindrical cages in anterior column reconstruction after thoracic and lumbar vertebral body resection. Spine. 2003;28:902–8.
16. Elsaghir H. Endoscopic medial parascapular approach to the thoracic spine. Surg Endosc. 2005;19: 389–92.
17. Elsaghir H. Extracoelomic mini approach for anterior reconstructive surgery of the thoracolumbar area. Neurosurgery. 2002;51(Suppl):118–22.
18. Faciszewski T, Winter RB, Lonstein JE, Denis F, Johnson L. The surgical and medical perioperative complications of anterior spinal fusion surgery in the thoracic and lumbar spine in adults: a review of 1223 procedures. Spine (Phila Pa 1976). 1995;20: 1592–9.
19. Faro FD, Marks MC, Newton PO, Blanke K, Lenke LG. Perioperative changes in pulmonary function after anterior scoliosis instrumentation: thoracoscopic versus open approaches. Spine. 2005;30: 1058–63.
20. Fessler RG, Sturgill M. Review: complications of surgery for thoracic disc disease. Surg Neurol. 1998;49: 609–18.
21. Graham III AW, Mac Millan M, Fessler RG. Lateral extracavitary approach to the thoracic and thoracolumbar spine. Orthopedics. 1997;20:605–10.
22. Hollinshead WH. Textbook of anatomy. 3rd ed. Hagerstown: Harper & Row; 1974. p. 496–501.
23. Huang TJ, Hsu RW, Li YY, Cheng CC. Minimal access spinal surgery (MASS) in treating thoracic spine metastasis. Spine. 2006;31:1860–3.
24. Isaacs RE, Hyde J, Goodrich JA, Rodgers WB, Phillips FM. A prospective, nonrandomized, multicenter evaluation of extreme lateral interbody fusion for the treatment of adult degenerative scoliosis: perioperative outcomes and complications. Spine (Phila Pa 1976). 2010;35:S322–30.
25. Jain AK, Dhammi IK, Jain S, Kumar J. Simultaneously anterior decompression and posterior instrumentation by extrapleural retroperitoneal approach in thoracolumbar lesions. Indian J Orthop. 2010;44: 409–16.
26. Kasliwal MK, Deutsch H. Minimally invasive retropleural approach for central thoracic disc herniation. Minim Invasive Neurosurg. 2011;54:167–71.

27. Khoo LT, Smith ZA, Asgarzadie F, Barlas Y, Armin SS, Tashjian V, et al. Minimally invasive extracavitary approach for thoracic discectomy and interbody fusion: 1-year clinical and radiographic outcomes in 13 patients compared with a cohort of traditional anterior transthoracic approaches. J Neurosurg Spine. 2011;14:250–60.
28. Kim DH, Jaikumar S, Kam AC. Minimally invasive spine instrumentation. Neurosurgery. 2002;51: S15–25.
29. Kim DH, O'Toole JE, Ogden AT, et al. Minimally invasive posterolateral thoracic corpectomy: cadaveric feasibility study and report of four clinical cases. Neurosurgery. 2009;64:746–52.
30. Kossmann T, Jacobi D, Trentz O. The use of a retractor system (SynFrame) for open, minimal invasive reconstruction of the anterior column of the thoracic and lumbar spine. Eur Spine J. 2001;10: 396–402.
31. Larson SJ, Holst RA, Hemmy DC, Sances Jr A. Lateral extracavitary approach to traumatic lesions of the thoracic and lumbar spine. J Neurosurg. 1976;45: 628–37.
32. Louis R. Surgery of the spine. New York: Springer; 1983. p. 228–31.
33. Maciejczak A, Barnas P, Dudziak P, Jagiello-Bajer B, Litwora B, Sumara M. Posterior keyhole corpectomy with percutaneous pedicle screw stabilization in the surgical management of lumbar burst fractures. Neurosurgery. 2007;60:232–41.
34. Mack MJ, Regan JJ, McAfee PC, Picetti G, Ben-Yishay A, Acuff TE. Video-assisted thoracic surgery for the anterior approach to the thoracic spine. Ann Thorac Surg. 1995;59:1100–6.
35. McAfee PC. Complications of anterior approaches to the thoracolumbar spine: emphasis on Kaneda instrumentation. Clin Orthop Relat Res. 1994;306: 110–9.
36. McCormick PC. Retropleural approach to the thoracic and thoracolumbar spine. Neurosurgery. 1995;37: 908–14.
37. Mirbaha MM. Anterior approach to the thoracolumbar junction of the spine by a retroperitoneal-extrapleural technique. Clin Orthop. 1973;91: 41–7.
38. Moskovich R, Benson D, Zhang ZH, Kabins M. Extracoelomic approach to the spine. J Bone Joint Surg Br. 1993;75:886–93.
39. Musacchio M, Patel N, Bagan B, Deutsch H, Vaccaro AR, Ratliff J. Minimally invasive thoracolumbar costotransversectomy and corpectomy via a dual-tube technique: evaluation in a cadaver model. Surg Technol Int. 2007;16:221–5.
40. Oskouian Jr RJ, Shaffrey CI, Whitehill R, Sansur CA, Pouratian N, Kanter AS, et al. Anterior stabilization of three-column thoracolumbar spinal trauma. J Neurosurg Spine. 2006;5:18–25.
41. Patterson Jr RH, Arbit E. A surgical approach through the pedicle to protruded thoracic discs. J Neurosurg. 1978;48:768–72.
42. Regan JJ, Mack MJ, Picetti III GD. A technical report on video-assisted thoracoscopy in thoracic spinal surgery: preliminary description. Spine (Phila Pa 1976). 1995;20:831–7.
43. Rosenthal D, Marquardt G, Lorenz R, Nichtweiss M. Anterior decompression and stabilization using a microsurgical endoscopic technique for metastatic tumors of the thoracic spine. J Neurosurg. 1996;84: 565–72.
44. Sasso RC, Renkens K, Hanson D, Reilly T, McGuire Jr RA, Best NM. Unstable thoracolumbar burst fractures: anterior-only versus short-segment posterior fixation. J Spinal Disord Tech. 2006;19: 242–8.
45. Scheufler KM. Technique and clinical results of minimally invasive reconstruction and stabilization of the thoracic and thoracolumbar spine with expandable cages and ventrolateral plate fixation. Neurosurgery. 2007;61:798–808.
46. Schmidt MH, Larson SJ, Maiman DJ. The lateral extracavitary approach to the thoracic and lumbar spine. Neurosurg Clin N Am. 2004;15: 437–41.
47. Shen FH, Marks I, Shaffrey C, Ouellet J, Arlet V. The use of an expandable cage for corpectomy reconstruction of vertebral body tumors through a posterior extracavitary approach: a multicenter consecutive case series of prospectively followed patients. Spine J. 2008;8:329–39.
48. Smith WD, Dakwar E, Le TV, Christian G, Serrano S, Uribe JS. Minimally invasive surgery for traumatic spinal pathologies: a mini-open, lateral approach in the thoracic and lumbar spine. Spine. 2010;35: S338–46.
49. Smith ZA, FesslerRG. Nature reviews neurology. doi:10.1038/nrneurol.2012.110
50. Stillerman CB, Chen TC, Couldwell WT, et al. Experience in the surgical management of 82 symptomatic herniated thoracic discs and review of the literature. J Neurosurg. 1998;88:623–33.
51. Sundaresan N, Shah J, Foley KM, Rosen G. An anterior surgical approach to the upper thoracic vertebrae. J Neurosurg. 1984;61:686–90.
52. Thiel W. Photographic atlas of practical anatomy. 2nd ed. New York: Springer; 2003.
53. Uchida K, Kobayashi S, Nakajima H, Kokubo Y, Yayama T, Sato R, et al. Anterior expandable strut cage replacement for osteoporotic thoracolumbar vertebral collapse. J Neurosurg Spine. 2006;4: 454–62.
54. Uribe JS, Dakwar E, Cardona RF, Vale FL. Minimally invasive lateral retropleural thoracolumbar approach: cadaveric feasibility study and report of 4 clinical cases. Neurosurgery. 2011;68:32–9.

55. Uribe JS, Smith WD, Pimenta L, Härtl R, Dakwar E, Modhia UM, et al. Minimally invasive lateral approach for symptomatic thoracic disc herniation: initial multicenter clinical experience. J Neurosurg Spine. 2012;16:264–79.
56. Vedantam R, Lenke LG, Bridwell KH, Haas J, Linville DA. A prospective evaluation of pulmonary function in patients with adolescent idiopathic scoliosis relative to the surgical approach used for spinal arthrodesis. Spine. 2000;25:82–90.
57. Verheyden AP, Hoelzl A, Lill H, Katscher S, Glasmacher S, Josten C. The endoscopically assisted simultaneous posteroanterior reconstruction of the thoracolumbar spine in prone position. Spine J. 2004;4:540–9.

Part V

Dealing with the Lumbo-Pelvic Junction

30 Mini-Open ALIF for Fusing the Lumbosacral Junction

Robert Watkins IV and Salvadore Brau

30.1 Indications

Anterior approaches to the lumbar spine have been used for decades, but it was in the early 1990s that they became much more popular because of the introduction of threaded cages and bone dowels for the performance of anterior lumbar interbody fusion (ALIF). The use of these cages declined in the late 1990s, but this was followed by the introduction of artificial discs that require an anterior approach for deployment. Today, although the interest in artificial discs is not as strong, new devices for stand-alone fusion have been introduced, which require an anterior approach as well.

Originally, these approaches were considered to be highly risky because of the possibility of injury to the iliac vessels and the superior hypogastric plexus. Since publication of the mini-open lateral approach and the mini-open anterior approach, both in 2000, hundreds of general and vascular surgeons have been trained in these techniques that result in a much lower incidence of these complications. These new approaches are muscle sparing, go via the retroperitoneal route, and can be performed quickly and safely providing the spinal surgeon with excellent exposure of the entire disc space. So the old, "shark bite," anterolateral incision and the traditional left "paramedian" incision have been abandoned in many spine surgery centers where these newer approaches have become the standard. More importantly, the need for revision surgery has become more common, and these mini-open approaches disrupt the retroperitoneal tissues much less than the older incisions and make it easier to return to either adjacent levels or the same level for revisions.

Spine surgeons should, therefore, avail themselves of a well-trained "access" surgeon if they have a significant number of patients who require an anterior approach. Unfortunately, there are no formal training programs that teach general or vascular surgery residents and fellows how to perform these procedures. There are, however, postgraduate courses and preceptorships sponsored by several device manufacturers and by postgraduate institutions that can help in the training of practicing general and vascular surgeons interested in performing access to the lumbar spine. Once the access surgeon is properly trained, then he or she needs to become familiar with the needs of the spine surgeon as well as the different devices that are used in order to determine what the best approach may be for any particular instrumentation. Once the access surgeons gain experience, they can become a resource to the spine surgeons to help design specific anterior approach plans for patients with difficult approach situations, such as in adjacent level degeneration, revisions of a previously instrumented level, and patients with prior

R. Watkins IV, M.D. (✉) • S. Brau, M.D., FACS
Marina Spine Center, Marina del Rey, CA, USA
e-mail: robertwatkinsmd@yahoo.com

M.Y. Wang et al. (eds.), *Minimally Invasive Spinal Deformity Surgery*,
DOI 10.1007/978-3-7091-1407-0_30,

retroperitoneal surgery. The access surgeons are also there to handle any of the complications such as iliac vein laceration or iliac artery thrombosis that may arise at the time of the original surgery. Their presence ensures that there will be no delay in both recognition and treatment of any of these problems, which can certainly lead to catastrophic outcomes when there is delay in diagnosis and treatment.

30.2 Contraindications

There are only relative contraindications to the performance of an anterior lumbar approach. In general, the presence of several comorbidities, such as diabetes, hypertension, heart disease, pulmonary disease, and obesity, in the same patient should trigger a consult to the access surgeon who can then determine if the risks are justifiable. Patients who have had prior retroperitoneal surgery, such as radical hysterectomy or prostatectomy with lymph node dissection, laparoscopic hernia repairs, ureteral surgery, radiation to the pelvis or retroperitoneum, and vascular reconstruction of the aorta or iliac vessels, whether open or endovascular, and patients with severe vascular occlusive disease or aneurysms present significant increase in the risk of complications and should be thoroughly evaluated by the access surgeon prior to any anterior lumbar surgery. Calcification of the iliac vessels and aorta, per se, is not a contraindication to anterior lumbar surgery; however, the access surgeon needs to educate the patient as to the higher risk of an arterial thrombosis and needs to alert the spine surgeon to have an alternative plan in case the full anterior exposure cannot be obtained so that devices are available that can be deployed from a more anterolateral direction.

30.3 Alternative Treatments

Although some devices, such as artificial discs, stand-alone fusion cages, and anterior plates, need to be deployed through a full anterior exposure so they can be aligned at the midline of the vertebral body, there are alternative devices that can be implanted into the disc space from a more anterolateral or direct lateral direction. The mini-open anterolateral approach, the anterolateral transpsoatic approach (ALPA), the anterolateral retroperitoneal approach (ARPA), and the extreme lateral approach can all be used to deploy these devices that do not require alignment with the midline. Nucleus replacement devices, femoral ring allografts, and lateral cages are examples of note.

30.4 Results

The results following ALIF and arthroplasty using the mini-open anterior approach have been remarkably good with approach complications remaining very low. A very large series of 2020 approaches in 2013 patients has shown an incidence of arterial injury of 0.29 % and of venous injury of 1.1 %. Only five patients in that series had any significant sequelae arising from these complications for an incidence of only 0.24 %. The incidence of retrograde ejaculation in the male patients of the series was 0. So the anterior approach can be done with significantly reduced approach risks and perhaps offers the possibility of a better result for the spinal procedure as well, be it arthrodesis or arthroplasty (Table 1).

30.5 Technique

30.5.1 Setup

The access surgeon and the spine surgeon need to discuss the planned procedure well in advance and become well aware of each other's needs. The access surgeon, in particular, needs to know which level needs exposure and which device is being used. The overall medical status of the patient, the age, the BMI, the gender, the presence or absence of pedal pulses, and the history of any prior retroperitoneal surgery are of importance. The A-P and lateral films of the spine and the CAT scan or MRI should be evaluated by the access surgeon to see if there are calcifications of the vessels, osteophytes, scoliosis or rotation of the spine, or aberrant locations of the iliac vessels in relation to the target level.

Place the patient in the supine position on an X-ray table with an inflatable bag under the lumbar region. Inflation of the bag will allow for extension of the spine at the time of discectomy and graft placement, if needed.

Place a pulse oximeter in the 1st or 2nd toe of the left foot. This will provide an early warning for left iliac artery thrombosis should the saturation not return to baseline levels after removal of the retractors, especially at L4–L5. The saturation levels are noted at the beginning of the operation as a baseline measurement. Upon placement of the retractors, especially at L4–L5, the saturation may fall to 0 in as many as 80 % of patients. Should this happen, the spine surgeon has 45–50 min to complete the spinal procedure. If that time is to be exceeded, the retractors need to be released and a few cardiac cycles allowed for return of the saturation to baseline levels. The retractors can then be reapplied and the spinal surgeon given another 30 min to complete the procedure. If necessary, this maneuver can be repeated every 30 min. If the saturation does not return to baseline levels and remains 8–10 points below that baseline, then further vascular investigation is necessary to determine the source of this deficit. The patient can be evaluated in the operating room with measurement of segmental pressures and an operative arteriogram and then treated as necessary via the same incision or through a femoral endovascular approach. Removing the patient from the operating room, especially to go to the X-ray department for angiography, will result in unnecessary delays in treatment, which will then give rise to further complications such as a compartment syndrome.

A naso- or orogastric tube is placed once the patient is under anesthesia. The tube is removed at the end of the procedure. Complete muscle relaxation is necessary throughout the procedure.

30.5.2 Instruments

No special instruments are required to perform this approach to the lumbar spine. It is preferable, however, to use a table-held retractor with reverse lip, anterior lumbar surgery (ALS) retractor blades that can be deployed once the exposure is completed. These retractors use the concept of a lever to provide adequate exposure through a small incision. They are also radiolucent so as not to interfere with fluoroscopic visualization of the posterior end plates. The use of sharp-tip retractor blades, such as a Homan's, or Steinmann pins is discouraged because of the potential for vessel injury when deploying or removing them, especially when less experienced surgeons are involved.

30.5.3 Procedure

The approach surgeon stands on the left and the assistant on the right. Transverse incisions are used for single-level approaches and vertical or slightly oblique incisions for multiple-level access. This incision needs to be localized depending on the angle of L5–S1 and the relationship of L4–L5 to the iliac crest as seen on a lateral plain film. The relationship of L4–L5 to the iliac crest allows the surgeon to place the incision precisely by palpating the iliac crest and then moving the incision site caudad or cephalad depending on that relationship. Proper placement of this small incision is crucial in placing the working sleeves, templates, and inserters at the proper angle parallel to the vertebral end plates. Fluoroscopy should be used for placement of the incision when the access surgeon has not had the experience to accurately do this by looking at the static films (Fig. 30.1a, b).

Begin the incision at the midline and carry it transversely to the lateral edge of the rectus muscle. For two-level exposure, the incision should be more oblique starting midline at the level of the lower disc and ending at the level of the upper disc at the lateral edge of the left rectus muscle. For three levels the obliquity increases. The incision may be vertical at the midline but never paramedian (Fig. 30.2).

Carry the incision to the anterior rectus sheath and then incise the rectus fascia from 1 cm. to the right of the midline to the edge of

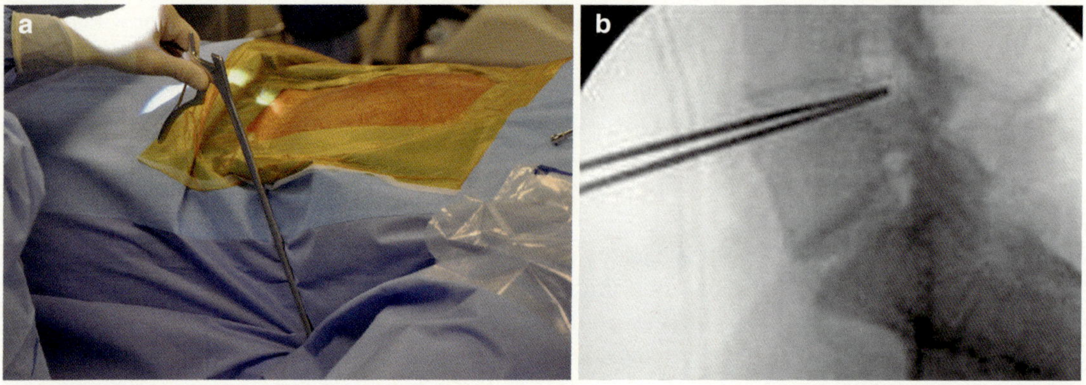

Fig. 30.1 (**a**) and (**b**) Radio-dense marker replicates the angle of the operative disc on the lateral fluoroscopic image to indicate the location of skin incision

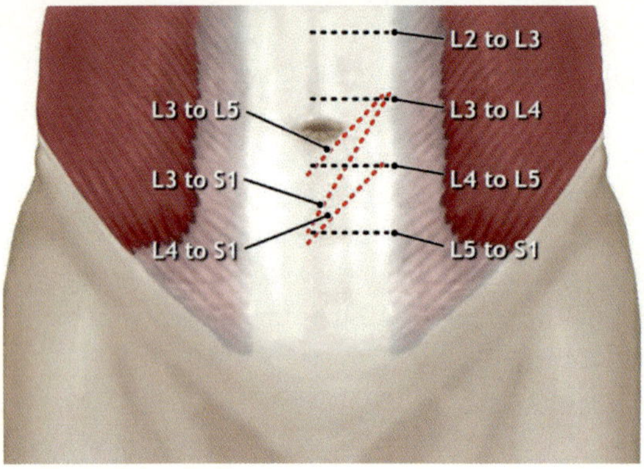

Fig. 30.2 Approximate location of incision depending on target level(s) to be exposed

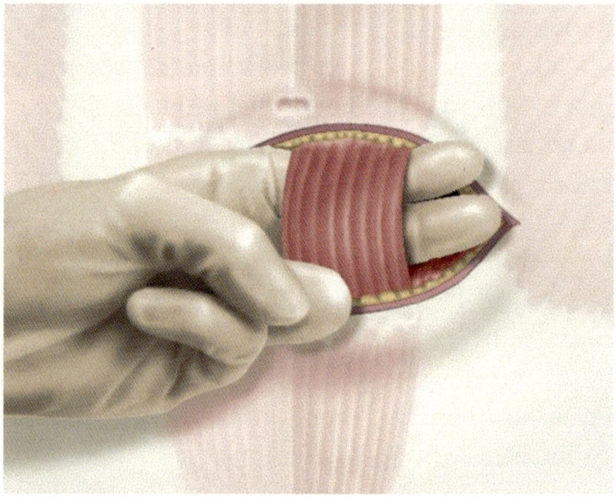

Fig. 30.3 Mobilization of the left rectus muscle for single-level approach

the rectus laterally. The anterior rectus sheath is then elevated anteriorly away from the muscle belly for a distance of 4–6 cm both superiorly and inferiorly to allow for full mobilization of the rectus muscle. This is an important step to keep this muscle from becoming an obstacle when the right-sided retractor is deployed. Medial, lateral, and posterior dissection of the muscle is then carried out taking great care to avoid injury to the inferior epigastric vessels. The rectus muscle is now easily retracted both medially and laterally (Fig. 30.3). This lateral dissection of the rectus muscle is only performed in single-level cases and does not result in rectus muscle paresis. In approaches involving 2 or more levels, lateral dissection of this muscle is not necessary because the incision is larger and the lateral aspect of the posterior rectus sheath can be accessed and incised with ease while retracting the muscle laterally from the midline.

With the rectus muscle initially retracted medially (for single-level cases only), incise the posterior sheath until the peritoneum is seen to shine through. Grasp the edges with a hemostat and very carefully dissect it from the peritoneum and incise it as far inferiorly and superiorly as possible. Carefully push the peritoneum posteriorly at the edge of the fascial incision, and slowly develop a plane between it and the undersurface of the internal oblique and transversus muscles and fascia. This will lead you into the retroperitoneal space (Figs. 30.4 and 30.5).

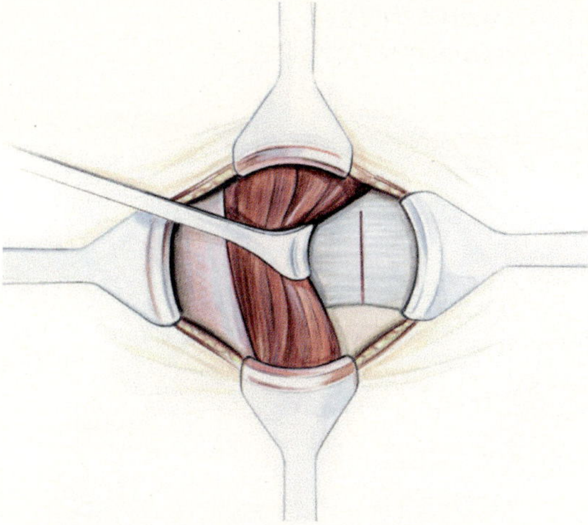

Fig. 30.4 Incision on posterior rectus sheath as lateral as possible

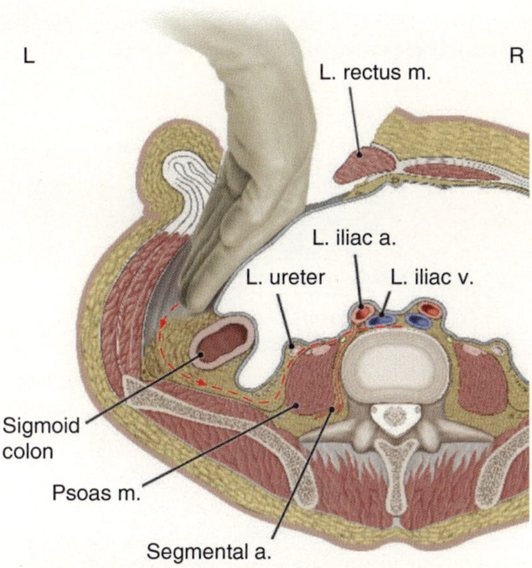

Fig. 30.5 Developing plane to elevate peritoneum and its contents away from retroperitoneal structures

Continue careful blunt finger dissection posteriorly and then start pushing medially trying to elevate the peritoneum away from the psoas muscle. The genitofemoral nerve can be easily identified over the psoas. The ureter can usually be identified as the peritoneum is lifted away from the psoas. Both of these structures should be preserved from injury.

Once the psoas is identified, a Harrington retractor is used to keep the peritoneal contents

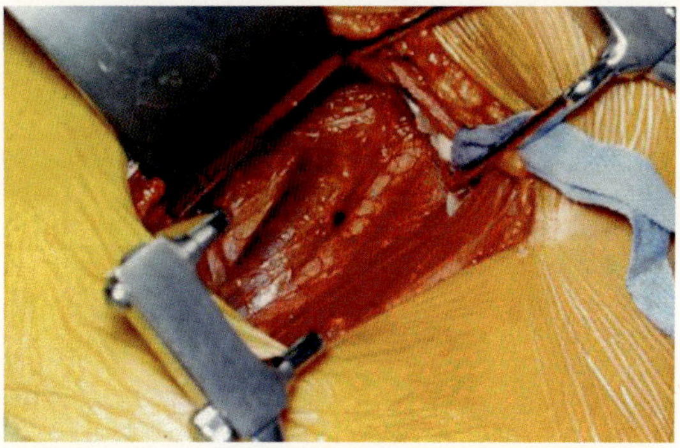

Fig. 30.6 Initial visualization of iliac vessels following elevation of peritoneum

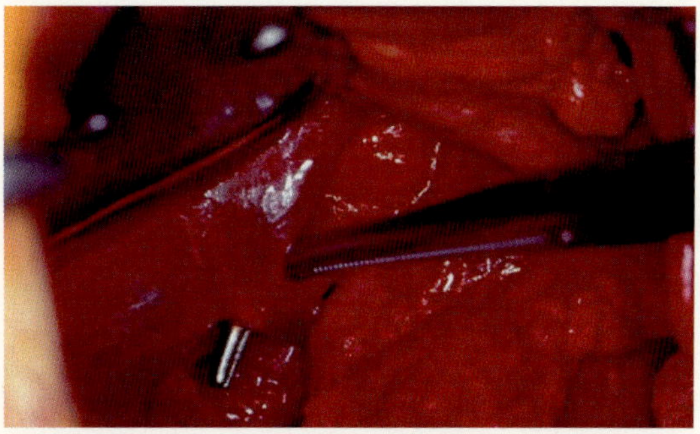

Fig. 30.7 Ileo-lumbar vein isolated and ready for ligature

away and allow further dissection. A Balfour retractor is then inserted to keep the incision open in the cranio-caudad plane. A dry lap sponge tucked above the upper blade of the Balfour is helpful in keeping retroperitoneal fat from creeping down and obscuring the field (Fig. 30.6).

For operations on L4–L5 or for operations that combine L4–L5 with either L3–L4 or L5–S1, the iliolumbar vein(s) must be ligated and cut. Expose the entire length of the common and external iliac arteries and mobilize them as far distally as possible. This is extremely important to prevent stretch to the artery when retracted to the right. The incidence of left iliac artery thrombosis can be reduced by this maneuver. After this, start careful blunt dissection along the lateral edge of the artery and expose the left common iliac vein just underneath it. Continue the dissection posteriorly to identify the iliolumbar vein(s), which crosses the body of L5 and dives into the

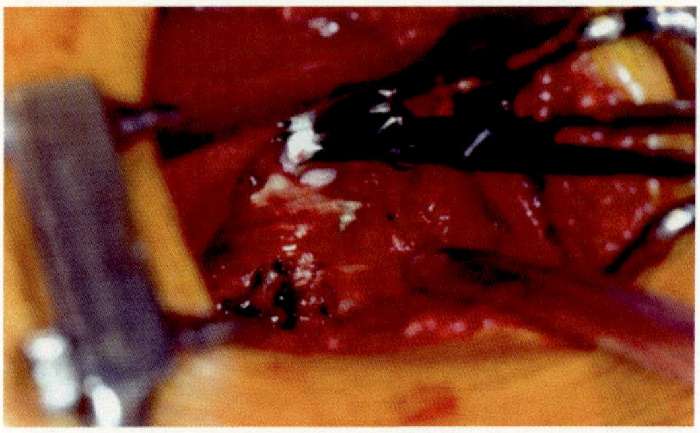

Fig. 30.8 Blunt dissection with peanut sponge toward right side of disc space at L4-5

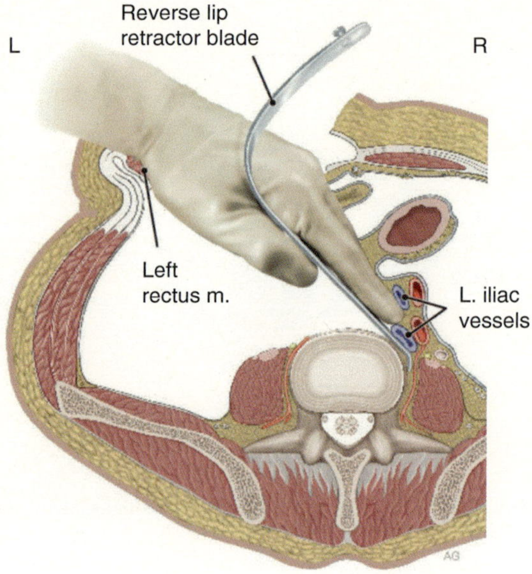

Fig. 30.9 Digital dissection under vessels guiding retractor blade toward right side of disc space

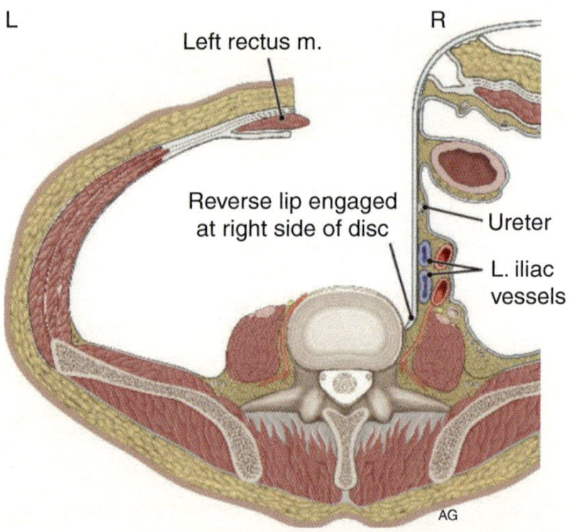

Fig. 30.10 Reverse lip blade deployed on right side protecting vessels and nerve plexus

left paraspinous area (Fig. 30.7). Ligation should be carried out in place prior to transection and not too close to the junction to the iliac vein itself in order to avoid injury to its sidewall. For any operation that involves L4–L5, these maneuvers are imperative to avoid avulsion of this vein.

The left iliac vein and artery can now be mobilized away from the spine using gentle, peanut sponge dissection. In most patients the vein "peels" away from the anterior surface of the spine easily (Fig. 30.8). In some patients, however, there is intense inflammatory reaction in the plane between the vein and the anterior longitudinal ligament, especially when osteophytes are present; so the dissection can be quite difficult and tedious.

All the vascular structures are thus swept from left to right providing adequate visualization of the disc involved. Once this part of the exposure is completed, the retractors (Balfour and Harrington) are removed.

The table-held retractor is then set up. The surgeon's left hand then reenters the retroperitoneal space with the rectus now moved laterally, and the fingers find their way to the right side of the spine following the planes previously dissected. A reverse lip, radiolucent, 1 in. blade of appropriate length is then placed on to the right side of the spine using the finger(s) as a guide (Fig. 30.9). This blade is then attached to table-held retractor system and then pushed to the right to elevate the vascular structures and expose the anterior surface of the spine (Fig. 30.10). The reverse lip keeps the blade anchored to the edge of the spine, prevents it from slipping anteriorly once tension is applied, and allows for leverage thus making a small incision possible.

Place a second such blade on the left side of the spine and attach to the table-held system to complete the exposure (Fig. 30.11). Commonly, additional retractor blades need to be placed superiorly or inferiorly to complete the exposure

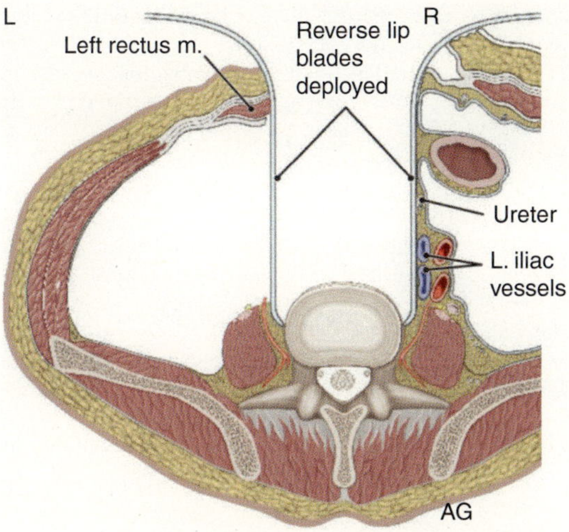

Fig. 30.11 Both reverse lip blades deployed

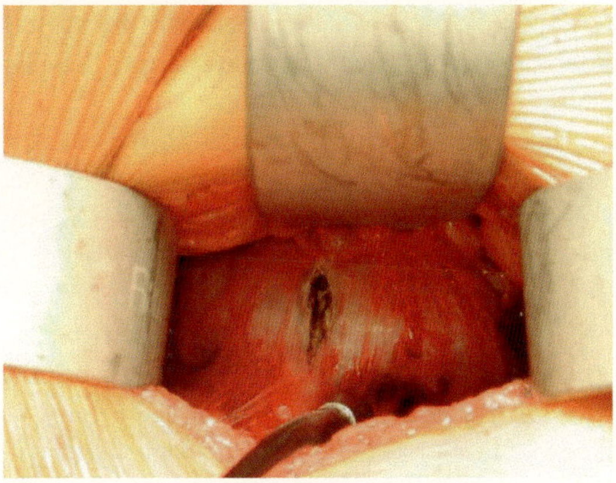

Fig. 30.12 Final exposure for a single-level L4-5

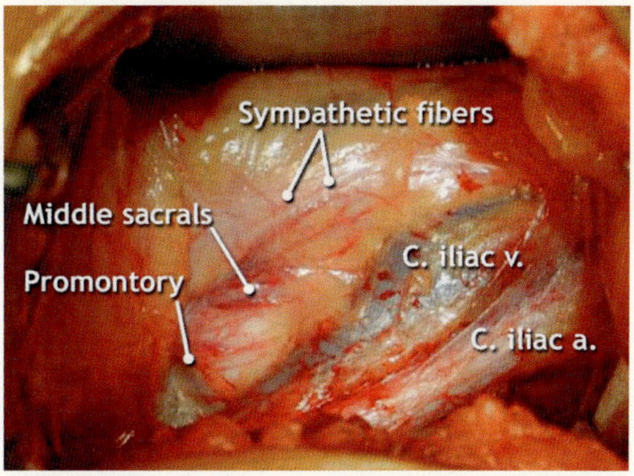

Fig. 30.13 Superior hypogastric plexus seen being elevated from promontory with peritoneum

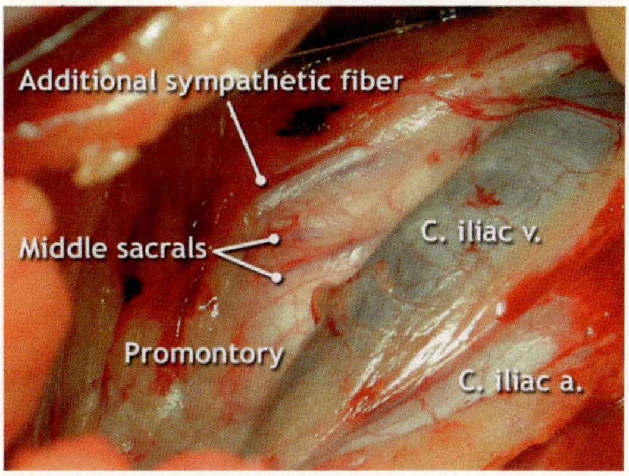

Fig. 30.14 Further mobilization of plexus fibers to right together with peritoneum to expose promontory

(Fig. 30.12). With these blades well anchored to the lateral wall of the vertebral column, the spine surgeon and his assistant can now work on the disc with relative security that vessels will not sneak around the retractors and expose themselves to injury.

For operations on L5–S1, exposure is usually between the iliac vessels below the aortic bifurcation. Blunt dissection is started anterior and medial to the left iliac artery toward the promontory. The L5–S1 disc is palpated and dissection carried toward it until the middle sacral vessels become apparent. At this point, the superior hypogastric plexus can be seen in most patients running with the peritoneum, much as the ureter does, as it is elevated away from the promontory (Figs. 30.13 and 30.14). Once the peritoneum is thus elevated and the middle sacral vessels are clearly identified, it is easy to continue pushing the peritoneum to the right carrying with it the nerve fibers and taking them away from possible injury. It is very important to look for this sympathetic plexus and for the approach surgeon to become familiar with its location if injury is to be avoided. The middle sacral vessels can then be cauterized with bipolar cautery or clipped and transected to further expose the disc space. The left iliac vein sometimes needs to be widely mobilized to allow adequate exposure. This vein is seen deep to the artery and can be swept further to the left with a peanut sponge to expose that

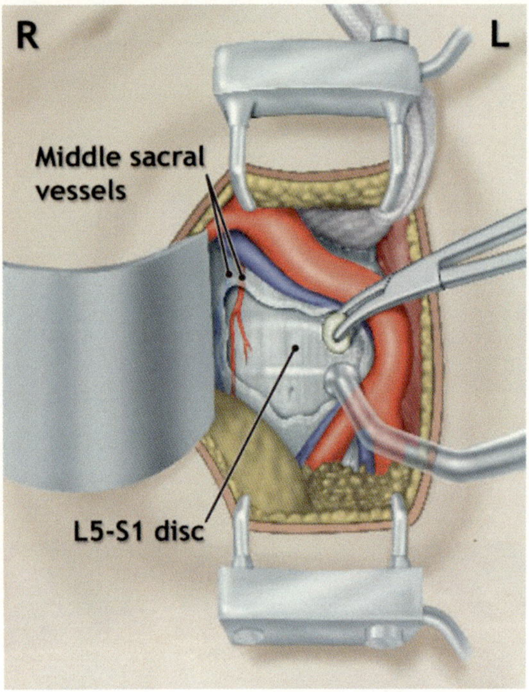

Fig. 30.15 Left iliac vessels mobilized to the left at L5–S1. Superior hypogastric plexus fibers are now safely behind the retractor on the right

side of the disc (Fig. 30.15). Dissection toward the right exposes that side of the disc, and a reverse-lipped retractor can be used to maintain exposure, protecting the superior hypogastric plexus by anchoring the lip on the lateral aspect of the spine. The iliac vessels are not usually visualized on the right side. A second reverse-lipped retractor is then deployed on the left side, and then the midline can be verified with X-rays. Additional blades are then placed superiorly and inferiorly to complete the exposure.

For operations of L3–L4 and L2–L3, mobilization of the iliac vessels is not necessary. This makes approaching these two levels somewhat easier, except that L2–L3 is extremely difficult to expose in the more obese patients and should only be attempted in normal weight patients.

When approaching both L4–L5 and L5–S1, it is usually necessary to get to L5–S1 between the vessels and to L4–L5 lateral to them. Occasionally L5–S1 can be exposed laterally if the bifurcation is low. In these cases you can actually see both levels simultaneously with only minimal adjustment of the retractor and its blades to provide optimal access. In some cases, it is possible to expose L4–L5 by going between the vessels after having completed the exposure of L5–S1. This requires a high bifurcation.

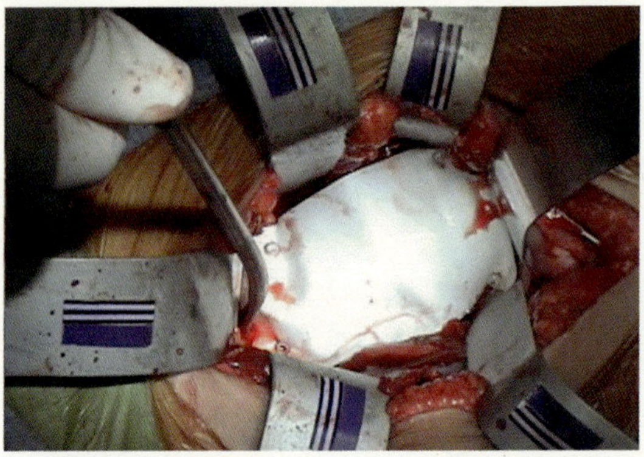

Fig. 30.16 Preclude Vessel Guard patch secured with tacks overlying L3–4 and L4–5 arthroplasties

Discectomy and instrumentation is then performed. Upon completion, a Preclude Vessel Guard patch (Gore Medical, Flagstaff, AZ) of appropriate size is secured with tacks over all arthroplasties, all arthrodeses at L4–L5 and above, and all anterior plates or tension bands. This is done to help the approach surgeon if a revision is needed for either the same level or adjacent level degeneration. This barrier will also help protect the vessels from injury or erosion if a plate or tension band is placed in such a way as to be in direct contact with the vessels (Fig. 30.16).

30.5.4 Wound Closure

The retractor blades are sequentially removed, leaving the right-sided blade for last. Check the integrity of the vessels thoroughly especially looking for arterial thrombosis or injury due to stretching. Remove the lap sponge and allow the tissues to fall back together anatomically. Check the distal pulses in the feet even though the oxygen saturation may have returned to baseline values.

The individual fascial layers are then closed separately with running absorbable sutures making sure that the anterior rectus sheath is well approximated. The posterior sheath need not be closed if it is tenuous and does not offer any significant strength to the closure. A thick, substantial posterior rectus sheath, however, should be closed. Subcutaneous tissues and skin are then closed as per surgeon's preference.

30.5.5 Postoperative Regimen

The postoperative protocol in these patients is left up to the spine surgeon including pain management. Prophylactic anticoagulation is not used. Clear liquid diet can usually be resumed the day after surgery unless there is any evidence of abdominal distention. Ambulation is started on post-op day 1 as well. Patients undergoing single-level arthroplasty or stand-alone anterior fusion are usually discharged in 1–2 days.

30.6 Avoiding Pitfalls and Complications

Optimal placement of the incision is important if it is to be kept small. Wide mobilization of the left rectus muscle keeps it from becoming an obstacle to exposure. Distal mobilization of the iliac artery reduces the stretch once it is retracted and reduces the incidence of thrombosis. Identify the superior hypogastric plexus while exposing L5–S1 to prevent injury to it. Ligation and transection of the iliolumbar vein will reduce the incidence of iliac vein laceration and is mandatory at L4–L5. Keep an eye on the pulse oximeter, especially while working at L4–L5. The saturation will drop to 0 in the majority of cases but the spine surgeon can continue to work for 45–50 min. After that time, the retractors must be released to allow 30 s of flow, and make sure the saturation returns to baseline levels. Once this is observed, the retractors can be reapplied and the spine surgeon given another 30 min. If necessary, repeat this every 30 min thereafter. Once the oxygen saturation returns to baseline levels after the spinal procedure and remains so upon discharge from the postanesthesia care unit, it would be extremely rare for an arterial thrombosis to present itself later. An orogastric tube should be used during the procedure to keep the stomach decompressed, and antiemetic agents should be prescribed for 24–48 h to reduce the incidence of ileus.

References

1. Baker JK, Reardon MJ, Heggeness MH. Vascular injury in anterior lumbar surgery. Spine. 1993;18:2227–30.
2. Brau SA. Mini-open approach to the spine for anterior lumbar interbody fusion, description of the procedure, results and complications. The Spine Journal. 2002; 2(3):216–23.
3. Brau SA. Prevention, diagnosis and management of complications in anterior lumbar spine surgery. Abstract Presentation, Spine Arthroplasty Society Annual Meeting, Montreal, May 8, 2006.
4. Brau SA, Delamarter RB, Schiffman ML, et al. Vascular injury during anterior lumbar surgery. The Spine Journal. 2004;4(3):409–12.
5. Brau SA, Delamarter RB, Schiffman ML, et al. Left iliac artery thrombosis during anterior lumbar surgery. Annals of Vascular Surgery. 2004;18(1):48–51.
6. Brau SA, Delamarter RB, Watkins RA, et al. Access strategies for revision in anterior lumbar surgery. Spine. 2008;33(15):1662–7.
7. Brau SA, Spoonamore MJ, Snyder L, et al. Nerve monitoring changes related to iliac artery compression during anterior lumbar spine surgery. Spine. 2003;3(4):351–5.
8. Faciszewski T, Winter RB, Lonstein JE, et al. The surgical and medical perioperative complications of anterior spinal fusion surgery in the thoracic and lumbar spine in adults. Spine. 1995;20(14):1592–99.
9. Khazim R, Boos N, Webb JK. Progressive thrombotic occlusion of the left common iliac artery after anterior lumbar interbody fusion. Eur Spine J. 1998;7: 239–41.
10. Mariscano J, Nirovsky Y, Remer S, et al. Thrombotic occlusion of the left common iliac artery after an anterior retroperitoneal approach to the lumbar spine. Spine. 1994;19(3):357–9.
11. Raskas DS, Delamarter RB. Occlusion of the left iliac artery after retroperitoneal exposure of the spine. Clin Orthop. 1997;338:86–9.
12. Regan JJ et al. Laparoscopic fusion of the lumbar spine: minimally invasive spine surgery. A prospective multicenter study evaluating open and laparoscopic spine fusion. Spine. 1999;24:402–11.
13. Regan JJ, Yuan H, McAfee PC. Laparoscopic fusion of the lumbar spine: minimally invasive spine surgery. Spine. 1999;24(4):402–11.
14. Watkins R. Anterior lumbar interbody fusion surgical complications. Clin Orthop. 1992;284:47–53.

31 Presacral Approach for Discectomy and Interbody Fusion in the Setting of Minimally Invasive Spine Surgery Deformity Correction

Neel Anand and Eli M. Baron

The presacral approach is a relatively recent approach that allows for discectomy and interbody fusion at L5–S1 and more recently at L4–L5 [1, 2]. Because of the unique properties of the AxiaLIF rod, it may obviate the need for pelvic fixation in certain cases. Thus, the procedure allows for a unique implant and approach in the minimally invasive treatment of spinal deformity. Advantages of this approach include sparing the surrounding musculature, ligaments, and annulus fibrosus and also the relatively short operative time associated with this procedure [3]. From start to finish this procedure typically takes under an hour and is considerably shorter than other posterior interbody approaches or anterior interbody approaches. Additionally, AxiaLIF may be associated with reduced risk when compared to traditional open anterior or even posterior procedures [4].

31.1 Indications for Fusion to the Sacrum in Deformity Correction

Bridwell described indications for fusing to the sacrum during deformity surgery [5]. These include L5–S1 spondylolisthesis, presence of previous L5–S1 laminectomy, any form of L5–S1 stenosis, oblique takeoff of L5–S1, and a significant L5–S1 disc degeneration (Fig. 31.1). All of these would be relative indications to fuse to the sacrum as opposed to stopping at L5 in terms of deformity correction. In order to achieve successful fusion to the sacrum in the setting of long-segment fusion, Bridwell further described the following factors as being necessary: (1) segmental fixation without gaps from the middle lumbar spine to the sacrum, (2) four-point fixation of the sacrum and pelvis to protect the sacral pedicle screws, (3) bicortical sacral screws, (4) anterior column support/anterior fusion of the distal lumbar spine, and (5) neutral or negative sagittal balance. AxiaLIF provides an ideal form of interbody fusion but also rigid fixation [5]. As detailed below, the Axial 3D screw may off-load the sacral screws and in many cases supplant the need for iliac fixation in deformity correction.

31.1.1 Surgical Anatomy

Between the visceral and parietal fascia, in front of the sacrum, is an area known as the presacral space. The sacrum itself is separated from the rectum by a layer known as the mesorectum. In this layer, adipose tissue, lymphatics, and blood vessels are found. There are blood vessels in this space also such as the middle sacral artery [3]. Yuan et al. noted in a cadaveric study that

N. Anand, M.D. (✉) • E.M. Baron, M.D.
Department of Surgery, Cedars Sinai Spine Center, Cedars Sinai Medical Center, 444 S. San Vicente Blvd., Suite 800, Los Angeles, CA 90048, USA
e-mail: neel.anand@cshs.org

M.Y. Wang et al. (eds.), *Minimally Invasive Spinal Deformity Surgery*,
DOI 10.1007/978-3-7091-1407-0_31, © Springer-Verlag Wien 2014

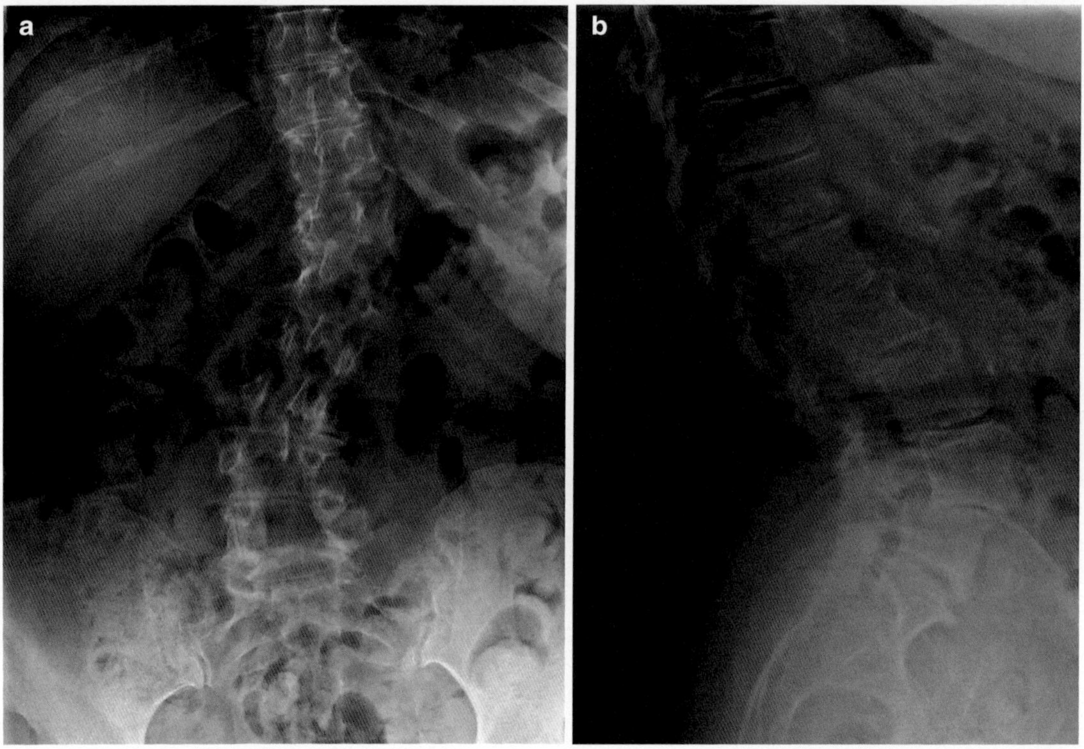

Fig. 31.1 (**a** and **b**) AP and lateral lumbosacral plain films of a 70-year-old female with degenerative scoliosis who underwent L4–L5 laminectomy elsewhere who presents with continued back pain and leg pain. Note the retrolisthesis at L3–L4, the spondylolisthesis at L4–L5, and the degenerated disc at L5–S1

there may be a safe zone along the anterior sacrum to perform a percutaneous approach [6]. They noted a distance along the anterior sacral margin to the rectum at the S3–S4 level as being approximately 1.2 cm on MRI and 1.3 cm on CT. They also noted a safe zone in terms of the distance between the right and left internal iliac vessels at S1–S2 of 6.9 cm on MRI and 6.0 cm on CT. They noted that the sacrum and its overlying parietal fascia provided a safe posterior border in which to potentially insert a blunt trocar to avoid structures anterior to the presacral space.

This corridor was actually first described by Cragg et al., where this corridor was used successfully for biopsy [1]. Eventually this was developed into a minimally invasive technique where discectomy and fusion could be performed [2]. Additionally, experience exists in the treatment of high-grade spondylolisthesis with transvertebral strut grafting, and this also influenced the design of this approach [7–9].

31.1.2 Device

To date, there is only one device available on the market for this approach. This is the AxiaLIF implant (Baxano Surgical, Raleigh, North Carolina). While initially the device was a single screw that was drilled into a channel through the sacrum, disc space, and L5 vertebral body over a guidewire, recent redesign has the device actually having four components. This allows selective internal distraction if necessary, by having a distraction rod internally rotate within the device with an S1 anchor and pushing on the shoulder with an L5 anchor to create distraction. Akesen et al. demonstrated rigid fixation for a single-level AxiaLIF supplemented with posterior instrumentation [10]. Similarly, Erkan et al. have shown rigid construct in presence of posterior fixation with a two-level AxiaLIF [11]. Most recently, Fleischer et al. compared S1 screw strain among four different constructs [12]. These included pedicle screws alone from L2 to S1, pedicle screws with anterior interbody fixation, pedicle screws with axial fixation, and pedicle screws with iliac screws. They showed that with pedicle screws alone, S1 screw strain was greatest. This was decreased by 38 % after anterior interbody augmentation, decreased by 75 % with axial fixation, and decreased by 78 % with pedicle screw and iliac screw fixation. This study demonstrated biomechanically that iliac screw fixation and AxiaLIF are quite similar in terms of the biomechanics with regard to protection of the S1 screw. Based on this biomechanical study, Boachie-Adjei et al. recommend using unilateral iliac screw for supplementation in spinal deformity correction when fusing to the sacrum and bilateral iliac screws for patients with osteoporosis [13]. However, they do not use any iliac screws for patients with normal bone mineral density where AxiaLIF is used in the setting of deformity correction. Our experience has been similar, where we also have not used iliac fixation for non-revision cases, where bone mineral density is within normal limits [14, 15].

31.2 Indications for the Presacral Approach for Discectomy and Fusion

Indications for using this approach include grade 1 degenerative spondylolisthesis, degenerative disc disease where fusion would be a consideration, interbody fusion in the setting of pseudarthrosis of a previous posterolateral fusion at L5–S1 or L4–L5 and L5–S1, and anterior column support in the setting of spinal deformity surgery. The approach to L4–L5 is also useful when the L4–L5 disc space is low and cannot be easily accessed via a transpsoas approach especially in deformity correction.

The presacral approach, however, has several important contraindications, including previous surgery in this region, history of prior colostomies, or pathology in the region of the rectum such as fistulas and also high-grade spondylolisthesis [3]. Any aberrant blood vessels in the region preclude this approach. Thus, a preoperative pelvic MRI is mandatory to exclude any aberrant midline vasculature at S1–S2 (Fig. 31.2).

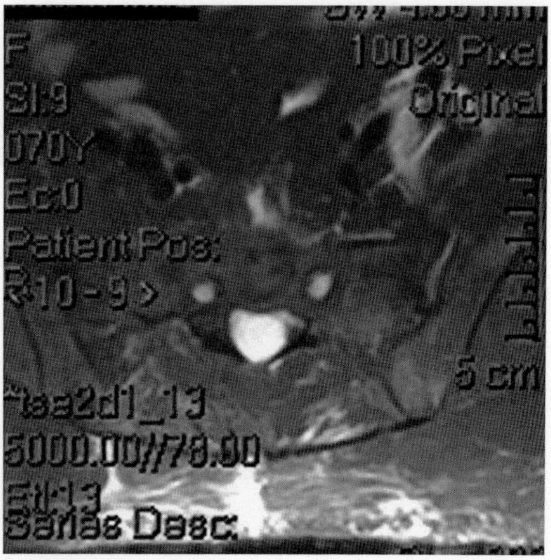

Fig. 31.2 Axial T2 MRI of the pelvis demonstrating normal midline at approximately the level of the S1–S2 segment: no midline flow voids are seen

Additionally, adhesions are excluded. Especially if the patient has a history of inflammatory bowel disease, pelvic CT with a rectal contrast should also be considered to rule out any adhesions or aberrant rectal/sacral anatomy that would necessitate a different approach [16].

31.2.1 AxiaLIF in the Setting of Deformity

Providing the decision is made as above, to fuse to the sacrum in the setting of deformity correction and a long fusion, we have suggested and agree with Boachie-Adjei et al. with regard to the AxiaLIF being a possible alternative to the use of iliac screws in cases of normal bone marrow density [13–15]. We confirm on 36-in. films the trajectory is appropriate. Additionally, preoperative sacral MRI is ordered to rule out aberrant pelvic vessels. If the history suggests any potential adhesions, our bias is not to do this procedure. All patients undergoing this procedure also undergo supplemental facet fusion. We use 2.1 mg of rhBMP-2 per disc space fused with this technique [17]. Additionally, in terms of the L5–S1 facets, we use approximately 1 mg of rhBMP-2 per facet-pars complex. Typically

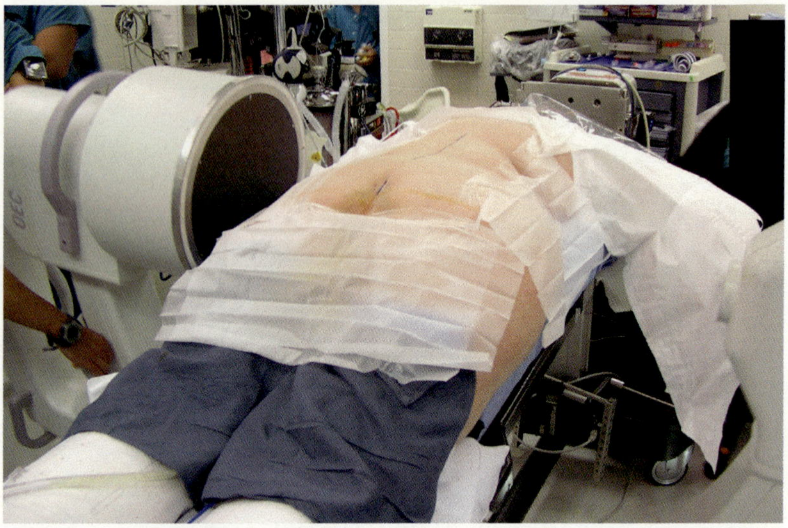

Fig. 31.3 Positioning for the AxiaLIF procedure. The patient is positioned prone on a Jackson table. The rectal area has been prepped and isolated from the field. Note that there is no thigh strap present that would limit excursion of the surgeon's hand

in our protocol for minimally invasive deformity correction, we will use a combination of three techniques [17–19]. These include the transpsoas discectomy and interbody fusion, the AxiaLIF if fusion extends to the sacrum, and multilevel percutaneous screws and rod placement. Typically, the AxiaLIF technique is performed prior to inserting pedicle screws unless there is preexisting lumbosacral junction obliquity. If there is obliquity present, we will typically correct it with screws prior to the transsacral fusion [18]. Additionally, we stress the importance of using tricortical pedicle screws as per Lehman et al [20]. We maximize the strength of our sacral fixation using a combination of this technique in addition to the AxiaLIF. In cases of revision surgery, or in the case of osteopenia, we have also used the S2 alar iliac technique to place collinear minimally invasive screws and avoid the need for extensive lateral dissection for iliac bolt placement [21, 22].

31.2.1.1 Procedure

The patient is positioned prone on a Jackson table. Extra padding is used to elevate the buttocks and legs. The legs are parted slightly to allow for the surgeon's hand to follow the correct trajectory to enter for the AxiaLIF technique. Great care is taken not to place the buttocks strap, which would limit the operator's excursion when performing this technique. The rectal area is prepped and isolated from the field (Fig. 31.3). Though others have recommended a bowel prep beforehand, we have not found this to be necessary [13, 23].

For the actual technique, a 1-in. incision is planned over the midline by the sacrococcygeal junction. The skin is incised. A blunt probe is then introduced along the paracoccygeal notch, and in a controlled manner the fascia is pierced and presacral space entered. The hand is immediately dropped down between the legs to keep the tip of the blunt probe against the ventral surface of the sacrum. Strict biplanar fluoroscopy is then used. The probe is advanced along the ventral surface of the sacrum. Great care is taken not to deviate laterally into the ventral sacral foramina. The blunt probe is rested on the S1–S2 junction to allow for appropriate trajectory across the disc space. A sharp guidewire is introduced into the probe through the sacrum and advanced into the bone with a slap hammer. Using Seldinger technique principles, serial dilators are placed into the sacrum. Eventually, a 10-mm dilator (assembled with a dilator sheath) is slid over the other dilators and anchored into the sacrum using a cannulated slap hammer. Subsequently, the dilators and guide pin are removed while the 10-mm dilator sheath is left in place. A 9-mm cannulated drill is then placed over the guidewire and drilled to the sacrum up to the level of the L5–S1 disc space. Subsequently, that drill is removed, twisting in a clockwise manner in order to save bone as local bone autograft.

A radical discectomy then ensues. This entails using a series of nitinol rasps, radial cutters,

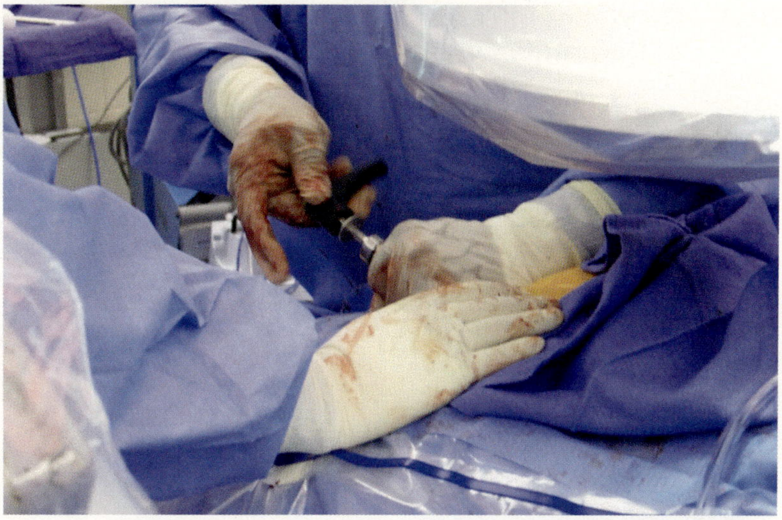

Fig. 31.4 Radial cutter being used to perform discectomy. Note that the surgeon's other hand holds the working cannula and maintains constant pressure against the face of the sacrum

and brush devices to remove disc material (Fig. 31.4). A thorough discectomy is performed. Subsequently, the disc space is irrigated out and grafted with local bone, demineralized bone matrix, and 2.1 mg of rhBMP-2 ACS using the manufacturer-supplied funnels [17].

Afterwards, a wire is reinserted into the disc space through the working 10-mm sheath. An 8-mm dilator is inserted, engaged with the 10-mm sheath, and together they are both removed while the wire is left in place.

A larger 12-mm dilator and dilator sheath assembly are inserted over the guidewire after removal of the 10-mm sheath. This is malleted into position with a slap hammer, and the sheath is left within the sacrum. The dilator is then removed. A larger 10.5-mm twist drill is then used to drill through the sacrum just past the S1 end plate. Subsequently, a 12-mm dilator tamp is placed over the wire. The sheath and tamp are advanced with a slap hammer to the inferior end plate of L5, as verified under lateral fluoroscopy. Afterwards, the tamp is removed. The 10.5-mm cannulated drill is placed over the guidewire and is used to drill 10–15 mm into the L5 vertebral body. The drill is removed in a counterclockwise fashion to make sure the bone graft remains in place. The guidewire is then removed.

The manufacturer then supplies a dilator trial to determine the length of the L5 and S1 components of the four-part piece screw. The screw is assembled and kept ready by the scrub technologist on a ratcheting screwdriver. Subsequently, the beveled guide pin is replaced. A 10-mm dilator is placed over the wire, and dilator and dilator sheath are removed while keeping the wire in place. An exchange system is then chosen where its angle approximates the face of the sacrum. This is actually a large channel that will be used for screw placement. An exchange bushing is placed over the guidewire and advanced with its longer side dorsally until it contacts the sacral face. This is then rotated 180° so the angle surface of the bushing matches the sacrum. This is also done with its corresponding tubular retractor. The retractor is then anchored to the sacral face using two fixation wires.

It is critical at this point to maintain constant forward pressure to make sure the exchange system does not lose contact with the sacrum. Afterwards, the titanium AxiaLIF screw assembly is inserted along the guidewire and screwed across the sacrum, across the L5–S1 disc space, into the L5 vertebral body. The L5 anchor is fully engaged in the L5 vertebral body, and the S1 one anchor is left with one or two threads proud to the sacral face. The driver is then removed. Distraction can be performed as needed across the L5–S1 disc space. Another fixation rod is then placed through the tube and engaged into the L5 anchor. This is all confirmed on biplanar fluoroscopy. The retractors are irrigated. The fixation wires are removed and the retractor is finally removed. The wound is irrigated and closed with three-layer closure. A similar technique is used for two-level AxiaLIFs.

31.3 Outcomes in Terms of Deformity Correction

We have reported outcomes of 97 patients undergoing AxiaLIF fusion at the end of long-segment constructs, primarily in the setting of deformity at two major spine centers (Fig. 31.5) [14]. Of these patients, only 14 had supplemental iliac bolt fixation. Mean follow-up is noted to be 24 months. No intraoperative complications were noted. There were two pseudarthroses at L5–S1; one late infection with nonunion and one

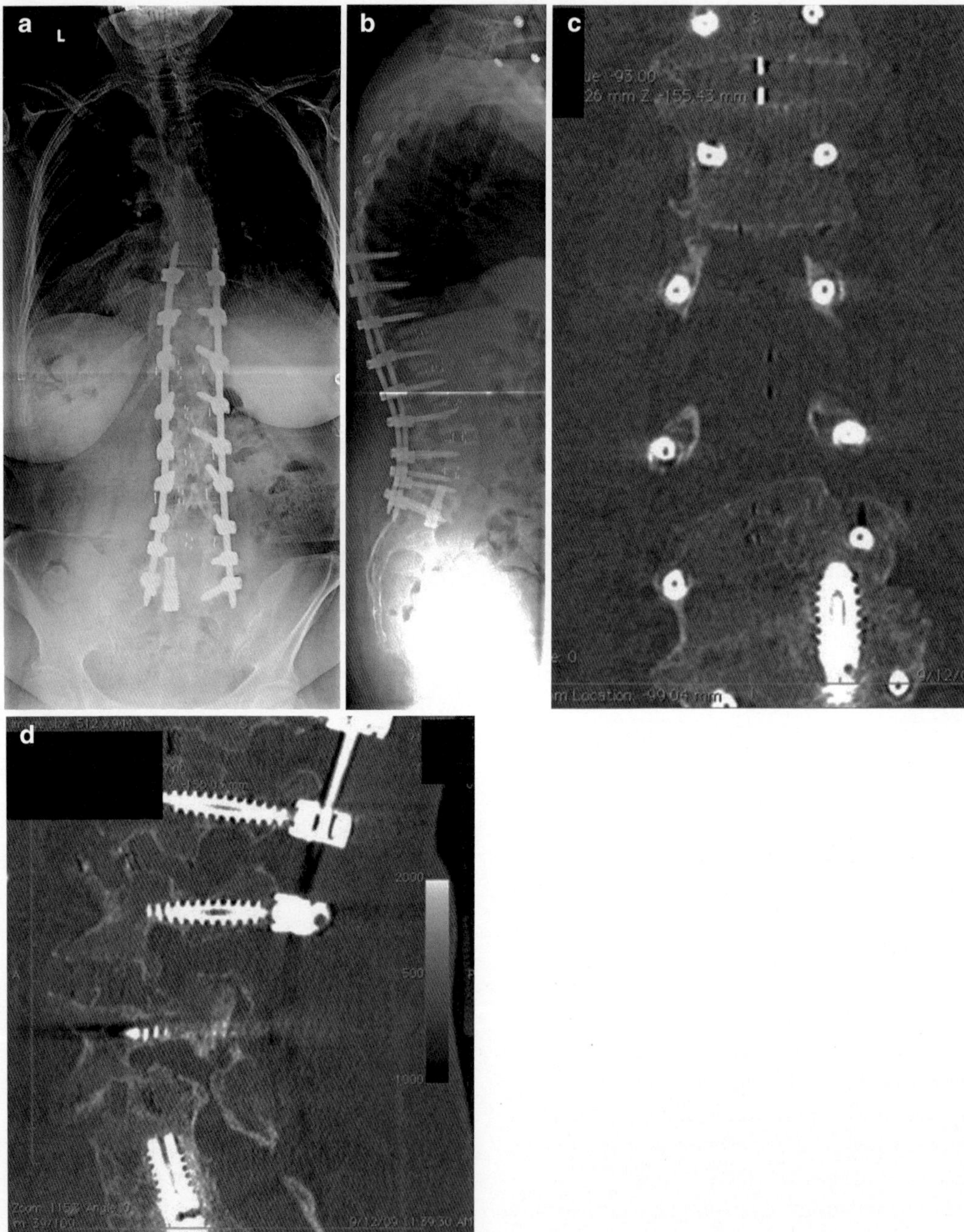

Fig. 31.5 (**a**, **b**) 36″ AP and lateral standing films at 1 year out reveal an excellent correction of the deformity using minimally invasive spine surgery techniques. Note the AxiaLIF screw at L5–S1. (**c** and **d**) Coronal and sagittal CT reconstruction shows a solid arthrodesis at the L5–S1 segment

sacral pedicle screw loosening were noted. No sacral insufficiency fractures were noted. AxiaLIF was concluded to be a viable alternative for providing anterior column support for long-segment fusion. Considerable experience now exists with outcomes for this technique in the setting of the degenerative spine with good results being reported by Tobler et al. and Gerszten et al [24, 25].

31.4 Complications

Surgeons remain hesitant to use this technique as they fear the possibility of bowel injury. In a review of 5,300 cases of TranS1 AxiaLIF being performed in the United States from January 2005 to 2009 per the US FDA Medical Device reporting data, we note an overall bowel injury rate of 0.47 % [4]. In our own experience of over 95 cases, we have not had a bowel injury. Lindley et al., however, noted a complication rate of 26.5 % [26]. They noted a rectal perforation rate of 2.9 % and superficial wound infection rate of 5.9 %. Should a bowel injury be suspected intraoperatively, one should consider rigid proctosigmoidoscopy or flexible sigmoidoscopy early on to identify the injury [23]. Other alternatives include Gastrografin enema. If the patient in the postoperative period presents with potential bowel injuries, CT of the abdomen and pelvis with rectal Gastrografin should be considered. Typically, injury to the sigmoid colon and intraoperative abdominal rectum presents with signs and symptoms of an acute abdomen. On the other hand, extraperitoneal rectal injuries may present less obviously with possibility of a localized abscess. If either of these are suspected, colorectal surgeon consultation is recommended [23]. If a vascular injury is suspected, typically venous bleeding will happen in the retroperitoneal space. Hematoma should thus not be drained as this may lead to massive bleeding or infection. Hematoma may be suspected if there is sacral pain or bloody drainage in the area. Any situation where there is an expanding hematoma or hemodynamic instability may require resuscitation and possibly angiography with embolization. We have shifted our incisions more laterally in the presence of extreme obesity or diabetes as incisional dehiscence may be a problem. Other complications reported included superficial wound infections, sacral fractures, pelvic hematoma, and transient nerve root irritation [26].

Conclusions

AxiaLIF is an excellent alternative for interbody fusion of L5–S1 and at times L4–L5 and L5–S1 especially in the setting of minimally invasive deformity correction and long construct fusions. L4–L5 is useful where a high-riding iliac crest may prevent access to the L4–L5 disc by other means. Additionally, in patients with good bone density, it may obviate the need for iliac bolts. Meticulous attention to technique and careful preoperative selection are necessary to avoid complications with this technique. The technique has shown promise in multiple centers with regard to avoiding other forms of interbody fusion and reducing the need for iliac bolt supplementation.

References

1. Cragg A, Carl A, Casteneda F, et al. New percutaneous access method for minimally invasive anterior lumbosacral surgery. J Spinal Disord Tech. 2004;17:21–8.
2. Marotta N, Cosar M, Pimenta L, et al. A novel minimally invasive presacral approach and instrumentation technique for anterior L5-S1 intervertebral discectomy and fusion: technical description and case presentations. Neurosurg Focus. 2006;20:E9.
3. Anand N, Baron EM. Presacral approaches for minimally invasive spinal fusion. In: Phillips F, Lieberman I, Polly D, editors. Minimally invasive spine surgery. Berlin: Springer; 2013. in press.
4. Anand N, Baron EM, Rosemann R, et al. Safety and complication profile of percutaneous lumbosacral interbody fusion. Congress of Neurological Surgeons. New Orleans, Louisiana; 2009.
5. Bridwell KH. Selection of instrumentation and fusion levels for scoliosis: where to start and where to stop. Invited submission from the Joint Section Meeting on Disorders of the Spine and Peripheral Nerves, March 2004. J Neurosurg Spine. 2004;1:1–8.
6. Yuan PS, Day TF, Albert TJ, et al. Anatomy of the percutaneous presacral space for a novel fusion technique. J Spinal Disord Tech. 2006;19:237–41.
7. Hanson DS, Bridwell KH, Rhee JM, et al. Dowel fibular strut grafts for high-grade dysplastic isthmic spondylolisthesis. Spine (Phila Pa 1976). 2002;27:1982–8.
8. Sasso RC, Shively KD, Reilly TM. Transvertebral transsacral strut grafting for high-grade isthmic

spondylolisthesis L5-S1 with fibular allograft. J Spinal Disord Tech. 2008;21:328–33.
9. Whitecloud 3rd TS, Butler JC. Anterior lumbar fusion utilizing transvertebral fibular graft. Spine (Phila Pa 1976). 1988;13:370–4.
10. Akesen B, Wu C, Mehbod AA, et al. Biomechanical evaluation of paracoccygeal transsacral fixation. J Spinal Disord Tech. 2008;21:39–44.
11. Erkan S, Wu C, Mehbod AA, et al. Biomechanical evaluation of a new AxiaLIF technique for two-level lumbar fusion. Eur Spine J. 2009;18:807–14.
12. Fleischer GD, Kim YJ, Ferrara LA, et al. Biomechanical analysis of sacral screw strain and range of motion in long posterior spinal fixation constructs: effects of lumbosacral fixation strategies in reducing sacral screw strains. Spine (Phila Pa 1976). 2012;37:E163–9.
13. Boachie-Adjei O, Cho W, King AB. Axial lumbar interbody fusion (AxiaLIF) approach for adult scoliosis. Eur Spine J. 2012;22(2):S225–31.
14. Anand N, Kahwaty S, Daroudi S, et al. Multicenter minimally, invasive AxiaLIF L5-S1 interbody fusion for anterior column support at the end of a long segment construct: feasibility, safety, complications, early and late 3 year outcomes. Sweden: International Society for the Study of the Lumbar Spine Gothenberg; 2011.
15. Anand N, Wupperman R, Rosemann R, et al. Minimally invasive AxiALIF L5-S1 interbody fusion For anterior column support at the end of a long segment fusion: early results. Miami: Spine Arthroplasty Society; 2008.
16. Botolin S, Agudelo J, Dwyer A, et al. High rectal injury during trans-1 axial lumbar interbody fusion L5-S1 fixation: a case report. Spine. 2010;35:E144–8.
17. Anand N, Rosemann R, Khalsa B, et al. Mid-term to long-term clinical and functional outcomes of minimally invasive correction and fusion for adults with scoliosis. Neurosurg Focus. 2010;28:E6.
18. Anand N, Baron EM. Minimally invasive approaches for the correction of adult spinal deformity. Eur Spine J. 2012;22(2):232–41 [Epub ahead of print].
19. Anand N, Baron EM, Thaiyananthan G, et al. Minimally invasive multilevel percutaneous correction and fusion for adult lumbar degenerative scoliosis: a technique and feasibility study. J Spinal Disord Tech. 2008;21:459–67.
20. Lehman Jr RA, Kuklo TR, Belmont Jr PJ, et al. Advantage of pedicle screw fixation directed into the apex of the sacral promontory over bicortical fixation: a biomechanical analysis. Spine. 2002;27: 806–11.
21. Matteini LE, Kebaish KM, Volk WR, et al. An S-2 alar iliac pelvic fixation. Technical note. Neurosurg Focus. 2010;28:E13.
22. O'Brien JR, Matteini L, Yu WD, et al. Feasibility of minimally invasive sacropelvic fixation: percutaneous S2 alar iliac fixation. Spine. 2010;35:460–4.
23. Lee S, Rivadeneira D, Hartl R. Best practices in avoidance detection and treatment of colorectal perforations during AxiaLIF surgery. Wilmington, NC: Trans1; 2009.
24. Gerszten PC, Tobler WD, Nasca RJ. Retrospective analysis of L5-S1 axial lumbar interbody fusion (AxiaLIF): a comparison with and without the use of recombinant human bone morphogenetic protein-2. Spine J. 2011;11:1027–32.
25. Tobler WD, Gerszten PC, Bradley WD, et al. Minimally invasive axial presacral L5-S1 interbody fusion: two-year clinical and radiographic outcomes. Spine. 2011;36:E1296–301.
26. Lindley EM, McCullough MA, Burger EL, et al. Complications of axial lumbar interbody fusion. J Neurosurg Spine. 2011;15:273–9.

Minimally Invasive Sacroiliac Joint Fusion

32

Yi Lu and Steven Wu

The sacroiliac joint is often an overlooked cause for low back pain. It is estimated that around 15–20 % of low back pain is caused by sacroiliac joint dysfunction [3, 22, 23]. This number may be even higher in patients with a history of lumbosacral fusion surgery, a history of posterior iliac crest bone graft harvesting, or in patients with sustained low back pain after spine surgery ("failed back syndrome") [6, 11, 15, 19, 24].

In addition to back pain, sacroiliac joint disease can manifest as buttock pain, trochanteric pain, pelvic pain, or dyspareunia [11]. Pain generated from the sacroiliac joint sometimes radiates to the lower limbs as well. Pain from sacroiliac joint degeneration could easily be confused with nerve root pain or facet joint pain. The most common location for sacroiliac joint pain is the upper medial part of the buttock at the junction of the sacrum. Several conditions contribute to the development of sacroiliac pain including degenerative and inflammatory arthritis, posttraumatic and postpartum instability, infection, and neoplastic disease.

The pathophysiology of sacroiliac joint pain is not completely clear. The sacroiliac joint could be considered as a shock absorber of the lower back. Natural movements in the joint are small in magnitude, but the direction of the motion is complex. Normally there is 2–4 mm gliding and 2°–4° of rotation in the sacroiliac joint. Significant individual variations in the direction and magnitude of the movements exist. The largest contributor to the nerve fibers supplying the sacroiliac joint is the dorsal part of the S1 roots. The L4 and L5 nerve roots and the superior gluteal nerve may be involved as well. In addition, pain generated from the sacroiliac joint could be from ligamentous or capsular tension, osteoarthritis, enthesis, or ligamentous sprain, etc. (Figs. 32.1 and 32.2).

Gender, age, and weight significantly influence the probability that a sacroiliac joint origin contributes to the patient's chronic low back pain [7]. Females are much more likely to suffer from sacroiliac joint pain than males likely due to the difference in anatomy as well as hormonal and structural changes related to pregnancy and childbirth. Older age correlates with an increased incidence of sacroiliac joint disease likely from

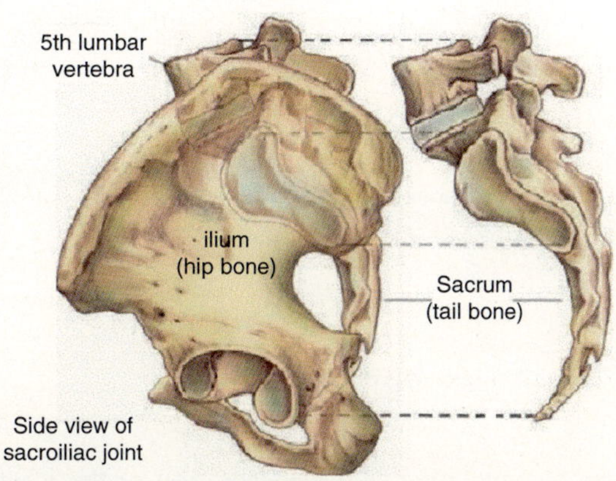

Fig. 32.1 Anatomy of sacroiliac joint

Y. Lu, M.D., Ph.D. • S. Wu
Department of Neurosurgery,
Brigham and Women's Hospital,
Harvard Medical School, Boston, MA, USA
e-mail: ylu4@partners.org

M.Y. Wang et al. (eds.), *Minimally Invasive Spinal Deformity Surgery*,
DOI 10.1007/978-3-7091-1407-0_32, © Springer-Verlag Wien 2014

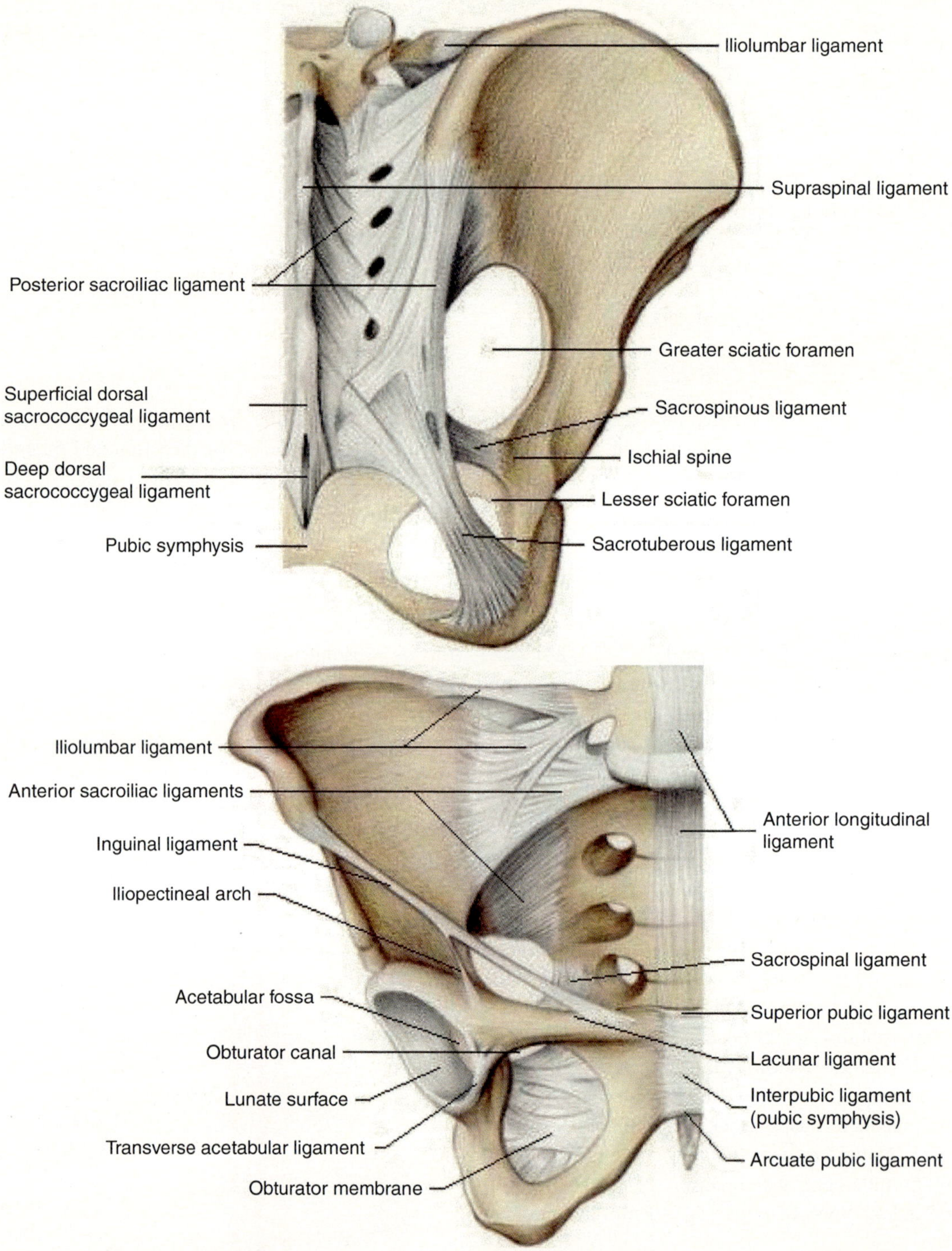

Fig. 32.2 Ligaments of sacroiliac joint

the accumulative slow degeneration of the joint with aging. Interestingly, lower BMIs are associated with higher probability of pain from sacroiliac joints if a patient presents with low back pain. This may be simply due to the lower incidence of other low back pain etiologies in patients with low BMIs. According to a multivariant analysis, for an elderly female who

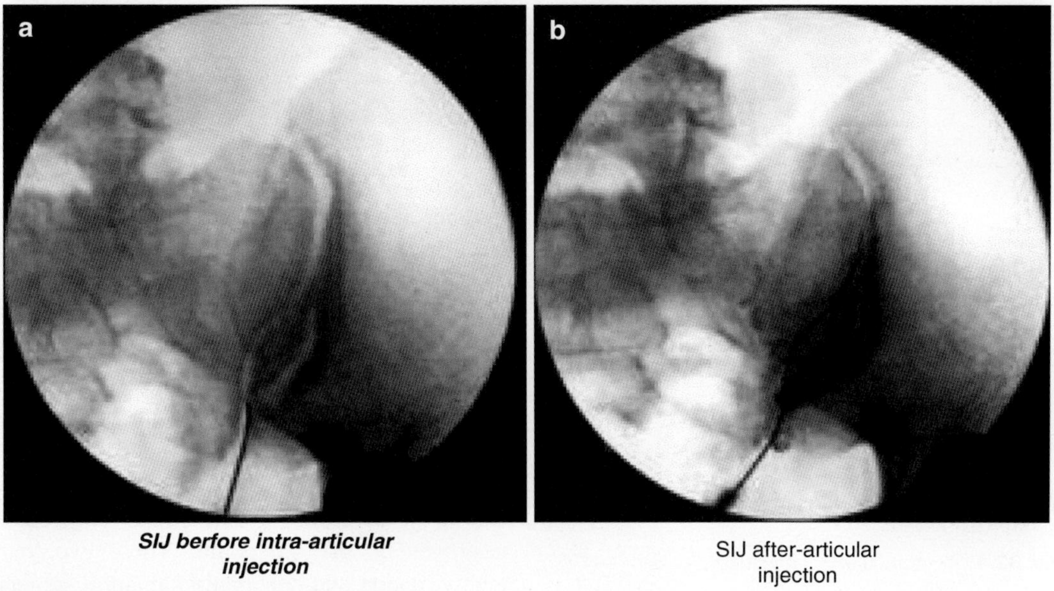

Fig. 32.3 (**a**) SIJ before intra-articular injection. (**b**) SIJ after intra-articular injection

presents with chronic low back pain, the chance of the pain originating from the sacroiliac joint could be well above 50 % [7].

Previous lumbosacral spine surgeries predispose patients to the development of sacroiliac joint disease [15, 27]. When lumbar fusion surgeries are extended to the sacrum, the sacral iliac joints are the adjacent joints to the fusion. Therefore, they experience the increased load and stress similar to other spinal adjacent joints after fusion surgery. The increased load and stress from the fused lumbosacral segments might expedite sacroiliac joint degeneration. It has been reported that the incidence of sacroiliac joint degeneration is higher in patients with fusion down to S1 than in patients with fusion down to L5 [15]. In biomechanical studies, it has been shown that posterior fusion of the lumbar spine leads to increased motion at the sacroiliac joint and increased stress across the sacroiliac articular surfaces [6, 16, 19].

A history of iliac crest bone graft harvesting also predisposes patients to sacroiliac joint degeneration. Harvesting cancellous bone was shown to induce pelvic instability [5]. In some studies, history of iliac bone graft harvesting correlated with increased sacroiliac joint degeneration [9].

The probability of chronic low back pain originating from sacroiliac joint degeneration is greater in patients diagnosed with failed back syndrome. Failed back syndrome is characterized by the occurrence or persistence of severe low back pain after spine surgery. A portion of patients with failed back syndrome may have had a misdiagnosis from the start with the sacroiliac joints being the source of pain instead of the lower lumbar spine. Some other patients may have developed new sacroiliac joint degeneration due to the increased stress from the lumbar fusion surgery. As a result, for patients who present with either persistent or new onset low back pain after lumbar surgeries, physicians must have a high suspicion whether the sacroiliac joints are the source of the low back pain.

One of the difficulties of treating sacroiliac joint disease is the lack of accurate diagnostic tests. Numerous sacroiliac joint provocative tests have been described to suggest the pain source, yet the specificity of those tests is generally low [8, 25]. Radiographic tests have been shown to have low sensitivity and specificity in diagnosing sacroiliac joint disease [10]. The most reliable diagnostic test for sacroiliac joint disease is the temporary pain relief after low-volume local anesthetic agents injection into the joint under fluoroscopic control [12, 13, 18, 23] (Figs. 32.3a, b and 32.4). Sacroiliac joint block is considered the gold standard for diagnosing

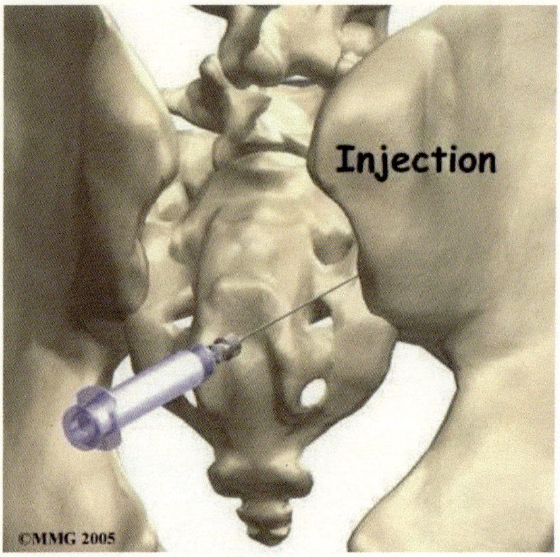

Fig. 32.4 Illustration of SIJ injection

sacroiliac joint disease. Yet, even the sacroiliac joint injection has been shown to be not very reliable. The effects of two consecutive injections are identical only 60 % of the time. One possible explanation for the inaccuracy of the sacroiliac joint injection is the diffusion of the anesthetic agents out of the sacroiliac joint during injection. The diffusion causes the anesthetic agents to come in contact with adjacent nerve trunks or roots, which leads to temporary pain relief even if the sacroiliac joint may not be the sources of pain. Injection of the anesthetic agents into the sacroiliac joint might relieve pain from numerous surrounding ligaments as well.

Given the uncertainty of diagnosing sacroiliac joint disease, it is without surprise that it is not easy to identify an effective treatment for the disease. The first-line treatments for sacroiliac joint pain are conservative treatments including analgesic and anti-inflammatory medications, physical therapy, and several types of injection treatments. When conservative therapies fail to relieve the symptoms and the physicians believe the pain is originating from the sacroiliac joint, more invasive treatment modalities are considered. Two such treatment options are surgical fusion of the sacroiliac joints or ablative therapy to denervate the joints. A systemic review of the published results from six fusion studies and five denervation ablative studies reported that the majority of patients were satisfied after receiving either treatment [2]. Both procedures reported efficacy in improving pain and functional outcome. However, the evidence was low to very low since all the studies were case series and the number of patients in those studies was generally low. In addition, the effects were relatively moderate. The mean rate of patient satisfaction was 57.6 % for fusion studies with great variations (range from 18 % to 100 %). The mean pain improvement in the studies that reported visual analog or numeric rating showed the improvement in the pain scale of 3.5 and 4.9 points, respectively. One study that documented Oswestry Disability Index (ODI) showed an improvement of 14.0 points. These two treatments (fusion and denervation ablation surgery) have comparable improvements in pain relief and functional outcome. The denervation ablation studies generally have a short follow-up of 6–12 months; therefore, it is unclear whether the denervation procedures provide durable pain relief. It is worth noting that many lumbar facet joint denervation ablation studies showed loss of efficacy after about 2 years.

When conservative treatment fails to relieve pain from suspected sacroiliac joint disease, fusion surgery becomes a treatment option. Various open fusion surgery techniques have been developed including the posterior or Smith-Petersen approach, the anterior approach, and the posterior midline fascia splitting approach [4, 14]. The results from the open sacroiliac joint fusion surgeries were mixed. Some reported great efficacy, yet some results were disappointing. In one study by Schutz et al., the nonunion rate with instability was 41.2 %, and more than 80 % of the patients still had significant pain after the surgery [21]. The open surgery itself is usually painful due to the extensive dissection needed for the surgery. The relatively high complications and nonunion rates of open surgeries encourage surgeons to search for alternatives with possible lower morbidities and higher efficacy.

In recent years, several minimally invasive sacroiliac joint arthrodesis techniques have been developed [1, 17, 20, 26]. Not all the techniques have clinical data to back up their effectiveness yet. However, the limited publications up to date indicated generally good clinical outcomes using minimally invasive sacroiliac joint fusion techniques in treating sacroiliac joint pain that had failed conservative treatments.

In 2008, Wise and Dall described a minimally invasive sacroiliac joint fusion procedure and published their series of 13 consecutive patients [26]. All the patients had no relief after more than 6 months of conservative therapy and completed exhaustive workups to rule out lumbar spine as the source of pain. A fluoroscopically guided intra-articular injection with a mixture of local anesthetic and corticosteroid was used to confirm the diagnosis of sacroiliac joint dysfunction. Their surgical technique involved inserting cages along the anterior-posterior (AP) axis of the sacroiliac joint percutaneously. The key for safe placement of the cages in the AP axis was the understanding of the safe cephalad and caudad margins of the sacroiliac joints and the depth of placement based on preoperative images. It is important to avoid placing the cage too deep through the anterior portion of the joint and into the pelvis. Preoperative CT scans of the bilateral sacroiliac joints with the patients in the prone position (same position as in the surgery) were used to determine the area with the most bony surface available on both sacral and iliac sides of the joint as the "safe zone" for cage placement. During surgery, with the patient in prone position, the starting point of the incision was made on the most prominent part of the posterior superior iliac spine (PSIS) and extended 1 cm caudad and 4 cm cephalad. The dissection was carried down to the PSIS, and a calibrated Steinman pin was tapped into the bone carefully. The placement of the Steinman pin was approximately 6–7 mm cephalad to the caudal margin of the safe zone. The depth of the Steinman pin advancement was carefully monitored using fluoroscopy so that it was within the preoperative measurements (usually between 4.5 and 6.5 cm). When the pin was at the predetermined position, a 9-mm cannulated drill was used to drill over the pin. The surgeon watched the lateral fluoroscopic images carefully to make sure the tip of the pin was not advancing with the drill to avoid its advancement into the pelvis. After palpation of the drilled hole, a threaded titanium cage, measuring 11 × 25 mm (Medtronic Sofamor Danek, Memphis, TN), was then packed with BMP and inserted in the hole with the open slots of the cage's sidewalls pointing to the sacrum and the ileum. After the first cage was placed, the second cage was inserted in a similar fashion, approximately 6–7 mm cephalad to the first cage. In their series of 13 consecutive patients, an 89 % fusion rate was achieved based on the 6-month CT scan. The low back pain improved by an average of 4.9 points on a ten-point visual analog scale. Leg pain improved by an average of 2.4 points, and dyspareunia improved by an average of 2.6 points. Seventy-seven percent of the patients reported satisfaction with the results of the surgery.

Al-khayer et al. from the UK published their method of percutaneous sacroiliac joint fusion and analyzed their outcomes from nine patients in the same year [1]. In their procedure, the authors used one single hollow modular anchorage (HMA) screw (Aesculap, Sheffield, UK), which is a hollow cylindrical implant made from one piece of titanium alloy and placed the screw perpendicular to and across the sacroiliac joint from the lateral side. The screw passed through the sacral alar to the body of S1 vertebra at the midpoint between the S1 neural foramina and the L5/S1 disc. Patients were placed supine on a radiolucent table. Four views (lateral, anteroposterior, inlet, and outlet) of the pelvis were obtained. A guidewire was placed percutaneously and advanced across the sacroiliac joint to the body of the S1 vertebra under fluoroscopic guidance. A cannulated 10-mm drill was then used to drill over the guidewire with the protection of a guide tube, also under fluoroscopic guidance. The guidewire was then removed, and a 10-mm tap was used to prepare for screw insertion. The HMA screw was then packed with the bone graft from the bone reaming obtained during drilling with demineralized bone matrix and screwed into the prepared tunnel. The usual length of the screw was about 40–50 mm.

The position of the screw was confirmed using the fluoroscope. In their series of nine patients with an average follow-up of 40 months, the mean VAS dropped from 8.1 preoperatively to 4.6 postoperatively. The mean ODI dropped from 59 to 45. The mean patient satisfaction was 6.8, and all the patients stated that they would undergo the same procedure again under the same circumstances. Placing the anchoring screws across the sacroiliac joint may have the benefits of immediate stabilization, before the fusion happens. Although the posteriorly placed grafts into the AP axis of the SI joints like the ones used by Wise and Dall may have the same effect functioning as a door wedge stabilizing a pivoting door.

Khurana et al. also reported their experience with 15 patients using the same hollow modular anchorage screws filled with demineralized bone matrix to treat the refractive sacroiliac joint disease [17]. In a mean follow-up of 17 months, the average Short Form-36 scores improved from 37 to 80 for physical function and from 53 to 86 for general health. Thirteen patients (87 %) had good to excellent outcomes.

There are several commercial minimally invasive sacroiliac joint fusion systems available on the market currently. Most of the systems were developed within the past several years; therefore, only limited data is available regarding the clinical efficacy of these systems.

1. iFuse®: The iFuse Implant System® from SI-BONE® places several (usually three) porous plasma-coated titanium implants across the sacroiliac joints laterally through an incision of approximately 3 cm (Fig. 32.5). The surgical technique includes initial placement of guidewire pins across the sacroiliac joint under fluoroscopic guidance. A drill and a triangular broach are then used to prepare the bone over the pins with the help of a soft tissue protector. The triangular implant is then inserted into the prepared tunnel with a mallet. Usually three implants are placed, in the sacral alar, above or adjacent to the S1 foramen, and between the S1 and S2 foramen, respectively (Figs. 32.6 and 32.7). There are several unique features of the iFuse system. The triangular implant profile minimizes rotations of the implant. The porous surface is designed to minimize micromotion of the implants and promotes bony overgrowth leading to eventual fusion. Usually three implants are placed in one sacroiliac joint; therefore, rotation movements of the sacroiliac joints with the single-threaded cage system

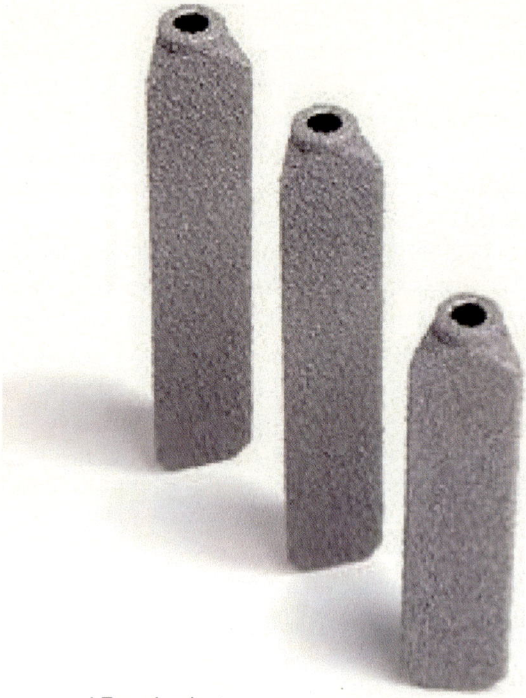

Fig. 32.5 iFuse® implant system

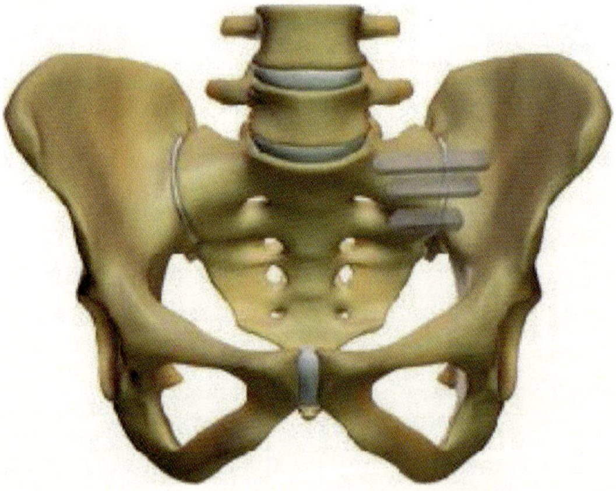

Fig. 32.6 iFuse® implants across the SI joints

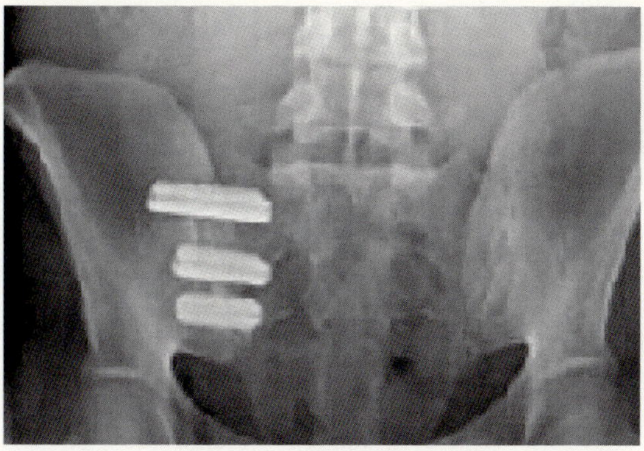

Fig. 32.7 X-ray image of iFuse® implants across SI joint

should be minimized, and strong immediate stabilization of sacroiliac joint is achieved. According to the company website, biomechanical studies demonstrated that the 7-mm triangular implant is three times stronger in shear and bending strength than an 8-mm cannulated screw. In the iFuse system, no autologous graft, allograft, or other fusion extenders were placed in the sacroiliac joints, nor does the sacroiliac joint be decorticated in preparation for fusion. The eventual bony fusion was therefore dependent upon the porous surface of the implants. Rudolf reported the use of iFuse for minimally invasive sacroiliac joint fusion on the first consecutive 50 patients treated [20]. Pain scale decreased from 7.6 to 3.3 at the 12-month follow-up and to 2.0 at the 24-month follow-up. Eighty-two percent of the patients reported satisfaction of the surgery. No radiographic outcomes about whether the implants led to fusion were discussed. Eleven patients (22 %) experienced complications including three cases of superficial cellulitis, one deep infection, two large buttock hematomas, one nondisplaced ilium fracture, and one delayed loosening of the implants causing recurrence of symptoms. Three patients were taken back to the OR for implant penetration into the sacral neural foramen or L5 neural foramen.

2. SI-LOK®: Globus Medical Inc. also developed a minimally invasive sacroiliac joint fixation system SI-LOK® (Fig. 32.8). SI-LOK® system places three hydroxyapatite-coated screws laterally through the sacroiliac joints (Figs. 32.9 and 32.10). The optional bone graft slots in the SI-LOK® screws allow surgeon to place bone grafts in the screws to promote fusion. Furthermore, the optional lag screw thread is designed to apply compression force across the SI joint during insertion, further improving chances of fusion. Clinical and biomechanical studies of the SI-LOK® system are currently underway.

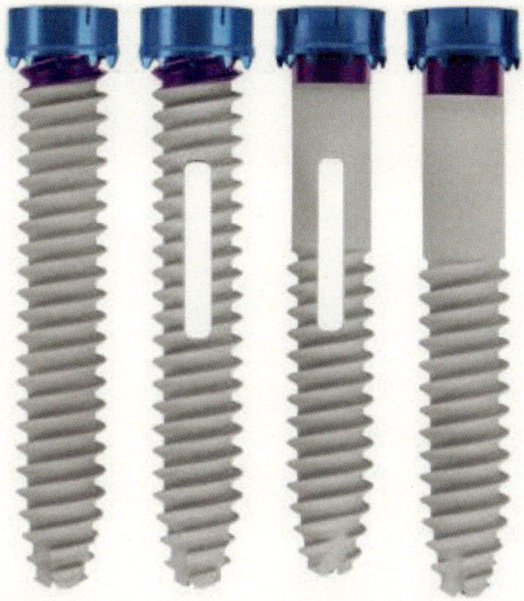

Fig. 32.8 SI-Lok® sacroiliac fixation system

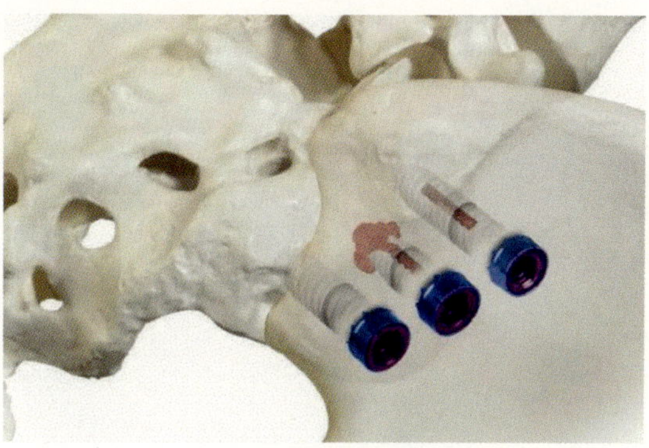

Fig. 32.9 SI-Lok® screws across the SI joints

3. SImmetry®: SImmetry® system from Zyga Technology Inc. places two cannulated titanium screws (one 12.5-mm and one 6.5-

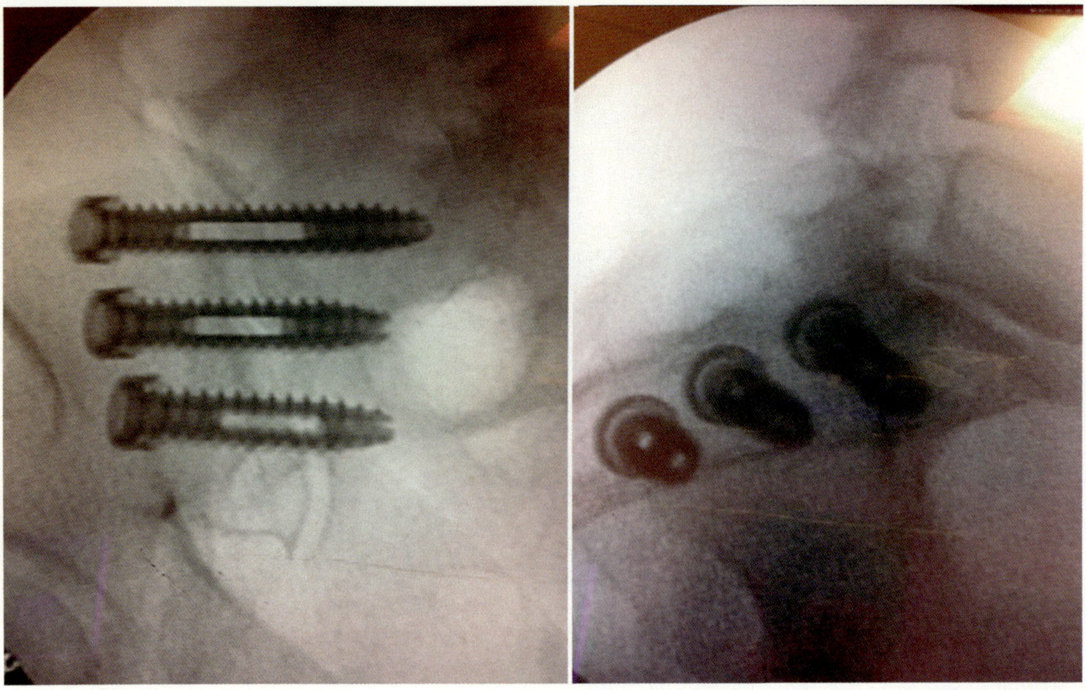

Fig. 32.10 Fluroscopic images of SI-Lok® screws placed across the SI joint

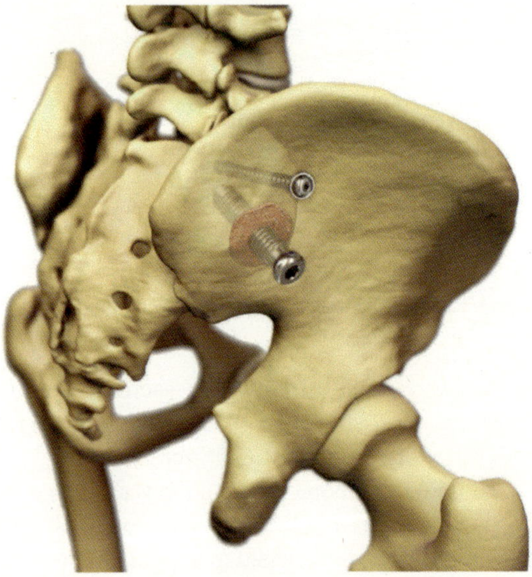

Fig. 32.11 SImmetry® sacroiliac joint fusion system

mm anti-rotation screw) across the sacroiliac joint laterally (Fig. 32.11). The screws are available from 30 to 70 mm in length. Unique features of SImmetry® include special steps for SI joint decortication using a series percutaneously placed stainless steel cutters and bone graft placement into the SI joints. These steps are designed to promote arthrodesis across the sacroiliac joints (Fig. 32.12).

Using the lateral fluoro view, a 6-mm dilator with obturator is advanced to the ilium at the planned trajectory and entry point. Obturator is then exchanged with the 3.2-mm guide pin, and the pin is driven into the outer ilium cortex slightly. Inlet- and outlet-oblique views are then used to confirm the correct trajectory of the guide pin. Under the outlet-oblique view, the guide pin is advanced to the joint. The lateral ilium cortex is then serially dilated with slap hammer and the 6-mm, 8-mm, and 9-mm dilators. After the guide pin is removed, a working cannula is tapped into the sacroiliac joint until the working cannula shoulder contacts the lateral ilium cortex. A 17-mm sleeve is then advanced over the working cannula. Scraper and serial special sacroiliac joint curettes are used to remove the cartilage and decorticate a portion of the

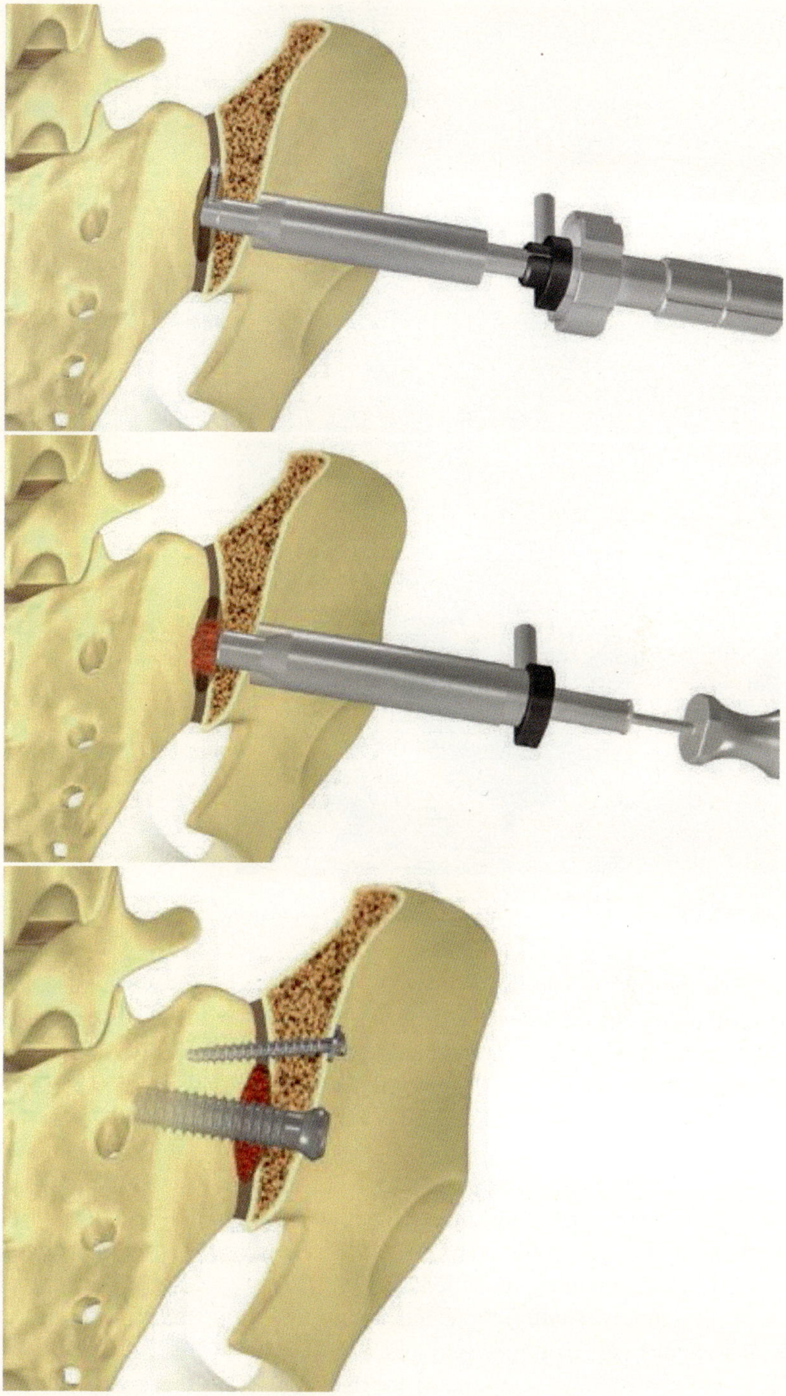

Fig. 32.12 SImmetry® system uses specials tools to decorticate the SI joints and place bone grafts into the SI joints

sacroiliac joint to create a bleeding bed for fusion (Fig. 32.12). A graft inserter loaded with 2-cc bone graft is then inserted into the working cannula just proximal to the joint. Pressing the back of the graft inserter extrudes bone graft into the denuded cavity in the sacroiliac joint (Fig. 32.12). A graft spreader is then used to spread the bone graft radially

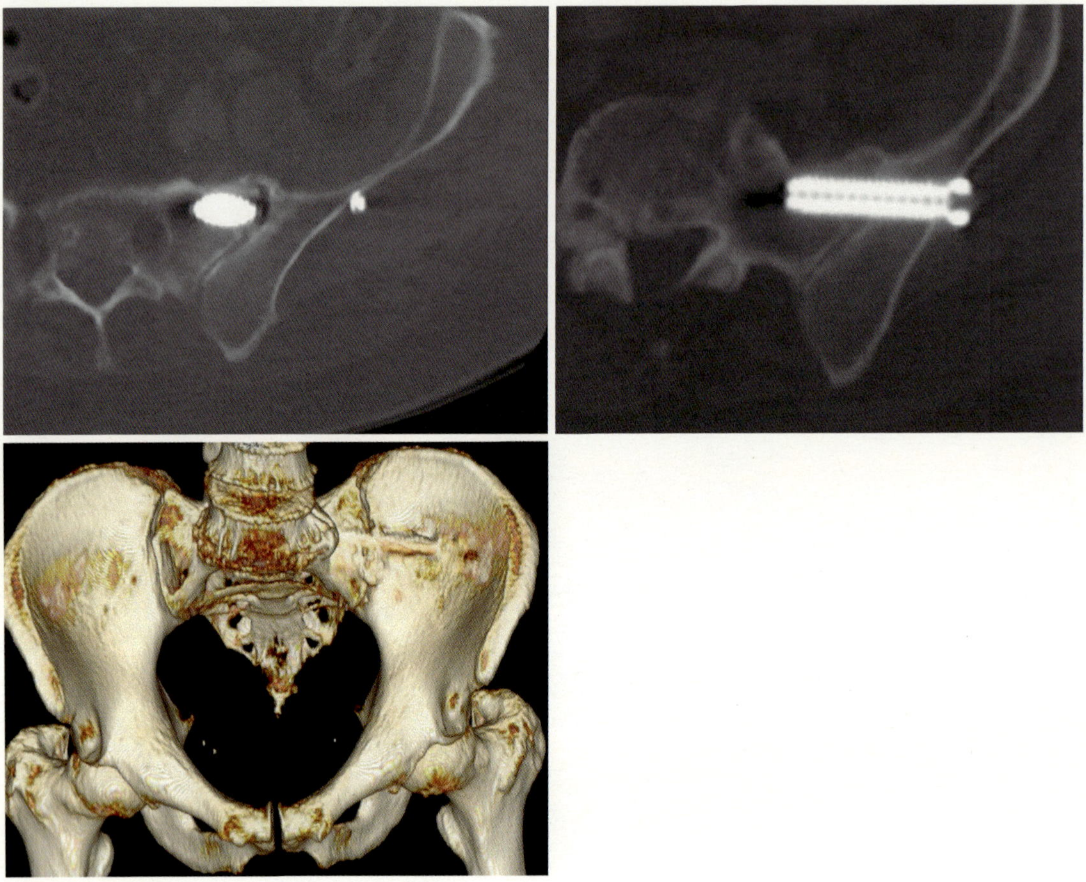

Fig. 32.13 12 month post-op CT scans showing fusion using SImmetry®

into the cavity. The uneven surface of the SI joints may cause some difficulty in the joint decortication and graft spreading. After the bone graft placement, 9-mm drill with the guide pin is replaced. Guide pin is advanced with a pin driver under fluoroscopic guidance. A 9-mm drill is then advanced into the sacrum cortex to the same depth and removed. A 12.5-mm fusion rod with the selected depth is advanced into the pre-drilled path with the 12.5-mm driver until fully seated. At this time, the fluoroscope is turned into lateral position, and a separate incision is made for the cephalad 6-mm anti-rotation screw. Similar techniques are used to place the 6-mm anti-rotation screw although there is no need to decorticate the sacroiliac joint here.

Currently Zyga Technology Inc. is conducting ongoing 12-month postoperative CT image studies with a third-party radiographic analysis group for all the patients who have received SImmetry® implants. The first few CTs showed solid fusion evidenced by extra-articular bone bridge, bone bridge immediately adjacent to the rod, and no radiolucency in the ilium or sacrum (Fig. 32.13).

4. SIFix®: SIFix®from Nutech Medical Inc. is the first commercial posterior minimally invasive sacroiliac joint system. It uses two carefully machinized threaded cancellous bone dowels measuring 22 mm × 11 mm (length × diameter) that are placed along the AP axis of SI joints to provide stabilization and fusion (Fig. 32.14). Because the SIFix® uses a midline posterior incision, surgeons can perform bilateral SI joint fusion through a single midline incision. Without repositioning the patient, the incision can also be easily extended to perform

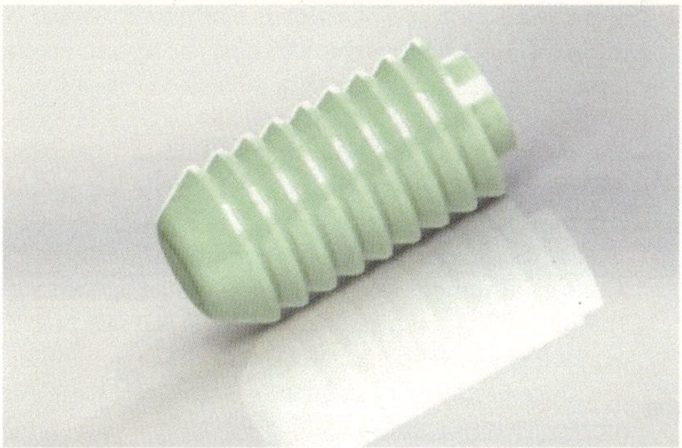

Fig. 32.14 SIFix® system

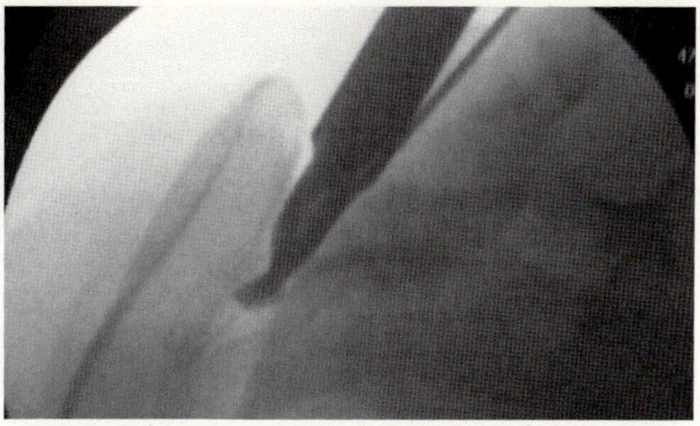

Fig. 32.16 Drill bit in the SI joint to decorticate the joint and create a void for the bone dowel

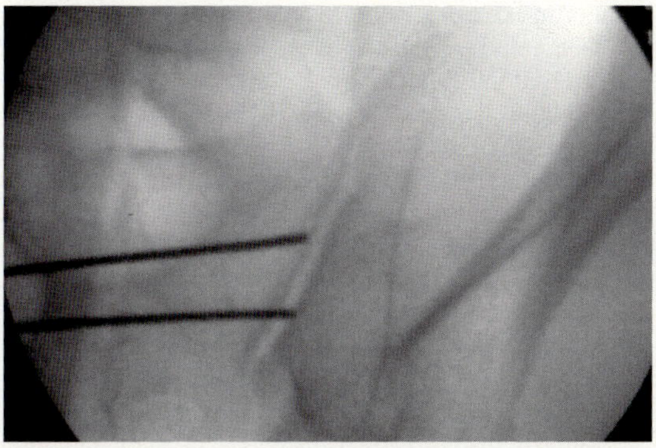

Fig. 32.15 Fluoroscopic assisted oblique view to visualize the SI joint

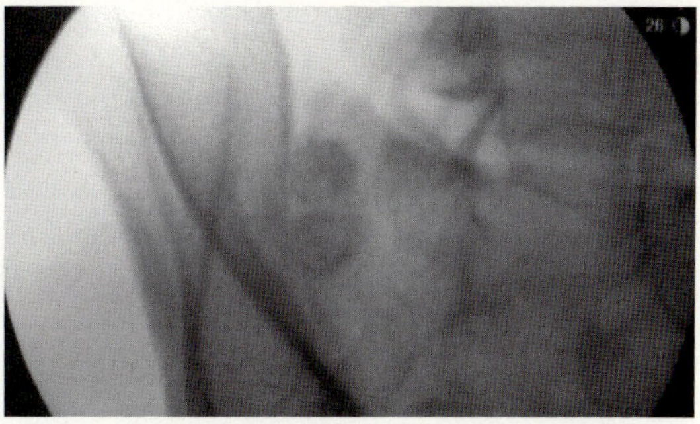

Fig. 32.17 Fluoroscopic image showing the placement of two SIFix® bone dowels along the AP axis of the SI joint

posterior spine procedures at the same time, if indicated. In SIFix®, the use of allograft bone dowel as the implant is designed to enhance bony ingrowth and fusion.

In SIFix® procedure, patient is placed in the prone position. An oblique view is obtained to visualize the SI joint (Fig. 32.15), and inferior and superior margin of the SI joint are identified. A single 4-cm midline incision is made to accommodate two planned bone dowels, and place guidewires into the SI joints under fluoroscopic guidance (Fig. 32.15). Serial dilators are used to create the path, and the SI drill guide is then placed through the final dilator to access the SI joint. Guidewire in the drill guide is then removed, and drill bit is used to create a void in the SI joint for implant placement (Fig. 32.16). Using the implant inserter, the implant is then inserted into the space. A second implant is placed in a similar fashion (Fig. 32.17). After the bone dowels have been countersunk into the SI joint, bone graft of choice can be packed into the socket to aid in fusion (Fig. 32.18).

In summary, minimally invasive sacroiliac joint fusion has seen significant advancement in the recent years. The advantages of minimally invasive sacroiliac joint fusion over the open fusion procedures are multifold. In addition to the minimal blood loss, shorter operation, and faster recovery time, minimizing damages to the surrounding ligaments preserved the intrinsic stability of the sacroiliac joint prior to fusion. In other words, using the minimally invasive techniques, there is no need to destabilize the sacroiliac joint first to promote eventual fusion. This might lead to better patient outcome; certainly there is less need to restraint patient's activity after the surgery. In comparison, in open SI fusion surgery, patients frequently need to be in no weight bearing status for 12 weeks.

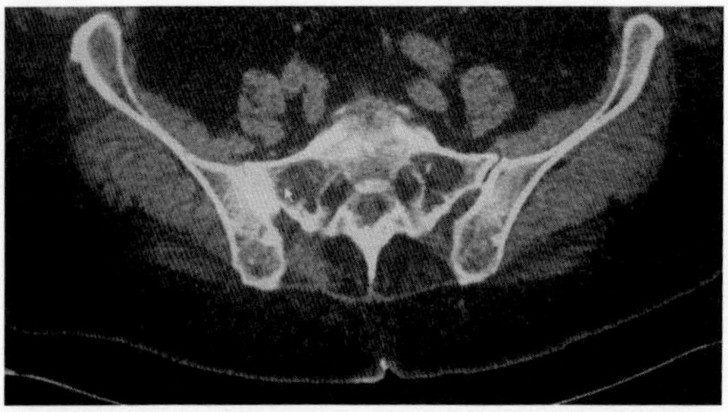

Fig. 32.18 CT scan showing evidence of SI joint fusion using SIFix

Traditionally, the benefit and risk/morbidity ratio does not favor much in the treatment of SI joint degenerative pain with open surgery. However, the advancement of the minimally invasive alternatives might change the balance and provide valid surgical options for patients with refractory degenerative SI joint disease. More clinical and radiographic data, however, is much needed to support the use of those new techniques and to prove their efficacy (Fig. 32.18).

References

1. Al-Khayer A, Hegarty J, Hahn D, Grevitt MP. Percutaneous sacroiliac joint arthrodesis: a novel technique. J Spinal Disord Tech. 2008;21:359–63.
2. Ashman B, Norvell DC, Hermsmeyer JT. Chronic sacroiliac joint pain: fusion versus denervation as treatment options. Evid Based Spine Care J. 2010;1:35–44.
3. Bernard Jr TN, Kirkaldy-Willis WH. Recognizing specific characteristics of nonspecific low back pain. Clin Orthop Relat Res. 1987;217:266–80.
4. Buchowski JM, Kebaish KM, Sinkov V, Cohen DB, Sieber AN, Kostuik JP. Functional and radiographic outcome of sacroiliac arthrodesis for the disorders of the sacroiliac joint. Spine J. 2005;5:520–8. discussion 529.
5. Chan K, Resnick D, Pathria M, Jacobson J. Pelvic instability after bone graft harvesting from posterior iliac crest: report of nine patients. Skeletal Radiol. 2001;30:278–81.
6. DePalma MJ, Ketchum JM, Saullo TR. Etiology of chronic low back pain in patients having undergone lumbar fusion. Pain Med. 2011;12:732–9.
7. DePalma MJ, Ketchum JM, Saullo TR. Multivariable analyses of the relationships between age, gender, and body mass index and the source of chronic low back pain. Pain Med. 2012;13:498–506.
8. Dreyfuss P, Dryer S, Griffin J, Hoffman J, Walsh N. Positive sacroiliac screening tests in asymptomatic adults. Spine (Phila Pa 1976). 1994;19:1138–43.
9. Ebraheim NA, Elgafy H, Semaan HB. Computed tomographic findings in patients with persistent sacroiliac pain after posterior iliac graft harvesting. Spine (Phila Pa 1976). 2000;25:2047–51.
10. Elgafy H, Semaan HB, Ebraheim NA, Coombs RJ. Computed tomography findings in patients with sacroiliac pain. Clin Orthop Relat Res. 2001;382:112–8.
11. Foley BS, Buschbacher RM. Sacroiliac joint pain: anatomy, biomechanics, diagnosis, and treatment. Am J Phys Med Rehabil. 2006;85:997–1006.
12. Fortin JD, Aprill CN, Ponthieux B, Pier J. Sacroiliac joint: pain referral maps upon applying a new injection/arthrography technique. Part II: Clinical evaluation. Spine (Phila Pa 1976). 1994;19:1483–9.
13. Fortin JD, Dwyer AP, West S, Pier J. Sacroiliac joint: pain referral maps upon applying a new injection/arthrography technique. Part I: Asymptomatic volunteers. Spine (Phila Pa 1976). 1994;19:1475–82.
14. Giannikas KA, Khan AM, Karski MT, Maxwell HA. Sacroiliac joint fusion for chronic pain: a simple technique avoiding the use of metalwork. Eur Spine J. 2004;13:253–6.
15. Ha KY, Lee JS, Kim KW. Degeneration of sacroiliac joint after instrumented lumbar or lumbosacral fusion: a prospective cohort study over five-year follow-up. Spine (Phila Pa 1976). 2008;33:1192–8.
16. Ivanov AA, Kiapour A, Ebraheim NA, Goel V. Lumbar fusion leads to increases in angular motion and stress across sacroiliac joint: a finite element study. Spine (Phila Pa 1976). 2009;34:E162–9.
17. Khurana A, Guha AR, Mohanty K, Ahuja S. Percutaneous fusion of the sacroiliac joint with hollow modular anchorage screws: clinical and radiological outcome. J Bone Joint Surg Br. 2009;91:627–31.
18. Maigne JY, Aivaliklis A, Pfefer F. Results of sacroiliac joint double block and value of sacroiliac pain provocation tests in 54 patients with low back pain. Spine (Phila Pa 1976). 1996;21:1889–92.
19. Maigne JY, Planchon CA. Sacroiliac joint pain after lumbar fusion. A study with anesthetic blocks. Eur Spine J. 2005;14:654–8.
20. Rudolf L. Sacroiliac joint arthrodesis – MIS technique with titanium implants: report of the first 50 patients and outcomes. Open Orthop J. 2012;6:495–502.
21. Schutz U, Grob D. Poor outcome following bilateral sacroiliac joint fusion for degenerative sacroiliac joint syndrome. Acta Orthop Belg. 2006;72:296–308.
22. Sembrano JN, Polly Jr DW. How often is low back pain not coming from the back? Spine (Phila Pa 1976). 2009;34:E27–32.
23. Simopoulos TT, Manchikanti L, Singh V, Gupta S, Hameed H, Diwan S, Cohen SP. A systematic evaluation of prevalence and diagnostic accuracy of sacroiliac joint interventions. Pain Physician. 2012;15:E305–44.
24. Slipman CW, Shin CH, Patel RK, Isaac Z, Huston CW, Lipetz JS, Lenrow DA, Braverman DL,

Vresilovic Jr EJ. Etiologies of failed back surgery syndrome. Pain Med. 2002;3:200–14. discussion 214–207.
25. Slipman CW, Sterenfeld EB, Chou LH, Herzog R, Vresilovic E. The predictive value of provocative sacroiliac joint stress maneuvers in the diagnosis of sacroiliac joint syndrome. Arch Phys Med Rehabil. 1998;79:288–92.
26. Wise CL, Dall BE. Minimally invasive sacroiliac arthrodesis: outcomes of a new technique. J Spinal Disord Tech. 2008;21:579–84.
27. Yoshihara H. Sacroiliac joint pain after lumbar/lumbosacral fusion: current knowledge. Eur Spine J. 2012;21:1788–96.

Part VI

Achieving Intersegmental Arthodesis

Bone Graft Extenders 33

Sonia Teufack, James Harrop, and Srinivas Prasad

33.1 Introduction

The goal of spinal arthrodesis is to eliminate pathologic motion between adjacent vertebral segments. Several spinal conditions which are managed and treated operatively after failure of conservative measures require surgical intervention such to achieve a solid fusion. Presently at the time of surgery intervention, spinal instrumentation is often used to further stabilize adjacent levels, but true arthrodesis is independent of the hardware and requires growth of bone across the immobilized spinal segments forming one unified structure. The use of autologous bone grafting has been shown to significantly improve the rate of spinal fusion [1–4]. However, presently, a wide variety of materials are used due to the morbidity of autologous bone graft harvesting either alone or in combination to facilitate fusion; these include autogenous graft, allogenic graft, dematerialized bone matrix, bone morphogenic proteins (BMP), synthetic graft extenders, and synthetic cages. In this chapter we will focus on bone graft extenders.

S. Teufack, M.D. • J. Harrop, M.D. (✉)
S. Prasad, M.D.
Department of Neurosurgery,
Thomas Jefferson University Hospital,
Philadelphia, PA, USA
e-mail: james.harrop@jefferson.edu

33.2 Bone Formation

Bone is a connective tissue primarily made of a mineralized matrix structure. Bone formation begins with osteoblasts producing type I collagen to form an osteoid matrix. Subsequently, osteoblasts secrete vesicles containing alkaline phosphatase that cleave phosphate groups and allow deposition of calcium and phosphate in the matrix. Over time, this process results in mineralization and hardening of the bone matrix with carbonated hydroxyapatite.

Four types of cells are involved in bone formation, maintenance, and healing. Osteoblasts produce bone matrix; osteocytes are mature osteoblasts that maintain the bone; osteoclasts are cells that breakdown and remove bone matrix; and bone lining cells cover bone surfaces.

Bone grafts can regenerate bone through three different processes: osteogenesis, osteoinduction, and osteoconduction. Osteogenesis is the formation of new bone by the osteoblasts within the graft material. Osteoinduction is a process by which chemical substances contained within the graft stimulate patients' osteoprogenitor cells to differentiate into osteoblasts to form new bone. Osteoconduction occurs when a graft provides a scaffold for new bone to grow. Successful arthrodesis relies on a combination of these processes.

M.Y. Wang et al. (eds.), *Minimally Invasive Spinal Deformity Surgery*,
DOI 10.1007/978-3-7091-1407-0_33, © Springer-Verlag Wien 2014

33.2.1 Autograft

Autograft, also known as autologous bone graft, has long been considered the "gold standard" for bone fusion in spine surgery [5, 6]. It can be obtained locally during the principal procedure or may require a separate incision for harvesting from another site, such as the iliac crest or fibula. Autograft is biologically ideal because it promotes all dimensions of bone regeneration without the risk of a foreign body. It typically contains a structural scaffold for osteoconduction, live osteoprogenitor cells in the marrow for osteogenesis, as well as intrinsic growth factors for osteoconduction. It is important to note that not all graft sites carry equivalent concentrations or proportions of these factors.

Nonetheless, the process of harvesting autologous bone graft comes with a few morbidities, namely, nerve or vascular injury during harvesting, pelvic fractures, wound infection, and significant postoperative acute and chronic pain [7–9]. Current technological advancement offers alternatives to autografts, with the intent to minimize surgical risk while maintaining similar rates of successful spinal fusion.

33.2.2 Allograft-Based Extenders

Allogenic graft, often referred to as allograft, is typically comprised of cadaveric donor bone used alone or in conjunction with other materials. Before allograft bone can be used, it goes through debridement of soft tissues, removal of blood products, and a sterilization process that destroys any live cells. The resulting product is a mineralized bone. Mineralized allograft is considered a bone graft replacement, as it maintains its mechanical strength; however the sterilization process renders then biologically inactive. Tricortical iliac crest and fibula allografts are successfully used in interbody fusion surgery as structural graft and promote bone fusion by osteoconduction. Mineralized allograft chips are also often used to supplement the patient's own bone (autograft) in a posterolateral intertransverse process fusion.

Allografts are available as mineralized structural strut or as demineralized bone matrix. Demineralized bone matrix (DBM) is allograft in which inorganic minerals have been removed. To prepare DBM allograft bone is first morselized then processed through acid demineralization and a few rounds of freeze-drying. The resulting demineralized bone powder is a composite of collagens, noncollagenous proteins and growth factors, a variable percent of residual calcium phosphate mineral, and some small percent cellular debris [10]. DBM can be formulated into putties, pastes, and flexible, preformed strips for implant use.

The process of demineralization significantly diminishes allograft mechanical properties but conversely increases its biological activity [10]. In 1965, following the work of Ray and Holloway [11], Urist published a landmark paper in *Science* [12] which demonstrated that ectopic osteogenesis occurred when demineralized bone was implanted into a non-bony site. DBM is now known to have both osteoconductive and osteoinductive properties that prompt bone regeneration. DBM is thought to contain bone morphogenic proteins (BMPs) and other bone growth-producing substances that stimulate bone development and fusion.

About 20 % of the $1 billion per year bone grafting market [13] is focused on DBM products in bone repair and regenerative strategies. There is a wide range of DBM products approved by the Food and Drug Administration for clinical use. Several factors regarding DBM as a human-derived tissue product are important to understand, as it is commonly used as a bone repair matrix and vehicle for delivering bioactive agents. Factors that influence the behavior of DBM include bone procurement techniques from human donors, donor age and gender, and the specific DBM composition and properties [14–17]. Examples of allograft-based bone graft extenders currently offered by pharmaceutical companies are listed in Table 33.1.

Table 33.1 Examples of commercially available allograft-based and mixed bone graft extenders

Company	Product name	Composition	Forms	Additional property	Human research
AlloSource	AlloFuse™	Heat sensitive copolymer with DBM	Injectable gel and putty	Osteoconduction Osteoinduction Bioresorbable	Case reports
Biomet Osteobiologics	InterGro®	DBM in a lecithin carrier	Paste, putty and mix with HA/CC composite granules	Osteoconduction Osteoinduction Bioresorbable	Case reports
Exactech	Optecure®	DBM in a hydrogel carrier	Dry mix kit with buffered saline	Osteoconduction	Case reports
	Optecure® + CCC	DBM + CCC in a hydrogel carrier	Dry mix kit with buffered saline	Osteoinduction Bioresorbable	Human studies
	Optefil®	DBM in gelatin carrier	Injectable bone paste, dry powder	Osteogenesis (when mixed with LAG)	
	Opteform®	DBM + CCC in gelatin carrier	Formable putty, dry powder		
Integra Orthobiologics/(IsoTis OrthoBiologic)	Accell Connexus®	DBM, Accell BM, Reverse phase medium	Injectable putty	Osteoconduction	Case reports
	Accell Evo3TM	DBM, Accell BM, Reverse phase medium	Injectable putty		
	Accell TBM®	DBM, Accell BM	Various sized strips	Osteoinduction	Human studies (Accell TBM, DynaGraft II,Ortho blast II)
	DynaGraft II	DBM, reverse phase medium	Injectable putty	Bioresorbable	
	OrthoBlast II	DBM, cancellous bone, reverse phase medium	Injectable putty		
LifeNet Health	IC Graft Chamber®	DBM particles and cancellous chips	Particles or chips in delivery chamber	Osteoconduction Osteoinduction	Case reports Human studies (optium)
	Optium DBM®	DBM in glycerol carrier	Formable putty and injectable gel	Bioresorbable Used with BMA or blood	
Medtronic Spinal & Biologics	Osteofil® DBM	DBM in porcine gelatin	Injectable paste and moldable strips	Osteoconduction	Case reports
	ProgenixTM Plus	DBM in type-1 bovine collagen and sodium alginate	Putty with demineralized cotical bone chips	Osteoinduction Bioresorbable	
	Progenix™ Putty	DBM in type-1 bovine collagen and sodium alginate	Injectable putty		
MTF/Orthofix	Trinity EvolutionTM	Viable cellular bone matrix	Multiple volumes available	Osteoconduction Osteoinduction Bioresorbable	Case reports

(continued)

Table 33.1 (continued)

Company	Product name	Composition	Forms	Additional property	Human research
MTF/Synthes	DBX®	DBM in sodium hyaluronate carrier	Paste, putty mix and strip	Osteoconduction Osteoinduction Bioresorbable	Case reports
NuVasive	Osteocel® Plus	Allograft cellular matrix w/ viable mesenchymal cells	Formable putty	Osteogenesis Osteoinduction Osteoconduction Bioresorbable	Case reports Human studies
Osteotech	GRAFTON® A-Flex®	DBM fiber technology	Round flexible sheet	Osteoconduction	Case reports
	GRAFTON® Crunch®	DBM fibers with demineralized cortical cubes	Packable graft	Osteoinduction	Human studies (level I-II evidence)
	GRAFTON® Flex®	DBM fiber technology	Various sizes of flexible sheets	Bioresorbable	
	GRAFTON® Gel	DBM in a syringe	MIS and Percutaneous injectable graft	Osteogenesis (when mixed with LAG or BMA)	
	GRAFTON® Matrix PLF	DBM fiber technology	Single and double troughs		
	GRAFTON® Matrix Scoliosis Strips	DBM fiber technology	Various sizes of strips		
	GRAFTON® Orthoblend Large Defect	DBM fibers with crushed cancellous chips	Packable graft		
	GRAFTON® Orthoblend Small Defect	DBM fibers with larger cancellous chips	Packable moldable graft		
	GRAFTON Plus® Paste	DBM in a syringe	Injectable MIS graft, resists irrigation		
	GRAFTON® Putty	DBM fiber technology	Packable moldable graft		
RegenerationTechnologies	BioSetTM	DBM combined with natural gelatin carrier	Injectable paste, & putty, strips and blocks with CCC	Osteoconduction Osteoinduction Bioresorbable	Case reports Human studies

Smith &Nephew	VIAGRAF	DBM combined with glycerol	Putty, paste, gel, crunch and flex	Osteoconduction Osteoinduction Bioresorbable	
Wright Medical Technology	ALLOMATRIX®	DBM with/without CBM in calcium sulfate powder	Injectable/formable putty	Osteoconduction Osteoinduction Bioresorbable	Case reports Human studies
	ALLOMATRIX® RCS	DBM with CACIPLEXTM technology in calcium sulfate powder	Various volumes of formable putty	IGNITE to be mixed with BMA	
	IGNITE®	DBM in calcium sulfate powder	Percutaneous graft		
	PRO-STIM™ Injectable Inductive Graft	40 % DBM, 50 % calcium sulfate, 10 % calcium phosphate	Injectable paste/formable putty		
Zimmer	Puros® DBM	Allograft DBM with same donor CCC	Putty and putty with chips	Osteoconduction Osteoinduction Bioresorbable	

Abbreviations: *CCC* cortical cancellous chips, *LAG* local autologous graft, *HA* hydroxyapatite, *BM* bome matrix, *DBM* demineralized bone matrix, *BMA* bone marrow aspirate

33.2.3 Growth Factor-Based Extenders

Growth factor-based bone graft substitutes are natural or recombinant growth factors that are used alone or in combination with other materials. They include transforming growth factor-beta (TGF-beta), platelet-derived growth factor (PDGF), fibroblast growth factor (FGF), insulin-like growth factor-1 (IGF-1), and bone morphogenetic proteins (BMP).

Naturally occurring growth factors and proteins in extracellular bone matrix are responsible for cell activity regulation. These factors interact with cell surface receptors, producing an intracellular cascade resulting in intra- and extracellular activity. TGF-beta and PDGF are growth factors that play crucial roles in tissue regeneration and remodeling, cell differentiation, and embryonic development. FGF is a "pluripotent" growth factor involved in angiogenesis, wound healing, and vertebral development [18, 19]. IGF-1 is a primary mediator of the effects of growth hormone (GH) that has growth-promoting effects on almost every cell in the body, including bone, cartilage, and hematopoietic cells. BMPs are a group of growth factors also known as cytokines and as metabologens that play a crucial role in induction of bone and cartilage formation [20, 21] BMPs are covered in more details in Chap. 38. The combined simultaneous action of these factors is responsible for controlled bone production, resorption, and remodeling.

Most of these proteins have been isolated and in some case synthesized by recombinant technology. Examples of preparations of growth factor-based bone graft extenders currently offered by pharmaceutical companies are listed in Table 33.2.

33.2.4 Cell-Based Extenders

Cell-based bone graft extenders facilitate in vitro generation of an osteoblastic cell lineage from progenitor mesenchymal stem cells. For instance, bone marrow stem cells grown in media enriched with growth factors such as TGF-beta and BMP as well as various additives such as dexamethasone, ascorbic acid, and beta-glycopyrrolate can be directed to differentiate into the osteoblast lineage. However, these mesenchymal stem cells also require the presence of a polymer scaffold such as bioactive ceramics. Commercially available cell-based extenders generally combine a progenitor cell for osteogenesis, growth factors for osteoinduction, and a scaffold for osteoconduction. Table 33.2 includes examples of cell-based bone graft extenders.

33.2.5 Ceramic-Based Extenders

A ceramic is an inorganic nonmetallic solid prepared by the action of high temperature followed by cooling; it may be crystalline, partly crystalline, or amorphous like glass. Sixty percent of commercially available bone graft extenders use ceramics as a primary component or adjunct. As they tend to be brittle, ceramics are frequently combined with other materials. Medical grade ceramic substitutes can be divided into three main categories based on their composition: calcium phosphate, calcium sulfate, and bioactive glass.

The use of ceramics was inspired by the fact that the primary inorganic component of bone is calcium hydroxyapatite, a subset of the calcium phosphate group. Calcium phosphates are thought to be osteoconductive, osteointegrative as they are incorporated in the new bone, as well as possibly osteoinductive. Examples of calcium phosphates currently used are tricalcium phosphate, synthetic hydroxyapatite, and coralline hydroxyapatite; these are available in pastes, putties, solid matrices, and granules.

Bioactive glass is a biologically active silicate-based glass. It is less frequently use, because it is very brittle and has to be used in combination with other materials such as polymethyl methacrylate to form bioactive bone cement or as a coating for metal implants. Table 33.2 includes examples of ceramic-based bone graft extenders.

Table 33.2 Examples of commercially available non-allograft-based bone graft extenders

Company	Product name	Composition	Forms	Additional property	Published research
ApaTech Limited	Actifuse	0.8 % silicate substituted calcium phosphate	Injectable, mixable granules, moldable strips and graft	Osteoconductive Osteoinduction Bioresorbable	Case reports
Biomet	ProOsteon 200R	Hydroxyapatite and calcium carbonate mix	Granules	Osteoconductive Bioresorbable	Case reports
Depuy Synthes	ChronOs	Beta-tricalcium phosphate and resorbable polymer mix	Granules, preform shapes and strips	Osteoconductive Osteoinductive Bioresorbable	Case reports
	Healos	Cross linked collagen fibers coated with hydroxyapatite	Mordable strips	Osteogenesis when mixed with BMA or blood	
Integra LifeSciences	MOZAIK™	80 % beta-tricalcium phosphate + 20 % type 1 collagen mix	Moldable strips	Osteoconductive Osteoinduction Bioresorbable	Case report
Integra Orthobiologics/ (Isotis Orthobiologics)	OsSatura TCP	75 % porous hydroxyapatite and beta-tricalcium phosphate mix	Granules	Osteoconductive Osteoinduction Bioresorbable	Case report
Medtronic Spinal & Biologics	INFUSE® Bone graft	rhBMP-2 soluble powder	1.5 mg/mL rhBMP-2 infused collagen sponge	Osteoinduction Require additional structural graft	Case reports
	AMPLIFY™ Matrix	rhBMP-2 with ceramic matrix (15:85 HA:β-TCP)	2 mg/mL rhBMP-2 infused graft	Osteoinduction Osteoconduction Bioresorbable	Human studies
NovaBone Products	Novabone	Silicate calcium phosphate matrix	MIS injectable and moldable putty, particles, morsels	Osteoconductive Osteoinduction Bioresorbable	Case report
Stryker	Hydroset	Self setting calcium phosphate cement	Formable and injectable paste	Osteoconductive Bioresorbable	Case report
	Vitoss®	90 % porous beta-tricalcium phosphate	Powder, pellets, moldable strip, injectable putty	Osteoconductive Osteoinductive Bioresorbable	Case reports
	Vitoss® BA	90 % porous beta-tricalcium phosphate with bioactive glass	Powder, pellets, moldable strip, injectable putty	Osteogenesis when mixed with BMA	Human studies (Level I-II evidence)
Wright Medical Technology	Osteoset	Calcium sulfate cement	Injectable pellets; formable paste	Osteoconductive Bioresorbable	Case reports

33.2.6 Polymer-Based Extenders

A polymer is a macromolecule composed of repeating structural units; it can be natural or synthetic. Polymers have a wider range of mechanical, physical, and chemical properties compared to other bone extenders. Degradable synthetic polymers are resorbed by the body, thus resulting in a fusion without any residual foreign body. Examples are polylactic acid and polylactic-co-glycolic acid; they can be used alone or in combination with autograft and allograft. Table 33.2 includes examples of polymer-based bone graft extenders.

33.3 Clinical Research

Spinal fusion surgery is paramount to the treatment of spinal instability resulting from degenerative disease, trauma, infection, neoplasm, or iatrogenic causes. In recent years, the number of spinal fusion surgery increased to an estimated 500,000 procedures annually in the United States alone [22]. Emerging biotechnologies are now focused on developing alternatives to autologous iliac crest bone graft in order to minimize the morbidity associated with spinal fusion while maintaining similar rates of fusion.

The majority of the work in osteobiology has focused around osteoinductive bone graft extenders such as demineralized bone matrix (DBM) and recombinant human bone morphogenic protein (rhBMP, rhBMP-7). Initial reports of serious complications with the use of rhBMP2 have fueled further research focused on the safety and efficacy of biologic and synthetic extenders.

Abdullah et al [6]. recently conducted a systematic review of 19 clinical human studies, including case series, cohorts, and randomized controlled trials, evaluating the use of BGEs in lumbar fusion surgery. Regarding demineralized bone matrix (DBM), only two studies of Class II level evidence were published [23, 24]. They both showed similar fusion rate between ICBG and ICBG + DBM in posterior lumbar fusion, suggesting that DBM can be used to supplement ICBG with the intent to decrease the size of the harvested autograft bone. No adverse events were reported with DBM. Beta-tricalcium phosphate (TCP) has been extensively reviewed. Two Level I studies using TCP in adolescent scoliosis surgery have been published [25, 26]. TCP combined with local allograft (LAG) had similar fusion rates compared to ICBG, with elimination of graft site complication and a trend toward lower blood loss.

Alsaleh et al [27]. published a systematic review focused on the use of osteoconductive bone graft extenders in posterolateral thoracolumbar spinal fusion for scoliosis and degenerative conditions. They evaluated 13 case control and randomized controlled trials comparing the use of BGEs mixed with local autograft (LAG) or bone marrow aspirate (BMA) versus ICBG alone or with LAG in 768 patients. The patients were evaluated for fusion at a minimum of 1 year postoperatively. Their conclusion was that BGEs had similar pooled fusion rates compared to ICBG for degenerative conditions but not scoliosis. Subgroup analysis revealed that beta-tricalcium phosphate (ß-TCP) alone and mixed with hydroxyapatite (HA) had similar pooled fusion rates as ICBG. However, calcium sulfate had a trend toward lower fusion rates compared to HA alone as well as ICBG. LAG and BMA were both used in the control and experimental arms. The review also showed a trend toward lower fusion rate when BMA was used alone to supplement BGEs as opposed to LAG alone or a combination of LAG + BMA. Overall they had a significantly lower incidence of adverse events in the BGE groups, including delayed wound healing, infection, and hematoma.

Conclusion

The ideal bone graft has properties of osteoconduction, osteoinduction, and osteogenesis. Autograft has been considered the "gold standard" of bone grafting; however the morbidity associated with the harvesting lessens its popularity. As technology develops there is an increased demand for an ideal bone graft substitute and extender. Several classes of bone graft extenders have been created and evaluated in spinal fusion. Combination products, particularly those using demineralized bone matrix, ceramic-based bone graft extenders, and local bone graft, have gained popularity and have been shown to offer similar rates of fusion with fewer complications compared to iliac crest bone graft in lumbar spine fusion. There still remains significant research to be conducted on the use of BGEs for specific pathologies, risks profiles, and long-term fusion rates.

References

1. Young WF, Rosenwasser RH. An early comparative analysis of the use of fibular allograft versus autologous iliac crest graft for interbody fusion after anterior cervical discectomy. Spine. 1993;18:1123–4.
2. Shapiro S. Banked fibula and the locking anterior cervical plate in anterior cervical fusions following cervical discectomy. J Neurosurg. 1996;84:161–5.
3. Bishop RC, Moore KA, Hadley MN. Anterior cervical interbody fusion using autogeneic and allogeneic bone graft substrate: a prospective comparative analysis. J Neurosurg. 1996;85:206–10.
4. An HS, Simpson JM, Glover JM, Stephany J. Comparison between allograft plus demineralized bone matrix versus autograft in anterior cervical fusion. A prospective multicenter study. Spine. 1995; 20:2211–6.
5. Glassman SD, Howard JM, Sweet A, et al. Complications and concerns with osteobiologics for spine fusion in clinical practice. Spine. 2010;35: 1621–8.
6. Abdullah KG, Steinmetz MP, Benzel EC, et al. The state of lumbar fusion extenders. Spine. 2011;36: E1328–34.
7. Heneghan HM, McCabe JP. Use of autologous bone graft in anterior cervical decompression: morbidity & quality of life analysis. BMC Musculoskelet Disord. 2009;10:158.
8. Kim DH, Rhim R, Li L, et al. Prospective study of iliac crest bone graft harvest site pain and morbidity. Spine J. 2009;9:886–92.
9. Silber JS, Anderson DG, Daffner SD, et al. Donor site morbidity after anterior iliac crest bone harvest for single-level anterior cervical discectomy and fusion. Spine. 2003;28:134–9.
10. Gruskin E, Doll BA, Futrell FW, Schmitz JP, Hollinger JO. Demineralized bone matrix in bone repair: history and use. Adv Drug Deliv Rev. 2012;64(12):1063–77 [Epub ahead of print].
11. Ray RD, Holloway JA. Preliminary report of an experimental study. J Bone Joint Surg. 1957;39A:1119.
12. Urist MR. Bone: formation by autoinduction. Science. 1965;150:893–9.
13. Group MR. US markets for orthopaedic. Biomaterials. 2004(2005).
14. Groessner-Schreiber B, Krukowski M, Lyons C, Osdoby P. Osteoclast recruitment in response to human bone matrix is age related. Mech Ageing Dev. 1992;62:143–54.
15. Aaboe M, Pinholt EM, Schou S, Hjorting-Hansen E. Incomplete bone regeneration of rabbit calvarial defects using different membranes. Clin Oral Implants Res. 1998;9:313–20.
16. Schwartz Z, Somers A, Mellonig JT, Carnes D, Dean D, Cochran D, Boyan B. Ability of demineralized freeze-dried bone allograft to induce new bone formation is dependent on donor age but not gender. J Periodontol. 1998;69:470–8.
17. Zhang M, Powers Jr RM, Wolfinbarger Jr L. A quantitative assessment of osteoinductivity of human demineralized bone matrix. J Periodontol. 1997;68: 1076–84.
18. Green PJ, Walsh FS, Doherty P. Promiscuity of fibroblast growth factor receptors. Bioessays. 1996; 18:639–46.
19. Böttcher RT, Niehrs C. Fibroblast growth factor signaling during early vertebrate development. Endocr Rev. 2005;26:63–77.
20. Reddi AH, Reddi A. Bone morphogenetic proteins (BMPs): from morphogens to metabologens. Cytokine Growth Factor Rev. 2009;20:341–2.
21. Bleuming SA, He XC, Kodach LL, Hardwick JC, Koopman FA, Ten Kate FJ, van Deventer SJ, Hommes DW, Peppelenbosch MP, Offerhaus GJ, Li L, van den Brink GR. Bone morphogenetic protein signaling suppresses tumorigenesis at gastric epithelial transition zones in mice. Cancer Res. 2007;67:8149–55.
22. Rajaee SS, Bae HW, Kanim LE, et al. Spinal fusion in the United States: analysis of trends from 1998 to 2008. Spine. 2012;37:67–76.
23. Cammisa Jr FP, Lowery G, Garfin SR, et al. Two-year fusion rate equivalency between grafton DBM gel and autograft in posterolateral spine fusion: a prospective controlled trial employing a side-by-side comparison in the same patient. Spine. 2004;29:660–6.
24. Schizas C, Triantafyllopoulos D, Kosmopoulos V, et al. Posterolateral lumbar spine fusion using a novel demineralized bone matrix: a controlled case pilot study. Arch Orthop Trauma Surg. 2008;128: 621–5.
25. Delecrin J, Takahashi S, Gouin F, et al. A synthetic porous ceramic as a bone graft substitute in the surgical management of scoliosis: a prospective, randomized study. Spine. 2000;25:563–9.
26. Lerner T, Bullmann V, Schulte TL, et al. A level-1 pilot study to evaluate of ultraporous beta-tricalcium phosphate as a graft extender in the posterior correction of adolescent idiopathic scoliosis. Eur Spine J. 2009;18:170–9.
27. Alsaleh KAM, Tougas CA, Roffey DM, Wai EK. Osteoconductive bone graft extenders in posterolateral thoracolumbar spinal fusion: a systematic review. Spine. 2012;37:E993–1000.

34 Minimally Invasive Wiltse Approaches for Posterolateral Fusion

Steve Ritland

34.1 Introduction

MISS approaches to the spine minimize requisite exposure to reduce morbidity associated with surgery, striving for that balance between minimizing anatomic compromise and optimizing surgical outcome. This chapter deals with a subset of approaches constrained by the posterior segmental muscles, with specific regard to their neurovascular supply. The local anatomy of the back supports an anatomic approach medial or lateral to the neurovascular and tendinous constraints about the superior articular process. Initial discussion addresses the fixed constraints about the articular complex in the back with subsequent attention to the more superficial elements constraining the approach.

Wiltse [9] described and popularized an intermuscular approach between the multifidus and erector spinae complex for posterior fusion. Approach along the multifidus and lateral to the mammillary process to the level of the transverse process avoids the tendons and fixed neurovascular elements essential to the integrity of the back muscles. Use of microsurgical technique and an understanding of the periarticular anatomy facilitate preservation of muscle integrity with segmental fixation and posterior fusion.

S. Ritland
Flagstaff Medical Center,
Flagstaff, AZ, USA
e-mail: stephenritland@gmail.com

A segmental approach along the lateral surface of the spinous process and over the lamina, constrained by the tendons inserting to the superior articular process, similarly respects the tensile and neurovascular integrity of the back muscles [7]. Medializing the screw construct allows for a decompression and/or fusion with a construct that underlies the segmental back muscles without compromise to the anatomic integrity of the muscles. Extending the approach with takedown of midline tendons and removal of bony elements may allow for better decompression and correction of deformity while still preserving the neurovascular integrity of the muscles.

Posterior and lateral fusion is variably anatomic. A robust facet fusion may be performed from a medial or lateral approach with no compromise of muscles. Extending to a posterolateral fusion incurs a variable cost in muscle attachments but may still be accomplished with no extension to adjacent segments. The decision to remove bone or muscle connections is then based on optimizing decompression, deformity correction, and the requisite bony exposure for adequate fusion.

I will review an intermuscular approach for fixation with a segmental approach to the facet joint for a muscle-sparing posterior fusion. I will then consider a medialized screw placement which provides an equally anatomic segmental approach, between fascicles of multifidus, for fixation and fusion. This provides the option of a facet fusion or decompression with an interbody fusion using an approach constrained by the

M.Y. Wang et al. (eds.), *Minimally Invasive Spinal Deformity Surgery*,
DOI 10.1007/978-3-7091-1407-0_34, © Springer-Verlag Wien 2014

tendons inserting to the superior articular process and respecting the associated segmental neurovascular supply.

34.2 Intermuscular Approach

Approach down the lateral aspect of the multifidus complex opens the intermuscular plane between longissimus laterally and the multifidus and lateral aspect of the superior articular process. Entry into the plane moves from adjacent to the spinous process at L1 laterally as the more distal multifidus fascicles are included in the medial muscle mass. The multifidus incorporates a common tendon of insertion to the superior articular process at each level, visible on the lateral aspect of the muscle complex. The lateral aspect of the articular process and the transition to the dorsum of the transverse process is free of attachments. The tendon of longissimus originates at each level on the accessory process. The tendon thins dorsally and may continue to the mammilloaccessory ligament and mammillary process. At progressively lower segments, the projection of tendons transitions from primarily caudal to a more dorsal trajectory consistent with the common tendon of the longissimus complex inserting to the iliac crest.

Figures 34.1 and 34.2 open the intermuscular plane and illustrate the muscle and neurovascular constraints about the mammillary process. This plane provides an elegant intermuscular placement of a fixation construct. Division of the segmental neurovascular supply occurs at or deep to the transverse process, allowing one to open between the multifidus and erector spinae complex with no compromise to the neurovascular supply to the back muscles. The medial branch of the dorsal ramus runs along the lateral articular process to turn medial through the mammilloaccessory notch, while the associated artery of the pars interarticularis, which supplies the corresponding muscle fascicle, runs medial to the intertransversarius medialis adjacent to the lateral aspect of the pars before turning over the laminar surface deep to the segmental multifidus. The lateral branch of the dorsal ramus and associated vessels enter the deep surface of the erector spinae fascicles. The lateral branch of the ramus and vessels are at risk with significant retraction over the transverse process.

A retractor engaging the lateral articular process retracts the longissimus traversing the transverse process and exposes bone for direct placement of a pedicle screw, with limited retraction of the longissimus. A screw entry point at the cephalad margin of the accessory process and 2–3 mm lateral to the lateral aspect of the mammillary process generally provides pedicle screw placement that respects the facet joint and mammilloaccessory notch.

Realizing that the spirit of MISS involves approaches preserving the anatomy rather than being defined by a skin incision, the illustrations reflect an anatomic approach opening intermuscular planes. This approach works for one or multiple segments and becomes easier with a multisegmental approach. While it is illustrated with a retractor engaging the articular process with limited retraction of the longissimus traversing from above, an awareness of the anatomy facilitates placement of a variety of retractors while taking advantage of an intermuscular construct placement. While the Wiltse approach has been used historically with decortication over the transverse process and articular complex, preservation of the back muscles is relatively straightforward. In a MISS situation, it may be appropriate to just decorticate inside the joint or extend the bony exposure along the lateral mass avoiding unnecessary neurovascular disruption.

It is my experience and impression that screw placement may respect the medial branch of the dorsal ramus most of the time. While it is difficult to visualize the nerve intraoperatively, an understanding of its course allows an entry generally sparing the mammilloaccessory notch and medial branch. There are certainly cases where maintaining an appropriate trajectory through the pedicle puts the nerve at risk, particularly in the upper lumbar spine, where divergence of the pedicles and articular complex necessitates encroaching to the region of the mammilloaccessory notch to avoid lateral compromise of the pedicle. With direct visualization and screw placement, it is appropriate to minimize Bovie use to preserve the nerve. Use of a cannulated screw with needle and wire to assist placement may also minimize risk to the nerve.

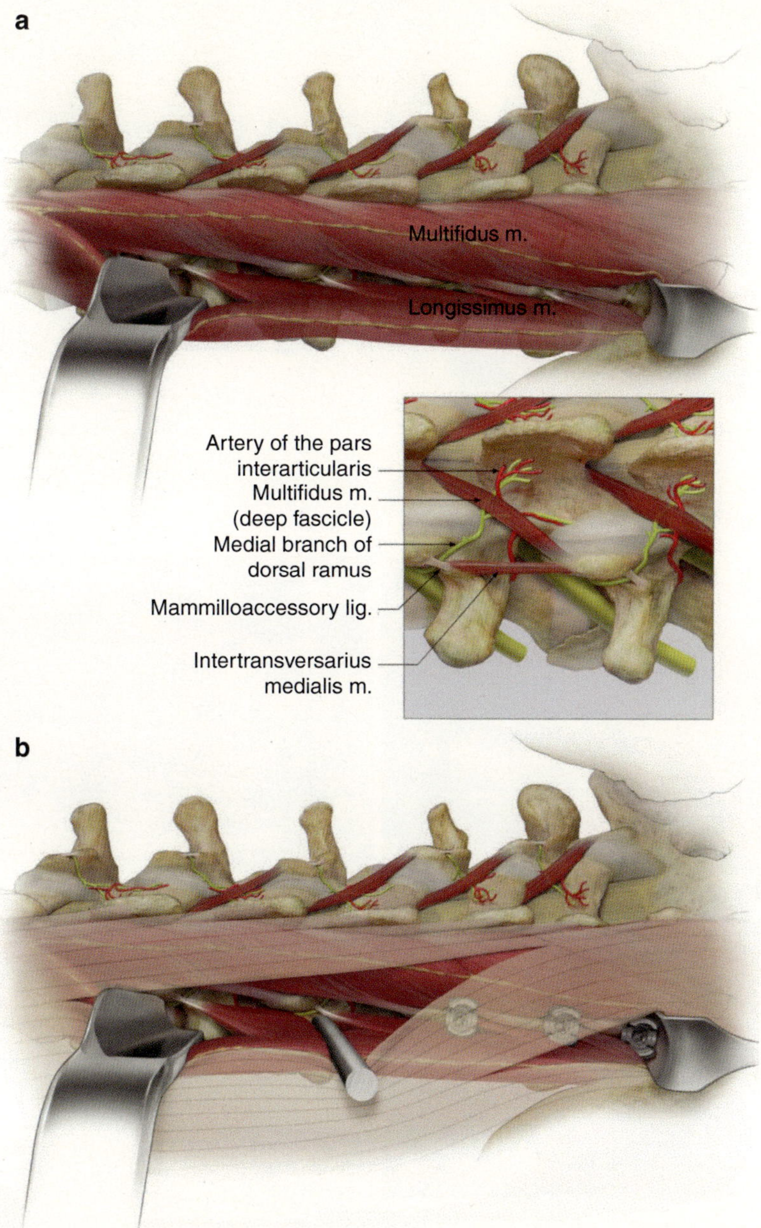

Fig. 34.1 (**a**) The intermuscular plane is opened from L2 through sacrum. The common tendon of multifidus is seen inserting to the superior articular process at each segment. The longissimus fascicle arising from each accessory process is seen projecting towards a common tendon of insertion to the medial superior iliac spine. A bit of fat typically defines the dorsum of the intermuscular plane, with the entry adjacent to the spinous process at L1 and just medial to the iliac crest at the sacrum. The inset shows anatomy important to consider during screw placement and fusion. It is generally possible to place a screw just caudal and lateral to the medial branch of the nerve by being aware of the anatomy. (**b**) A right angle retractor may be used to engage the lateral articular process and retract the longissimus arising from the cephalad segment. The entry point for screw placement is seen on L2 just inferior to and lateral to the mammilloaccessory notch and nerve and at the upper margin of the tendon arising on the accessory process. Tap placement is seen at L3, with screw placement L4 to sacrum. The erector spinae aponeurosis is opened and retracted as necessary. (**c**) Screws are placed L2 through sacrum. The tendon and proximal longissimus lie between screw heads and may at times require a bit of division of the most dorsal portion of the tendon extending from the accessory process onto the mammilloaccessory ligament, to allow the rod to seat fully without unduly stretching the muscle and tendon. The assembled construct lies lateral to the multifidus complex with minimal impingement against back muscles

Fig. 34.1 (continued)

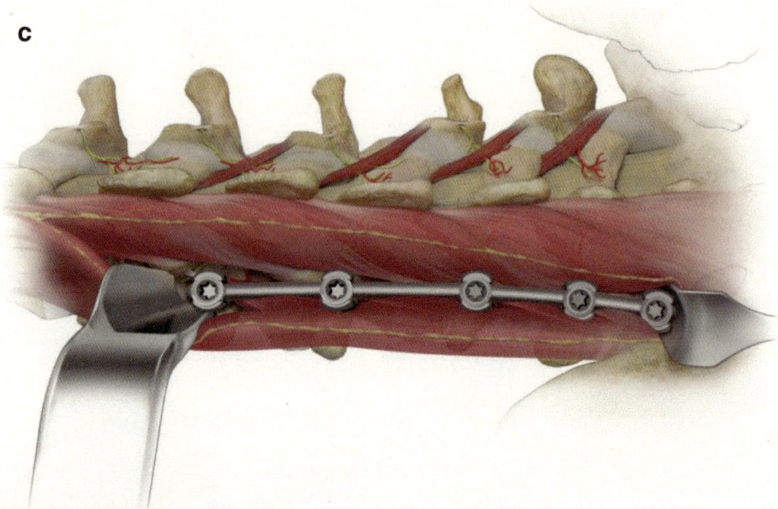

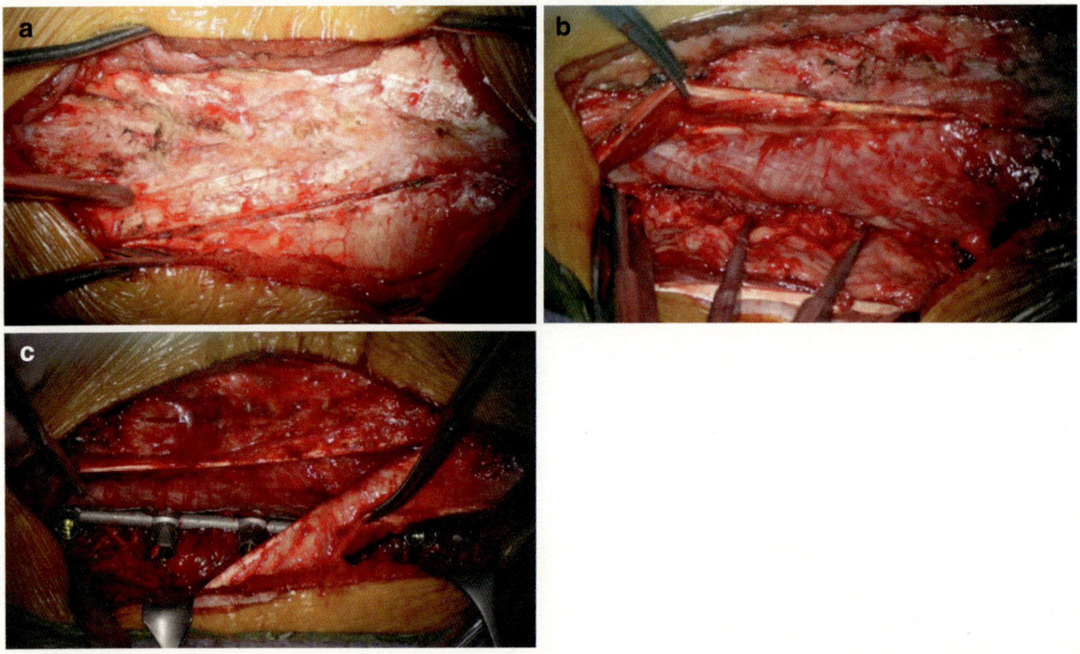

Fig. 34.2 (**a**) A midline skin incision has been made, with the dorsolumbar fascia reflected from L1 to the sacrum. The tendons of the ESA are seen projecting caudally to insertions on the dorsum of the spinous processes. The opening of the ESA is seen between tendons inserting to L4 and L5. (**b**) The upper medial ESA is reflected medially. The intermuscular plane is seen with the upper opening occurring near spinous process, adjacent to the spinous process. The tendons of the multifidus are seen forming on the lateral aspect of the multifidus to insert to the superior articular process (*SAP*). The retractor is seen engaged against the L1 SAP. Taps are in place in the pedicles L1 through L4. A bit of fat is appreciated in the deep plane between fascicles of longissimus. (**c**) The final construct is in place. Screws are seen in L1 through L3. The L4 screw underlies intervening ESA. The L5 and S1 screws are seen through a second opening in the ESA

The erector spinae aponeurosis (ESA) is the tendon complex of the thoracic fascicles of longissimus and iliocostalis. This overlies the local back muscles with a medial trajectory to insertions on the dorsum of the spinous processes and across the distal sacrum and ilium.

These tendons cross the intermuscular plane obliquely. Dividing the fibers over the underlying intermuscular plane generally allows easy exposure of three or four segments. A second parallel opening generally allows exposure of the entire lumbar spine with minimal difficulty encountered working under the preserved intervening tendons.

The dorsolumbar fascia is the aponeurosis of the latissimus dorsi. Reflecting this from adjacent to the spinous process provides a generous exposure for opening between the tendons of the ESA. A mediolateral opening along its fibers opens up the plane over the ESA and provides easy exposure for one or two segments. Exposing the entire lumbar intermuscular plane generally requires three or more openings in the dorsolumbar fascia if one wishes to avoid reflecting and reclosing this layer.

The skin incision is less critical in minimizing morbidity to lumbar muscles. At L3 and above mobilizing a midline incision for intermuscular approach is generally straightforward. When the dorsolumbar fascia is mobilized along the spinous process, retraction occurs over the ESA, avoiding a potential space for fluid collection or seroma superficial to the fascia. At L5–S1 and to a lesser extent at L4–5 mobilizing a short midline incision is more difficult because of the relatively lateral entry to the intermuscular plane, and short paramedian incisions are simpler for a short-segment construct.

34.3 Facet Fusion

The multifidus has a common tendon of insertion to each superior articular process. Figure 34.3 illustrates approach at the dorsal margin of the common tendon over the mammillary process that allows retraction of muscle traversing the lamina and facet capsule to caudal insertions. Opening the capsule of the joint allows decortication of the articular surfaces, with direct graft placement. This provides a robust facet fusion with no compromise of segmental muscle integrity. Extending decortication from the articular process to the lateral pars and base of the pedicle above, or to the laminar surface below, increases fusion, area with limited muscle disruption. For many years I have used a facet fusion only, when the articular processes have not been compromised and interbody grafting has been deemed unnecessary.

Retraction is generally straightforward and I continue to use a variety of retractors to maintain visualization in the intermuscular plane. A malleable brain retractor may be bent slightly to engage the rod and folded at the skin to open the plane. An appropriate handheld retractor such a Langenbeck may then be used to retract muscle over the facet capsule for appropriate decortication and fusion in the joint.

While a facet fusion is adequately robust much of the time (Fig. 34.4), it is straightforward to extend through the inferior articular process to a transforaminal fusion. This may be done from the same opening used for the joint, or approach through the multifidus or down the lateral margin of the spinous process may provide a more medial, segmental approach while still preserving the muscles over the articular process.

34.4 Medialized Segmental Approach to Fixation

A medial approach constrained by the muscle insertions to the superior articular process provides a complementary and equally anatomic approach to fixation and fusion. It is a segmental approach, rather than exposing the length of the lumbar spine, when the multifidus origins are preserved. In many cases, correction of deformity dictates osteotomies removing portions of spinous process or inferior articular process. Intervention is variably muscle sparing, however, and midline muscle disconnection optimizes exposure. In this situation the neurovascular integrity of the muscle is still preserved, and fixation across multiple segments is facilitated without exposure extending lateral to the superior articular process.

At each segment the multifidus arises from a common tendon of origin along the lateral caudal margin of the spinous process, with a deep subfascicle coming off of the deep spinous process and medial laminar margin to insert on the

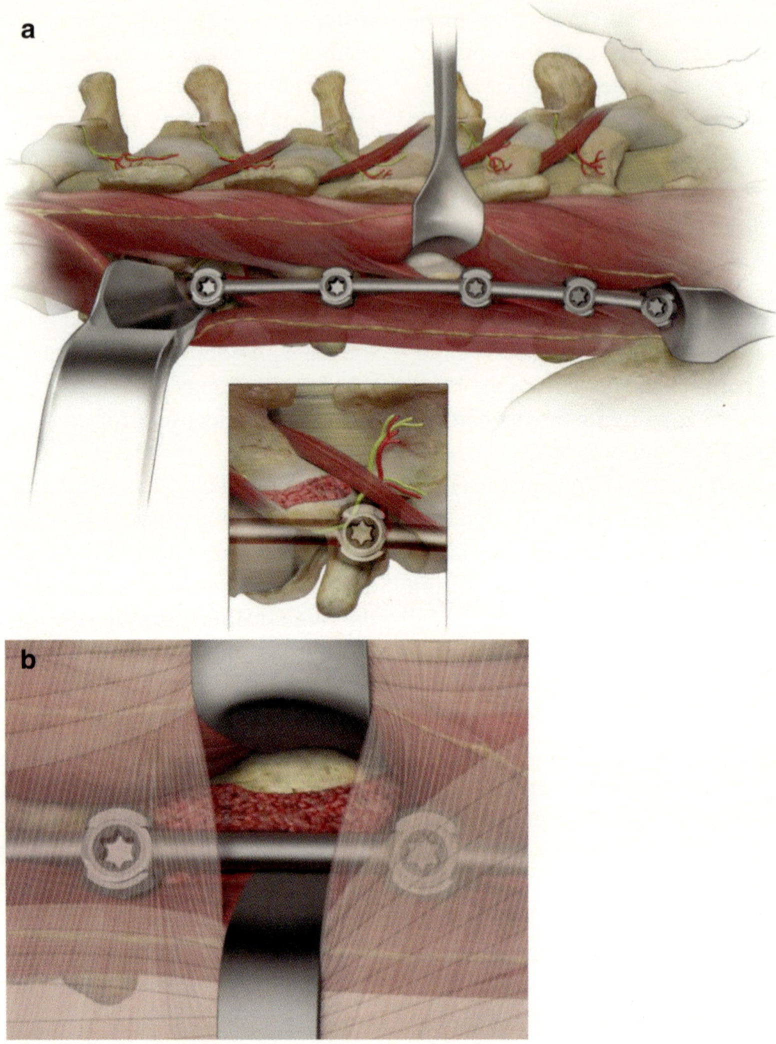

Fig. 34.3 (**a**) Approach at the caudal margin of the common tendon inserting to the SAP allows retraction of multifidus complex traversing to caudal levels. The retractor exposes the capsule of the facet joint and the lateral margin of the lamina and inferior articular process. The capsule of the facet joint is opened. This allows decorticating the facet joint with preservation of the integrity of the articular processes. The trajectory from the intermuscular plane allows optimal preparation of the joint for grafting. Bone graft is packed into the prepared joint before releasing the overlying muscle. (**b**) Disconnection of adjacent tendons on the SAP and accessory and transverse processes allows extending the graft for a more conventional lateral fusion in the situation where it is felt that sacrificing muscle is warranted for a more generous bony fusion. This view demonstrates both the ESA tendons separated to provide access to the joint and a mediolateral opening through the dorsolumbar fascia, preserving significant integrity to this layer with a segmented approach

superior articular process two segments caudal (i.e., L2 spinous process to L4 superior articular process). Figure 34.5 illustrates opening the plane along the spinous process and engaging the segmental multifidus. This exposes the lamina, inferior articular process, and facet capsule. Figure 34.6 illustrates the deep subfascicle of multifidus inserting to the superior articular process. The retractor can engage the tendon inserting to the adjacent SAP and muscle traversing to lower levels without disrupting or compromising the segmental neurovascular

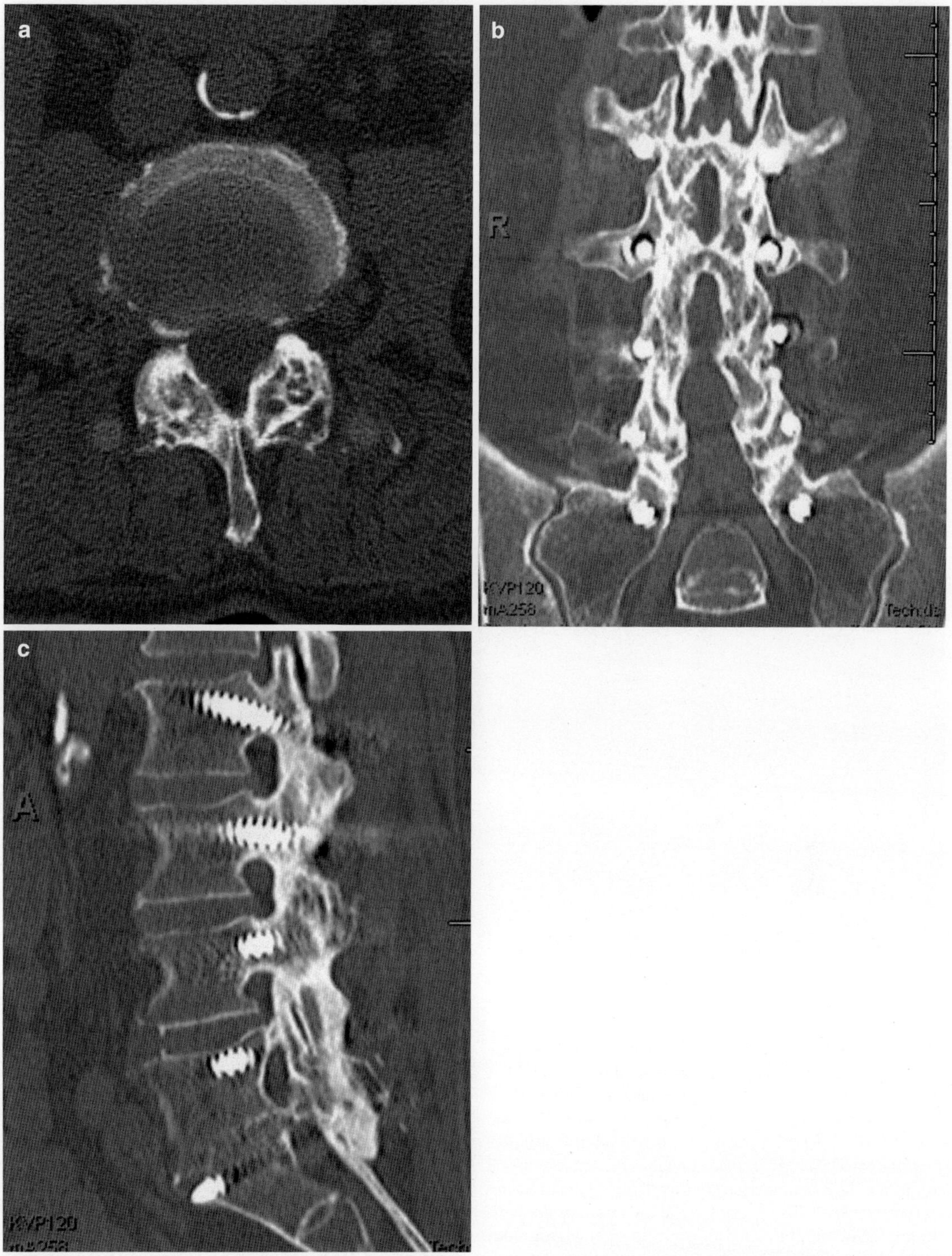

Fig. 34.4 (**a**) Axial section through a facet fusion. Peek rods are seen in cross section adjacent to the dorsal joint, in the intermuscular plane between multifidus and longissimus. (**b**) Dorsal view of reconstruction, demonstrating facet fusion along the articular complexes. (**c**) Lateral reconstruction demonstrating the robust fusion along the articular complex, with an interbody fusion at L5–S1

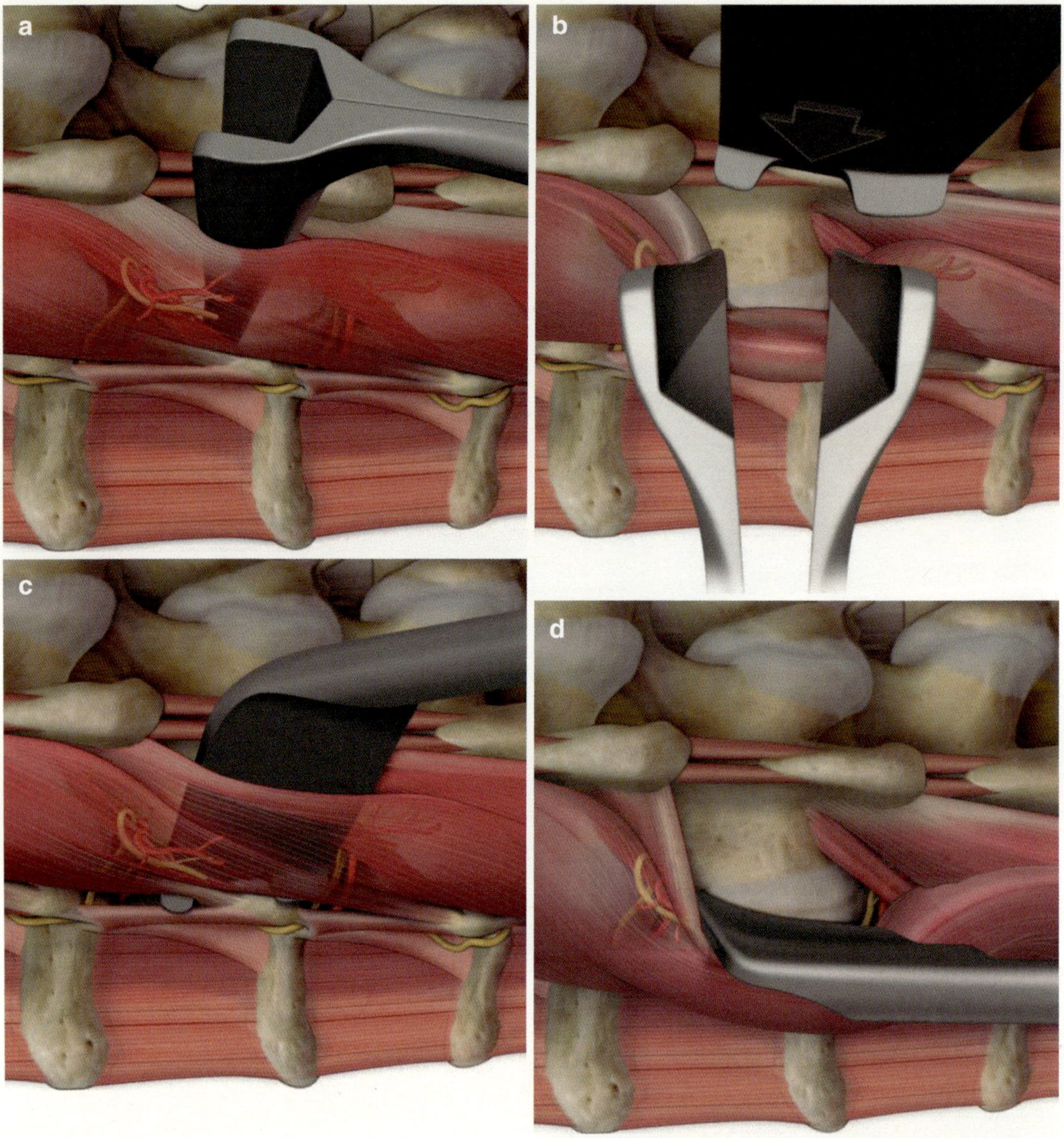

Fig. 34.5 (**a**) View of medial approach. Inserting a speculum along the spinous process elevates the muscle from the lateral spinous process and lamina. (**b**) Opening the speculum provides a protected path for inserting the retractor blade to the dorsum of the lamina and articular process. (**c**) The retractor blade engages the tendon inserting to the SAP and the muscle traversing to insert at the next caudal level. The asymmetry in the retractor tip, with the cephalad margin being longer, allows engaging both the tendon to the SAP and the muscle and tendon traversing to the caudal level. (**d**) The retractor is in place and open. This exposes the IAP and the capsule of the joint. Medially, the fascicle of multifidus from the adjacent spinous process is preserved. The segmental nerve and vessel retract with the muscle from the process above, while the segmental neurovascular supply to the segment below runs below the joint to the segmental muscle arising on the adjacent process. The deep subfascicle arising from the transition of spinous process to the laminar margin is seen. This subfascicle frequently needs to be at least partially sacrificed for decompression in the canal or interbody fusion. There is frequently a bit of fat over the lamina and articular process which may be removed as necessary. (**e**) Opening and decorticating the joint allows for a robust facet fusion if the integrity of the articular process is respected. Medializing screw placement to the base of the superior articular process avoids risking the neurovascular elements inferiorly. (**f**) The facet joint is packed with graft and is ready for screw placement. (**g**) Final screw construct in place

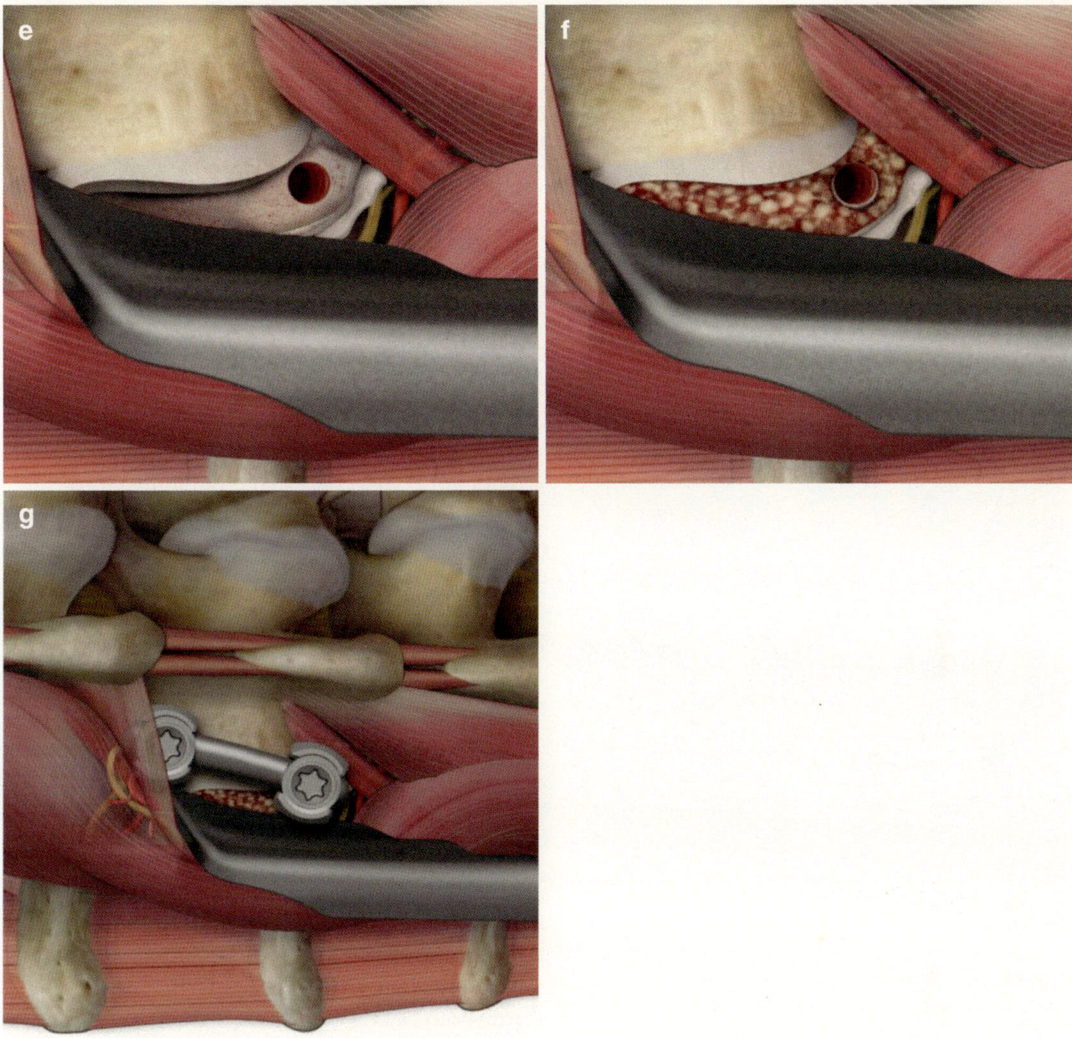

Fig. 34.5 (continued)

supply. When a speculum is used to open this plane for retractor placement, the cephalad blade is constrained by the tendon arising from the spinous process above and the caudal blade elevates the multifidus complex from the fascicle arising on the process adjacent. A retractor blade is contoured to follow the facet surface and with projections to engage the tendon to the SAP, and the muscle traversing to caudal segments minimizes risk of compromise to muscle integrity. With a symmetric exposure, mild divergence of the blades provides secure retractor positioning without a mechanical support arm being required. Figures 34.7 and 34.8 illustrate operative approach with retention of tendon layers and exposure over the lamina.

There are considerations for detaching midline muscles. These include access for better decompression of neural elements, bone removal or osteotomies for better correction of deformity, and harvesting bone for grafting. While this may interrupt the tensile integrity of the muscle, it does not devitalize the muscle and is relatively anatomic compared to conventional and some expanding tube approaches which sacrifice anatomy about the articular complex. This makes the approach particularly useful in multisegment exposure for deformity correction.

34.5 Medialized Screw Fixation

Medializing screw placement allows fixation respecting the neurovascular and tendon constraints along the superior articular process.

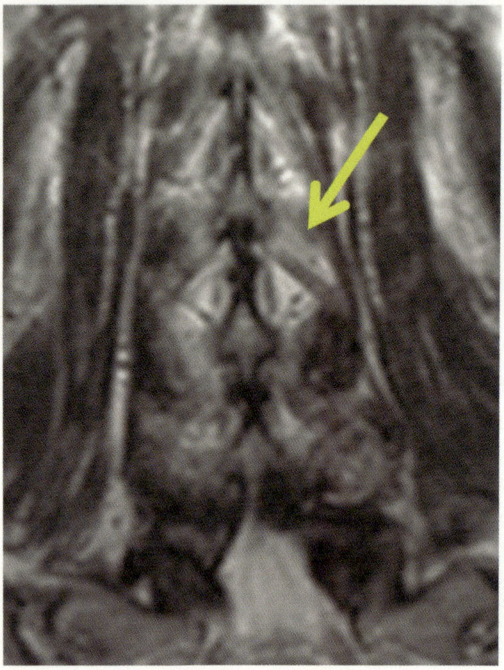

Fig. 34.6 A coronal MRI reconstruction demonstrates the course of the deep subfascicle of multifidus from the margin of the spinous process and lamina to the SAP. This insertion is a portion of the common tendon of insertion of multifidus to the articular process. Engaging this tendon helps elevate the deep muscle and associated neurovascular segments to allow for screw placement

Exposure and retraction constrained at the SAP allows for a comfortable screw fixation respecting the neurovascular integrity of the back muscles.

Richard Hynes pioneered the use of medially placed screws with a relatively cortical trajectory traversing the pars interarticularis and was involved in investigating the biomechanics of medial fixation. Lab testing demonstrated comparable strength comparing a traditional pedicle trajectory with a medialized, relatively more cortical trajectory for screw placement [8]. Experience in more than 1,000 cases over the past 14 years has demonstrated clinical efficacy (Richard Hynes, personal communication).

For a single-segment fusion, there are slightly different constraints for a cephalad or caudal screw respecting the local anatomy. While a medialized placement may be made from a range of cephalad to caudal trajectories, preservation of segmental neurovascular integrity constrains placement further. The cephalad screw may be placed deep and medial to the multifidus with an entry point on the dorsum of the pars interarticularis below the joint for the segment above. For the caudal screw, if the muscle origins on the adjacent spinous process are preserved, placing a screw entry point at the inferior margin of the articular surface of the SAP avoids transecting the medial branch of the dorsal ramus and the artery supplying the corresponding multifidus.

When preserving the muscles from the segment above, there is limited exposure of very

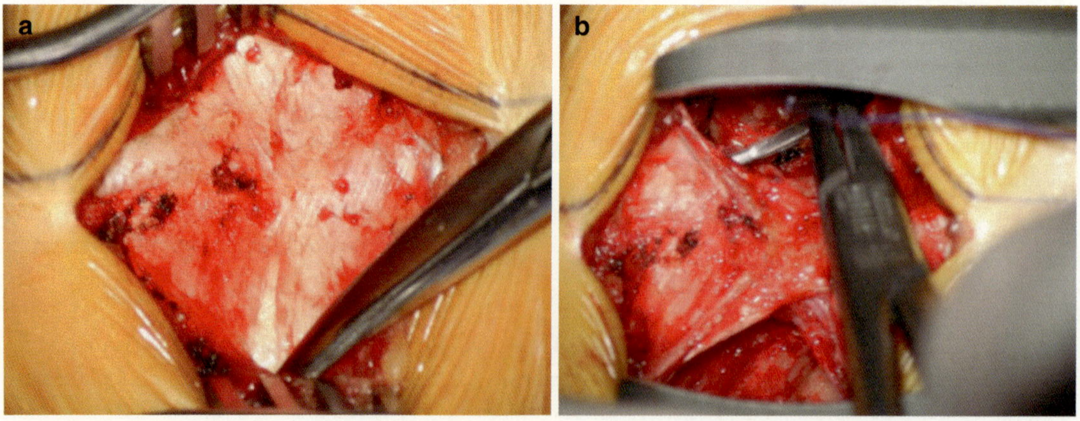

Fig. 34.7 (**a**) Opening the dorsolumbar fascia along the course of its fibers minimizes compromise while allowing access for segmental approach for decompression and fusion. (**b**) Once the dorsolumbar fascia and ESA have been opened and retractor blades placed, a suture may be placed to hold open the surgical field

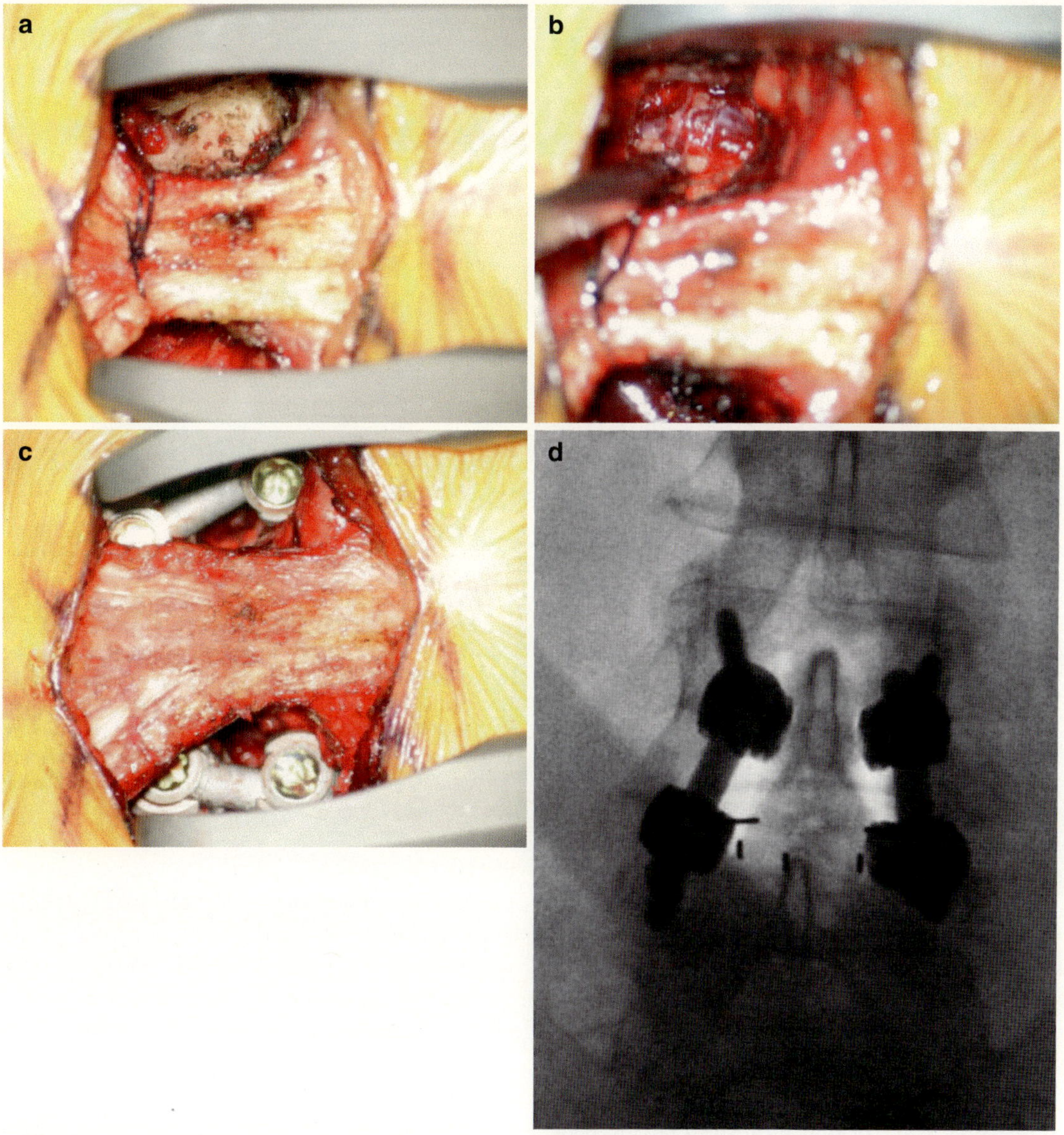

Fig. 34.8 (**a**) The lamina and inferior articular process of L4 are exposed, with the retractor engaging the tendon inserting to the articular process of L5 and traversing to sacral insertions. The multifidus arising from the spinous process is seen caudally. The retraction suture holds the cephalad margin of the exposure open, retracting the ESA medially. The dorsolumbar fascia has been freed along the spinous process and reflected laterally over the ESA. (**b**) The inferior articular process is removed. The medial superior articular process has been removed. The foraminal venous complex overlying the disk is seen with a window for discectomy and fusion with minimal or no retraction of neural elements. (**c**) Screw construct is in place after interbody work is complete. The suture retaining the ESA has been removed allowing the tendons to relax towards normal position. (**d**) AP x-ray view demonstrating preservation of midline muscles

reliable surface anatomy to assist in screw placement (Fig. 34.9). There is an arcuate fossa between the lateral margin of the pars and the accessory process that I find critical for anatomic placement of screws. Richard Hynes has used it to assist in his screw placement and for reasons of description and history I consider it Rick's fossa. The fossa defines the inferior dorsum of the pedicle, with a transition to the accessory process and longissimus lateral, and transition to the pars interarticularis and lamina medial. Approach over the surface of the lamina to the edge of

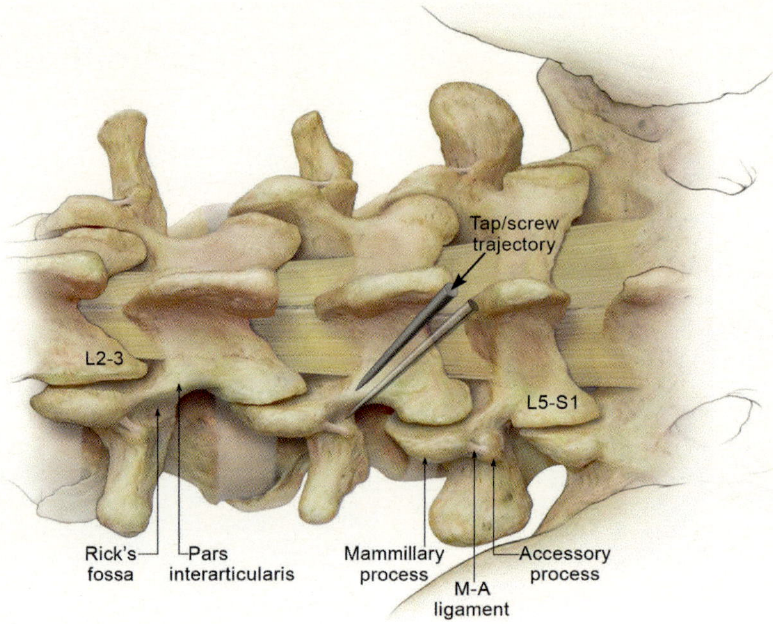

Fig. 34.9 Landmarks for medial screw placement traversing pars. There is a keel of cortical bone running from the mammillary process to the of inferior articular process that defines the transition from dorsal surface to lateral margin of the pars interarticularis. There is an arcuate fossa between the keel and lateral pars and the accessory process that defines the dorsal and inferior margin of the pedicle (Rick's fossa). Palpation of the surface of the fossa defines a plane of transition for screw trajectory across the pedicle. Moving medial on the surface of the pars shifts the screw course to a tract through more cortical bone and one that places the construct adjacent to the spinous process, better underlying the muscle from segment above

the pars elevates the overlying muscle and neurovascular supply. Identifying the lateral margin of the pars defines a screw entry slightly medial that maintains the course of the screw in bone while accessing a relatively cortical trajectory to traverse the pars into the pedicle. Palpating over the margin of the pars into Rick's fossa defines the plane of transition from pars to pedicle, with relatively certain definition of craniocaudal placement of the screw entry point to avoid an inferior breach of the screw on the pedicle to pars transition.

I use a high-speed burr to make the initial entry through the pars and convert to a tap once the burr reaches the cancellous bone in the pedicle. I feel the margin of the pars and into Rick's fossa to define the trajectory of the screw in the sagittal plane and then rotate the trajectory to place the screw entry on the dorsum of the pars for a much stronger and more cortical screw placement than starting in the fossa would provide. The trajectory approximates 25° cranial and 15° lateral to the axial and sagittal plane, respectively (Fig. 34.10). Full dimension tapping is important to avoid fracturing out the cortical pars with an oversized screw. A cortical thread screw of 4.5–5.5 mm diameter optimizes thread pitch and minor diameter to most effectively engage the bone and maximize screw strength. Screw length is typically 25–35 mm.

In advanced degenerative cases, a combination of factors may obscure surface anatomy. Settling of the disk brings the superior articular process into contact with the inferior margin of the pedicle and Rick's fossa. Hypertrophic arthropathy with capsular and bony overgrowth of the joint further obscures the keel of lamina and pars. Opening the facet joint allows one to follow the inferior articular process to the keel of the pars and Rick's fossa.

The caudal screw presents slightly different limitations. With a short exposure, I use a

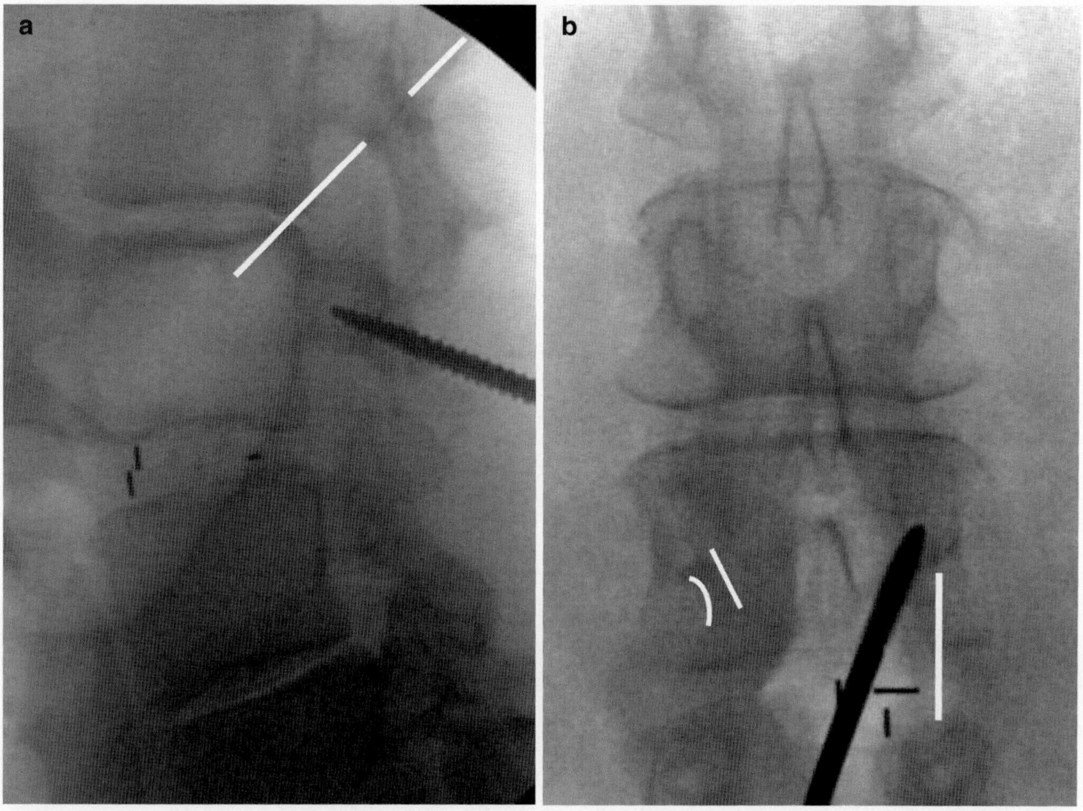

Fig. 34.10 (**a**) A lateral x-ray demonstrates the sclerotic cortical surface of the accessory process and Rick's fossa and defining a transition to pedicle. The white lines indicate margins of the sclerotic bone visualized on image. The tap is seen with tip projecting across cortical density into pedicle but is rotated to traverse the pars rather than the cortical surface of the fossa. (**b**) AP x-ray image with initial tap placement demonstrating trajectory to pedicle. On the *left*, the line segments define the lateral border of the pars transitioning to Rick's fossa and a segment with ends defining the entry to laminar surface and tip position corresponding to tap. On the *right*, a line segment defines a direct placement trajectory. Rotating the trajectory to a medial entry over the laminar surface corresponds to the alignment of the tap

medialized trajectory entering through the articular surface. The capsule of the facet provides some protection to the segmental nerve and vessel just inferior to the joint, supplying the adjacent multifidus. I enter typically at the base of the articular surface between middle and lateral third, with an AP or slightly lateral trajectory that allows the screw to engage the vertebral endplate and lateral body junction for maximal security (Fig. 34.11). If the canal has been decompressed, direct confirmation of the medial pedicle confirms anatomy. If the muscle has been detached for exposure, placement analogous to the cephalad screw is straightforward but requires a slightly longer incision to achieve the desired trajectory.

L5 is unique in that the pars interarticularis is foreshortened relative to cephalad levels, with a less well-developed cortical portion than levels above and with a transition to the pedicle and body providing somewhat less margin to inferomedial pedicle compromise. In surgery it is frequently not easy to directly palpate the lateral pars and into Rick's fossa directly. Opening the sacral facet joint allows one to follow the inferior articular process of L5 to the fossa and inferior pedicle and define screw entry.

Sacrum presents a different issue. An analogous trajectory lacks the same cortical development seen at levels above, which relates to the stresses across the lamina and pars associated

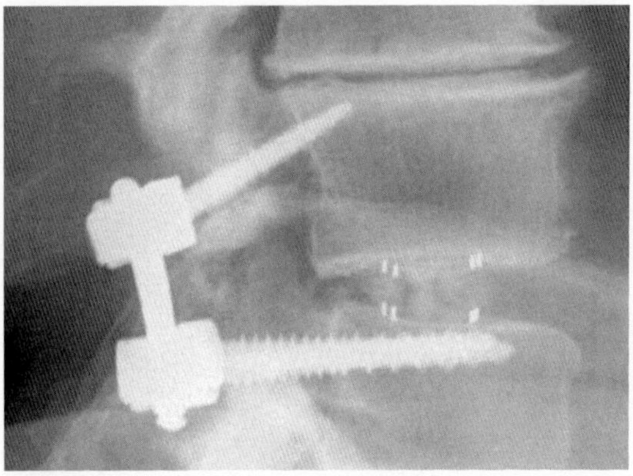

Fig. 34.11 Medializing a pedicle screw at the caudal segment, with entry at the lower margin of the articular surface, provides adequate fixation with a trajectory minimizing skin incision. When the segmental muscle origins are preserved, this avoids extending across the medial ramus and artery just below the facet

with the dynamics of the motion segment disk complex. I frequently place a pedicle screw directly, or through the muscle with a medial trajectory, to optimize placement in the better bone under the sacral endplate and to engage the sacral apex anteriorly. A short side connector facilitates lining up with the cephalad construct, if necessary. A sacral alar screw provides an elegant and secure solution in many cases and places the head of the screw in relatively better alignment with a medial construct.

With two or three segments, it is possible to pass the rod under or through the segmental multifidus; however detachment of the midline muscles may facilitate and optimize surgery while still preserving the neurovascular integrity of the muscles (Fig. 34.12).

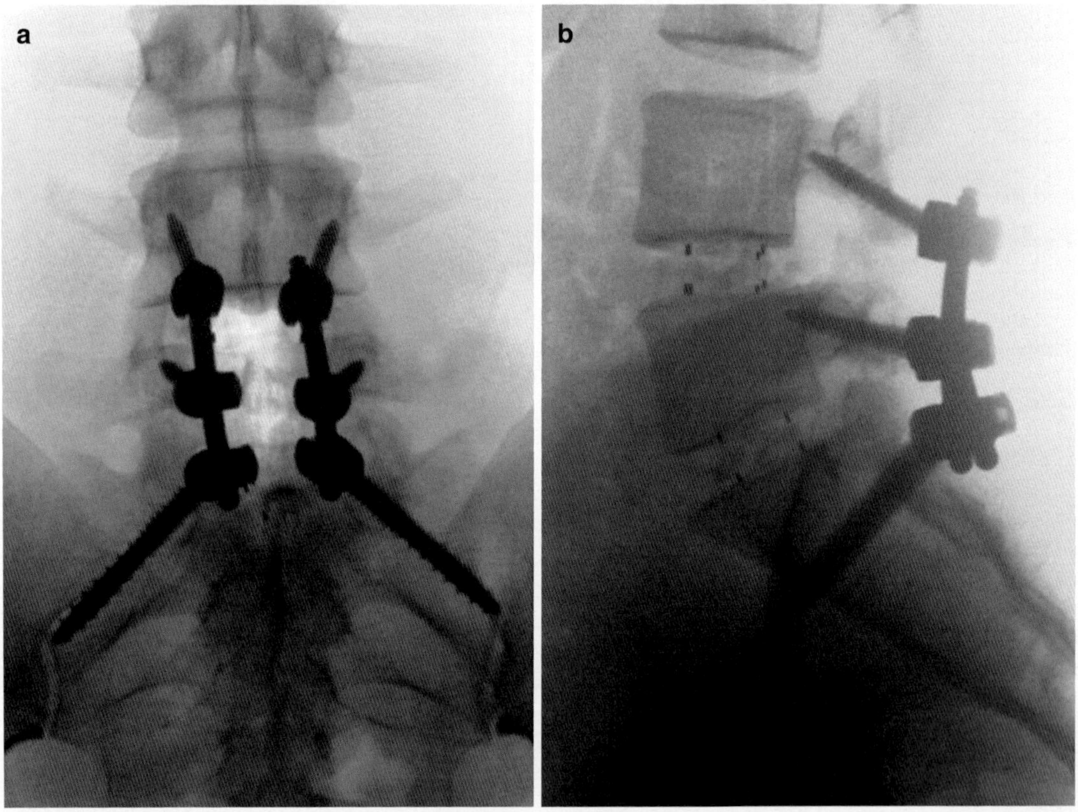

Fig. 34.12 (**a**) Medial screw construct with laminar exposure L4 to sacrum. Detachment of midline muscle attachments provides generous access for decompression and bone harvest while still preserving the neurovascular integrity of the muscles. The screws are placed deep to the muscle arising on the L3 spinous process and remain medial to tendon and neurovascular constraints along the articular processes. Placing a sacral alar screw avoids disrupting multifidus insertions to the sacrum (**b**) A lateral view of the construct shows the cephalad trajectory traversing the pars interarticularis and pedicle

34.6 Discussion

Anatomic approach about the muscles of the back provides a muscle sparing, naturally minimal approach to the back. Historically, many approaches simply disconnected muscles of the spine for exposure as desired. Caspar [2] introduced the use of the operating microscope to lumbar discectomy, with a slightly paramedian approach through the ESA, and retraction of the multifidus from the cephalad segment to avoid local muscle compromise. Ritland [5, 6] described a microsurgical intermuscular fusion or micro-TLIF, working about the muscle constraints with an intermuscular approach to construct placement, and a segmented intermuscular approach to the lamina for decompression and interbody fusion. Foley [3] initiated a parallel approach to MISS with percutaneous screw fixation and a transmuscular approach to the spine. This provided a limited approach but one frequently extra-anatomic in regard to the tendon and neurovascular elements in the back.

To the extent that MISS involves not just the skin incision, but preservation of the muscular integrity of the back, there is a compelling argument for approaches that respect the integrity of the back muscles and work about rather than through muscle fascicles. Engaging and respecting the segmental muscles in the back has the potential to preserve muscle integrity at risk with transmuscular or expanding retraction. In the situation of deformity and multisegmental correction, an intermuscular approach provides a muscle-sparing approach to placing fixation and seats the construct between the major back muscles. Combined with a segmented approach to facet or interbody fusion, it is possible to fully preserve the back muscle integrity. It places the construct between muscle groups with minimal impact on segmental muscle function. A midline approach for fixation with medialized screw placement is similarly anatomic. Midline muscle detachment may provide a more generous approach to the spine and spinal canal while still preserving the neurovascular integrity of the midline back muscles.

An understanding of the segmental muscles of the back enables and facilitates anatomic approaches to the back which preserve or minimally impact the functional integrity of the back. It is reasonable to consider approaches which detach muscles only as required to optimize deformity correction, neurologic decompression, or as necessitated for fusion.

Acknowledgments The artwork has been developed with Scott Bodell over a period of years. It is meant to illustrate the most relevant surgical anatomy. For purposes of illustration and clarity, some details such as interspinales and intertransversarii have been variably omitted. It expands on work previously published with Hoh [4]. I reference Bogduk [1] for anatomic nomenclature.

References

1. Bogduk N. Clinical anatomy of the lumbar spine and sacrum. 4th ed. Edinburgh: Churchill-Livingstone; 2005.
2. Caspar W. A new surgical procedure for lumbar disk herniation causing less tissue damage through a microsurgical approach. In: Wullenweber R, Brock M, Hamer JN, editors. Advances in neurosurgery. Berlin: Springer; 1977. p. 74–7.
3. Foley KT, Holly LT, Schwender JD. Minimally invasive lumbar fusion. Spine. 2003;28(15):S26–35.
4. Hoh DJ, Wang MY, Ritland S. Anatomic features of the paramedian muscle-splitting approaches to the lumbar spine. Neurosurgery. 2010;66(3 Suppl Operative):13–24.
5. Ritland, S. Microsurgical intermuscular lumbar arthrodesis. Poster Session, Congress of Neurological Surgeons, Annual Meeting, San Antonio, Texas, September, 2000.
6. Ritland, S. Micro-TLIF™ a mini-open and intermuscular transforaminal lumbar interbody fusion. DePuy AcroMed Inc, Surgical Technique, October, 2002.
7. Ritland S. Intermuscular approaches for lumbar fixation and arthrodesis. Semin Spine Surg. 2003;15(4):420–9.
8. Santoni BG, Hynes RA, et al. Cortical bone trajectory for lumbar pedicle screws. Spine J. 2009;5:366–73.
9. Wiltse LL, Hutchinson RH. Surgical treatment of spondylolisthesis. Clin Orthop Relat Res. 1964;35:116–35.

Minimally Invasive Thoracolumbar Facet Joint Fusion

35

Oliver Tannous, Kelley Banagan,
and Steven C. Ludwig

35.1 Introduction

For minimally invasive spine surgery to be successful, it is mandatory that it achieves the same goals that open surgical procedures achieve. By avoiding collateral damages to anatomic structures, the purported advantages of minimally invasive techniques include reduction in postoperative pain, length of hospitalization, blood loss, and medical and surgical complications. During the past several years, surgeons have been expanding the indications for minimally invasive techniques from degenerative procedures to more complex spinal disorders, including thoracolumbar deformity, trauma, tumor, and infections. Paramount to successful results of treatment of many thoracolumbar pathological conditions is achieving a solid biological fusion.

A variety of techniques have been advocated for achieving the fusion goal, including minimally invasive posterior interbody fusions, lateral interbody fusions, and anterior interbody fusions. With the advent of implementing minimally invasive techniques for more complex disorders, performing interbody approaches can become an arduous task when spanning multiple spinal segments. A different option for minimally invasive fusion would thus take advantage of fusing the facet joint with the addition of pedicular fixation to stabilize and fuse the thoracolumbar segments.

Lumbar transfacet fixation was first introduced by King [1] in 1948. He described the fusion technique with the use of short screws inserted horizontally across the facet joint. The screw member entered the inferior articular process and crossed the joint into the ipsilateral superior articular process [2]. In 1959, Boucher [3] described a modification of King's technique. He used the same starting point but directed the screw with a more vertical trajectory to penetrate the base of the ipsilateral pedicle with the tip of the screw to obtain greater body purchase. Another modification of transfacet fusion was introduced by Magerl [4] in 1984, who described the use of a translaminar facet screw entering the contralateral base of the spinous process, traversing through the lamina and entering the ipsilateral facet joint. With recent advances in minimally invasive techniques, facet fusions can be accomplished with posterior pedicular fixation as an alternative to the use of transfacet screws to achieve biological fusion.

35.2 Indications and Contraindications

Indications for minimally invasive posterior facet fusion with transfacet or transpedicular fixation include lumbar degenerative disorders,

O. Tannous, M.D. • K. Banagan, M.D.
S.C. Ludwig, M.D. (✉)
Department of Orthopaedics,
University of Maryland, 22 S. Greene Street,
Suite S11B, Baltimore, MD 21201, USA
e-mail: sludwig@umoa.umm.edu

M.Y. Wang et al. (eds.), *Minimally Invasive Spinal Deformity Surgery*,
DOI 10.1007/978-3-7091-1407-0_35, © Springer-Verlag Wien 2014

thoracolumbar fusions for deformity, trauma, infection, and tumor reconstruction. Relative contraindications to minimally invasive instrumentation include advanced osteoporosis and active sepsis.

35.3 Surgical Technique Section

When performing minimally invasive posterior facet fusions, the principles of minimally invasive posterior pedicle screw instrumentation are applied and adhered to. The facet joints to be fused are determined preoperatively. The pedicles associated with the chosen facets are cannulated in a minimally invasive manner. The pedicles are visualized on a true anteroposterior view intraoperative radiograph, with the endplates of the vertebral body parallel to the floor. Once a true anteroposterior view radiograph has been obtained, Kirschner wires (K-wires) are placed over the skin and horizontal and vertical lines are drawn on the skin through the center of the pedicle. The intersection of the lines represents the approximate starting point for the pedicle screws. Based on the starting point, an incision is made overlying the pedicle and vertebral body through skin, subcutaneous tissues, and fascia. A Jamshidi needle is then introduced into the incision and placed at the 3 o'clock and 9 o'clock positions of the pedicle. Placement of the Jamshidi needle is confirmed with intraoperative fluoroscopic imaging. Once the needle is in an acceptable position, it is advanced to the pedicle-vertebral body junction and positioning is again confirmed with intraoperative imaging. A K-wire is then introduced through the cannulated Jamshidi needle. The K-wire is advanced into the vertebral body.

K-wire placements at the respective levels are confirmed with fluoroscopic guidance (Fig. 35.1). Once the K-wires are deemed to be in acceptable positions, the trajectories for the pedicle screws are tapped over the K-wires (Fig. 35.2). The sizes of the screws and the taps to be used are determined based on preoperative CT. Once the screw trajectory has been tapped, dilators are placed over the K-wires in a sequential manner.

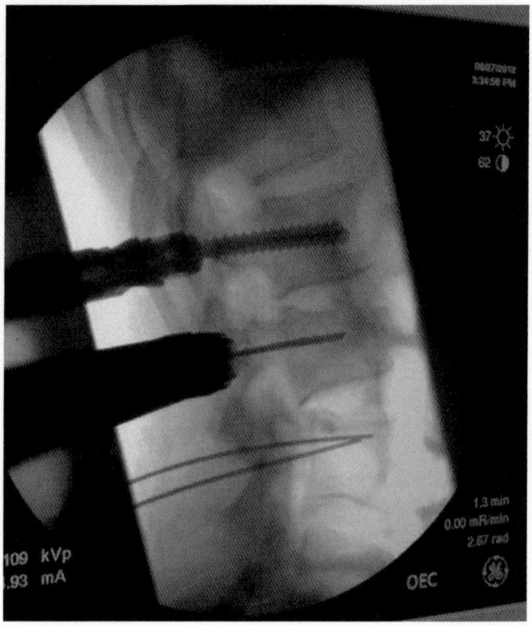

Fig. 35.1 Intraoperative fluoroscopic image of K-wire insertion into the pedicle and vertebral body with overlying dilator

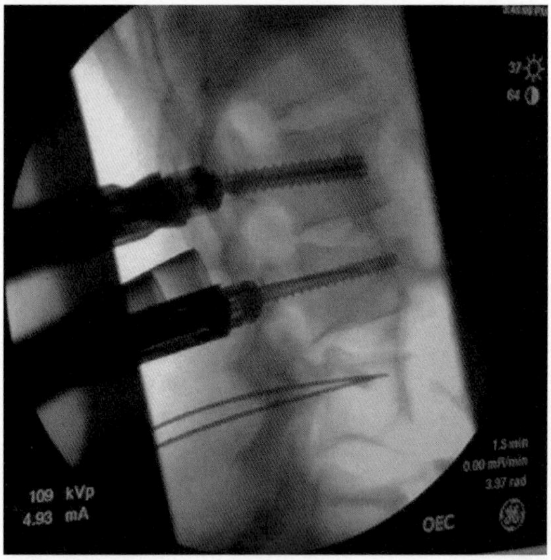

Fig. 35.2 Fluoroscopic image of screw placement after facet fusion

The dilators are used not only to create a field in which to perform the facet fusion but, when used in a wand-type manner, to clear the overlying soft tissue from the facet joint (Fig. 35.3). Once the appropriate sized dilator is placed over the facet joint, the surgeon should assess that optimal visualization of the facet joint has been obtained (Fig. 35.4). This often requires the use of a headlight and loops if a microscope is not introduced into the field. Bovie electrocautery is used to clear the facet joint of overlying soft tissue and capsule. This material is removed with a pituitary rongeur. Once the facet joint is cleared of overlying soft tissue and is adequately visualized, a high-speed cutting burr is introduced into the tube. Lateral view intraoperative fluoroscopic imaging can be used with the burr in place to confirm correct placement at the facet joint (Fig. 35.5). The facet joint is then decorticated with a high-speed burr. Next, bone graft material of the surgeon's choice is introduced through the dilator and packed around the facet (Fig. 35.6). The dilator tube is removed, and the screw is inserted over the K-wire. The K-wire is then removed. This procedure is performed in sequence, bilaterally, at all facet joints to be addressed.

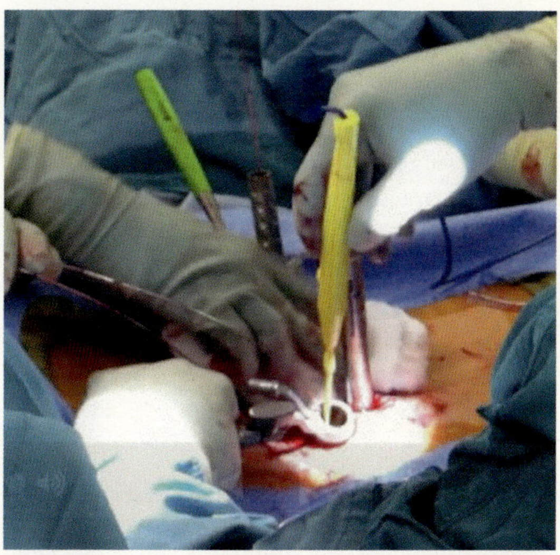

Fig. 35.3 Intraoperative photograph of the dilator over the facet joint

35.4 Clinical Data

Most of the clinical data regarding facet-mediated fusions are based on open techniques [1, 3, 5–7]. King [1] described a fusion rate of 91 % in his original series of 55 patients, with only one patient experiencing nerve root irritation secondary to screw placement. Other surgeons [5], however, reported pseudarthrosis rates of up to 55 % with transfacet screw fixation using the King's technique. Boucher [3], with his modified technique, reported a 100 % fusion rate in patients undergoing single-level fusion for degenerative disc disease and a 92 % fusion rate in patients undergoing fusion for spondylolisthesis. In more recent years, El Masry et al. [6] reported a 100 % fusion rate, with 89 % of patients in this cohort having excellent or good results and no neurological complications. Margulies and Seimon [7] similarly reported that 91 % of their patients had excellent clinical results after single-level fusion with the open Boucher technique.

Magerl's variation of open transfacet fixation using a translaminar facet screw has also been shown to be a successful technique with few complications and favorable clinical outcomes [4, 8–11]. Jacobs et al. [8] reported a 91 % fusion rate with favorable clinical results in 93 % of their cohort undergoing lumbosacral fusion. Humke et al. [9] obtained a 94 % fusion rate using translaminar facet screw fixation for posterior fusion, achieving good or excellent clinical results in 97 % of their patients. One of 173 patients in this series had temporary quadriceps

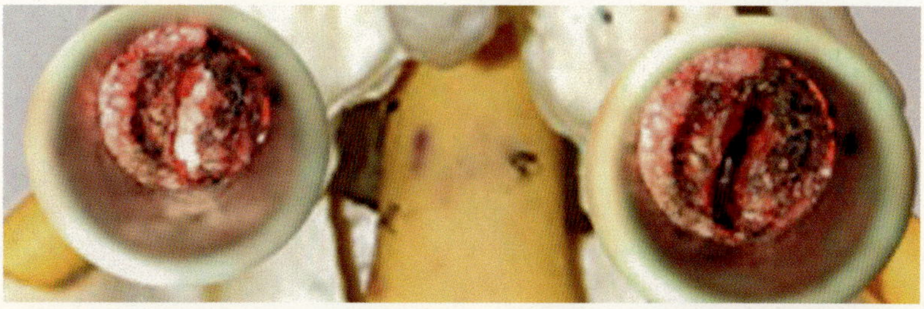

Fig. 35.4 View of the decorticated facet joint through the dilator tube

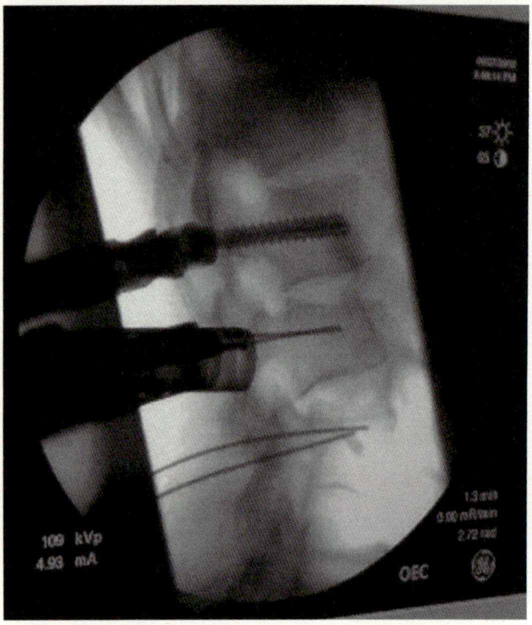

Fig. 35.5 Fluoroscopic image of the burr inserted through the dilator to the level of the facet joint

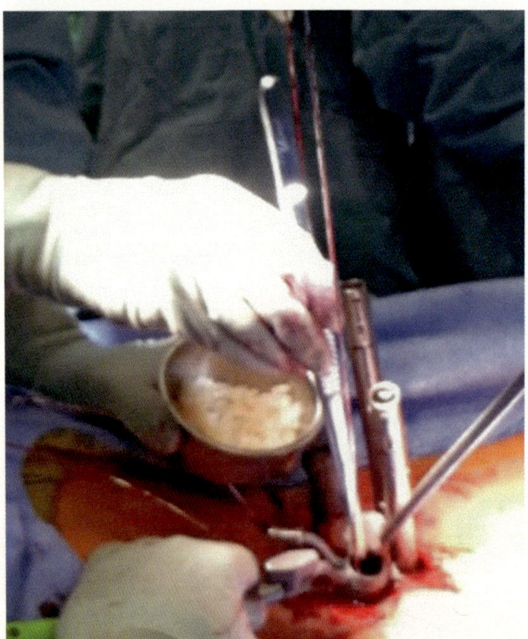

Fig. 35.6 Intraoperative photograph showing placement of bone graft through the dilator tube

weakness that resolved within 6 months after fusion and decompression at L2–L3. Three of 173 had symptomatic nerve root irritation that resolved at minimum final follow-up of 52 months. Other studies [10, 11] using open translaminar facet fixation have reported fusion rates exceeding 94 % with good or excellent results achieved in a high percentage of patients.

Best and Sasso [12] also presented a cohort of patients who underwent circumferential lumbar fusion. The authors compared the reoperation rate of translaminar facet screw fixation with that of pedicle screw fixation. In this series, two of 43 patients (4.7 %) with translaminar facet fusion and none of 24 patients (37.5 %) with pedicle screw instrumentation required a second operation at the index level. Operative re-exploration revealed that the pseudarthrosis rate was 2.3 % in the translaminar facet screw population, compared with 4.2 % in the pedicle screw population. Interestingly, the single patient in the translaminar facet screw group with pseudarthrosis had additionally undergone an intertransverse process fusion, using pedicle screws, without removal of the facet screws. All patients in the pedicle screw group who underwent reoperation required removal of the screws and rods.

To date, no study of open or minimally invasive surgery has analyzed the results of performing thoracolumbar fusion with just a facet or mediated fusions with pedicle screws. Whether historical data regarding transfacet screw fixation with facet fusion is generalizable to minimally invasive facet fusions with pedicle screws is unknown. Thus, data to champion this technique as a viable option is based on anecdotal experiences.

Conclusion

With advances in minimally invasive spine surgery, percutaneous facet fusion is becoming an attractive alternative for posterior lumbar fusion. The percutaneous procedures offer numerous advantages compared with open techniques, including less blood loss [13–15], less soft-tissue disruption [16–18], less postoperative pain [16, 19, 20], and less risk of infection [14, 21, 22]. Radiation exposure is a concern; however, it can be minimized with virtual fluoroscopy and CT-guided techniques [23, 24].

Percutaneous facet fusion is a promising technique. The clinical studies available to date, however, are comparative and non-comparative case series with no randomized controlled trials with a different type of surgical technique. Nevertheless, percutaneous facet fusion with pedicular fixation is a feasible alternative for obtaining fusion through a minimally invasive surgical approach.

References

1. King D. Internal fixation for lumbosacral fusion. J Bone Joint Surg Am. 1948;30:560–5.
2. Ferrara LA, Secor JL, Jin BH, Wakefield A, Inceoglu S, Benzel EC. A biomechanical comparison of facet screw fixation and pedicle screw fixation: effects of short-term and long-term repetitive cycling. Spine (Phila Pa 1976). 2003;28:1226–34.
3. Boucher HH. A method of spinal fusion. J Bone Joint Surg Br. 1959;41:248–59.
4. Magerl FP. Stabilization of the lower thoracic and lumbar spine with external skeletal fixation. Clin Orthop Relat Res. 1984;189:125–41.
5. Thompson WA, El R. Pseudarthrosis following spine fusion. J Bone Joint Surg Am. 1949;31:400–5.
6. El Masry MA, McAllen CJ, Weatherley CR. Lumbosacral fusion using the Boucher technique in combination with a posterolateral bone graft. Eur Spine J. 2003;12:408–12.
7. Margulies JY, Seimon LP. Clinical efficacy of lumbar and lumbosacral fusion using the Boucher facet screw fixation technique. Bull Hosp Jt Dis. 2000;59:33–9.
8. Jacobs RR, Montesano PX, Jackson RP. Enhancement of lumbar spine fusion by use of translaminar facet joint screws. Spine (Phila Pa 1976). 1989;14:12–5.
9. Humke T, Grob D, Dvorak J, Messikommer A. Translaminar screw fixation of the lumbar and lumbosacral spine: a 5-year follow-up. Spine (Phila Pa 1976). 1998;23:1180–4.
10. Grob D, Humke T. Translaminar screw fixation in the lumbar spine: technique, indications, results. Eur Spine J. 1998;7:178–86.
11. Reich SM, Kuflik P, Neuwirth M. Translaminar facet screw fixation in lumbar spine fusion. Spine (Phila Pa 1976). 1993;18:444–9.
12. Best NM, Sasso RC. Efficacy of translaminar facet screw fixation in circumferential interbody fusions as compared to pedicle screw fixation. J Spinal Disord Tech. 2006;19:98–103.
13. Wild MH, Glees M, Plieschnegger C, Wenda K. Five-year follow-up examination after purely minimally invasive posterior stabilization of thoracolumbar fractures: a comparison of minimally invasive percutaneously and conventionally open treated patients. Arch Orthop Trauma Surg. 2007; 127:335–43.
14. Schmidt OI, Strasser S, Kaufmann V, Strasser E, Gahr RH. Role of early minimal-invasive spine fixation in acute thoracic and lumbar spine trauma. Indian J Orthop. 2007;41:374–80.
15. Merom L, Raz N, Hamud C, Weisz I, Hanani A. Minimally invasive burst fracture fixation in the thoracolumbar region. Orthopedics. 2009;32.
16. Kim DY, Lee SH, Chung SK, Lee HY. Comparison of multifidus muscle atrophy and trunk extension muscle strength: percutaneous versus open pedicle screw fixation. Spine (Phila Pa 1976). 2005;30:123–9.
17. Regev GJ, Lee YP, Taylor WR, Garfin SR, Kim CW. Nerve injury to the posterior rami medial branch during the insertion of pedicle screws: comparison of mini-open versus percutaneous pedicle screw insertion techniques. Spine (Phila Pa 1976). 2009;34: 1239–42.
18. Lehmann W, Ushmaev A, Ruecker A, Nuechtern J, Grossterlinden L, Begemann PG, Baeumer T, Rueger JM, Briem D. Comparison of open versus percutaneous pedicle screw insertion in a sheep model. Eur Spine J. 2008;17:857–63.
19. Charles Y, Zairi F, Vincent C, Fuentes S, Bronsard N, Court C, Huec J-C. Minimally invasive posterior surgery for thoracolumbar fractures: new trends to decrease muscle damage. Eur J Orthop Surg Traumatol. 2012;22:1–7.
20. Rampersaud YR, Annand N, Dekutoski MB. Use of minimally invasive surgical techniques in the management of thoracolumbar trauma: current concepts. Spine. 2006;31(11):S96–102.
21. Ni WF, Huang YX, Chi YL, Xu HZ, Lin Y, Wang XY, Huang QS, Mao FM. Percutaneous pedicle screw fixation for neurologic intact thoracolumbar burst fractures. J Spinal Disord Tech. 2010;23:530–7.
22. Palmisani M, Gasbarrini A, Brodano GB, De Iure F, Cappuccio M, Boriani L, Amendola L, Boriani S. Minimally invasive percutaneous fixation in the treatment of thoracic and lumbar spine fractures. Eur Spine J. 2009;18(1):71–4.
23. Kang HY, Lee SH, Jeon SH, Shin SW. Computed tomography-guided percutaneous facet screw fixation in the lumbar spine: technical note. J Neurosurg Spine. 2007;7:95–8.
24. Sasso RC, Best NM, Potts EA. Percutaneous computer-assisted translaminar facet screw: an initial human cadaveric study. Spine J. 2005;5:515–9.

Part VII

Future Directions

Clinical Research in MIS Surgery: Current State and Future Challenges

36

Christina L. Goldstein and Y. Raja Rampersaud

36.1 Introduction

Spinal fusion is an accepted method of treatment for a wide variety of spinal pathologies requiring stabilization, including spinal deformity. Unfortunately, traditional open techniques are associated with extensive soft tissue dissection and retraction required to identify anatomic landmarks for appropriate placement of instrumentation and adequate preparation of the fusion bed. The morbidity associated with these open surgical exposures may include substantial blood loss [1], high complication rates [2], prolonged hospital stays [3], increased postoperative low back pain, and decreased trunk muscle strength [4].

The demonstration of improved outcomes and decreased morbidity associated with minimally invasive techniques in other surgical specialties [5–8], coupled with technical advances in magnification, illumination and access, and surgical instrumentation, has led to a desire to apply MIS techniques to spinal fusion surgery. However, before widespread adoption of these techniques can occur, the safety and efficacy of MIS spine surgery compared to currently accepted and commonly used techniques for open spinal fusion must be examined. In addition, with the higher up-front costs typically associated with new surgical technology, the decision to adopt MIS techniques must include a consideration of cost-effectiveness.

Using the current evidence pertaining to posterior MIS lumbar spine fusion as an example, this chapter aims to outline the current state of the literature regarding MIS fusion surgery, identify shortcomings of the evidence to date, and suggest possible directions and challenges to be addressed as future research is undertaken.

36.2 Current State of the Literature: Comparative Effectiveness Research

Prior to adoption of a novel surgical technique, its relative worth, utility, and importance must be compared to standard interventions. This need has been highlighted by the Institute of Medicine (IOM) and is addressed through the completion of comparative effectiveness research (CER). As per the IOM, "comparative effectiveness research is the generation and synthesis of evidence that compares the benefits and harms of alternative methods to prevent, diagnose, treat, and monitor or improve the delivery of care.

C.L. Goldstein, M.D., FRCSC
Toronto Western Hospital Spine Program,
Division of Neurosurgery, Toronto Western Hospital,
University of Toronto, 399 Bathurst Street,
WW 4-418, Toronto, ON M5T 2S8, Canada
e-mail: drcgoldstein@gmail.com

Y.R. Rampersaud, M.D., FRCSC (✉)
Krembil Neuroscience – Spine Program,
Division of Orthopaedics, Toronto Western Hospital,
University of Toronto, University Health Network,
399 Bathurst Street, EW 1-441, Toronto, ON
M5T 2S8, Canada
e-mail: raja.rampersaud@uhn.ca

M.Y. Wang et al. (eds.), *Minimally Invasive Spinal Deformity Surgery*,
DOI 10.1007/978-3-7091-1407-0_36, © Springer-Verlag Wien 2014

The purpose of CER is to assist consumers, clinicians, purchasers, and policy makers to make informed decisions that will improve health care at both the individual and population levels" [9].

Surgeons have traditionally understood CER to mean the demonstration of equivalent or superior safety and efficacy of one intervention compared to another. According to this basic understanding of CER, MIS fusion techniques must be shown to be at least as safe and effective as traditional open methods of spinal fusion. Thus, until recently, the evidence in support of new MIS fusion procedures, conducted primarily by surgeons, has been limited to case series, cohort studies, comparative observational studies, and, rarely, randomized controlled trials, examining outcomes such as surgical time, blood loss, length of stay, complication rate, and fusion rate [10].

36.3 Comparative Effectiveness of MIS Lumbar Fusion

The number of studies comparing open to MIS posterior lumbar fusion techniques for degenerative conditions has increased significantly in recent years. These studies examine techniques such as direct lateral or extreme lateral interbody fusion (DLIF/XLIF), axial lumbar interbody fusion (AxiaLIF), and MIS anterior lumbar interbody fusion (ALIF). A detailed account of the current evidence pertaining to all these techniques is beyond the scope of this chapter. We will instead focus on comparative effectiveness research comparing posterior MIS lumbar fusion to traditional midline open posterior spinal fusion for degenerative lumbar conditions. For a summary of the indications and outcomes of the lateral transpsoas approach, we would direct the reader to an excellent review recently published by Arnold et al. [11].

We have recently completed a systematic review of the literature to determine the comparative effectiveness of MIS versus open posterior fusion for degenerative lumbar conditions (Goldstein and Rampersaud – 2012, submitted for peer review). Medline, EMBASE, Web of Science, and Cochrane databases were queried. The MeSH terms used were derivatives of "Minimally invasive"/"Minimal access" and "Lumbar spine"/"Lumbar vertebrae" or "Fusion"/"Surgical Procedures." PubMed was searched using the phrase "Minimally invasive spine surgery," and a hand search of reference lists was also performed. Article titles, abstracts, and full-text versions were reviewed by two independent assessors to identify randomized controlled trials or comparative cohort studies including ten or more patients in each group undergoing open or MIS fusion for degenerative pathology and reporting at least one of (1) clinical outcome measure, (2) perioperative outcome measure, (3) radiographic outcome, (4) complications, or (5) economic analysis. Study quality was assessed using the GRADE protocol [12]. In cases of disagreement, a third surgeon was involved to assess suitability for study inclusion and GRADE rating. A meta-analysis was conducted on outcomes data when appropriate.

We identified 25 comparative cohort studies [13–37] and one prospective randomized trial [38] meeting our inclusion criteria. According to the GRADE protocol, all studies were rated as low or very low quality due to multiple factors including but not limited to, patient and surgical heterogeneity, small sample size, methodological flaws, and/or small treatment effect size. In these 26 studies, 856 patients with a mean age of 54.9 years underwent MIS lumbar fusion and 806 patients with a mean age of 56.7 years underwent traditional open instrumented fusion. The indications for surgery among the studies were mixed; in the 14 studies reporting on preoperative diagnosis, more than half of the patients underwent surgery for degenerative or isthmic spondylolisthesis with the remainder suffering from spinal stenosis, degenerative disc disease, or other spinal pathology.

36.3.1 Perioperative Outcome Measures

As demonstrated in Table 36.1, except for radiation exposure, meta-analysis of perioperative

Table 36.1 Meta-analysis of results for perioperative outcome measures comparing MIS vs. open TLIF

Outcome	No. of studies	No. of patients	Mean difference (MIS – open fusion) [95 % CI]	*p*-value
Operative time [minutes]	15	1,016	−2.49 [−19.66, 14.68]	0.78
Length of stay [days]	13	891	−2.87 [−3.82, −1.91]	<0.0001
Estimated blood loss [mL]	17	1,091	−260.11 [−332.69, −187.54]	<0.0001
X-ray time [s]	6	481	55.93 [36.12, 75.75]	<0.0001
Time to ambulation [days]	4	330	−3.52 [−5.52, −1.51]	0.0006

outcome measures favors MIS fusion compared to open surgery. No significant difference was observed in operative time between the open and MIS cohorts, though as expected an MIS approach exposed patients to an average of 56 more seconds of intraoperative radiation (95 % confidence interval (CI) 36.12–75.75, $p<0.0001$). In the 17 studies reporting on intraoperative blood loss, patients undergoing MIS fusion lost on average 260 mL less blood (95 % CI 187.54–332.69, $p<0.0001$). Patients undergoing MIS fusion were also able to ambulate an average of 3.5 days faster than patients in the open cohort (95 % CI 1.51–5.52, $p=0.0006$) and were discharged a mean of 2.9 days sooner (95 % CI 1.91–3.82, $p<0.0001$).

These results are similar to those demonstrated in a previous literature review by Karikari et al. [10] including seven comparative cohort studies examining MIS versus open TLIF or PLIF. As in our review, all comparative studies reviewed ($n=7$) demonstrated that the MIS subgroup performed better than the open group with regard to estimated blood loss and length of stay. No significant difference was observed in operative time in these seven studies (MIS 156.2–348.2 min; open 142.8–312.2 min).

36.3.2 Complication Rates

Demonstration of safety of new surgical techniques is also required prior to widespread implementation of MIS techniques for lumbar spine fusion. Complications of spinal fusion have been shown to be more common in the elderly and patients with multiple comorbidities [39]. This is particularly relevant as the percentage of people over the age of 65 increases and the number of patients suffering from degenerative spinal conditions grows. Thus, a comparative effectiveness study of MIS vs. open spinal fusion would not be complete without an analysis of complication rates.

In 2010 Wu et al. performed a review of the literature and meta-analysis of fusion rates reported in cohort and comparative studies, including a single RCT, examining open and/or MIS TLIF [40]. Open TLIF was performed on 716 patients in 16 studies and 312 patients underwent MIS TLIF in 8 studies. Among these patients no significant difference in fusion rates was observed (open: 90.9 % [95 % CI: 86.4–94.0 %]; MIS: 94.8 % [95 %CI: 85.4–98.3 %]). The authors also noted a trend towards lower complication rates in the MIS cohort (7.5 % [95 % CI: 3.0–17.3 %]) compared to the open cohort (12.6 % [95 % CI: 7.5–20.3 %]). It should be noted, however, that there was significant variability in the method of reporting and defining what was a complication and that a significantly higher percentage of patients in the MIS cohort underwent fusion with BMP (50 % vs. 12.2 % in the open cohort).

In a more recent publication, Parker et al. performed a systematic review of the literature to identify studies in which rates of surgical site infections (SSIs) were reported to examine the difference between open and MIS TLIF [41]. The authors identified 10 MIS studies and 20 open studies enrolling 362 and 1,133 patients, respectively. Pooled analysis from these 30 studies demonstrated a significantly lower rate of SSI in the MIS cohort at 0.6 % compared to 4.0 % in the open cohort ($p=0.0005$).

In our systematic review of the literature, 23 of the 26 studies reported on at least one type of

Table 36.2 Meta-analysis of complications rates comparing MIS vs. open TLIF

Outcome	No. of studies	No. of patients	Risk ratio [95 % CI]	*p*-value
Dural tear	16	1,009	0.71 [0.39, 1.30]	0.27
Infection	13	852	0.66 [0.32, 1.36]	0.26
Surgical complications	15	991	0.72 [0.42, 1.21]	0.21
Medical complications	13	854	0.39 [0.23, 0.69]	0.001
Nonunion	8	455	0.97 [0.35, 2.63]	0.95
Reoperation	9	640	0.99 [0.40, 2.44]	0.97
All complications	23	1,420	0.63 [0.47, 0.85]	0.002

complication including nonunion, with the meta-analysis of complication rates summarized in Table 36.2. As per Wu et al. [40], no significant difference was found in fusion rates between the open and MIS cohorts in the eight studies in which union was addressed (RR = 0.97 [95 % CI 0.35–2.63]; $p = 0.95$). Unlike the findings of Parker et al. [41], our meta-analysis failed to identify a difference in deep and superficial infection rates between the two surgical treatment groups (RR = 0.66 [95 % CI = 0.32–1.36]; $p = 0.26$). However, this difference is possibly due to variation in definitions of surgical site infection as well as the exclusion of studies without a comparative cohort from our systematic review. Further analysis revealed no difference in surgical complication rates between open and MIS lumbar fusion, including dural tear, implant malposition, neurologic injury, or postoperative hematoma (RR = 0.72 [95 % CI 0.42–1.21], $p = 021$). However, significantly more patients undergoing open surgery suffered from a medical complication including urinary tract infections, respiratory complications, and cardiac complications (RR = 0.39 [95 % CI 0.23–0.69], $p = 0.001$). Transfusion rates were also significantly higher in open fusion patients (RR = 031 [95 % CI = 0.10–0.93], $p = 0.04$).

Although there is currently no comparative literature meeting our inclusion criteria regarding complications or outcomes following MIS versus open treatment of multilevel coronal plane deformity, this growing area warrants specific mention. The prevalence of spinal deformity in patients over the age of 60 is almost 70 % [42] with up to 50 % of patients hospitalized with a primary diagnosis of spinal deformity being 65 years of age or older [43]. Given the increased burden of comorbid disease in this patient population and the association between preoperative pulmonary, renal, and cardiac testing and perioperative complications involving these organ systems [44], increased application of MIS techniques to adult deformity surgery has the potential to translate into significant improvement in clinical outcomes in this patient population. Published case series would suggest that other than specific complications associated with a transpsoas approach, MIS techniques result in an overall reduction in other (i.e., medical) complications [11]. Furthermore, with an estimated cost of $10,000 USD per in-hospital complication experienced by a spine patient [39], the economic impact of decreased complication rates with MIS surgery would be substantial.

36.3.3 Patient-Reported Outcome Measures

While perioperative outcome measures and complication rates are an important component of determining safety and efficacy of a new surgical technique, these outcomes tend to have greater meaning for surgeons than patients and thus may not accurately reflect comparative effectiveness from the patient's perspective. Instead, administration of patient-centered outcome measures including parameters most important to the patient (e.g., pain, function, return to work) is an important way of documenting the comparative effectiveness of different treatment strategies for spinal conditions.

The most common patient-reported outcome measures used in the study of lumbar disorders are the Oswestry Disability Index (ODI), the Medical Outcomes Study 36-item Short-Form

General Health Survey (SF-36), and the EuroQoL (EQ)-5D. Of the 26 studies identified in our systematic review, 22 included at least 1 patient-reported outcome with 10 employing the ODI [13, 16, 22–24, 27, 28, 34–36], 3 utilizing the SF-36 [17, 22, 31], and only a single study administering the EQ-5D [13]. Other patient-reported outcome measures identified in our review included a Visual Analogue Scale pain score for back or leg pain, the McGill pain score, perceived stress and profile of mood, the Japanese Orthopaedic Association (JOA) score, the Roland-Morris Disability Questionnaire (RMQ), the North American Spine Society score, the AAOS score, Short-Form 12 (SF-12), and the Prolo Scale.

Details of the results of the patient-reported outcome measures utilized in the 22 studies identified in our systematic review are outlined in Table 36.3. Meta-analysis of patient-reported outcome results was limited to change in ODI score due to the small number of studies utilizing the other outcome measures (Fig. 36.1). Pooled analysis of the change in ODI comparing MIS to open fusion from ten studies resulted in a statistically significant mean difference favoring MIS surgery (MD = 3.32 [95 % CI 1.33–5.32], $p = 0.001$). However, this observed difference between the groups does not approach the minimal clinically important difference or threshold for substantial clinical benefit for the ODI [45]. Thus, the results from this limited pooled analysis as well as those demonstrated in Table 36.2 qualitatively demonstrate clinical equivalence between MIS and open fusion for degenerative lumbar conditions at up to 2 years or more of follow-up with no study reporting inferior clinical results in an MIS cohort.

36.4 Shortcomings of the Current Comparative Effectiveness Literature

While current comparative effectiveness research for MIS vs. open lumbar fusion suggests compelling evidence for the clinical equivalence of the two techniques, limitations in study design prevent strong recommendations from being made based on these studies. As stated earlier, only one prospective randomized controlled trial exists comparing single-level open vs. MIS lumbar fusion in patients with a mixture of lumbar degenerative disorders [38]. At a minimum follow-up time of 2 years, clinical equivalence in patient-reported outcomes (ODI and VAS) was observed. However, no significant difference in intraoperative estimated blood loss or length of stay was seen between the cohorts, likely due to the study being underpowered with only 79 patients enrolled (MIS $n = 41$, open $n = 38$). Further design limitations including failure to mention allocation concealment, the number of patients screened, and lack of blinding of outcome assessors led to a downgrading of this RCT from an initial GRADE level of evidence rating of high to one of low. Similarly, the remaining prospective and retrospective cohort studies identified in our systematic review were graded as low or very low quality.

The heterogeneity of diagnoses included in most of the current studies comparing open and MIS lumbar fusion also impacts pooled analysis of results. As opposed to degenerative or isthmic spondylolisthesis, specific criteria by which patients are diagnosed with degenerative disc disease or discogenic back pain do not exist. As a result, heterogeneous populations of patients are lumped together for the purpose of assessing treatment effects, with the resultant outcomes providing little insight into the efficacy of the treatment for specific spinal pathologies. As has been previously demonstrated, clinical outcome of lumbar fusion is dependent on primary diagnosis, with improved 2-year changes in health-related quality of life seen in patients with a diagnosis of spondylolisthesis or scoliosis compared to disc pathology, stenosis, or post-discectomy revision [46]. Thus, the clinical equivalence observed in our systematic review between MIS and open fusion for lumbar degenerative disorders may be a result of heterogeneity of diagnoses rather than a true lack of superiority of MIS fusion.

Finally, a lack of clear definitions of adverse events and absence of standardized methods of

Table 36.3 Summary of results of patient-reported outcomes in comparative studies of MIS vs. open fusion

Study (origin)	Diagnosis	Outcome measure	Follow-up period 6–12 weeks Outcome	6 months Outcome	1 year Outcome	≥2 years Outcome
Park and Ha [25] (Korea)	Mixed	VAS back		MIS	MIS	
		Prolo scale			Equivalent	
Scheuffler et al. [28] (Switzerland)	Mixed	RMQ		MIS	MIS	
		AAOS score		MIS	MIS	
Dhall et al. 2008 [15] (USA)	Mixed	Modified Prolo scale				Equivalent
Starkweather et al. [31] (USA)	Instability	McGill pain score	MIS			
		Perceived stress	MIS			
		Profile of mood	MIS			
		SF-36	MIS			
Peng et al. [53] (Singapore)	Degenerative spondylolisthesis	VAS		Equivalent		Equivalent
		NASS score		Equivalent		Equivalent
		ODI		Equivalent		Equivalent
Schizas et al. [30] (Switzerland)	Mixed	VAS				Equivalent
		ODI				Equivalent
Tsutsumimoto et al. [32] (Japan)	Degenerative spondylolisthesis	JOA	Equivalent		Equivalent	Equivalent
Fan et al. [16] (China)	Mixed	VAS back		Equivalent	Equivalent	
		ODI		Equivalent	Equivalent	
Gahreman et al. [17] (Australia)	Isthmic or degenerative spondylolisthesis (<50 % slip)	VAS leg			Equivalent	
		VAS back			Equivalent	
		SF-36			Equivalent	
Ntoukas and Muller [24] (Germany)	Degenerative spondylolisthesis	VAS	MIS	Equivalent	Equivalent	
		ODI	Equivalent	Equivalent	Equivalent	
Villavicencio et al. [33] (USA)	Mixed	VAS				Equivalent
		MacNab's Criteria				Equivalent
Wang, Cummock et al. [34] (USA)	Mixed	Prolo scale			MIS (1-level)	
Wang Zhou et al. [35] (China)	Isthmic or degenerative spondylolisthesis	ODI				Equivalent

Adogwa et al. [13] (USA)	Degenerative spondylolisthesis	VAS leg				Equivalent
		VAS back				Equivalent
		ODI				Equivalent
		EQ-5D				Equivalent
Harris et al. [18] (USA)	Degenerative spondylolisthesis	VAS leg	Equivalent		Equivalent	
		ODI	Equivalent		Equivalent	
Wang Lu et al. [38] (China)	Mixed	VAS	Equivalent	Equivalent	Equivalent	Equivalent
		ODI	Equivalent	Equivalent	Equivalent	Equivalent
Wang Zhou et al. [36] (China)	Mixed	VAS back				Equivalent
		VAS leg				Equivalent
		ODI				Equivalent
Kotani et al. [20] (Japan)	Degenerative spondylolisthesis	JOA	MIS	MIS	MIS	MIS
		ODI	MIS	MIS	MIS	MIS
		RMQ				MIS
Rampersaud et al. [28] (Canada)	Isthmic or degenerative spondylolisthesis (<50 % slip)	ODI			MIS	
Lee et al. [22] (Singapore)	Mixed	VAS leg		Equivalent		Equivalent
		VAS back		Equivalent		Equivalent
		SF-36		Equivalent		Equivalent
		ODI		Equivalent		Equivalent
		NASS score		Equivalent		Equivalent
Mobbs et al. [23] (Australia)	Mixed	VAS			Open	
		ODI			Equivalent	
		SF-12			Equivalent	
Pelton et al. [26] (USA)	Mixed	VAS		MIS		
Wang Zhou et al. [37] (China)	Mixed	VAS back				Equivalent
		VAS leg				Equivalent
		ODI				Equivalent

Study or subgroup	MIS Mean	MIS SD	MIS Total	Open TLIF Mean	Open TLIF SD	Open TLIF Total	Weight	Mean difference IV,Random, 95 % CI
Adogwa 2011	−21.2	2.82	15	−17.2	3.85	15	9.1 %	−4.00 [−6.42, −1.58]
Fan,Hu,zaho 2010	−58.5	3.41	28	−48	3.38	31	9.7 %	−10.50 [−12.24, −8.76]
Lww2012	−26.7	3.31	72	−23.7	2.88	72	10.2 %	−3.00 [−4.01, −1.99]
Mobbs 2012	−31.59	4.25	36	−24.29	4.46	29	9.4 %	−7.30 [−9.44, −5.16]
Ntoukas 2010	−59	1.43	20	−54	1.5	20	10.3 %	−5.00 [−5.91, −4.09]
Peng 2009	−29	0.91	29	−30.2	0.92	29	10.5 %	1.20 [0.73, 1.67]
Rampersaud 2011	−17.99	3.84	37	−17.65	3.85	41	9.8 %	−0.34 [−2.05, − 1.37]
Wang,zhou 2010	−30.4	1.14	42	−26.4	1.28	43	10.2 %	−4.00 [−4.52, −3.48]
Wang,zhou 2011	−27.3	2.14	25	−26.4	1.77	27	10.2 %	−0.90 [−1.97, 0.17]
Wang,zhou 2012	−22.9	1.83	42	−22.8	1.01	30	10.3 %	−0.10 [−0.92, −0.72]
Total (95 % CI)			**346**			**346**	**100.0 %**	**−3.32 [−5.32, −1.33]**

Heterogeneity: $Tau^2 = 9.87$; $Chi^2 = 426.39$, df = 9 (P<0.0000); $I^2 = 98\ \%$
Test for overall effect Z = 3.26 (P = 0.001)

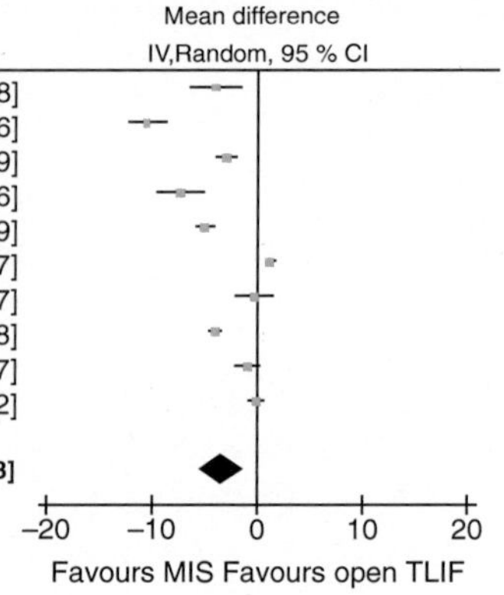

Fig. 36.1 Forest plot demonstrating pooled analysis of change in ODI in patients undergoing MIS vs. open TLIF

diagnosis impact the accuracy of the results reported in the studies included in our systematic review. A recent report on the rigorous prospective assessment of minor and major adverse events in 942 patients undergoing major spine surgery utilizing standardized definitions and multiple data collection methods identified a complication rate of 87 %, including a 73.5 % rate of postoperative complications [47]. This rate is significantly higher than the rate of 23 % that was previously observed at the authors' institution prior to implementation of the prospective reporting process and is also higher than the complication rates identified in our systematic review. Thus, the retrospective nature of the majority of the studies comparing open to MIS lumbar fusion may underestimate the difference in complication rates observed between the cohorts and thus the benefits of MIS lumbar fusion.

36.5 Future Direction of the Literature: Cost-Effectiveness Research

Despite the identified limitations, current CER literature suggests improved perioperative outcomes with equivalent 2-year clinical outcomes comparing MIS and open fusion for the treatment of degenerative lumbar conditions. However, widespread adoption of MIS spinal fusion based solely on procedural quality and health outcomes with no knowledge of the costs associated with these techniques risks adopting an approach to health service delivery that will quickly become unsustainable.

In 2008 Martin et al. identified that the $86 billion dollars spent annually in the USA to treat back and neck problems had reached levels comparable to diabetes, cancer, and non-spine arthritis [48]. As the population continues to age, with more than 50 % of US adults estimated to be over the age of 65 by 2030 [49], spine surgeons can no longer afford to view comparative effectiveness research and health economic research as mutually exclusive. A comprehensive review of methods of health economic evaluation (HEE) is outside the scope of this chapter; however a basic understanding of HEE is required to understand current HEE pertaining to MIS lumbar spine fusion and appreciate the shortcomings of this literature and future challenges faced by spine researchers.

Several types of HEE exist, though they are not interchangeable or of equal value when applied to health care decision-making. In order to balance the priorities of the "payer" as well as the "patient," a cost-effectiveness analysis (CEA), which simultaneously examines comparative clinical effectiveness and the costs of alternative interventions, is the ideal method of HEE [50]. The goal of a CEA is to measure the incremental cost and effects resulting from choosing one intervention over another [51]. The need to conduct a CEA can be determined by the nature

Table 36.4 Approach to determination of the need for a cost-effectiveness analysis (CEA)

		Cost of new treatment	
		Higher	Lower
Effectiveness of new treatment	More effective	Perform CEA	New treatment is superior – ADOPT
	Less effective	New treatment is inferior – ABANDON	Perform CEA

of the relationship between cost and effectiveness as illustrated in Table 36.4.

In 1996 recommendations regarding the key components of study design required for a high-quality CEA were put forward [52]. First, the CEA should be performed from the societal perspective, incorporating both direct (i.e., procedure and complication related) and indirect (i.e., loss of productivity of the patient or caregiver) costs. Next, measurement of clinical utility should be performed using validated general and disease-specific health outcome measures. For lumbar spine conditions, both the ODI and EuroQoL-5D or SF-6D should be used [49]. Uncertainties in cost should also be acknowledged with a sensitivity analysis, in which statistical analysis is performed using higher costs and decreased clinical benefits. The CEA should also include discounting of costs and benefits to account for the assumption that patients place more value on money spent on health care today than on that spent in the future. Finally, an appropriate comparison group must be included to allow for the proper incremental comparisons to be made across treatment strategies.

While a CEA informs decision-making regarding alternative treatment options for a single condition (e.g., operative vs. nonoperative treatment or open vs. MIS fusion for degenerative spondylolisthesis), the information obtained cannot be used to aid payers and policy-makers when comparing cost-effectiveness of interventions for competing pathologies (e.g., spinal stenosis vs. hip arthritis) such that decisions regarding health resource allocation can be made. Determination of the relative value of treatment of different conditions instead requires a different type of HEE, a cost utility analysis (CUA) [53].

In a CUA a generic health utility score is used to measure treatment outcomes in terms of a universal unit, the quality-adjusted life-year (QALY). A QALY is a generic measure of the impact of disease on life reflecting both the quality and quantity of life lived and is calculated by multiplying the utility score of a treatment of interest by the duration of treatment effect [45]. The utility score can be derived from a variety of generic health-related quality of life measures, including the SF-36, Health Utilities Index, and EQ-5D, and is expressed as a value in the range from 0 to 1 with 0 representing death and 1 representing a perfect health state [53]. Once the cost of an intervention and its utility score are known, the incremental cost utility ratio (ICUR), or cost required to obtain one QALY, can be determined. It is the ICUR that allows comparison of relative value of treatment across disease states with values between $50 and $100 K USD being considered a reasonable cost for the utility gained [54].

36.6 Cost-Effectiveness of MIS Lumbar Fusion

The increasing importance of value of treatment options for spinal disorders has been demonstrated by the 70 % increase in articles related to the lumbar spine including a CEA from 2004 to 2009 compared to 1999 to 2004 [45]. Despite this, during the latter time period, less than 1 % of articles published on the lumbar spine included a CEA [45]. More recently, Kepler et al. performed a systematic review of the Tufts Medical Center Institute for Clinical Research and Health Policy CEA Registry Database and the National Health Service Economic Evaluation Database to identify studies related to the spine that included a CUA [55]. Between 1976 and 2010, 33 studies including a CUA were found with only 4 of the articles (12 %) meeting all the key recommendations for performance of a high-quality CEA put forward by the US Panel of Cost-Effectiveness in Health and Medicine [52]. None of those four

Table 36.5 Summary of current cost-effectiveness data for MIS vs. open TLIF

Study	Type of cost	MIS	Open	Favors
Pelton et al. [26]	Hospital direct cost (USD)	WCB $19,705 +/− 5,391	$24,115 +/− 3,313	MIS
	Direct cost implant (USD)	Non-WCB $19,429 +/− 8,179	$26,804 +/− 1,208	MIS
	Direct cost surgical (USD)	WCB $13,798 +/− 4,260	$14,702 +/− 2,689	Equivalent
	Total direct cost (USD)	Non-WCB $14,658 +/− 4,802	$13,527 +/− 4,221	Equivalent
		WCB $3,756 +/− 1,211	$6,513 +/− 1,818	MIS
		Non-WCB $3,824 +/− 742	$6,673 +/− 1,172	Equivalent
		WCB $28,060	$33,862	MIS
		Non-WCB $29,429	$32,998	MIS
Wang et al. [37]	Covariate adjusted total cost (USD)	1-level $29,187 +/− 461	$29,947 +/− 324	Equivalent
		2-levels $33,879 +/− 521	$35,984 +/− 269	MIS
McGirt et al. [56]	Surgical site infection treatment direct cost (USD)	1-level $684	$724	Equivalent
		2-levels $756	$1,140	MIS
Rampersaud et al. [28]	Direct cost (CAD)	$14,182	$18,633	MIS
	Cost/QALY (1 year, CAD)	$128,936	$232,912	MIS
	Cost/QALY (2 years, CAD)	$70,915	$122,585	MIS
	Cost/QALY (4 years, CAD)	$37,720	$67,510	MIS
Wang Cummock et al. [34]	Acute hospital charges (USD)	1-level $70,159	$78,444	MIS
		2-levels $87,454	$108,843	Equivalent

articles involved MIS treatment of spinal disorders.

To date no prospective randomized controlled trials comparing open to MIS fusion and including a CEA have been performed. Instead, the literature pertaining to the health economics of MIS versus open fusion is limited to three comparative cohort studies identified by our systematic review [26, 28, 34] and two retrospective reviews of a large American surgical database [36, 56]. Data from these five studies is summarized in Table 36.5. According to the GRADE rating, these five studies were of low [28, 34] or very low quality [26, 36, 41].

In the earliest assessment of cost-effectiveness of MIS lumbar fusion, Wang et al. performed a retrospective comparative study including a cost analysis (CA) of hospital charges (not true cost) for 1- and 2-level MIS and open posterior interbody fusion for lumbar spondylosis, disc degeneration, and spondylolisthesis [35]. No assessment of patient-reported clinical outcome was performed. Patients with unilateral symptoms were treated with MIS fusion ($n=52$) and those with bilateral symptoms underwent open fusion ($n=22$). No significant difference in cost was identified in patients undergoing 2-level fusions; however in the single-level comparison, the mean cost of an MIS procedure was $70,159 compared to $78,444 for an open surgery ($p=0.027$). While the authors attributed the cost difference to an increased length of stay and higher complication rate in the open cohort, a formal statistical assessment of predictors of increased cost was not performed.

In a more recent retrospective study by Pelton et al., MIS and open TLIF were compared in 66 patients suffering from degenerative disc disease or spondylolisthesis who were or were not involved in workers' compensation claims [26]. Intraoperative, immediate postoperative, and financial outcomes were examined in both groups. Administrative databases were used to determine individual case costs from the perspective of the hospital, including transfusion, imaging, surgical implants, laboratory, pharmacy, allied health, hospital stay, and surgical services. Compensation status was not found to impact perioperative outcomes, including operative time, blood loss, and length of stay, in either group. However, a significant difference in these outcomes, as well as 6-month pain scores, favoring MIS over open surgery, was found in both compensation and non-compensation cohorts. Despite the 10 % increased cost associated with MIS implants, a statistically significant difference in total costs associated with decreased utilization of the other hospital resources was observed between the patients in the compensation group undergoing MIS versus open TLIF (\$28,060 vs. \$33,862, respectively; $p=0.03$).

In the only published cost utility study performed to date examining open vs. MIS TLIF, Rampersaud et al. retrospectively reviewed 78 consecutive patients undergoing 1- or 2-level open or MIS TLIF for degenerative or isthmic spondylolisthesis to determine the direct economic impact of surgical technique [28]. Direct case costing from the perspective of the hospital included operative costs, nursing, allied health, imaging, laboratory, and pharmacy. While the two groups (MIS = 37, open = 41) were the same with regard to demographic data including age, sex, medical comorbidities, and body mass index, patients undergoing MIS surgery had a significantly lower baseline ODI (MIS 36.90 ± 15.04 vs. open 51.33 ± 15.85; $p=0.001$) and fewer patients underwent 2-level fusions (MIS = 12 vs. open = 20). Consistent with the findings of other studies, the authors found that estimated blood loss, transfusion rate, and length of stay were significantly lower in the MIS cohort. Furthermore, the observed complication rate was also lower in the MIS group (10.8 % vs. 29.3 %; $p=0.02$). While both cohorts exhibited significant improvement in clinical status at 1 year, a nonsignificant trend in favor of MIS surgery was observed in 1-year SF-36 and ODI scores ($p=0.08$). The authors further identified an almost 24 % reduction in total direct cost between the open and MIS treatment groups (\$18,633 vs. \$14,183; $p=0.0009$). As a result of the equivalence in the 1-year utility scores, and study limitation, this cost savings translated into what was considered to be relatively equivalent cost utility between the two surgical techniques at the 1-year postoperative time point.

36.7 Clinical Research in MIS Surgery: Future Challenges

To date, these three low-quality retrospective comparative cohort studies have all demonstrated lower direct hospital costs associated with the index surgical procedure in favor of MIS lumbar spinal fusion compared to open surgery. This cost savings occurs due to decreased perioperative resource utilization despite additional surgical costs associated with MIS implants and increased use of fluoroscopy, with the most consistent cost savings coming from a reduced length of hospital stay [28]. However, several limitations in these studies preclude the drawing of definitive conclusions regarding the value of MIS techniques in lumbar fusion surgery. With the exception of the study by Rampersaud et al. [28], these economic evaluations do not take clinical outcome into account and therefore represent simple cost analysis studies. Based on the current comparative effectiveness research, which demonstrates equivalent clinical outcomes for MIS and open fusion for degenerative lumbar pathology, these studies support the use of MIS surgery as a method to minimize the direct hospital costs associated with surgical treatment of these disorders (i.e., cost minimization under the assumption of equal clinical benefit of two interventions).

As previously stated, the value of a health care intervention is equal to the quality of the intervention divided by the cost of the intervention over time. As these studies involve short follow-up periods and cost savings demonstrated in the perioperative period alone, our ability to draw conclusions regarding the value of MIS lumbar spine fusion is limited at best. For MIS spinal fusion to be a valuable health care intervention for degenerative spinal pathology, it must be found to be associated with either prolonged improvements in clinical outcome compared to open spinal fusion or continued cost savings in the postoperative period or both. Thus, in order to demonstrate prolonged clinical and economic benefit, future studies comparing MIS to open spinal fusion must involve longer follow-up periods and an ongoing analysis of indirect health care costs.

The importance of long-term follow-up is demonstrated by the results of the cost utility analysis performed by Rampersaud et al. of MIS versus open TLIF [28]. Despite the trend towards improved cost utility of the MIS procedures, both open and MIS TLIF were found to cost more than $100,000 per QALY gained, more than the threshold considered to be of reasonable value for a surgical intervention [54]. The authors estimated that at 2- and 4-year follow-up, the cost utility would fall below this threshold with a single-level MIS TLIF costing $37,720 CAD/QALY gained. In order to attain this level of value, however, prolonged improvements in clinical outcome must be demonstrated for MIS lumbar fusion.

In our systematic review, pooled analysis of ODI results from ten studies demonstrated clinical equivalence at a median follow-up of 24 months (mean difference (MIS – open)=–3.32 [95 % CI, –5.32 to –1.33]; $p=0.001$). In a recent study, Rouben et al. demonstrated that the clinical improvements observed in a cohort of 169 patients undergoing 1–2 level MIS TLIF were sustained at a minimum follow-up of 3 years (mean follow-up=49 months, mean % improvement in ODI=41 %) [57]. In 27 patients with 5-year follow-up, Simon and Rampersaud have shown that changes in ODI and SF-36 seen at 2 years in patients following MIS TLIF for low-grade degenerative or isthmic spondylolisthesis are maintained at 5-year follow-up [58]. Though these limited studies do not present substantial evidence in support of long-term clinical improvements with MIS TLIF, they suggest that with increased follow-up time the cost benefit of MIS lumbar fusion may be sustained. This will only be the case, however, if the costs associated with MIS fusion in the postoperative period are lower than in open fusion patients during this same follow-up period.

While no current study has examined ongoing resource utilization following MIS lumbar spine fusion, limited evidence exists to support the assumption that it is decreased. One example of this relates to the costs associated with the treatment of complications of spinal fusion, the rates of which have been shown to be lower in MIS procedures. In 2011, Parker et al. performed a systematic review of the literature and retrospective review of 120 open TLIF cases to determine the incidence of surgical site infection (SSI) following open and MIS TLIF and direct hospital cost associated with treating these SSIs [41]. Pooled analysis of the results revealed that the incidence of SSI was significantly lower in the 20 MIS cohorts than the 10 open cohorts (0.6 % vs. 4.0 %, $p=0.0005$), with a mean cost of treatment of an SSI being $29,110 at the authors' institution. This 3.4 % decrease in the rate of SSI translated into a cost savings of $98,974 per 100 MIS TLIF procedures performed.

Future studies including the economic impact of loss of productivity are also likely to demonstrate cost savings associated with MIS spinal fusion. In their small ($n=30$) comparative study of open versus MIS TLIF for grade I degenerative spondylolisthesis, Adogwa et al. included return to work as one of their primary outcome measures [13]. The two cohorts were similar with regard to the percentage of patients involved in sedentary occupations (MIS=7 [46.7 %], open=9 [60.0 %]; $p=0.72$). Despite the small sample size, a 50 % decrease in time to return to work was observed, with patients treated with MIS TLIF returning to work an average of 8.5 weeks earlier than their open counterparts (8.5 [4.4–21.4] vs. 17.1 [1.7–35.9] weeks; $p=0.02$). Based on this difference, Parker et al. estimated an indirect cost savings of $10,147 per employee undergoing MIS TLIF [41]. Recently, Dagenais et al. have suggested that economic costs related to loss of productivity and early retirement constitute a median of 85 % of the total cost associated with the treatment of low back pain [59]. Thus, it is reasonable to believe that the inclusion of indirect costs associated with return to work in future economic evaluations of spinal fusion will demonstrate additional cost savings in support of MIS techniques.

Conclusion

Current comparative effectiveness research examining open versus MIS lumbar fusion for degenerative conditions suggests midterm clinical equivalence with improved perioperative outcomes such as estimated blood loss, length of stay, and a trend towards decreased complication rates in patients undergoing MIS surgery. In addition, limited evidence from cost analysis studies has shown decreased direct hospital costs associated with the index surgical procedure in favor of MIS lumbar fusion. However, significant limitations in study design, outcome assessment, and comprehensive health economic analysis preclude definitive overall conclusions regarding favorable comparative effectiveness and value of MIS and open lumbar fusion from being drawn. However, we can conclude that MIS fusion does not appear to be inferior to open fusion.

Future studies comparing open to MIS lumbar fusion require many improvements in study design. A multicenter randomized controlled trial enrolling an adequate number of patients, stratified to homogeneous diagnostic categories (e.g., isthmic spondylolisthesis, degenerative spondylolisthesis, and degenerative disc), and including a comprehensive CEA as well as long-term follow-up would be ideal. However, as proven by the enrollment challenges and fatal flaws (e.g., high crossover) of the SPORT studies, the reality and generalizability of this are unlikely. Rather, prospective multicenter observational studies that allow for patient and surgeon preference as well as regional variation or appropriately robust surgical registries with patient level outcome data are more ideally suited to assess the question of MIS versus open lumbar fusion. Valid, reliable, and responsive health-related quality of life instruments capable of calculating a utility score, such as the SF-6D, ODI, or EQ-5D, should be used to assess patient-reported outcomes. The definitions of adverse events should be determined a priori with data pertaining to adverse event rates being collected in a prospective manner. Follow-up time should be long enough to demonstrate the durability, or lack thereof, of clinical improvements associated with lumbar spine fusion. Evaluation of the economics of MIS and open lumbar fusion must include both direct and indirect costs, in particular post-discharge costs associated with treatment of complications, ongoing resource utilization, and loss of productivity of patients and caregivers.

With the implementation of these suggested changes in future studies comparing MIS to open lumbar fusion, definitive conclusions could be drawn regarding the comparative effectiveness and value of these different treatment strategies. If current findings of equivalent or improved clinical outcomes coupled with lower complication rates, decreased direct hospital cost, less postoperative resource utilization, and faster return to work are borne out, the true clinical and cost-effectiveness of MIS lumbar fusion is likely to be realized.

References

1. Cho KJ, Suk SI, Park SR, et al. Complications in posterior fusion and instrumentation for degenerative lumbar scoliosis. Spine. 2007;32(20):2232–7.
2. Carreon LY, Puno RM, Dimar 2nd JR, et al. Perioperative complications of posterior lumbar decompression and arthrodesis in older adults. J Bone Joint Surg Am. 2003;85-A(11):2089–92.
3. Thomsen K, Christensen FB, Eiskjaer SP, et al. Volvo award winner in clinical studies. The effect of pedicle screw instrumentation on functional outcome and fusion rates in posterolateral lumbar spinal fusion: a prospective, randomized clinical study. Spine. 1997;22:2813–22.
4. Gejo R, Matsui H, Kawaguchi Y, et al. Serial changes in trunk muscle performance after posterior lumbar surgery. Spine. 1996;21:941–4.
5. Bosch F, Wehrman U, Saeger HD, et al. Laparoscopic or conventional cholecystectomy: clinical and economic considerations. Eur J Surg. 2002;168(5):270–7.
6. Topcu O, Karakayali F, Kuzu MA, et al. Comparison of long-term quality of life after laparoscopic and open cholecystectomy. Surg Endos. 2003;17(2):291–5.
7. Garry R, Fountain J, Mason S, et al. The eVALuate study: two parallel randomized trials, one comparing laparoscopic with abdominal hysterectomy, the other comparing laparoscopic with vaginal hysterectomy. BMJ. 2004;328(7432):129–35.

8. Pace KT, Dyer SJ, Stewart RJ, et al. Health-related quality of life after laparoscopic and open nephrectomy. Surg Endos. 2003;17(1):143–52.
9. O'Leary TJ, Slutsky JR, Bernard MA. Comparative effectiveness research priorities at Federal Agencies: the view from the Department of Veterans Affairs, National Institute on Aging, and Agency for Healthcare Research and Quality. J Am Geriatr Soc. 2010;58:1187–92.
10. Karikari IO, Isaacs RE. Minimally invasive transforaminal lumbar interbody fusion. A review of techniques and outcomes. Spine. 2010;36(26S):S294–301.
11. Arnold PM, Anderson KK, McGuire Jr RA. The lateral transpsoas approach to the lumbar and thoracic spine: a review. Surg Neurol Int. 2012;3(3):S198–215. Epub 2012 Jul 17.
12. Brozek JL, Akl EA, Alonso-Coello P, et al. Grading quality of evidence and strength of recommendations in clinical practice guidelines. Part 1 of 3. An overview of the grade approach and grading quality of evidence about interventions. Allergy. 2009;64:669–77.
13. Adogwa O, Parker SL, Bydon A, et al. Comparative effectiveness of minimally invasive versus open transforaminal lumbar interbody fusion. 2-year assessment of narcotic use, return to work, disability and quality of life. J Spinal Disord Tech. 2011;24(8):479–84.
14. Bagan B, Patel N, Deutsch H, et al. Perioperative complications of minimally invasive surgery (MIS): comparison of MIS and open interbody fusion techniques. Surg Technol Int. 2008;17:281–6.
15. Dhall SS, Wang MY, Mummanenni PV. Clinical and radiographic comparison of mini-open transforaminal lumbar interbody fusion with open transforaminal lumbar interbody fusion in 42 patients with long-term follow-up. J Neurosurg Spine. 2008;9:560–5.
16. Fan S, Hu Z, Zhao F, et al. Multifidus muscle changes and clinical effects of one-level posterior lumbar interbody fusion: minimally invasive procedure versus conventional open approach. Eur Spine J. 2010;19:316–24.
17. Gahreman A, Ferch RD, Rao PJ, et al. Minimal access versus open posterior lumbar interbody fusion in the treatment of spondylolisthesis. Neurosurgery. 2010; 66(2):296–304.
18. Harris EB, Sayadipour A, Massey P, et al. Mini-open versus open decompression and fusion for lumbar degenerative spondylolisthesis with stenosis. Am J Orthop. 2011;40(12):E257–61.
19. Isaacs RE, Podichetty VK, Santiago P, et al. Minimally invasive microendoscopy-assisted transforaminal lumbar interbody fusion with instrumentation. J Neurosurg Spine. 2005;3:98–105.
20. Kotani Y, Abumi K, Ito M, et al. Mid-term clinical results of minimally invasive decompression and posterolateral fusion with percutaneous pedicle screws versus conventional approach for degenerative spondylolisthesis with spinal stenosis. Eur Spine J. 2012;21:1171–7.
21. Lau D, Lee JG, Han SJ, et al. Complications and perioperative factors associated with learning the technique of minimally invasive transforaminal lumbar interbody fusion (TLIF). J Clin Neurosci. 2011;18:624–7.
22. Lee KH, Yue WM, Yeo W, et al. Clinical and radiological outcomes of open versus minimally invasive transforaminal lumbar interbody fusion. Eur Spine J. 2012;21(11):2265–70 [ePub ahead of print].
23. Mobbs RJ, Sivabalan P, Li J. Minimally invasive surgery compared to open spinal fusion for the treatment of degenerative lumbar spine pathologies. J Clin Neurosci. 2012;12:829–35.
24. Ntoukas V, Muller A. Minimally invasive approach versus traditional open approach for one level posterior lumbar interbody fusion. Minim Invasive Neurosurg. 2010;53(1):21–4.
25. Park Y, Ha JW. Comparison of one-level posterior lumbar interbody fusion performed with a minimally invasive approach or a traditional open approach. Spine. 2007;32(5):537–43.
26. Pelton MA, Phillips FM, Sing K. A comparison of perioperative costs and outcomes in patients with and without workers' compensation claims treated with MIS or open TLIF. Spine. 2012;37(22):1914–9 [ePub ahead of print].
27. Peng CWB, Yue WM, Ph SY, et al. Clinical and radiological outcomes of minimally invasive versus open transforaminal lumbar interbody fusion. Spine. 2009;34(13):1385–9.
28. Rampersaud YR, Gray R, Lewis SJ, et al. Cost-utility analysis of posterior minimally invasive fusion compared with conventional open fusion for lumbar spondylolisthesis. SAS J. 2011;5:29–35.
29. Scheuffler K, Dohmen H, Vougiokas VI. Percutaneous transforaminal lumbar interbody fusion for the treatment of degenerative lumbar instability. Operat Neurosurg. 2007;60(ONS Suppl 2):ONS-203–13.
30. Schizas C, Tzinieris N, Tsiridis E, et al. Minimally invasive versus open transforaminal lumbar interbody fusion. Evaluating initial experience. Int Orthop. 2009;33(6):1683–8.
31. Starkweather AR, Witek-Janusek L, Nockels RP, et al. The multiple benefits of minimally invasive spinal surgery: results comparing transforaminal lumbar interbody fusion and posterior lumbar fusion. J Neurosci Nurs. 2008;49(1):32–9.
32. Tsutsumimoto T, Shimogata M, Ohta H, et al. Mini-open versus conventional open posterior lumbar interbody fusion for the treatment of lumbar degenerative spondylolisthesis. Spine. 2009;34(18):1923–28.
33. Villavicencio AT, Burneikiene S, Roeca CM, et al. Minimally invasive versus open transforaminal lumbar interbody fusion. Surg Neurol Int. 2010;1:12.
34. Wang MY, Cummock MD, Yu Y, et al. An analysis of the differences in the acute hospitalization charges following minimally invasive versus open posterior lumbar interbody fusion. J Neurosurg Spine. 2010;12: 694–9.
35. Wang J, Zhou Y, Zhang ZF, et al. Comparison of one-level minimally invasive and open transforaminal lumbar interbody fusion in degenerative and isthmic

spondylolisthesis grades 1 and 2. Eur Spine J. 2010; 19:1780–4.
36. Wang J, Zhou Y, Zhang ZF, et al. Minimally invasive or open transforaminal lumbar interbody fusion as revision surgery for patients previously treated by open discectomy and decompression of the lumbar spine. Eur Spine J. 2011;20:623–8.
37. Wang J, Zhou Y, Zhang ZF, et al. Comparison of clinical outcome in overweight or obese patients after minimally invasive versus open transforaminal lumbar interbody fusion. J Spinal Disord Tech. 2012;May 17 [ePub ahead of print].
38. Wang H, Lu F, Jiang J, et al. Minimally invasive lumbar interbody fusion via MAST Quadrant retractor versus open surgery: a prospective randomized clinical trial. Chin Med J. 2011;124(23):3868–74.
39. Kalanithi PS, Patil CG, Boakye M. National complication rates and disposition after posterior lumbar fusion for acquired spondylolisthesis. Spine. 2009;34: 1963–9.
40. Wu RH, Fraser JF, Hartl R. Minimal access versus open transforaminal lumbar interbody fusion. Meta-analysis of fusion rates. Spine. 2010;35(26): 2273–81.
41. Parker SL, Adogwa O, Witham TF, et al. Post-operative infection after minimally invasive versus open transforaminal lumbar interbody fusion (TLIF): literature review and cost analysis. Minim Invas Neurosurg. 2011;54:33–7.
42. Schwab F, Dubey A, Gamez L, et al. Adult scoliosis: prevalence, SF-36, and nutritional parameters in an elderly volunteer population. Spine. 2005;30:1082–5.
43. Jo DJ, Jun JK, Kim KT, et al. Lumbar interbody fusion outcomes in degenerative lumbar disease. Comparison of results between patients over and under 65 years of age. J Korean Neurosurg Soc. 2010;48:412–8.
44. Drazin D, Shirzadi A, Rosner J, et al. Complications and outcomes after spinal deformity surgery in the elderly: review of the existing literature and future directions. Neurosurg Focus. 2011;31(4):E3.
45. Rihn JA, Berven S, Allen T, et al. Defining value in spine care. Am J Med Qual. 2009;29(S6):4S–14.
46. Glassman SD, Carreon LY, Djurasovic M, et al. Lumbar fusion outcomes stratified by specific diagnostic indication. Spine J. 2009;9:13–21.
47. Street JT, Lenehan BJ, DiPaola CP, et al. Morbidity and mortality of major adult spinal surgery. A prospective cohort analysis of 942 consecutive patients. Spine J. 2012;12:22–34.
48. Martin BI, Deyo RA, Mirza SK, et al. Expenditures and health status among adults with back and neck problems. JAMA. 2008;299(6):656–64.
49. Allen RT, Garfin SR. The economics of minimally invasive spine surgery. The value perspective. Spine. 2010;35(26S):S375–82.
50. Detsky AS, Naglie IG. A clinician's guide to cost-effectiveness analysis. Ann Int Med. 1990;113:147–54.
51. Detsky AS, Laupacis A. Relevance of cost-effectiveness analysis to clinicians and policy makers. JAMA. 2007;298(2):221–4.
52. Siegel JE, Weinstein MD, Russell LB, et al. Recommendations for reporting cost-effectiveness analysis. Panel on cost-effectiveness in health and medicine. JAMA. 1996;276:1339–41.
53. Barnett DB. Assessment of quality of life. Am J Cardiol. 1991;67:41C–4.
54. Laupacis A, Feeny D, Detsky AS, et al. How attractive does a new technology have to be to warrant adoption and utilization? Tentative guidelines for using clinical and economic evaluations. CMAJ. 1992;146:473–81.
55. Kepler CK, Wilkinson SM, Radcliff KE, et al. Cost-utility analysis in spine care: a systematic review. Spine J. 2012;12(8):676–90.
56. McGirt MJ, Parker SL, Lerner J, et al. Comparative analysis of perioperative surgical site infection after minimally invasive versus open posterior/transforaminal lumbar interbody fusion: analysis of hospital billing and discharge data from 5170 patients. J Neurosurg Spine. 2011;14:771–8.
57. Rouben D, Casnellie M, Ferguson M. Long-term durability of minimally invasive posterior transforaminal lumbar interbody fusion: a clinical and radiographic follow-up. J Spinal Disord Tech. 2011;24(5):288–96.
58. Harris SA, Rampersaud YR. Minimally invasive surgery lumbar fusion for low-grade isthmic and degenerative spondylolisthesis: 2- to 5-year follow-up. Can J Surg. 2012;55(Suppl):S45.
59. Dagenais S, Haldeman S, Polatin PB. It is time for physicians to embrace cost-effectiveness and cost utility analysis research in the treatment of spinal pain. Spine J. 2005;5:357–60.

37 MIS in Adolescent Deformity

Firoz Miyanji

The prevalence of adolescent idiopathic scoliosis (AIS) is reported to be 2–3 %, with approximately less than 0.1 % of all adolescents having curves greater than 40°. The goals of surgical treatment in the setting of AIS remain threefold: (1) to prevent progression of the deformity by obtaining a solid arthrodesis, (2) to limit the extent of the fusion, and (3) to obtain a three-dimensional correction of the deformity to achieve a balanced spine in all three planes.

To date surgical options include open posterior instrumented fusion, open anterior instrumented fusion, and thoracoscopic techniques. Although the goals of AIS treatment are achieved with these techniques, each with its own reported advantages and disadvantages, any emphasis on approach-related morbidity with these conventional procedures is minimal. The primary debate between anterior and posterior surgery for AIS is centered around concerns of crankshaft for the very young patient, the distal extent of the fusion, the ability to restore and maintain the sagittal plane, and when faced with severe, rigid deformities. Thoracoscopic techniques have reported more favorable postoperative lung function compared to open anterior thoracotomies [1–3]; however, the perioperative morbidity with single-lung ventilation should not be overlooked [4, 6]. In addition, anterior thoracoscopic instrumented fusions rely on a single anterior rod with most surgeons favoring a postoperative bracing protocol due to reports of significant pseudarthrosis rates in some studies [4–6].

Conventional open spine procedures for AIS are often associated with significant blood loss, soft tissue disruption, prolonged recovery, and postsurgical pain. A number of authors have reported on the significant soft tissue and muscle morbidity offered by standard open spine procedures possibly leading to increased perioperative morbidity and long-term pain [7–24]. The rationale for MIS in the setting of AIS is therefore to try and minimize the approach-related morbidity inherent in the current available surgical options for this patient population.

37.1 Indications for MIS in AIS

The surgical indications for AIS remain a thoracic curve reaching 50° or greater in skeletally mature patients for risk of progression into adulthood. In patients with thoracolumbar/lumbar curves, a magnitude of 40–45° is generally an indication for surgical stabilization. Although firm curve characteristics exist to guide intervention, patient factors are equally as important when deciding about surgery in the setting of idiopathic scoliosis. Once the decision for surgery is made, the indications for MIS rely heavily on curve magnitude, flexibility, and patient factors. Generally curves less than 70°, which on

F. Miyanji, MD, FRCSC
Department of Orthopedics, British Columbia Children's Hospital, University of British Columbia, Vancouver, BC, Canada
e-mail: fmiyanji@cw.bc.ca

M.Y. Wang et al. (eds.), *Minimally Invasive Spinal Deformity Surgery*,
DOI 10.1007/978-3-7091-1407-0_37, © Springer-Verlag Wien 2014

side-bending films correct below 30–35°, can be considered for MIS. The Lenke curve type or the extent of the fusion is not a contraindication for MIS. Patient factors that suggest poor protoplasm, fusion concerns (e.g., smoking), or compliance issues with the slow graduated postoperative return to activity protocol should be very carefully evaluated prior to embarking on MIS in these instances.

37.2 Technique of MIS in AIS

Three individual midline skin incisions are planned using fluoroscopy. (Fluoroscopy is limited to preoperative planning of the incisions.) The skin is then undermined laterally to allow for paramedian fascial incisions approximately one fingerbreadth from midline. A blunt muscle-sparing approach is used down to the facet joints, which are visualized using handheld retractors. Pedicles are then cannulated using the freehand technique after performing wide facetectomies (Fig. 37.1a, b). Once cannulated, the pedicles remained localized by placement of the guidewires available on the VIPER II system (Depuy, J&J). The facet joints are then meticulously decorticated using a high-speed burr, and bone graft is laid down *prior* to screw placement to help augment fusion. Once the grafting material is laid down (which consisted of freeze-dried allograft bone), the appropriate size pedicle screw is inserted and the guidewire is removed.

Once the screws are placed at all levels, an appropriate length rod contoured to the appropriate sagittal profile is introduced. The rod is passed from distal to proximal below the soft tissues and under the skin bridges utilizing the elongated slots designed on the VIPER II cylinders (Depuy, J&J) (Fig. 37.2). The cylinders are made collinear prior to placement of the rod allowing for the majority of the deformity correction. The rod is reduced to the pedicle screws using the reduction instruments and secured using setscrews. Further correction is obtained with rod derotation into the appropriate sagittal plane. Prior to placement of the second rod en bloc, direct vertebral apical derotation is performed using the VIPER II cylinders. The second convex rod is then under-contoured in the sagittal plane and also placed from distal to proximal. Under-contouring of this rod allows for further deformity correction in the axial plane (Fig. 37.3). All rods are cobalt chrome and 5.5 mm in diameter. Uniaxial screws are primarily used (Fig. 37.4a, b).

Currently data focusing on outcomes of MIS techniques in AIS is limited. Anand and colleagues [25] reported on a series of 12 adult patients with degenerative scoliosis who had on average 3.64 segments fused. They reported a feasibility study in which patients underwent a lateral retroperitoneal approach followed by

a

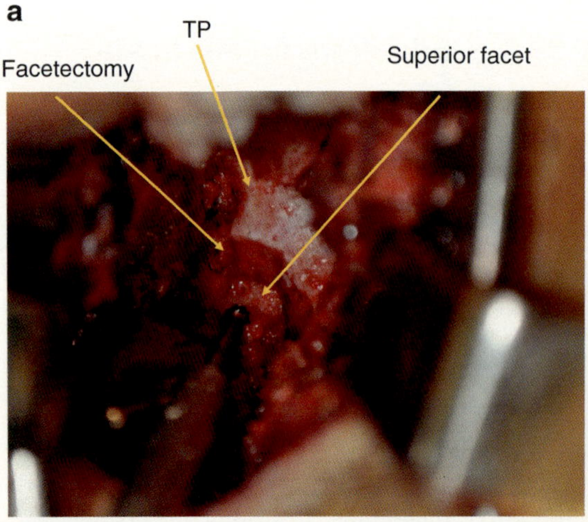

b

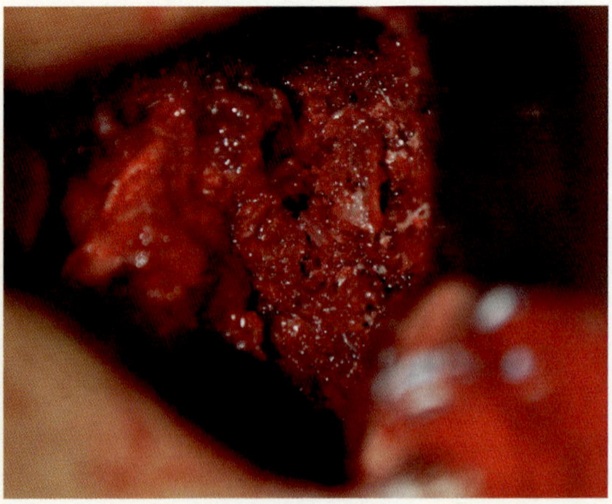

Fig. 37.1 (**a**) Facetectomy and pedicle screw cannulation. (**b**) Morselized bone graft prior to screw placement

percutaneous pedicle screw placements. Functional or long-term data was not available in this series. Similarly Hsieh and colleagues [26] have described MIS procedures on a heterogeneous group of patients with complex spine disorders, but only one patient was treated for deformity. Samdani et al. [27] retrospectively reviewed their experience with MIS in 15 patients and had on average a preoperative major Cobb angle of 54° correcting to 18°, noting a 67 % correction. The average blood loss in their series was 254 cc and OR time was on average 470 min.

Our recent prospective comparison of MIS to open standard posterior techniques in the setting of AIS aimed at comparing curve correction and perioperative variables between the two groups [28]. The study found near-equivalent curve correction between the two groups (63 % open group; 68 % MIS group) (Fig. 37.5). The advantages of MIS over open posterior procedures were a significantly lower blood loss on average and decreased length of hospital stay. However, the operative time was significantly longer in patients treated with MIS. This may be the effect of a learning curve when applying new techniques but should be emphasized as a potential limitation of MIS in the setting of deformity.

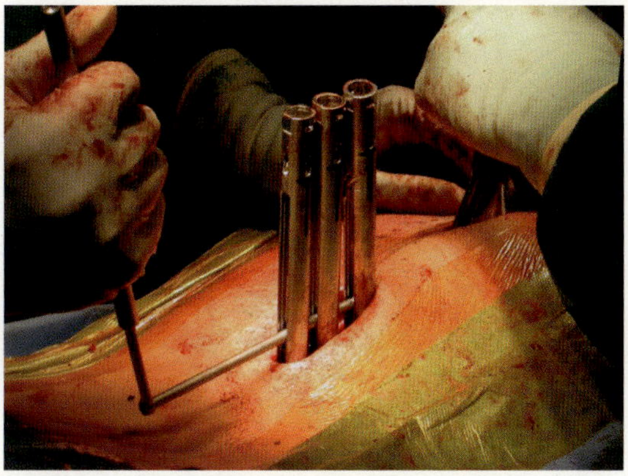

Fig. 37.2 Rod passage distal to proximal

37.3 Limitations and Future Trends

Curve correction, fusion, rod passage, and length of operative time have been raised as theoretical concerns of MIS. Although a number of deformity correction techniques exist for open procedures, not all are available to apply in the setting of MIS. There is greater emphasis on rod rotation, deferential rod contouring, distraction, compression, and intraoperative traction with MIS cases.

The fusion model in pediatric patients is different than adults and appears to be more

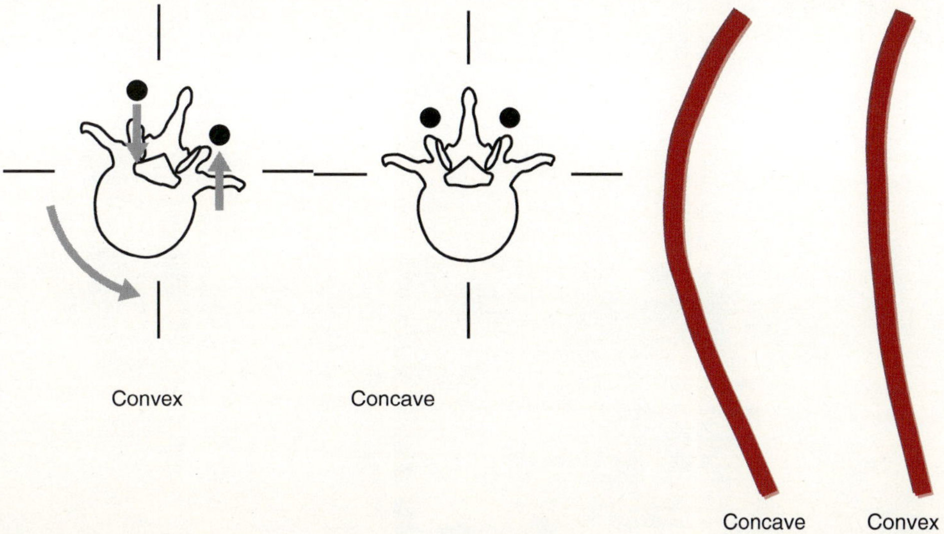

Fig. 37.3 Differential rod contouring (Courtesy Peter O. Newton)

favorable [29, 30]. However, fusion rates and/or time to fusion has not been reported for AIS treated with MIS techniques and should be the focus of much-needed prospective longer-term follow-up studies to assess these principal goals of AIS treatment and demonstrate the true clinical benefits of MIS in the setting of adolescent deformity.

The evolution of MIS as an effort to decrease the rate of approach-related morbidity associated

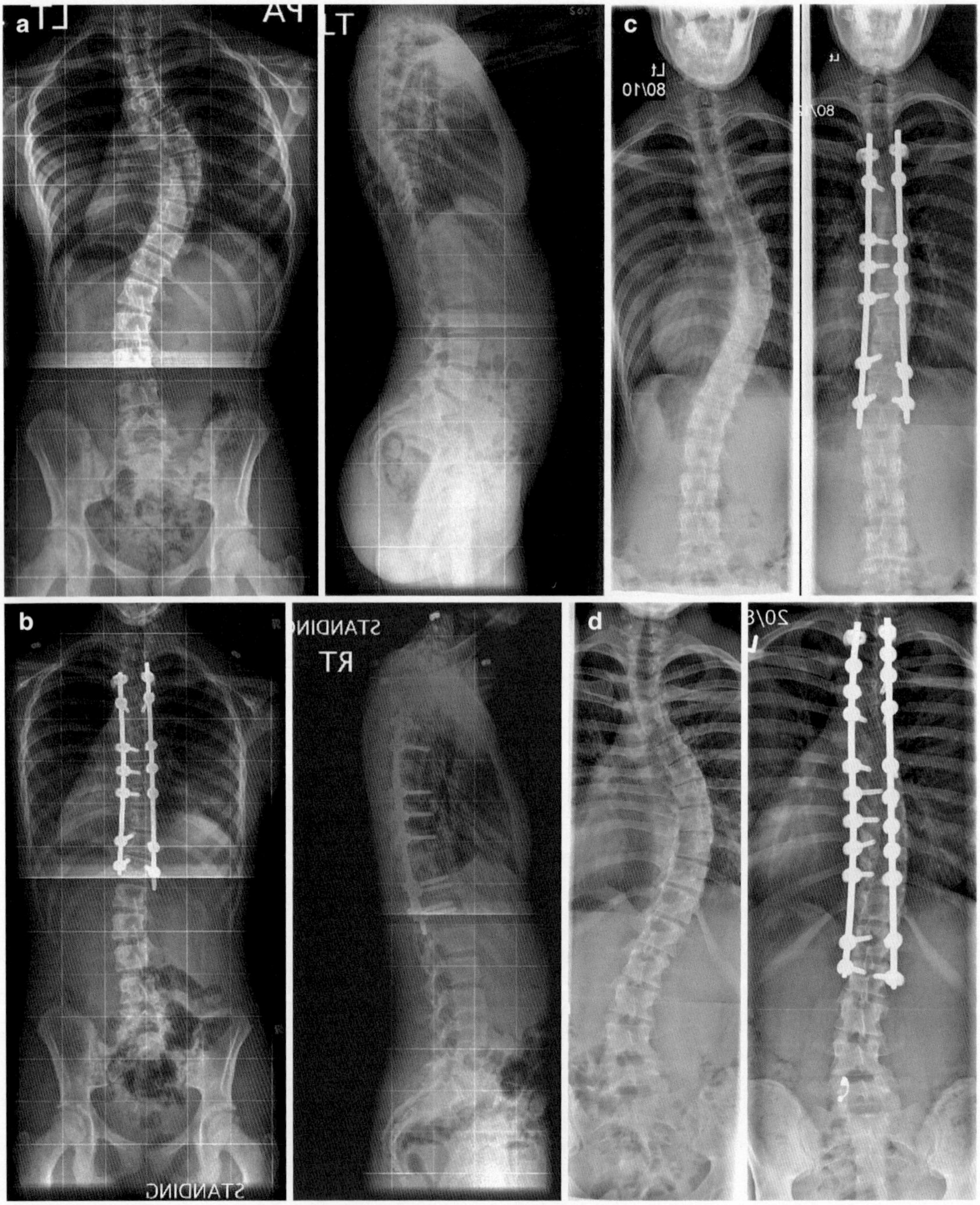

Fig. 37.4 (**a–d**) Pre and postoperative case examples of MIS in AIS

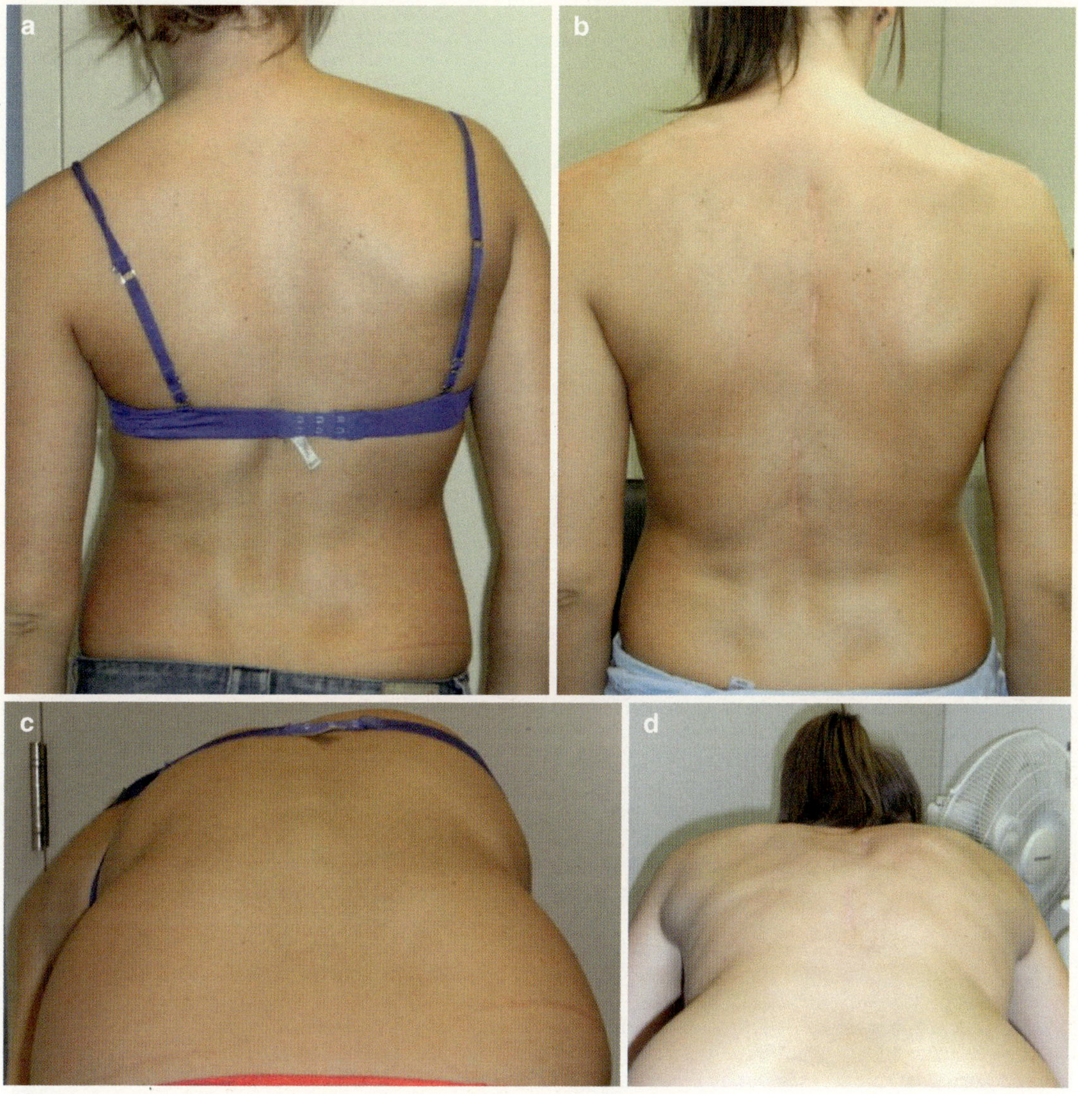

Fig. 37.5 Pre and 18 months post-operative clinical images. (**a**) Pre-operative clinical deformity, (**b**) Post-operative clinical result, (**c**) Pre-operative rib hump deformity, (**d**) Post-operative rib hump correction

with conventional open procedures certainly has shown potential for AIS at least in the short term, giving both surgeons and patients additional options to consider when planning surgical treatment for AIS.

References

1. Kishan S, Bastrom T, Betz RR, Lenke LG, Lowe TG, Clemets D, D'Andrea L, Sucato DJ, Newton PO. Thoracoscopic scoliosis surgery affects pulmonary function less than thoracotomy at 2 years postsurgery. Spine. 2007;32(4):453–8.
2. Lonner BS, Auerbach JD, Estreicher MB, et al. Pulmonary function changes after various anterior approaches in the treatment of AIS. J Spinal Disord Tech. 2009;22(8):551–8.
3. Newton PO, Perry A, Bastrom TP, et al. Predictors of change in postoperative pulmonary function in adolescent idiopathic scoliosis: a prospective study of 254 patients. Spine. 2007;32(17):1875–82.
4. Reddi V, Clarke Jr DV, Arlet V. Anterior thoracoscopic instrumentation in adolescent idiopathic scoliosis: a systematic review. Spine. 2008;33(18):1985–94.
5. Newton PO, Upasani VV, Lhamby J, et al. Surgical treatment of main thoracic scoliosis with thoracoscopic anterior instrumentation a five-year follow-up study. J Bone Joint Surg Am. 2008;90(10):20077–89.

6. Wong HK, Hee HT, Yu Z, et al. Results of thoracoscopic instrumentation and fusion versus conventional posterior instrumented fusion in AIS undergoing selective thoracic fusion. Spine. 2004; 29(18):2031–8.
7. German JW, Adamo MA, Hoppenot RG, et al. Perioperative results following lumbar discectomy: comparison of minimally invasive discectomy and standard microdiscectomy. Neurosurg Focus. 2008;25(2):E20.
8. Ryang YM, Oertel MF, Mayfrank L, et al. Standard open microdiscectomy versus minimal access trocar microdiscectomy: result of a prospective randomized study. Neurosurgery. 2008;62:174–81.
9. Righesso O, et al. Comparison of open discectomy with microendoscopic discectomy in lumbar disc herniations: results of a randomized controlled trial. Neurosurgery. 2007;61(3):545–9.
10. Peng CW, et al. Clinical and radiographic outcomes of minimally invasive versus open transforaminal lumbar interbody fusion. Spine. 2009; 34(13):1385–9.
11. Katayama Y, Matsuyama Y, Yoshishara H, et al. Comparison of surgical outcomes between macro discectomy and micro discectomy for lumbar disc herniation: a prospective randomized study with surgery performed by the same spine surgeon. J Spinal Disord Tech. 2006;19:344–7.
12. Rampersaud YR, Annand N, Dekutoski MB. Use of minimally invasive surgical techniques in the management of thoracolumbar trauma: current concepts. Spine. 2006;31(11):S96–104.
13. Smith JS, Ogden AT, Fessler RG. Minimally invasive posterior thoracic fusion. Neurosurg Focus. 2008; 25(2):E9.
14. Kawaguchi Y, Matsui H, Tsuji H. Back muscle injury after posterior lumbar spine surgery. A histologic and enzymatic analysis. Spine. 1996;21:941–4.
15. Kawaguchi Y, Matsui H, Tsuji H. Back muscle injury after posterior lumbar spine surgery. Part 1: Histologic and histochemical analyses in rats. Spine. 1994;19: 2590–7.
16. Kawaguchi Y, Matsui H, Tsuji H. Back muscle injury after posterior lumbar spine surgery. Part 2: Histologic and histochemical analyses in humans. Spine. 1994;19:2598–602.
17. Kawaguchi Y, Yakubi S, Styf J, et al. Back muscle injury after posterior lumbar spine surgery. Topographic evaluation of intramuscular pressure and blood flow in the porcine back muscle during surgery. Spine. 1996;21:2683–8.
18. Kim DY, Lee SH, Chung SK, et al. Comparison of multifidus muscle atrophy and trunk extension muscle strength: percutaneous versus open pedicle screw fixation. Spine. 2005;30:123–9.
19. Macnab I, Cuthbert H, Godfrey CM. The incidence of denervation of the sacrospinalis muscle following spinal surgery. Spine. 1977;2:294–8.
20. Mayer TG, Vanharanta H, Gatchel RJ, et al. Comparison of CT scan muscle measurements and isokinetic trunk strength in postoperative patients. Spine. 1989;14:33–6.
21. Rantanen J, Hurme M, Falck B, et al. The lumbar multifidus muscle five years after surgery for a lumbar intervertebral disc herniation. Spine. 1993;18:568–74.
22. Sihvonen T, Herno A, Paljärvi L, et al. A local denervation atrophy of paraspinal muscles in postoperative failed back syndrome. Spine. 1993;18:575–81.
23. Styf JR, Willén J. The effects of external compression by three different retractors on pressure in the erector spine muscles during and after posterior lumbar spine surgery in humans. Spine. 1998;23:354–8.
24. Weber BR, Grob D, Dvorák J, et al. Posterior surgical approach to the lumbar spine and its effect on the multifidus muscle. Spine. 1997;22:1765–72.
25. Anand N, Baron EM, Thaiyananthan G, et al. Minimally invasive multilevel percutaneous correction and fusion for adult lumbar degenerative scoliosis: a technique and feasibility study. J Spinal Disord Tech. 2008;21:459–67.
26. Hsieh PC, Koski TR, Sciubba DM, et al. Maximizing the potential of minimally invasive spine surgery in complex spinal disorders. Neurosurg Focus. 2008;25(2):E19.
27. Samdani AF, Asghar J, Miyanji F, et al. Minimally invasive treatment of pediatric spinal deformity. Semin Spine Surg. 2011;23(1):72–75.
28. Miyanji F, Samdani AF, Marks M, et al. Minimally invasive surgery for AIS: an early prospective comparison with standard open posterior surgery. J Spine. 2013;2(4):S5–001.
29. Cahill PJ, Marvil S, Cuddihy L, et al. Autofusion in the immature spine treated with growing rods. Spine. 2010;35:E1199–203.
30. Betz RR, Petrizzo AM, Kerner PJ, et al. Allograft versus no graft with a posterior multisegmented hook system for the treatment of idiopathic scoliosis. Spine. 2006;31:121–7.

The Future of MIS Spine Surgery 38

Richard G. Fessler

38.1 Introduction

So many factors affect where minimally invasive spine surgery (*MISS*) will go in the immediate and near future that it is hazardous, and probably foolhardy, to make predictions. Many of these factors, if not most, have little to do with surgery, medicine, or even health care. To consider this issue systematically, however, let's first define what we mean by "minimally invasive spine surgery" and then consider the question of "Where *should MISS* surgery go, in a perfect world?" Then let's examine the question, "What factors could alter the pathway of where *MISS* should go?" Finally, by combining the information learned from the answers to both of those questions, let's consider the final question, "Where is *MISS likely* to go in the future?"

38.2 What Is MISS?

Recently, there has been great debate over exactly what surgery qualifies as *MISS* and what doesn't. Is a 2 cm skin incision *MISS*? 3 cm? 4 cm? 25 cm? Or is the size of the skin incision irrelevant? Does MISS require complete sparing of the muscles and other soft tissues? Must it be done through a tubular retractor? Must you use an endoscope? Does a procedure in which only a limited paraspinal muscle dissection is performed qualify as *MISS*? [1, 2] If a vertebrectomy is performed through a small incision using soft tissue sparing technique, is that *MISS*? Clearly, the variety of operations proposed as *MISS*, and the variability of pathology approached (from a small disc herniation to intradural tumors and major scoliosis), complicates attempts to establish a firm definition. I would propose, however, that every *MISS* procedure be judged upon the equivalent operation if performed open. Thus, one possible definition for a *MISS* operation is:

> *a spine surgical procedure which produces significantly reduced, approach related, soft tissue destruction when compared to the equivalent open surgical procedure*

Note that this does not define any specific type of equipment, approach, amount of blood loss, skin incision, etc. Moreover, it is still somewhat vague in specifics. However, in some ways, the question here seems a little like the question regarding the definition of obscenity. As proclaimed by Justice Potter Stewart in 1964, "I shall not today attempt further to define {obscenity}; and perhaps I could never succeed in intelligibly doing so. But I know it when I see it…" [3]. The above definition at least gives you the tools to "know it when you see it."

R.G. Fessler, M.D., Ph.D.
Department of Neurosurgery,
Northwestern University, Chicago, IL, USA
e-mail: rfessler@rush.edu

M.Y. Wang et al. (eds.), *Minimally Invasive Spinal Deformity Surgery*,
DOI 10.1007/978-3-7091-1407-0_38, © Springer-Verlag Wien 2014

38.3 Where *Should* MISS Go in the Future?

Several years ago, while writing a chapter conjecturing on this same topic, I made the statement: "*MISS MUST* progress and become the mainstream technique of performing spinal surgery" [4]. I based that statement on the belief that *MISS* would most closely achieve the "goals" of spine surgery. Thus, where *MISS* needs to "go" is that place where it most successfully achieves the desired surgical result, with the least possible pain, anatomical destruction, complications, and cost. That is the ideal but will vary depending upon the specific surgical procedure involved. In this text, we have considered surgery for spinal deformity; therefore, let's consider the ideal future for deformity surgery. The "ideal" goal of deformity surgery includes (1) perfect correction of sagittal, coronal, and axial deformity, (2) 100 % fusion rate, (3) 0 % complications, (4) relief of pain, (5) maintenance of normal paraspinal soft tissue anatomy, (6) minimal blood loss, and (7) immediate return to normal activities of daily living with excellent quality of life.

Is this an achievable goal? There is now an accumulating literature demonstrating that spinal surgery performed with *MISS* technique has similar long-term outcomes compared to open equivalents but results in less pain and less use of pain medicine [5, 6], less blood loss [7, 8], lower infection rates [9], less requirement for intensive care [10], and less hospitalization [7, 8]. Physiologic stress is reduced [11]. Complication rates are lower [12]. Muscle atrophy is reduced [13] and normal motion is more accurately preserved [14]. Fusion rates are reported in the 80–95 % range [8, 15]. So, is the "ideal" suggested above achieved? No. But, significant improvements are evident in many areas, such as complications, relief of pain, soft tissue anatomy and blood loss, and rate of return to normal activities.

Progress is also being made in the ability to correct deformity using MISS techniques. Anand et al. reported 12 patients in whom coronal Cobb angle was corrected from a mean of 18.93° (SD 10.48) to 6.19° (SD 7.20) [16]. More recently, Wang reported on a "hybrid" *MISS* technique in which he reported correction of preoperative coronal Cobb angles from 29.2° to 9.0°, improvement of lumbar lordosis from 27.8° to 42.6°, and improvement of spinal vertebral angle (*SVA*) from 7.4 to 4.3 cm [1]. Clinical outcomes, as measured by visual analog scale (VAS) and Oswestry Disability Index (*ODI*), were similar to those achieved with open correction of deformity.

In my own personal series of patients with at least 2-year follow-up (i.e., my first deformity patients done with pure MISS technique), preoperative coronal Cobb angle improved from 25.9° to 8.3°. Lumbar lordosis slightly improved from 27.9° to 33.6°. Pelvic tilt improved from 25.7° to 18° and *SVA* minimally worsened from 5.1 to 5.7 cm. Thus, although coronal deformity significantly improved, lumbar lordosis, pelvic tilt, and SVA were minimally altered. However, as techniques and technologies have evolved, data collected on more recent patients is markedly better. In the last five patients operated on, coronal Cobb angle improved from 33.1° to 9.3°, lumbar lordosis improved from 14° to 34.9°, pelvic tilt improved from 29.6° to 19.1°, and *SVA* improved from 8.1 to 4.0 cm. Thus, even in a short period of time, results of *MISS* correction of sagittal plane deformity have dramatically improved. It seems highly likely that as experience, techniques, and instrumentation continue to improve, these results will likewise continue to improve. Finally, it should be noted that even in the early patients, in whom radiographic results were not as acceptable as patients operated on using open technique, results of *VAS*, *OSI*, and SF-36 were not significantly different between the groups (unpublished data) and the classical advantages of *MISS* techniques were still maintained with significantly shorter hospitalization, blood loss, CSF leaks, wound infections, and interestingly junctional kyphosis!

38.4 What Factors Could Alter the Pathway of Where MISS Should Go?

38.4.1 Patient Demand

As public awareness increases, demand for *MISS* procedures will increase. This is particularly true for traditionally "large" operations associated with prolonged and severe pain, high complication rates, and lengthy recoveries, such as scoliosis correction. This is going to be compounded by patients becoming increasingly more informed via the Internet. Furthermore, as more and more patients who have received *MISS* procedures are available to give testimony to their friends and neighbors, public awareness will increase, as will requests for *MISS* technique.

38.4.2 Skill Level and Education

The success of any surgical procedure depends upon the ability of surgeons to perform it safely and successfully. That, in turn, depends upon the inherent difficulty of the operation and the skill level of the surgeon. Thus, education and training are of paramount importance for increasing the use of *MISS* technique in deformity. Currently, surgeons versed in the techniques of *MISS* are not experienced in performing correction of scoliosis and *vice versa*. For surgeons bringing either skill set, to excel at performing *MISS* correction of deformity, it will be necessary to acquire the skills of the "other" group as well. For *MISS* surgeons, this means understanding the pathobiology of the causes and natural history of kyphoscoliosis, as well as the detailed biomechanics of occipital-spinal-sacral/pelvic balance, and the surgical techniques necessary to achieve spinal axis balance. For scoliosis surgeons, it means becoming comfortable with an entirely new set of instruments, perhaps learning the visual and proprioceptive skills necessary to operate in a two-dimensional visual field (i.e., endoscopic), learning to work in the restricted space of expandable tubular working channels (therefore working in parallel rather than triangulation), and performing complex procedures such as hemostasis and dural closure in very restricted spaces.

In general, new technologies take one to two generations to become widely adopted. This is partly a result of what must be learned but is also influenced by the nature of graduate and postgraduate education. Surgical residents, who are being trained in programs in which *MISS* deformity surgery is already being practiced, will simply learn these skills as part of their armamentarium. As more and more institutions have skilled faculty, this will become standard of care, similar to the way in which spinal instrumentation was adopted in the United States over the last 25–30 years. Given this rate of adoption, it is likely that spinal surgeons approaching the end of their active career will never need to learn these techniques. However, that leaves a group of surgeons who were not trained in *MISS* deformity during residency, but who have long careers ahead of them, and will need to learn the techniques to continue to perform "state-of-the-art" surgery. Since this is not the type of surgery that can be adequately learned in a weekend course, the question is: How do these surgeons learn these techniques?

Current recommendations to acquire this training include a series of educational steps. First, trained deformity surgeons should attend one or more didactic courses to learn the indications, contraindications, theory, and basic techniques for MISS procedures. Similarly, trained *MISS* surgeons should do the same to learn the basics of deformity surgery. Second, hands-on training, on both foam bone models and cadavers, should be completed. Although early in its development and implementation, computer simulation might also play a role in this training. Third, the student-surgeon should observe several procedures being performed by an experienced *MISS* deformity surgeon. Finally, if the opportunity exists, it would also be reasonable for the lesser experienced *MISS* deformity surgeon to "scrub" on several cases for proctoring prior to independently engaging in the procedures. It is the later suggestion that is particularly problematic for surgeons, as few centers are available where this is actually possible. In addition to the traditional industry and professional society educational courses, the Society for Minimally Invasive Spine Surgery (*SMISS*) is specifically creating a defined curriculum to teach both basic and advanced MISS procedures.

38.4.3 Instrumentation

Perhaps first among the challenges of *MISS* is visualization of the surgical field. Limitations exist whether the technology is endoscopic or microscopic. On the one hand, endoscopic visualization gives one the advantage of excellent image quality of the working area and the tips of the instruments without the instrument handles and surgeon's hand obstructing the view of the operative field and without the "hassle" of bumping the instruments into the microscope lens when entering or exiting the wound. The price paid for this advantage, however, is the necessity of working in a two-dimensional visual field with a moderately bulky camera lens obstructing part of the working channel. To circumvent this frustration many surgeons chose to use microscopic visualization. This solved the problem of working in a two-dimensional visual field but, as indicated above, created the problems of having the surgeon's hands and shaft of the instrument in the relatively narrow visual field, thus obstructing a clear view of the surgical site. To partially address this problem, bayoneted instruments were developed. These did help remove the surgeon's hands, but not the instruments shaft, from the visual field. In many cases, surgeons have opted for limited magnification, but ease of use, by utilizing loupes rather than either the endoscope or microscope.

The second challenge of *MISS* deformity surgery is in the instruments themselves. Although basic instrumentation has come a long way since our early attempts at *MISS*, available "tools" for advanced *MISS* procedures still have significant limitations. For example, correction of coronal deformity is quite good using the *MISS* lateral, retroperitoneal approach to the lumbar spine. However, instrumentation to manipulate the vertebral bodies from that approach could be improved. Moreover, rotational deformity is only minimally affected with current instrumentation for this approach. Although the lateral approach can also be used in the thoracic spine and at the thoracolumbar junction, the technical skill required to work in these areas is greater than that of the lumbar spine. Thus, one wonders if improved instrumentation would make surgery in these areas less daunting.

Whether using open or *MISS* technique, posterior deformity correction usually requires a combination of surgical procedures, including facet fusions, Smith-Petersen osteotomies, pedicle subtraction osteotomies, and occasionally even vertebrectomy. All these procedures can be completed using *MISS* technique. However, the retractors and instruments used to perform these procedures are "first generation." Although they work well in the lumbar spine, where the musculature is predominantly parallel to the spine, they do not work well in more complicated anatomical environments. For vertebrectomies, drills need to be slimmed down and modified to extend slightly longer. Furthermore, protective sleeves need to be readily available for each drill bit head design, to protect the surrounding structures in limited visual fields. Micro-instruments need to be designed to be used through tubes and yield the same delicacy as when used under a microscope. Instruments need to be designed to easily close the dura. Thus, although technically feasible with current instruments, improvements designed specifically for the completion of these procedures would make their completion both faster and easier.

Similarly, although instruments have been developed to place percutaneous rods and pedicle screws, our ability to create complex bends, either before or after passing the rods, is very limited. Our ability to correct coronal deformity from the posterior approach is also limited by the equipment available. As a result, the extent of correction is also limited. To perform these more complicated procedures, therefore, instrumentation needs to be modified specifically for these procedures. In major reconstructive cases such as correction of scoliosis, MISS de-rotation instruments, compression and distraction devices, and *in situ* bending instruments need to be developed.

38.4.4 Image Guidance

Three-dimensional knowledge of the spine, and its intraspinal and surrounding soft tissue structures, is critical to safely performing *MISS*. In complex, rotational deformity, understanding this anatomy is particularly difficult, and accurate imaging of the spine can be very challenging. For example, to image the pedicles using fluoroscopy alone often requires turning the surgical table to extremes, which can place the patient at risk for sliding off the table. Furthermore, even when acceptable images can be obtained, the transfer of two-dimensional fluoroscopic imaging to three-dimensional anatomy is not easy for all surgeons. In addition, the amount of radiation exposure to the surgical team has become a major concern.

Intraoperative "navigation" and intraoperative CT imaging have significantly impacted these challenges. Kim et al. recently reported that "total" exposure to radiation time was decreased from 147 to 57 s using "Fluoro-Navigation" versus standard fluoroscopy [17]. Similarly, using CT-based image guidance, Florian et al. reported a decrease from 177 to 75 s of total radiation time [18].

In addition to reducing exposure to radiation, accuracy and reliability have increased significantly. However, these imaging modalities are also limited. Accuracy is still dependent upon the fixation, and lack of movement, of the reference frame during the entire time image guidance is used. The size of the surgical field in which the reference frame is accurate is relatively small and usually requires moving the frame at least once during the procedure (thus necessitating a second CT scan). Other areas in which improvements will help the surgeons are (1) improved and more widely available "guidable" instruments, which accurately reflect the typical working instruments needed to complete the surgical procedure, (2) image technology which does not rely on "line of sight" imaging between the camera and imaging array, (3) less bulky equipment (e.g., the "O-arm"), and (4) more time "efficient" technology.

38.4.5 Cost, Quality of Life (QOL)

Over the past decade, it seems that emphasis on patient-perceived outcomes, quality of life, and cost has exceeded interest in advancing the art and science of medicine and surgery in particular. Although this may have negative implications for the rate at which medical knowledge expands, it has had positive effects on how closely we've looked at our own surgical outcomes. At this time, minimal data has been published on the long-term QOL outcomes versus cost of scoliosis surgery. However, progress is being made in this area. Age-gender normative data, for example, has been collected and published through the Scoliosis Research Society [19]. This will serve as a baseline upon which further studies can be designed and compared. Similarly, Glassman et al. has defined parameters of minimal perceived clinical benefit in lumbar arthrodesis [20]. In their analysis, to perceive clinical benefit, back pain must improve 41 %, leg pain must improve 38 %, SF-36 must improve 31.5 %, and Oswestry Disability Scores must improve 36 %. Moktar et al. have reported 1-year health-related *QOL* (*HRQOL*) for repair of degenerative spondylolisthesis to be equivalent to that achieved with either hip or knee replacement [21].

Similar progress is being reported in the MISS literature, although the quantity of literature available is substantially smaller than that from the open literature. Parker et al. reported equivalent QOL outcomes in patients undergoing MISS versus open repair of degenerative spondylolisthesis, with $8,731 2-year cost savings [22]. Their conclusion was that MISS was a cost-reducing technology. Similar results and conclusions were reported by Wang et al. [23]. In a literature review published in 2010, Allen and Garfin concluded that "although the cost effectiveness of *MIS* surgery is yet to be carefully studied, the few economic studies that do exist suggest that *MIS* has the potential to be a cost effective intervention…" [24]. They further suggested that the most important features differentiating several *MIS* procedures included fewer infections, fewer approach and possibly surgery-related complications, less blood loss, shorter *LOS*, less early narcotic pain medicine requirements, and a more rapid return to work and productivity. Preliminary data from our research suggests an approximately 50 % decrease in overall complications in scoliosis surgery performed using MISS technique compared to open. This is accompanied by dramatically less blood loss and fewer infections (manuscript in preparation). A cost-effectiveness and *QOL* evaluation is also currently underway.

38.4.6 Health-Care Policy

All of the above discussion focuses on medical, technological, and educational aspects of the delivery of medical care, which can be evaluated, understood, and altered in relatively predictable fashions. Each of these would predict the slow, but progressive, expansion of the use of MISS surgery for most spinal procedures, including deformity procedures. What is less certain, however, is the impact of recent changes national health-care policy will have on the delivery of health care in the United States, particularly as it relates to surgery. Implementation of the massive *Patient Protection and Affordable Care Act (PPACA)* will undoubtedly change the delivery of spine surgical care to patients, but all claims of improvement or deteriorization are mere speculation, devoid of any real information upon which to make a claim. The thousands of new regulations being implemented, many of which compete with one another, could result in any variety of alterations. For example, the health insurance exchanges and new laws regulating the behavior of insurance companies could be suggested to increase the number of patients who would have access to health care. On the other hand, potential decisions by the Independent Payment Advisory Board (IPAB), early directions of the Comparative Effectiveness Research Committee, and payment "punishments" for the so-called never events would all seem to conspire to restrict advanced medical care to those patients who are sickest and most in need of care. Advanced deformity patients would certainly fall into this category. One potential scenario, for example, could be that rather than insurance companies denying surgery to a potential candidate (where upon the patient has legal recourse), IPAB could pass a national policy determining that that same patient was not eligible for payment for that surgery (whereupon the patient had *no* recourse). Thus, the question has to be asked, "Exactly what" medical care "will" be available to these patients? Frequent visits to their primary care physician will not likely render them the care they most need.

Another unpredictable change in the landscape is the rapid transformation of private practice medicine into "Accountable Care Organizations" (ACOs) and the consequent possible alteration of the mechanism of payment for the delivery of health care. There is no disguising in the fact that ACOs are vehicles for rationing health-care dollars. In the context of "teams" of health-care professionals from multiple disciplines participating in the CMS-administered "Shared Savings Program," there is little doubt that the one-time high cost of surgery will be disproportionately minimized, despite the accumulating evidence that long-term costs are less than prolonged, marginally effective nonsurgical care.

Although the current list of uncertainties in the health-care environment seems endless, one other factor which will impact the development and delivery of health care to American patients deserves particular mention. Most medical devices which ultimately reach the patient are jointly developed by entrepreneurial physician/scientists and industry. Few of these research and development health-care dollars come from federal agencies such as the National Institutes of Health (NIH). The recent imposition of a 2.3 % medical device tax is certain to negatively impact research and development of new devices and thus also negatively impact improvements in the delivery of health care.

38.5 Where Is MISS *Likely* to Go in the Future

Without considering outside factors, as experience, techniques, and technology continue to evolve, it seems highly likely that a greater percentage of scoliosis correction will be performed using MISS techniques. This already seems certain for primary lumbar curves. It is less certain for primary thoracic curves or "double major" scoliotic curves. Although it is only recently that prospective, multicenter trials are being organized to specifically compare outcome and cost-effectiveness of open versus *MISS* correction of deformity, enough retrospective data has accumulated from numerous spinal procedures to make this statement with relative assurance. This will happen even with the less than ideal technology and techniques currently available to the MISS surgeon and will more rapidly expand as the issues discussed above are resolved.

That being said, medicine does not live in an isolated and protected world. The framework for medical rationing is now firmly in place, the capital for investment in medical device development has been on the decline for more than several years, and the federal government has recently instituted a punishing tax on medical devices which will further slow technological development. These factors will certainly play important roles in the manner in which medical care is rendered in the United States and the role which MISS will play in that framework. In a system in which health-care dollars are rationed, it is likely that elective spine surgery will experience an overall decline. Furthermore, it is likely that the rate of medical innovation will similarly decline. If, in this context, MISS is found to deliver better, equivalent or near-equivalent QOL results, for less cost, it will continue to expand its share of the spine surgical procedures as they exist in this new future. Factors such as fewer infections, fewer complications, less blood loss, and less pain will virtually guarantee this. If, on the other hand, it is found not to be cost-effective or that the cost and outcomes are the same as open surgery, then other factors such as education, technical familiarity, and procedural difficulty will negatively impact the development of *MISS*. In that case, *MISS* will continue to be practiced by a subset of dedicated surgeons, but will not likely reach the mainstream of surgical technique.

References

1. Wang M. Improvement of sagittal balance and lumbar lordosis following less invasive adult spinal deformity surgery with expandable cages and percutaneous instrumentation. J Neurosurg Spine. 2013;18:4–12.
2. Shaffrey CI, Smith JS. Editorial: minimally invasive spinal deformity surgery. J Neurosurg Spine. 2013;18:1–2.
3. Potter, Stewart: Jacobellis v. Ohio *378 U.S. 184,* 1964.
4. Fessler RG. Promising advances in minimally invasive spine surgery. In: Sandhu FA, Voyadzis JM, Fessler RG, editors. Decision making for minimally invasive spine surgery. New York: Thieme Medical Publishers; 2011. p. 2071–206.
5. Fessler RG, Khoo LT. Minimally invasive cervical Microendoscopic Foraminotomy (MEF): an initial clinical experience. Neurosurgery. 2002; 51(5, Supplement):37–45.
6. O'Toole JE, Sheikh J, Eichholz KM, Fessler RG, Perez-Cruet MJ. Endoscopic posterior cervical foraminotomy and discectomy. Neurosurg Clin N Am. 2006;17:411–22.
7. Khoo LT, Palmer S, Laich DT, Fessler RG. Minimally invasive percutaneous posterior lumbar interbody fusion. Neurosurgery. 2002;51(5):S166–71.
8. Peng CWB, Yue WM, Poh SY, Mphyty WY, Tan SB. Clinical and radiological outcomes of minimally invasive vs open transforaminal lumbar interbody fusion. Spine. 2009;34:1385–9.
9. O'Toole JE, Eichholz KM, Fessler RG. Surgical site infection rates after minimally invasive spinal surgery. J Neurosurg Spine. 2009;11:471–6.
10. Eichholz KM, O'Toole JE, Fessler RG. Thoracic microendoscopic discectomy. Neurosurg Clin N Am. 2006;17:441–6.
11. Huang TJ, Hsu RW, Li YY. Less systemic cytokine response in patients following microendoscopic versus open lumbar discectomy. J Orthop Res. 2005;23:406–11.
12. Rosen DS, O'Toole JE, Eichholz KM, et al. Minimally invasive lumbar spinal decompression in the elderly: outcomes in 50 patients aged 75 years and older. Neurosurgery. 2007;60:503–9.
13. Bresnahan I, Fessler RG, Natarajan RN. Evaluation of change in muscle activity as a result of posterior lumbar spine surgery using a dynamic modeling. Spine. 2010;35:E761–7.
14. Bresnahan L, Ogden AT, Natarajan RN, Fessler RG. A biomechanical evaluation of graded posterior element removal for treatment of lumbar stenosis: comparison of a minimally invasive approach with two standard laminectomy techniques. Spine. 2009;34:17–23.
15. Lauber S, Schulte TL, Liljenqvist U, Halm H, Hackenberg L. Clinical and radiologic 2–4 year results of transforaminal lumbar interbody fusion in degenerative and isthmic spondylolisthesis grades 1 and 2. Spine. 2006;31:1693–8.
16. Anand N, Baron EM, Thaiyananthan G, Khalsa K, Goldstein TB. Minimally invasive multilevel percutaneous correction and fusion for adult lumbar degenerative scoliosis: a technique and feasibility study. J Spinal Disord Tech. 2008;21:459–67.

17. Kim CW, Lee Y, Taylor W, Oygar A, Kim WK. Use of navigation-assisted fluoroscopy to decrease radiation exposure during minimally invasive spine surgery. Spine J. 2008;8:584–90.
18. Florian TG, Kraus MD, Schneider E, Liener UC, Kinzl L, Arand M. Does computer-assisted spine surgery reduce intraoperative radiation doses? Spine. 2006;31:2024–7.
19. Baldus C, Bridwell K, Harrast J, Shaffrey C, Ondra S, Lenke L, Schwab F, Mardjetko S, Glassman S, Edwards C, Lowe T, Horton W, Polly D. The Scoliosis Research Society health-related quality of life (SRS-30) age-gender normative data. Spine. 2011;36:1154–62.
20. Glassman SD, Copay AG, Berven SH, Polly DW, Subach BR, Carreon LY. Defining substantial clinical benefit following lumbar spine arthrodesis. J Bone Joint Surg Am. 2008;90:1839–47.
21. Moktar SA, McCombe PF, Williamson OD, White MD, Gavin J, Sears WR. Health related quality of life: a comparison of outcomes after lumbar fusion for degenerative spondylolisthesis with large joint replacement surgery and population norms. Spine J. 2010;10:306–12.
22. Parker SL, Adogwa O, Bydon A, Cheng J, McGirt MJ. Cost-effectiveness of minimally invasive versus open transforaminal lumbar interbody fusion for degenerative spondylolisthesis associated low back and leg pain over two years. World Neurosurg. 2012;78:178–84.
23. Wang MY, Commock MD, Yu Y. An analysis of the differences in the acute hospitalization charges following minimally invasive versus open posterior lumbar interbody fusion. J Neurosurg Spine. 2010;12:694–9.
24. Allen RT, Garfin SR. The economics of minimally invasive spine surgery. Spine. 2010;35:S375–82.

Index

M.Y. Wang et al. (eds.), *Minimally Invasive Spinal Deformity Surgery*,
DOI 10.1007/978-3-7091-1407-0, © Springer-Verlag Wien 2014

Printed by Printforce, the Netherlands